Pulmonary Vascular Disease

Pulmonary Vascular Disease

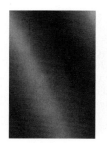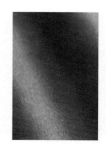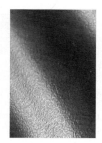

Edited by

Jess Mandel, M.D.
Director, Pulmonary Hypertension Program
Associate Professor of Medicine and Assistant Dean
The University of Iowa Roy J. and Lucille A. Carver College of Medicine
Iowa City, Iowa

Darren Taichman, M.D., Ph.D.
Director, Medical Intensive Care Unit
Associate Director, Pulmonary Vascular Disease Program
Penn Presbyterian Medical Center
Assistant Professor of Medicine
University of Pennsylvania School of Medicine
Philadelphia, Pennsylvania

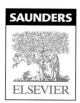
SAUNDERS
ELSEVIER

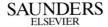

1600 John F. Kennedy Blvd.
Ste 1800
Philadelphia, PA 19103-2899

Pulmonary Vascular Disease

ISBN-13: 978-1-4160-2246-6
ISBN-10: 1-4160-2246-5

Notice

Knowledge and best practice in this field are constantly changing. As new research and experience broaden our knowledge, changes in practice, treatment and drug therapy may become necessary or appropriate. Readers are advised to check the most current information provided (i) on procedures featured or (ii) by the manufacturer of each product to be administered, to verify the recommended dose or formula, the method and duration of administration, and contraindications. It is the responsibility of the practitioner, relying on their own experience and knowledge of the patient, to make diagnoses, to determine dosages and the best treatment for each individual patient, and to take all appropriate safety precautions. To the fullest extent of the law, neither the Publisher nor the Editors assumes any liability for any injury and/or damage to persons or property arising out or related to any use of the material contained in this book.

The Publisher

Library of Congress Cataloging-in-Publication Data

ISBN-13: 978-1-4160-2246-6
ISBN-10: 1-4160-2246-5

Acquisitions Editor: Dolores Meloni
Developmental Editor: Kristina Oberle

Printed in The United States of America

Last digit is the print number: 9   8   7   6   5   4   3   2   1

Working together to grow
libraries in developing countries

www.elsevier.com | www.bookaid.org | www.sabre.org

ELSEVIER   BOOK AID International   Sabre Foundation

To Meg, Emily, and Jonathan
Jess Mandel, M.D.

To Lilach, Elya, Mira, and Rebecca
Darren Taichman, M.D., Ph.D.

Preface

Historically, the pulmonary vasculature has proven to be difficult to evaluate clinically and challenging to investigate by radiographic and hemodynamic methods. For these and other reasons, study of the pulmonary circulation has largely existed at the fringes of cardiology, pulmonology, and other disciplines. Most diseases of the pulmonary circulation have been considered esoteric, highly lethal, and virtually untreatable, leading many to question the necessity of vigorously pursuing an antemortem diagnosis.

However, after centuries of little or no progress in the understanding and treatment of this challenging group of disorders, the last 15 years have witnessed a proliferation of breakthroughs in the scientific and clinical approaches to pulmonary vascular disease. The field has moved from one of relative stasis to one where important advances now occur with such regularity that even experts in the area are hard pressed to keep abreast. Many of these key developments reflect the tenacity of a relatively small group of investigators that began to coalesce in the 1980s and 1990s, and continues to serve as a model for rigorous research methods, international collaboration, and the rapid translation of basic science insights into useful clinical tools.

This textbook was prepared with the aim of disseminating useful information about the rapidly evolving field of pulmonary vascular disease into the hands of those who are called upon to care for patients with this difficult group of diseases. Research is only useful to society if its hard-won victories can be applied to the populations that can benefit from them. Our hope is that this book will assist physicians, nurses, medical trainees, and others who are confronted with any of the myriad problems that can develop in the care of patients with pulmonary vascular disease, and ultimately benefit the patients themselves.

Many thanks are due to those who helped make this book possible. Steve Weinberger recognized the need for a book of this type, and provided us with consistent inspiration to help us complete it. Todd Hummel, Dolores Meloni, and Kristina Oberle at Elsevier, and Jeff Somers at Graphic World Publishing Services helped translate our ideas into a finished work. The tireless efforts of Peggy Hegarty and Traci Stewart have been invaluable. Giuseppe Pietra was extremely charitable in providing pathologic images, and he and his family were marvelously generous with their time, support, and hospitality. Completion of the book would not have been possible without the chapters from our contributing authors, and we cannot thank them enough for taking on these additional tasks above and beyond their already numerous academic responsibilities. We thank the Pulmonary Hypertension Association for its enthusiasm, and its members who share their personal experiences in the final chapter of this book. Our families have been wonderfully encouraging to us throughout the preparation of the book, and we will always be grateful for their support and their belief in us which many times exceeded our own.

This book would not exist without the efforts of our many outstanding teachers, including but not limited to Al Fishman, Steve Weinberger, Rich Schwartzstein, Gary Hunninghake, John Hansen-Flaschen, Harold Palevsky, Jeff Drazen, Woody Weiss, Gregory Tino, Robert Kotloff, Mike Laposata, Morris Swartz, James Shinnick, Bob Glickman, Bob Moellering, and Bud Rose. Finally, our patients have been among our most important teachers, and we remain profoundly touched by their courage and dignity in the face of the extreme challenges they face on a daily basis.

Jess Mandel, M.D.
Iowa City, Iowa

Darren Taichman, M.D., Ph.D.
Philadelphia, Pennsylvania

Historical Perspective

Alfred P. Fishman, M.D.

In 1628, in a small town in Germany (Frankfurt), a little book issued by a second-rate publisher announced one of the great biological discoveries of all time (1-3). The book, written in Latin, and entitled "Exercitatio Anatomica de Motu Cordis et Sanguinis in Animalibus" was destined to become the linch pin of circulatory physiology and medicine. And the author of this little book, usually referred to as "De Motu Cordis," William Harvey, was to be immortalized as the discoverer of the circulation of the blood (3).

Before William Harvey, observations on the heart and blood vessels were isolated, fragmentary and, as a rule, misinterpreted (4-5). The views of Galen, an Asiatic Greek who had come to the great medical school in Alexandria, Egypt, dominated thinking about the motion of blood in the vessels (Figure 1). Galen was an inspiring teacher and his ideas, set forth in his book "De usu partium," Book VI, Chapter 10, had quickly gained currency and spread widely. Unfortunately, Galen's teachings were flawed by several misconceptions, including two particularly erroneous ideas: 1) that blood can pass from one ventricle to the other via pores in the ventricular septum and 2) that the pulmonary vein is a conduit for air, rather than aerated blood. These misconceptions were destined to endure for 1500 years (4, 5) and to become the starting point from which others set out to discover the pulmonary circulation.

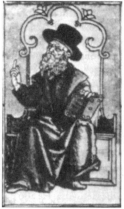

Fig. 1

Galen of Pergamon (131-200 AD). Personal physician to the Emperor Marcus Aurelius and a foremost physician of the Roman Empire. He conducted experiments and is often regarded as the founder of experimental physiology.

Although greatly influenced by Galen's ideas, Ibn Nafis, in the thirteenth century, came to realize that blood had to traverse the lungs to get from the right side of the heart to the left simply because the ventricular septum had no pores by which blood could get from one side to the other. Another pre-Harvean insight into the circulation came by way of theology rather than science. In a book written in Latin, with the title translated as "Restitution of Christianity," Michael Servetus (1511-1553) provided the first written description of the pulmonary circulation. He pictured the pulmonary circulation as the distributing system by which the soul, after entering the body via the airways, is distributed throughout the body. Servetus took exception to the notion that the pulmonary artery was a nutrient vessel on the grounds that it was simply too large, and carried too much blood, to serve this limited function. For his rebellious interpretations of passages in the bible, Servetus became a "hunted heretic" and was advised by Calvin to stay away from Geneva where Calvin was holding forth. Servetus paid no heed to this warning. He was spotted in the audience, captured, and burned at the stake in 1553.

A much more staid individual was Mateo Realdo Colombo (1516-1559), an Italian anatomist who in the course of his dissections of the heart, came to realize that the ventricular septum had no pores (4, 5). Moreover, contrary to Galen's schema, which called for air in the pulmonary veins, Colombo's dissections consistently revealed blood in the pulmonary veins of both living and dead animals. Fabricius of Aquapendente provided support for the idea of unidirectional flow towards the heart in the illustrations of venous valves in his book "On the Valves of the Veins" (1574). However, he did not synthesize his observations on venous valves into a conception of the circulation.

William Harvey (1578-1657) was strongly influenced by the works of Fabricius and Colombo (2, 3) (Figure 2). Harvey had attended Fabricius' lectures at Padua and realized that the valves

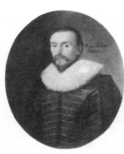

Fig. 2
William Harvey (1578-1657). His book, written in Latin, usually referred to by its abbreviated title, "de Motu Cordis," not only demonstrated the circulation of the blood but also revolutionized physiology and essential bases of medical practice.

that Fabricius portrayed implied that blood in the veins had to flow towards the heart. He was also familiar with Colombo's book, "De re Anatomica" which the advent of printing had made widely available. The dissections on living animals described in Colombo's text had consistently revealed blood in the pulmonary veins rather than the air which Galen had postulated. For Colombo, the finding of blood rather than air in the pulmonary veins was convincing evidence that blood must be traversing the lungs to get to the left side of the heart. Nevertheless, despite this seminal observation, he did not follow through with the idea of the circulation of the blood (1).

The conception of the circulation of the blood originated with William Harvey and was set forth in "De Motu Cordis" (3). This book was destined to become a classic for three reasons: 1) it provided a clear and accurate description of the laws that govern the motion of the heart and blood, 2) it undermined the Galenic concept that envisaged pores in the ventricular septum and the to-and-fro movement of the blood in the great vessels and 3) it demonstrated the superiority of observation and experimentation over philosophical reasoning in solving a biological problem. In essence, "De Motu Cordis" marked the transition from a period of philosophical speculation to one of clinical evaluation, anatomical observation and physiological experimentation. In doing so, it redirected the course of biology from unrewarding quests and fruitless discussions to unforeseen discoveries and new horizons.

Harvey's biological studies were in step with the remarkable progress in science that Western Europe was then experiencing (1, 4, 5). Indeed, it was an age of scientific revolution, the age of Copernicus, Fracastoro, Galileo, Vesalius and Fabrizio. Harvey was part and parcel of this age of discovery. The advent of printing spread the message of this age far and wide.

Two centuries were to elapse after Harvey before the function of the heart began to be explored systematically (6). Catheterization of the heart paved the way. In the 1840s, Claude Bernard used catheters made of lead to record cardiac pressures in the horse, and thereby settle the question, hotly debated by Antoine Lavoisier and Gustav Magnus, whether body heat was generated in the lungs during breathing or in the tissues. In 1861, Auguste Chauveau and Étienne-Jules Marey used cardiac catheterization to obtain records of the relationship between the apex beat and the movement of the atria and ventricles. Their experiments provided a model for subsequent studies because of the accuracy of their pressure recordings and the comprehensive description and interpretation of pressure recordings in the left ventricle and aorta (1). Major contributions to the understanding of central circulatory functions and its relationships to fluid exchange at the capillary level were made subsequently by Ernest Henry

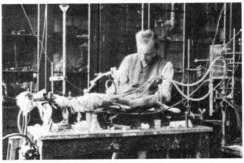

Fig. 3
Ernest Henry Starling (1866-1927). One of the most influential physiologists of the twentieth century. His contributions include the "law of the heart," the functional significance of serum proteins, the stimulation of pancreatic secretion of secretin (with W. M. Bayliss), and the reabsorption of water by the renal tubules (with E. B. Verney).

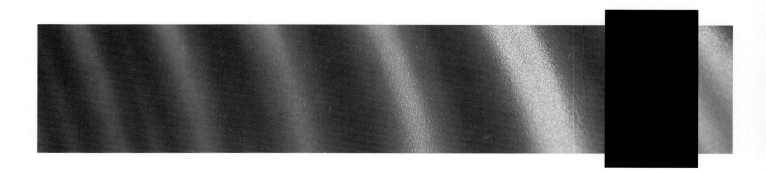

Starling (1866-1927) (Figure 3). Starling's contributions provided both the gateway and unifying theme for contemporary concepts of circulatory organization and operation. Starling's experiments focused on the mechanical properties of the heart which determined its basic functions. Intrinsic, self-regulatory mechanisms that automatically direct mixed venous blood to well-ventilated alveoli, were explored in anesthetized cats by Euler and Liljestrand (Figure 4) and soon thereafter by Motley and Cournand in humans under natural conditions.

Early in the twentieth century, Forssmann showed that cardiac catheterization could be safely applied in humans. He did so by passing a ureteral catheter via a peripheral vein into his own heart (7). To illustrate the safety of the procedure, he repeated the self-catheterization on several different occasions. In his book, "Experiments on Myself," he reflects on the motivation for his self-catheterization. As a surgeon, he was seeking a direct route to the heart for cardiac resuscitation other than cannulation of a large neck vein or direct cardiac puncture. The idea of catheterizing the human heart under natural conditions came to him from a picture in a textbook of physiology which showed a horse standing quietly with a cardiac catheter in the right atrium. In the report of his experiment, which appeared in the Klinische Wochenschrift in 1929, Forssmann included a picture of the catheter tip in his own right atrium. The report generated much more enthusiasm for the procedure in medical centers throughout Europe and abroad than in Germany. Forssmann, disappointed with the cool reception in his own country, retreated to Eberwalde, a small town on the outskirts of Berlin, where he set up a practice in urology (4, 5).

Although the local impact of Forssmann's demonstrations fell short of his expectations, ripples from the demonstration of the safety of right heart catheterization spread far and wide. In the Cardiopulmonary Laboratory at Bellevue Hospital in New York City, where direct measurement of the cardiac output had become an almost impossible dream, Forssmann's demonstration pointed the way to obtaining mixed venous blood for application of the Fick principle. In short order, André F. Cournand and Dickinson W. Richards, Jr. adopted Forssmann's technique of right heart catheterization, convinced a manufacturer to improve and adapt the ureteral catheter for its new application, standardized the procedure for measuring the cardiac output by the Fick principle and applied the technique not only for physiological studies but also for studies of acquired and congenital heart diseases (8).

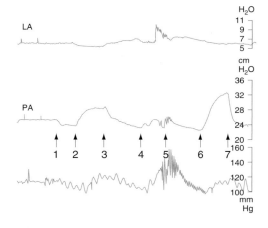

Fig. 4

Responses of pulmonary arterial (PA) and left arterial (LA) pressures to different inspired mixtures in an open-chest cat anesthetized with chloralose.

$1=O_2$; $2=6.5\%$ CO_2; $3=O_2$; $4=18\%$ CO_2 in O_2; $5=O_2$; $6=10\%$ O_2 in N_2; $7=O_2$.

From: Observations on the Pulmonary Arterial Blood Pressure in the Cat, by U.S. von Euler and G.L. Liljestrand, Acta Physiol Scand. 12:301-320, 1946.

Among the diseases that illustrate the remarkable insights afforded by cardiac catheterization is the rare entity called "primary pulmonary hypertension," an intrinsic disease of the pulmonary arteries and arterioles (9). This disease had been described in 1891 in a case report by Ernest Romberg, a distinguished physician and pathologist who failed, despite intensive search, to find an etiologic basis for his histopathological findings. After Romberg's publication, others took up the search for etiology. An intensive effort was made in the 1920s by clinicians of the Argentinian School. They designated the disease as "Ayerza's Disease," in honor of the master clinician who headed their program and pinpointed the treponema pallidum as the etiologic agent. However, the idea of a syphilitic etiology was laid to rest in the 1940s by Oscar Brenner, a British cardiologist. After an exhaustive review of the literature and of the records of patients in Paul D. White's cardiac clinic at the Massachusetts General Hospital, Brenner could find no evidence that the spirochete is involved in the pathogenesis of the disease. Since then, the search for the etiology and pathogenesis of primary (or idiopathic) pulmonary hypertension has continued, handicapped by the fact that the disease becomes manifest clinically only when far advanced.

Originally, the diagnosis of primary pulmonary hypertension amounted to a death sentence, destined to be fulfilled within two years after diagnosis. The grim outlook began to brighten in the 1950s, with the demonstration by David Dresdale that a vasodilator agent, tolazoline, administered intravenously, could lower pulmonary arterial pressures in primary pulmonary hypertension. However, tolazoline was not an ideal pulmonary vasodilator since it is also a systemic vasodilator, thereby raising the possibility that decreases in pulmonary arterial pressures might be secondary to the systemic hypotensive effects of the drug. This uncertainty about the pulmonary vascular site of action was dispelled in subsequent studies designed to confine the vasodilator effect to the pulmonary circulation. This was accomplished by the intravenous infusion of acetylcholine, a pulmonary vasodilator with effects limited to the pulmonary circulation (9). Since then, therapeutic options for primary pulmonary hypertension, now termed "idiopathic pulmonary arterial hypertension" (IPAH) have increased dramatically. For example, instead of vasodilator agents delivered by continuous intravenous infusions, medications taken by mouth exert their effects by blocking receptor sites on the blood vessel lining.

In recent years, observations on familial pulmonary arterial hypertension (FPAH) have provided fresh insights into the pathogenesis of the disease (10-15). Genetic factors influence both the susceptibility and heritability of pulmonary arterial hypertension. The role of susceptibility is reflected in the relatively small numbers of individuals who were affected during both the aminorex and fen-phen epidemics; the role of heritability is reflected in the 6% incidence of familial pulmonary arterial hypertension in the 187 patients in the National Institutes of Health registry of primary pulmonary hypertension.

The pattern of inheritance seems to be autosomal dominant with incomplete penetrance, resulting in the development of the disease in up to 20 percent of individuals at risk (10,11). Mutations in two different genes have been identified (13). Both are TGF-β receptor genes (Bone Morphogenetic Protein Receptor II [BMPR2] and Activin-Receptor-like Kinase 1) and both seem to operate separately to influence vascular cell growth: a mutation in *BMPR2* leads to FPAH by inducing smooth muscle proliferation whereas a mutation in Activin-Receptor-Like Kinase 1 leads to endothelial cell proliferation. Germline mutations in *BMPR2* have also been identified in

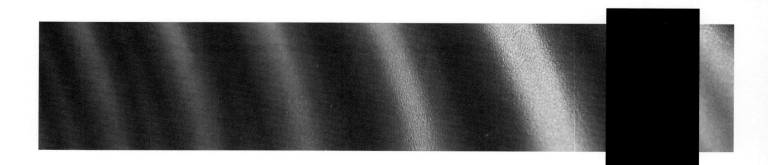

patients with apparently sporadic PAH. These germline mutations are inherited in some cases but some arise de novo. It is possible that mutation in other genes may predispose to the development of pulmonary arterial hypertension (13).

Interest is high in how the endothelial receptors exert their effects. The members of the TGF-β receptor family connect with transmembrane signaling molecules by various signaling and transcriptional pathways. A mutation in *BMPR2* may lead to a loss of the inhibitory action of BMPR on the growth of vascular smooth muscle cells in the pulmonary vasculature, leading to smooth muscle proliferation. A missense mutation — such as the substitution of guanine for thymine in Exon 3 of *BMPR2* — has been found in affected family members (10-13). Other mutations in *BMPR2* have also been found to run in families.

The association of incomplete penetrance of FPAH and the finding that only about one quarter of patients have a mutation in *BMPR2* suggest that non-heritable factors influence phenotypic expression or there are other (undisclosed as yet) genetic determinants. Genetic anticipation also suggests that disease-modifying genes influence phenotype (i.e. the disease becomes increasingly severe with succeeding generations or occurs at an earlier age) — especially since the mutations in *BMPR2* in families with FPAH are in the coding region of the gene and are invariant among generations in an affected family (10).

A new perspective has recently been provided by families in whom pulmonary arterial hypertension is associated with Hereditary Haemorrhagic Telangiectasia (HHT) (16, 17). HHT is an autosomal dominant disorder characterized by vascular dilatations which are presumably endothelial in nature. HHT is caused by mutations in endoglin or Activin-Like Kinase 1, both of which are involved in the endothelial transforming growth factor-β signaling pathways. The mutations are in genes located on chromosomes 12 and 9, respectively, both of which code for receptor members of the TGF-β pathway. In patients with coincident familial PAH and HHT, mutations have been found in the gene for Activin-Receptor-Like Kinase 1, a gene which is abundant in endothelial cells.

The present volume provides a comprehensive overview of issues related to pulmonary hypertension from a variety of causes. These diseases become clinically manifest at different stages in their evolution and each affords distinctive features which, taken together, afford a broad perspective of the pathogenesis and clinical management of pulmonary vascular disease. The present volume affords the reader a synthesis of what is currently known about pulmonary vascular disease and a vantage for viewing what lies ahead.

References

1. Fulton, JF. Selected Readings in the History of Physiology. Springfield, IL: Charles C. Thomas. Second Edition. 1966.
2. Keynes, G (ed.) The Anatomical exercises of Dr. William Harvey: The First Edition Text of 1653. London, 1928, page 197.
3. Willis, R (Translator) The Works of William Harvey. Philadelphia, PA: University of Pennsylvania Press. 1989.
4. Singer, C. The Discovery of the Circulation of the Blood. London: G. Bell and Sons, Ltd. 1922.
5. Singer, C. From Magic to Science. New York: Dover. 1958.
6. Fishman, AP. A Century of Pulmonary Hemodynamics. *Am J Respir Crit Care Med* 170:109–113, 2004.
7. Forssmann, W. Die Sondierung des Rechten Herzens. *Klin Wohrschr* 8:2085–2087, 1929.
8. Cournand, A, Ranges, HA. Catheterization of right auricle in man. *Proc Soc Exp Biol Med* 46:462–466, 1941.
9. Fishman, AP. Primary Pulmonary Arterial Hypertension: A Look Back. *J Am Col of Cardiology* 43 (Suppl 2–4. 2004.)
10. Loyd, JE, Newman, J. Familial primary pulmonary hypertension: clinical patterns. *Am Rev Resp Dis* 129:194–197, 1984.
11. Loyd, JE, Slovis, B, Phillips, JA 3rd, Butler, MG, Foroud, TM, Conneally, PM, Newman, JH. The presence of genetic anticipation suggests that the molecular basis of familial primary pulmonary hypertension may be trinucleotide repeat expansion. *Chest* 111(6 Suppl):82S-83S, 1997.
12. Loyd, JE, Butler, MG, Foroud, TM, Conneally, PM, Phillips, JA 3rd, Newman, JH. Genetic anticipation and abnormal gender ratio at birth in familial primary pulmonary hypertension. *Am J Resp Crit Care Med* 152:93–97, 1995.
13. Deng, Z, Morse, JH, Slager, SL, et al. Familial primary pulmonary hypertension (gene PPH1) is caused by mutations in the bone morphogenetic protein receptor-II gene. *Am J Hum Gen* 67:737–744, 2000.
14. Newman, JH, Trembath, RC, Morse, JA, et al. Genetic Basis of Pulmonary Arterial Hypertension: Current Understanding and Future Directions. *J Am Coll Cardiol* 43:(Suppl 8):33S–39S, 2004.
15. Morse, JH. Genetic Studies of Pulmonary Arterial Hypertension. *Lupus* 12:209–212, 2003.
16. Begbie, ME, Wallace, GMF, Shovlin, CL. Hereditary haemorrhagic telangiectasia (Osler-Weber-Rendu syndrome): a view from the 21st century. *Postgrad Med J* 79:18–24, 2003.
17. Fuchizaki, U, Miyamori, H, Kitagawa, S, Kaneko, S, Kobayashi, K. Hereditary haemorrhagic telangiectasia (Osler-Weber-Rendu disease). *Lancet* 362:1490–1494, 2003.

List of Contributors

Vivek N. Ahya, M.D.
Assistant Professor of Medicine
University of Pennsylvania School of Medicine
Medical Director, Lung Transplantation Program
Pulmonary, Allergy, and Critical Care Division
Hospital of the University of Pennsylvania
Philadelphia, Pennsylvania

Christine Archer-Chicko, M.S.N., C.R.N.P.
Coordinator, Pulmonary Vascular Disease Program
Pulmonary, Allergy and Critical Care Division
Penn Presbyterian Medical Center
Philadelphia, Pennsylvania

Alix Ashare, M.D.
Assistant Professor
Department of Internal Medicine
Division of Pulmonary, Critical Care, and
Occupational Medicine
University of Iowa Carver College of Medicine
Iowa City, Iowa

James Carroll, M.D.
Assistant Professor
Department of Internal Medicine
Division of Pulmonary, Critical Care, and
Occupational Medicine
University of Iowa Carver College of Medicine
Iowa City, Iowa

Kelly M. Chin, M.D.
Pulmonary and Critical Care Division
University of California, San Diego Medical Center
San Diego, California

C. Gregory Elliott, M.D.
Professor of Medicine
Chief, Pulmonary Division
Medical Director, Respiratory
LDS Hospital Pulmonary Division
University of Utah School of Medicine
Salt Lake City, Utah

Eliot B. Friedman, M.D.
Pulmonary, Allergy and Critical Care Division
Hospital of the University of Pennsylvania
Philadelphia, Pennsylvania

Peter F. Fedullo, M.D.
Clinical Professor of Medicine
Pulmonary and Critical Care Division
Director, Medical Intensive Care Unit
University of California, San Diego Medical Center
San Diego, California

Alfred P. Fishman, M.D.
Professor of Medicine and Senior Associate Dean
University of Pennsylvania School of Medicine
Philadelphia, Pennsylvania

Alicia Gerke, M.D.
Department of Internal Medicine
Division of Pulmonary, Critical Care, and
Occupational Medicine
University of Iowa Carver College of Medicine
Iowa City, Iowa

Mark T. Gladwin, M.D.
Vascular Medicine Branch
National Heart Lung and Blood Institute
Critical Care Medicine Department
Clinical Center
National Institutes of Health
Bethesda, Maryland

Dayna J. Groskreutz, M.D.
Department of Internal Medicine
Division of Pulmonary, Critical Care, and
Occupational Medicine
University of Iowa Carver College of Medicine
Iowa City, Iowa

Traci Housten-Harris, R.N., M.S.
Program Manager
Johns Hopkins Pulmonary Hypertension Program
The Johns Hopkins Hospital
Baltimore, Maryland

D. Dunbar Ivy, M.D.
Chief and Selby's Chair of Pediatric Cardiology
Director, Pediatric Pulmonary Hypertension
Program
Pediatric Heart Lung Center
The University of Colorado Health Sciences
Center, and
The Children's Hospital
Denver, Colorado

Maren E. Jeffery, M.D.
Cardiovascular Division
Hospital of the University of Pennsylvania
Philadelphia, Pennsylvania

Peter Lloyd Jones, Ph.D.
Associate Professor
Institute for Medicine and Engineering
Department of Pathology and Laboratory Medicine
University of Pennsylvania School of Medicine
Philadelphia, Pennsylvania

Robert M. Kotloff, M.D.
Professor of Medicine
University of Pennsylvania School of Medicine
Chief, Section of Advanced Lung Disease and
Lung Transplantation
Pulmonary, Allergy, and Critical Care Division
Hospital of the University of Pennsylvania
Philadelphia, Pennsylvania

Michael J. Krowka, M.D.
Professor of Medicine
Division of Pulmonary and Critical Care
Mayo Clinic College of Medicine
Mayo Clinic
Rochester, Minnesota

Roberto F. Machado, M.D.
Vascular Medicine Branch
National Heart Lung and Blood Institute
Critical Care Medicine Department
Clinical Center
National Institutes of Health
Bethesda, Maryland

Jess Mandel, M.D.
Associate Professor and Assistant Dean
Director, Pulmonary Hypertension Program
Department of Internal Medicine
Division of Pulmonary, Critical Care, and
Occupational Medicine
University of Iowa Carver College of Medicine
Iowa City, Iowa

Emilio Mazza Jr., M.D., Ph.D.
Pulmonary, Allergy and Critical Care Division
Hospital of the University of Pennsylvania
Philadelphia, Pennsylvania

Giora Netzer, M.D.
Pulmonary, Allergy and Critical Care Division
Hospital of the University of Pennsylvania
Philadelphia, Pennsylvania

Harold I. Palevsky, M.D.
Professor of Medicine
University of Pennsylvania School of Medicine
Chief, Pulmonary, Allergy and Critical Care Division
Director, Pulmonary Vascular Disease Program
Penn Presbyterian Medical Center
Philadelphia, Pennsylvania

Giuseppe G. Pietra, M.D.
Professor Emeritus
Department of Pathology and Laboratory Medicine
University of Pennsylvania School of Medicine
Philadelphia, Pennsylvania

Asrar Rashid, MBChB, MRCP, MRCPCH, DTM&H
Consultant Paediatric Intensivist
Department of Paediatric Intensive Care
Queens Medical Centre
Nottingham
University Hospital NHS Trust
United Kingdom

Jeffrey S. Sager, M.D., M.S.C.E.
Assistant Professor of Medicine
University of Pennsylvania School of Medicine
Associate Medical Director, Lung Transplantation
Program
Pulmonary, Allergy, and Critical Care Division
Hospital of the University of Pennsylvania
Philadelphia, Pennsylvania

Jennifer L. Snow, M.D.
Pulmonary, Allergy and Critical Care Division
Hospital of the University of Pennsylvania
Philadelphia, Pennsylvania

Karen L. Swanson, D.O.
Assistant Professor of Medicine
Division of Pulmonary and Critical Care
Mayo Clinic College of Medicine
Mayo Clinic
Rochester, Minnesota

Darren B. Taichman, M.D., Ph.D.
Assistant Professor of Medicine
University of Pennsylvania School of Medicine
Director, Medical Intensive Care Unit
Associate Director, Pulmonary Vascular Disease
Program
Pulmonary, Allergy and Critical Care Division
Penn Presbyterian Medical Center
Philadelphia, PA

Karl W. Thomas, M.D.
Assistant Professor
Department of Internal Medicine
Division of Pulmonary, Critical Care, and
Occupational Medicine
University of Iowa Carver College of Medicine
Iowa City, Iowa

Contents

Contents (continued)

COLOR PLATES

PLATE 1

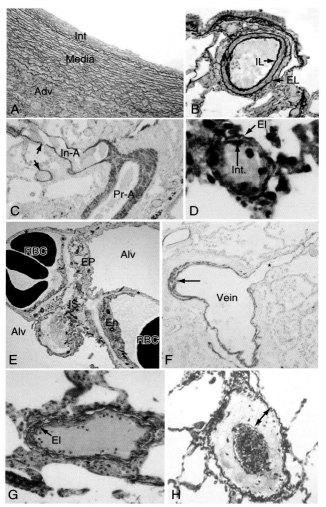

Figure 2-1. Normal Pulmonary Vessels. **A.** The media of an elastic pulmonary artery is composed of a latticework of coarse elastic laminae. A narrow strip of the intima (*Int*) overlying the media is visible. A normal adventitia (*Adv*) is also seen. **B.** Cross-section of a pre-acinar muscular pulmonary artery revealing a thin muscular media (*M*) bounded by internal (*IL*) and external (*EL*) elastic laminae. **C.** Branching off of an intra-acinar artery (*In-A*) from a pre-acinar artery (*Pr-A*). The media of the vessels has been decorated with anti-smooth muscle actin antibody (*rust color*) to show the marked decrease in medial muscle as the caliber of the arteries decreases. The *arrows* point to a partial loss of the medial muscle in the vessel walls. **D.** Nonmuscular intra-acinar artery composed of intima (*Int*) and elastic lamina (*EL*). **E.** Electron micrograph of an alveolar septum showing the subdivision of the interstitial space (IS) into thin (***) and thick (*IS*) zones by the eccentric course of the alveolar capillary. *RBC,* red blood cell; *EP,* Type 1 pneumocyte; *En,* endothelium; *Alv,* alveolar space. **F.** Intra-acinar venule (***) draining into an interlobular vein (*vein*). Smooth muscle actin staining reveals the irregular distribution of the medial muscle in the venous wall (*arrow*). **G.** Cross-section of an interlobular vein showing the single elastic lamina (*El*) separating the media from the adventitia. **H.** Cross-section of an interlobular vein showing age-related fibrous thickening of the intima (*double arrow*). (Stains: **A, B, D, G,** and **H**: Verhoeff-van Gieson; **C** and **F**: Smooth muscle actin; **E**: Uranyl acetate-lead citrate.)

Figure 2-4. Low-power view of an elastic pulmonary artery from a patient with idiopathic pulmonary arterial hypertension showing a calcified atheromatous plaque. (Hematoxylin and eosin stain.)

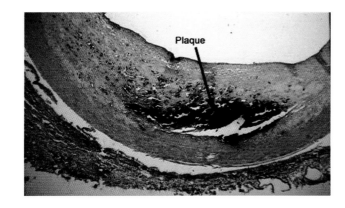

PLATE 2

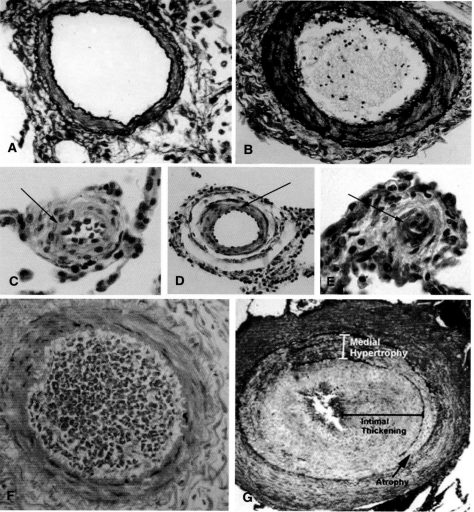

Figure 2-5. Medial Hypertrophy. As compared with a normal vessel (**A**), an increase in the medial smooth muscle is seen in the pulmonary artery of a patient with pulmonary hypertension (**B**). High-power photomicrographs showing extension of muscularization to involve small intra-acinar pulmonary arteries (**C**, **D**, **E**, *arrows*). Medial hypertrophy can occur as an isolated lesion (**F**) or in association with intimal fibrosis (**G**). Panel **G** shows a photomicrograph of a muscular pulmonary artery (approximately 20 microns) with marked nonlaminar concentric intimal thickening. Medial hypertrophy and segmental atrophy with partial destruction of the internal elastic lamina are seen. (Stains: **A**, **B**, **G**: Verhoeff-van Gieson; **C**, **D**, **E**, **F**: Hematoxylin and eosin.)

PLATE 3

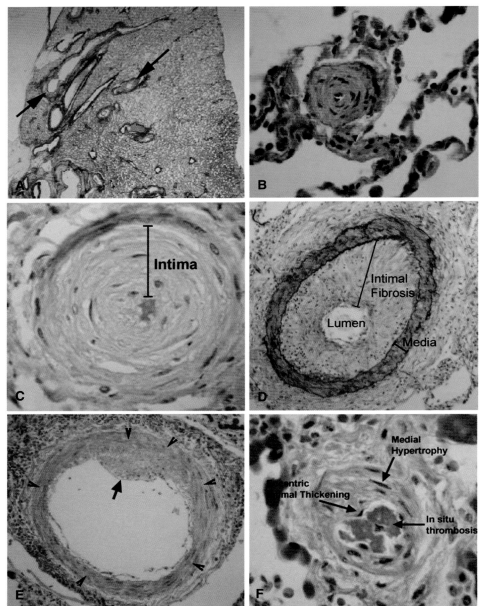

Figure 2-6. Intimal Thickening. **A.** Whole lung section from a patient with exposure to the appetite suppressant aminorex. Enlargement and thickening of the pulmonary arterial structures can be seen (*arrows*). **B.** Concentric laminar intimal thickening in an intraacinar pulmonary artery of a patient with human immunodeficiency virus (HIV) infection. He did not meet criteria for a diagnosis of acquired immunodeficiency syndrome (AIDS) when pulmonary arterial hypertension was diagnosed. **C.** Pre-acinar pulmonary artery with marked concentric intimal thickening ("onion skinning") and resultant narrowing of the vessel lumen in a patient with systemic sclerosis and focal pulmonary fibrosis. This patient did not have pulmonary hypertension. The vascular lesions were localized to the areas of pulmonary fibrosis. **D** and **E.** Nonlaminar intimal thickening can be concentric (**D**) or eccentric (**E,** *arrow*) as seen in these pre-acinar muscular arteries. Medial hypertrophy is also seen (*arrow heads* and *label*). **F.** High-power photomicrograph showing an intra-acinar pulmonary artery with eccentric nonlaminar intimal thickening, medial hypertrophy, and *in situ* thrombosis. (Stains: **A, D**: Verhoeff-Van Gieson; **B, C, E, F**: Hematoxylin and eosin.) (Reproduced with permission from Pietra GG: The pathology of primary pulmonary hypertension. In: Rubin LJ, Rich S, editors: *Primary pulmonary hypertension,* New York, 1997, Marcel Dekker, pp 19-61; Pietra GG, Capron F, Stewart S, et al: Pathologic assessment of vasculopathies in pulmonary hypertension. *J Am Coll Cardiol* 43(12 Suppl S):25S-32S, 2004.)

PLATE 4

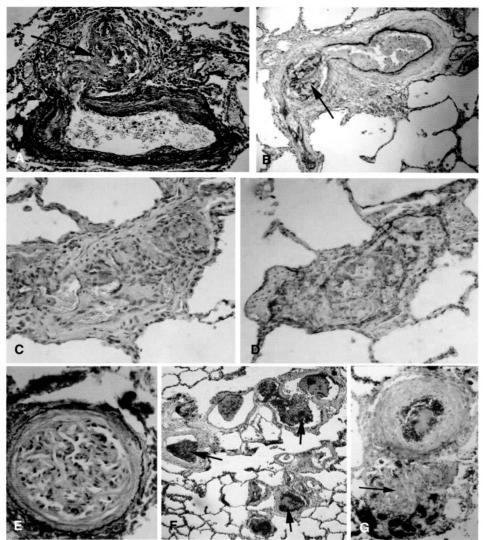

Figure 2-7. A and **B.** Plexiform lesions (*arrows*) often are located at the origin of a pulmonary artery at its branching point from a parent vessel. In (**A**), the vessel wall has been destroyed locally and is filled with small channels of blood and granulation tissue. Immunostaining for CD31 (*rust color*) reveals endothelial cells lining the parent vessel and within the plexiform lesion (**B**). **C** and **D.** Endothelial and smooth muscle cells within a plexiform lesion involving an intra-acinar pulmonary artery in a patient with idiopathic pulmonary arterial hypertension. Anti-factor VIII immunostaining (*rust color*) outlines endothelial cells (**C**) and anti-smooth muscle actin outlines smooth muscle cells (**D**) within the same plexiform lesion. **E.** A pre-acinar pulmonary artery displaying recanalized thrombus, giving rise to a "colander-like" lesion (often confused with plexiform lesions). **F.** Low-power photomicrograph showing dilation lesions (*arrows*) consisting of thin-walled sinusoidal channels within the alveolar-capillary network. These lesions usually are found distal to plexiform lesions and may result in hemoptysis if rupture occurs. **G.** Low-power photomicrograph showing a plexiform lesion (*arrow*) and dilation lesions in a patient with portopulmonary hypertension. (Stains: **A**: Verhoeff-Van Gieson; **F, G**: Hematoxylin and eosin.) (Reprinted with permission from [A] Pietra GG: The histopathology of primary pulmonary hypertension. In: Fishman AP, editor: *The pulmonary circulation: Normal and abnormal. Mechanisms, management, and the National Registry,* Philadelphia, 1990, University of Pennsylvania Press, pp 459-472; [F] Pietra GG, Capron F, Stewart S, et al: Pathologic assessment of vasculopathies in pulmonary hypertension. *J Am Coll Cardiol* 43[12 Suppl S]:25S-32S, 2004.)

PLATE 5

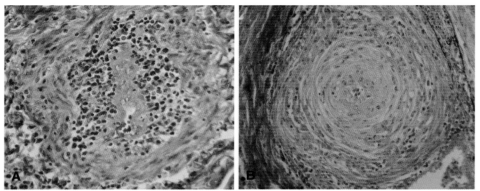

Figure 2-8. **A.** Medium-power photomicrograph of a pre-acinar pulmonary artery in a patient with pulmonary hypertension showing an inflammatory infiltrate in the vessel wall. (Hematoxylin and eosin stain.) **B.** A pre-acinar pulmonary artery with lymphocytic arteritis. (Verhoeff-Van Gieson stain). (Reproduced with permission from [**B**] Pietra GG, Capron F, Stewart S, et al: Pathologic assessment of vasculopathies in pulmonary hypertension. *J Am Coll Cardiol* 43[12 Suppl S]:25S-32S, 2004.)

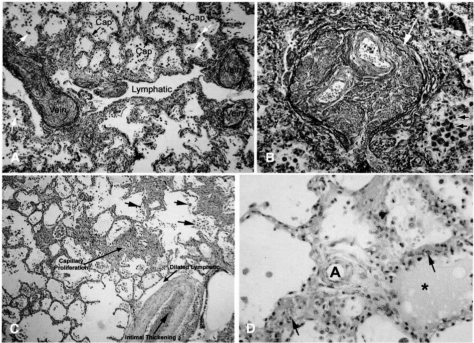

Figure 2-9. Pulmonary Obstructive Venopathy and Pulmonary Microvasculopathy. **A.** Low-power photomicrograph showing near-total obstruction of pulmonary veins, lymphatic dilation, capillary congestion (*Cap, black arrows),* and accumulation of hemosiderin-laden macrophages (*white arrows*) in pulmonary obstructive venopathy. (Verhoeff-Van Gieson stain.) **B.** High-power photomicrograph showing obstruction and recanalization of a pulmonary vein. Note also the arterialization characterized by medial muscle hypertrophy and the double elastic laminae (*white arrow*). Hemosiderin-laden macrophages fill the alveolar spaces (*black arrows*). This patient's clinical diagnosis was pulmonary veno-occlusive disease. (Verhoeff-Van Gieson stain.) **C.** Low-power photomicrograph showing pulmonary microvasculopathy, with patchy capillary proliferation and accumulation of hemosiderin-laden macrophages (*short arrows*) in the alveoli and interstitium. Intimal thickening within the artery as well as lymphatic dilation are seen. (Hematoxylin and eosin stain.) **D.** Low-power photomicrograph revealing the presence of more than one capillary (*arrows*) in the widened alveolar septa, indicative of pulmonary microvasculopathy seen here in a patient with pulmonary capillary hemangiomatosis. Also seen is an intra-acinar artery (*A*) with medial hypertrophy. Note that in the normal adult lung, only one capillary is seen in cross-sections of the alveolar septa; a double layer of capillaries here is an important histopathologic feature of pulmonary microvasculopathy. (Hematoxylin and eosin stain.) (Reproduced with permission from [A] Pietra GG, Capron F, Stewart S, et al: Pathologic assessment of vasculopathies in pulmonary hypertension. *J Am Coll Cardiol* 43[12 Suppl S]:25S-32S, 2004.)

PLATE 6

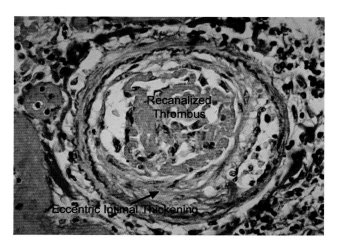

Figure 2-10. *In situ* thrombosis. Photomicrograph showing *in situ* thrombosis with organization and recanalization within a pre-acinar muscular artery with eccentric intimal thickening. (Verhoeff-Van Gieson stain.)

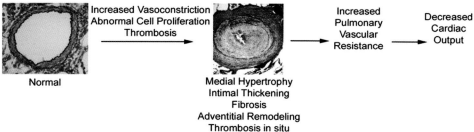

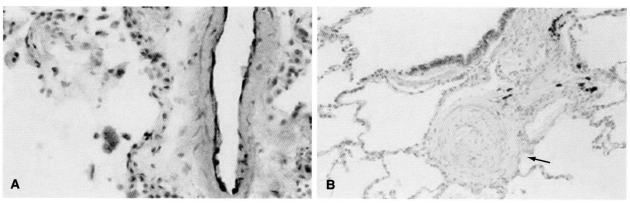

Figure 3-1. Schematic depiction of key pathobiologic processes involved in pulmonary arterial hypertension. Multiple factors contribute to abnormal vasoconstriction, cellular proliferation, and thrombosis. These changes result in an elevated resistance to the transit of blood through the pulmonary circulation and eventual right heart failure with impaired cardiac output. (Histologic images courtesy of G.G. Pietra, MD.)

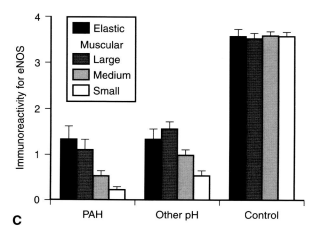

Figure 3-2. Decreased expression of endothelial nitric oxide synthase (eNOS) in the lungs of patients with pulmonary hypertension. Immunostaining (*rust color*) identifies eNOS on a muscular pulmonary artery from a normal (non–pulmonary hypertensive) lung (**A**). In the lung of a patient with pulmonary arterial hypertension (**B**), however, immunoreactivity for eNOS is seen on bronchial epithelial cells but not on an adjacent pulmonary artery (*arrow*), where intimal fibrosis and medial hypertrophy are found. Panel **C** shows a semi-quantitative assessment eNOS immunoreactivity on elastic and muscular pulmonary arteries from patients with pulmonary arterial hypertension (PAH) and non-PAH forms of pulmonary hypertension. For all vessel types and sizes, eNOS immunoreactivity was reduced as compared with that seen on vessels from normal (control) lungs. (Reproduced with permission from Giaid A, Saleh D: Reduced expression of endothelial nitric oxide synthase in the lungs of patients with pulmonary hypertension. *N Engl J Med* 333[4]:214-221, 1995.)

PLATE 7

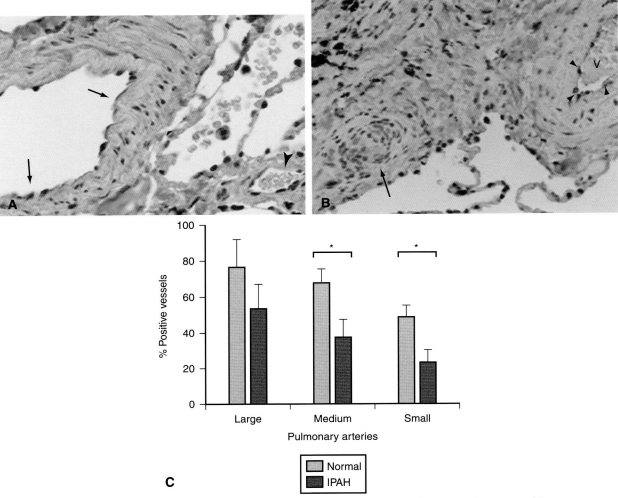

Figure 3-3. Decreased vascular expression of prostacyclin synthase in the lungs of patients with severe pulmonary arterial hypertension (PAH). Immunostaining *(rust color)* identifies the presence of prostacyclin synthase on the vessels of lung tissue from a patient without pulmonary hypertension *(arrows,* **A**). In a patient with idiopathic PAH (IPAH) (**B**), prostacyclin synthase expression is seen on histologically normal vessels *(V, arrowheads),* while absent on most endothelial cells within abnormal vessels, such as those within plexiform lesions *(arrow).* Although the frequency of large vessels expressing prostacyclin synthase was the same in lung tissue from patients with IPAH as compared with non–pulmonary hypertensive samples, there was a significant reduction on medium and small vessels from patients with IPAH (**C;** *P < .05). (Adapted with permission from Tuder RM, Cool CD, Geraci MW, et al: Prostacyclin synthase expression is decreased in lungs from patients with severe pulmonary hypertension. *Am J Respir Crit Care Med* 159[6]:1925-1932, 1999.)

PLATE 8

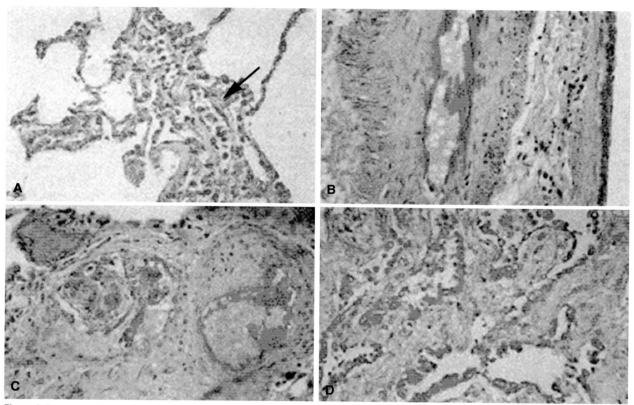

Figure 3-5. Increased expression of endothelin-1 in the lungs of patients with pulmonary hypertension. Immunostaining with an antibody to endothelin-1 decorates vascular endothelial cells in a normal (non–pulmonary hypertensive) lung (**A**, *rust color, arrow*). Markedly increased endothelin-1 expression is seen on pulmonary arteries of patients with idiopathic pulmonary arterial hypertension (**B** and **C**), including within plexiform lesions (**C**). Increased endothelin expression is also found in the lungs of patients with other forms of pulmonary hypertension, as well as on nonvascular cell populations such as on Type 2 alveolar pneumocytes (**D**). (Reproduced with permission from Giaid A, Yanagisawa M, Langleben D, et al: Expression of endothelin-1 in the lungs of patients with pulmonary hypertension. *N Engl J Med* 328[24]:1732-1739, 1993.)

PLATE 9

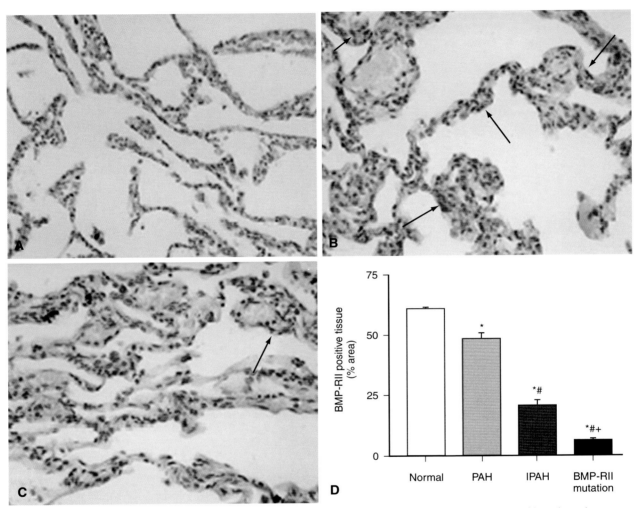

Figure 3-7. Expression of BMP-RII in normal and lung with pulmonary arterial hypertension (PAH). Immunostaining of lung tissue demonstrating the expression BMP-RII (*rust color*) in a control subject (**A**). Reduced expression is seen in the lung of patient with congenital heart disease—associated PAH (**B**) and markedly reduced in a patient with PAH and a mutation in the *BMP-RII* gene (**C**). The graph shows a semi-quantitative assessment of *BMP-RII* expression in normal lungs and those from patients with PAH associated with *BMP-RII* mutations, idiopathic (IPAH) and other forms of PAH. The reduction in staining in the tissue carrying *BMP-RII* mutations was not due to a reduction in the number of endothelial cells, because no difference was seen upon staining with an endothelial cell marker (CD31, not shown). *P < .05 compared with control; #P < .05 compared with PAH; +P < .05 compared with IPAH. (Adapted with permission from Atkinson C, Stewart S, Upton PD, et al: Primary pulmonary hypertension is associated with reduced pulmonary vascular expression of type II bone morphogenetic protein receptor. *Circulation* 105[14]:1672-1678, 2002.)

PLATE 10

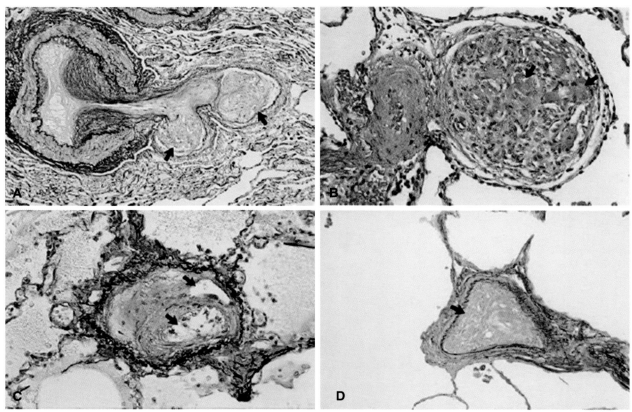

Figure 9-2. Pathologic findings in the pulmonary vasculature in portopulmonary hypertension: (**A**) plexogenic type (plexiform lesions: *arrows*); (**B**) obstructive plexiform lesion with occluding platelet-fibrin thrombi (*arrows*); (**C**) thrombotic type: muscular pulmonary arteriole obstructed by recanalized thrombus (*arrows*); (**D**) fibrotic type: pulmonary arteriole obstructed by dense fibrin plug. (From Krowka MJ, Edwards WD: A spectrum of pulmonary vascular pathology in portopulmonary hypertension. *Liver Transpl* 6:241-242, 2000.)

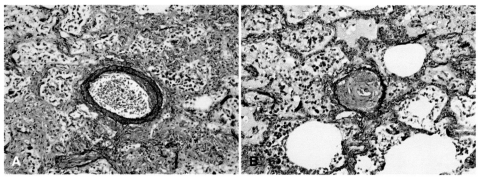

Figure 11-1. Pulmonary Veno-occlusive Disease. Elastic stain distinguishes a small artery (A) from an involved small vein (B) (20). (Courtesy of Michelle Bianco, MD.)

Figure 11-2. Pulmonary Veno-occlusive Disease. Hematoxylin and eosin staining shows obstructive intimal fibrosis of small vein (thin arrow) and extensive hemosiderin-laden intraalveolar macrophages (thick arrow) (20). (Courtesy of Michelle Bianco, MD.)

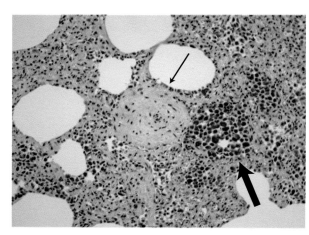

PLATE 11

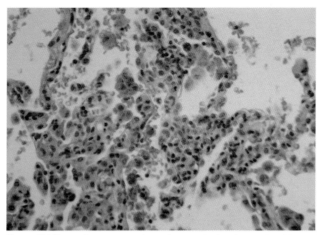

Figure 15-2. Medium-power photomicrograph showing capillaritis and hemorrhage in a patient with systemic lupus erythematosus. The inflammatory infiltrate consists primarily of neutrophils. (Hematoxylin and eosin stain.) (Courtesy of Dr. Giuseppe G. Pietra.)

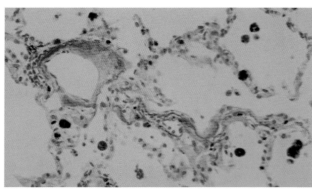

Figure 15-4. Photomicrograph showing blue areas of siderosis of a pulmonary vein and alveolar capillary in a patient with Goodpasture syndrome. (Prussian blue stain.) (Courtesy of Dr. Giuseppe G. Pietra.)

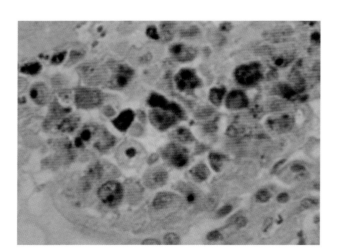

Figure 15-3. Photomicrograph showing hemosiderin-laden macrophages (staining blue due to their iron content) in a patient with Goodpasture syndrome. (Prussian blue stain.) (Courtesy of Dr. Giuseppe G. Pietra.)

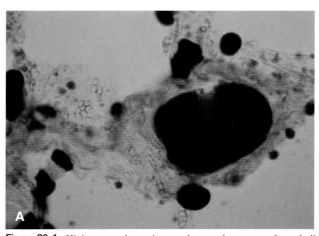

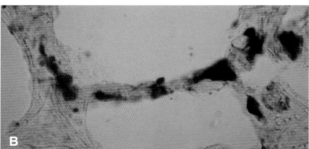

Figure 20-1. High-power photomicrographs reveal numerous fat emboli within pulmonary capillaries. The patient was an unrestrained driver in a high speed motor vehicle accident and suffered multiple fractures. (Sudan III stain.) (Courtesy of Dr. Giuseppe G. Pietra.)

Chapter 1

Functions and Control of the Pulmonary Circulation

Emilio Mazza Jr., MD, PhD,

Darren B. Taichman, MD, PhD

Anatomy of the Pulmonary Circulation

The blood supply of the lung consists of the pulmonary and bronchial circulations. The pulmonary circulation, which originates with deoxygenated blood from the right ventricle, allows for gas exchange with the alveoli in which the pulmonary capillaries run. The bronchial circulation, which consists of systemic arterial branches from the aorta, ensures the vitality of the gas-exchanging units and the conducting airways of the lung. The pulmonary circulation is an intricate and complex system, with properties and adaptive control systems quite distinct from those of the systemic circulation and well suited to the physiologic role of blood gas homeostasis.

The pulmonary circulation begins with the main pulmonary artery, then divides and enters each lung at the hilum adjacent to its respective mainstem bronchus. From there it travels adjacent to and branches with each airway generation to the level of the respiratory bronchiole; these are the so-called "axial arteries." However, there are more arteries than bronchi because of the presence of supernumerary arteries[1] that branch off axial arteries and perfuse alveolar parenchyma in a nongeographic manner. In contrast, the axial arteries branch at the terminal bronchus, supplying a specific volume of respiratory tissue or lobule. Unlike in the systemic circulation in which arteries branch into arterioles, capillaries, and venules, the pulmonary arteries at the level of the alveoli branch into precapillary arteries leading to a diffuse network of capillaries that traverse several alveoli,

then drain into postcapillary veins. Pulmonary veins each drain portions of several lobules and are not associated with the airways until the level of the hilum, where they associate with the mainstem bronchi and pulmonary artery in a loosely organized connective tissue sheath (FIGURE 1-1).

The lung can triple its volume when expanding from functional residual capacity to total lung capacity. This change in lung volume has opposing effects on the alveolar vessels (capillaries) and the conduit or extra-alveolar vessels (arteries and veins).[2] As the lung expands, the diameter of the extra-alveolar vessels increases secondary to the radial traction created by the expanding alveoli (FIGURE 1-2). In contrast, the diameter of alveolar capillaries decreases as the lung expands and the alveolar septae lengthen. The exceptions to the latter are alveolar vessels termed "corner vessels."[3,4] These corner vessels differ from other alveolar capillaries in their ability to resist the effects of high alveolar pressures that cause the closure of most alveolar septal capillaries.

As in the systemic circulation, the wall structure of the pulmonary arteries and their smooth muscle content differ according to their location in the pulmonary vascular tree.[5] For any given caliber, however, the medial smooth muscle layer of a pulmonary artery is thinner than that of the systemic vasculature, reflecting the lower pressures seen by the normal pulmonary circulation. The larger elastic arteries have an adventitial, muscular, and intimal layer. The muscle layer is bounded by internal and external elastic laminae and accounts for 1-2 percent of the external diameter. The muscular arteries, which are smaller in size and lack an internal elastic lamina, have a thick muscle layer

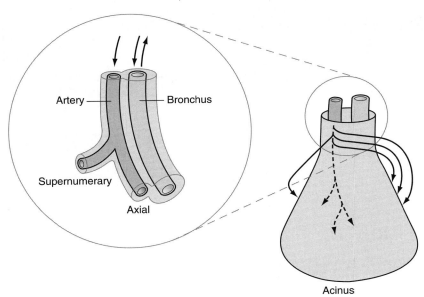

Figure 1-1. Diagram showing the arrangement of the arteries in relation to bronchi and acini. The pulmonary artery travels adjacent to and branches with each airway generation to the level of the respiratory bronchiole. These are called "axial arteries." There are supernumerary arteries that branch off axial arteries and perfuse alveolar parenchyma in a nongeographic manner (interrupted arrows). (From Gil J, Ciurea D: Functional structure of the pulmonary circulation. In: Peacock AJ, editor: *Pulmonary circulation. A handbook for clinicians,* London, 1996, Chapman and Hall Medical, pp 3-84.)

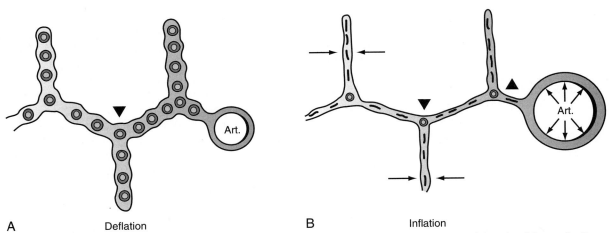

A   Deflation   B   Inflation

Figure 1-2. Effects of inflation and deflation of the lung on extraalveolar, alveolar, and corner *(arrowheads)* vessels diameter. Extra-alveolar vessel (Art) size increases with lung inflation, due to radial traction exerted by the surrounding alveolar tissue. In contrast, the diameter of alveolar capillaries decrease with inflation *(large arrows).* Note that corner vessel diameter stays relatively constant (arrowheads). (From Gil J, Ciurea D: Functional structure of the pulmonary circulation. In: Peacock AJ, editor: *Pulmonary circulation. a handbook for clinicians,* London, 1996, Chapman and Hall Medical, pp 3-84.)

that is 2-5 percent of the external diameter. More distal in the pulmonary artery tree are partially muscularized arteries with an incomplete muscle layer. Finally, in the nonmuscular arteries the smooth muscle layer is replaced by pericytes. It has been suggested that pericytes may produce and organize the surrounding matrix and basement membrane. In addition, pericytes may differentiate into smooth muscle cells and constitute the site of vascular remodeling in pulmonary hypertension.[6]

Functional Correlates of the Pulmonary Circulatory Anatomy

The blood-gas barrier of the lung consists of the alveolar-capillary interface. The capillary surface area is approximately 125 m[2] and approximately 86 percent of the alveolar surface area. An individual capillary is approximately 7-10 μm in diameter (roughly the size of a single erythrocyte and smaller than many white blood cells). The microvascular bed consists of a network of capillaries where erythrocytes flow through each sheet in single file exposed to gas exchange surfaces on either side.[7] Alveolar capillaries have a thin and thick side. The thin side (approximately 0.2-0.3 μm thick) is the gas exchange interface, made up of the capillary endothelial cell, an apposing alveolar epithelial cell (Type 1 pneumocyte), and their fused basement membranes. The thick side, which provides structural support to the parenchyma, is approximately 2 μm thick and contains type I collagen, fibroblasts, and pericytes (FIGURE 1-3).

Optimal gas exchange is facilitated by the extremely short distance for diffusion at the thin side of the blood-gas barrier. This minimal distance required for diffusion, however, comes at the cost of strength. The thin side of the blood-gas barrier allows for optimal gas exchange. The integrity of the blood-gas barrier is dependent on the "lamina densa," the fused basement membrane of the lining cells. The lamina densa is comprised of type IV collagen and its thickness is dependent on the amount of tension placed upon it. In situations of high vascular wall tension, the lamina densa can thicken in order to increase the strength of this interface; this, however, increases the diffusion distance required for gas exchange. Despite such protective thickening of the lamina densa, elevation in capillary pressure can ultimately lead to alveolar damage via disruption of the endothelial and epithelial lining. In an isolated perfused rabbit lung model, Tsukimoto and colleagues[8] observed that increases in capillary pressures to 24-40 mmHg for 4 minutes could result in disruption of the blood-gas barrier. Increased lung volumes can further worsen the disruptive effect of high capillary pressure.

The precise anatomic arrangement of the pulmonary vasculature with the airways and alveoli is in keeping with the closely coordinated relationship between ventilation and perfusion. Very little gas exchange occurs prior to the alveolar capillaries. Accordingly, although larger vessels of the lung contain the majority of blood volume, most of the

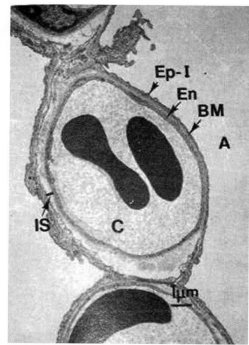

Figure 1-3. Transmission electron micrograph of a rat pulmonary capillary *(C)* illustrating the fused basement membrane *(BM)* of an endothelial *(En)* and type I epithelial *(Ep-I)* cell. A, alveolar space; *IS*, interstitial space. (Image courtesy of Dr. Guissepe Pietra. Reproduced with permission from Pietra GG, Ruttner JR, Wust W, et al: The lung after trauma and shock. Fine structure of the alveolar-capillary barrier in 23 autopsies (Fig 1). *J Trauma* 21:454-462, 1981.)

vascular surface area is contained within smaller vessels involved in gas exchange (FIGURE 1-4).

The distribution of blood flow increases almost linearly from the top to the bottom of the lung (FIGURE 1-5). This distribution of blood flow has been further divided into three functional zones based upon the interaction between the alveolar (P_A), arterial (P_a), and venous (P_v) pressures.[9] In Zone 1 of the upright lung, pulmonary alveolar pressure exceeds pulmonary arterial pressure, which in turn exceeds pulmonary venous pressure $(P_A > P_a > P_v)$, resulting in minimal blood flow because most alveolar capillaries are collapsed. Blood flow through extra-alveolar vessels is unaffected. Blood flow through part of Zone 1 is also maintained to some degree through corner vessels that remain patent despite P_A, as well as during systole due to the pulsatile nature of pulmonary arterial flow.[10] In the upright lung, Zone 1 has the smallest topographic distribution (as compared

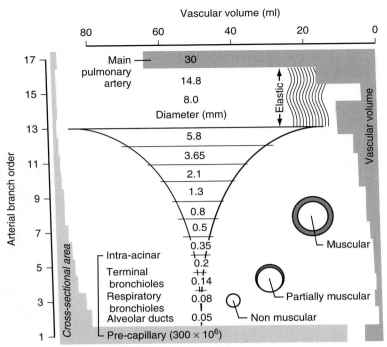

Figure 1-4. Diagram of the pulmonary artery tree in relation to blood volume, cross-sectional area, diameter, and wall structure. Note that although larger diameter vessels contain the greatest blood volume, smaller vessels account for most of the vascular surface area. Numerically lower branch order represents a more distal vessel. (From Hughes LMB, Morrell NW: Vascular structure and function. In: Hughes LMB, Morrell NW, eds, *Pulmonary Circulation. From basic mechanisms to clinical practice,* London, 2001, Imperial College Press, pp 14-30.)

with Zones 2 and 3, described below), occurring only at the apices of the lung. In the horizontal lung gravitational forces allow for an increase in P_a and Zone 1 is nonexistent.

In Zone 2, pulmonary arterial pressure exceeds pulmonary alveolar pressure, which in turn exceeds pulmonary venous pressure ($P_a > P_A > P_v$) (see FIGURE 1-5). In this setting, the outflow pressure is the pulmonary alveolar pressure and the driving force to blood flow is the difference between P_a and P_A. This creates a waterfall effect in that blood flow is independent of the downstream pressure. The driving force to blood flow increases further down along the lung due to the effect of gravity. Changing interactions between the P_A and P_v, as occurs with increasing venous pressure from left-sided heart failure for example, can shift outflow pressures from P_A to P_v and back.

In Zone 3 of the lung, pulmonary arterial pressure exceeds pulmonary venous pressure and both exceed pulmonary alveolar pressure ($P_a > P_v > P_A$) (see FIGURE 1-5). Therefore, this is the only zone of the lung where the use of a flow-directed, balloon-tipped catheter (commonly termed a "Swan-Ganz catheter") to measure pulmonary capillary occlusion pressure (representing transmitted left atrial pressures) and calculate pulmonary vascular resistance (PVR) is valid. Most of the blood flow is in Zone 3 in both the upright and horizontal lung. The driving force to blood flow in Zone 3 is the difference between the P_a and P_v pressures, and this difference remains constant down to the bottom of the lung. Increases in blood flow from the top to the bottom of Zone 3, therefore, are reflective of decreases in PVR resulting from the distention of blood-filled pulmonary arteries (discussed further below).

In the upright lung, a fourth zone is described where vascular pressures are at their highest but blood flow is reduced.[11] This zone of reduced blood flow is located at the base of the lung and is present at residual volume but disappears with deep inspiration. Decreases in pulmonary blood flow are hypothesized to be caused by loss of the tethering effect of the lung parenchyma at smaller lung volumes, resulting in a decrease in the caliber of extra-alveolar vessels. In addition, increasing

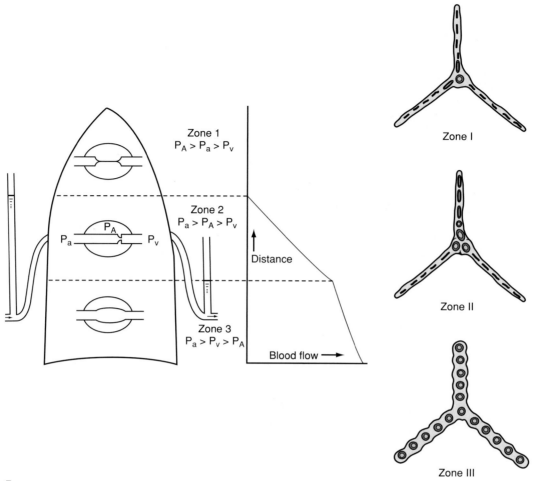

Figure 1-5. Theoretical zones of blood flow in the upright lung. In Zone 1 of the lung, alveolar pressure exceeds arterial vessel pressure, with resultant collapse of alveolar capillaries. In Zone 2 arterial pressure is greater than alveolar pressure, but alveolar pressure exceeds venous pressure. This causes a waterfall effect, with the pressure gradient causing flow equal to the arterial-alveolar pressure. In Zone 3 venous pressure exceeds alveolar pressure and the collapsible vessels are held open. The pressure gradient for blood flow is now arterial-venous pressure. Blood flow progressively increases from the top of Zone 2 to the bottom of Zone 3 because of gravitational effects on venous pressure. *PA*, alveolar pressure; *Pa*, arterial pressure; *Pv*, venous pressure. (From West JB, Dollery CT, Naimark A: Distribution of blood flow in isolated lung; relation to vascular and alveolar pressures. *J Appl Physiol* 19:713-724, 1964; and Gil J, Ciurea D: Functional structure of the pulmonary circulation. In: Peacock AJ, editor; *Pulmonary circulation: A handbook for clinicians*, London, 1996, Chapman and Hall Medical, pp 3-84.)

interstitial pressure may also contribute to a reduction in the caliber of extra-alveolar vessels.

The concept of lung zones presented above is a functional rather than an anatomic construct, and the extent of the zones described can change in a dynamic manner depending upon the physiologic or pathophysiologic state. As an example, with exercise, increases in P_a tend to increase the size of functional Zone 2 while decreasing Zone 1. An elevation in pulmonary venous pressures, as in states of impaired left heart function, will increase functional Zone 3.

Regional Control of Blood Flow

Basic Principles of Pulmonary Vascular Resistance

The pulmonary circulation is a low-pressure, low-resistance system as compared with the systemic circulation. In the lung, regional blood flow is determined by the driving pressure (arterial-venous or arterial-alveolar pressure difference) and the vascular resistance. In the pulmonary circulation, almost half of the resistance to flow occurs in the alveolar capillaries.[12] In addition, resistance is regulated by vasomotor activity of small muscular precapillary arteries.[13] The contribution of the pulmonary veins, although small, is less well characterized.

Clinically, PVR has been determined through the use of a flow-directed balloon-tipped pulmonary artery catheter (Swan-Ganz catheter).[14] Assuming a steady state, PVR can be calculated using Ohm's law:

$$PVR = \text{Driving Pressure} (P_{inflow} - P_{outflow}) \div \text{Flow}$$

Using data obtained from the pulmonary artery catheter, P_{inflow} is the measured mean pulmonary artery pressure (mPAP), $P_{outflow}$ the pulmonary artery occlusion pressure (PAOP), and Flow is the cardiac output. PVR is expressed in mmHg/L/min (Wood units) as calculated above, or approximated to dynes/sec $\times$ cm^5 by multiplying by 80. This calculation of PVR requires that measurements are made in Zone 3 of the lung, where the determinant of blood flow is the difference between arterial and venous pressures. Here, with the catheter in a "wedged" position by virtue of its balloon having been inflated, the measured pressure is reflective of the pulmonary venous system (and as discussed above, is representative of left atrial pressure). In non-Zone 3 conditions, P_A exceeds P_v, causing collapse of alveolar vessels, and the measured pressure erroneously reflects alveolar pressures. It should also be noted that measuring PVR in this fashion represents an oversimplification because it ignores the pulsatile nature of the pulmonary circulation. When interpreted properly and with an understanding of these shortcomings, however, this method of measuring PVR is facile and yields values that can be clinically useful.

To understand how the anatomy of the pulmonary circulation plays a role in determining PVR, one can apply Poiseuille's law to determine resistance. Assuming that blood is a Newtonian fluid (one that has a constant viscosity regardless of shear rate), then with laminar flow through a smooth, nondistensible tube, resistance and flow are related as the following:

$$\text{Resistance} = (P_{inflow} - P_{outflow}) \div \text{Flow} = 8 \times 1 \times \eta \div (\pi \times r^4)$$

where l is the length of the tube, η is the viscosity coefficient, and r is the radius of the tube. Assuming that blood viscosity is constant, it is apparent that PVR is exquisitely sensitive to changes in pulmonary vascular radius. Again, as with the use of Ohm's law, the use of Poiseuille's law to determine PVR has important limitations. First, blood flow through the pulmonary circulation is not laminar because of several factors, including the amount of branching of the pulmonary vessels. Second, blood is not a Newtonian fluid but rather made up of varying amounts of cellular and noncellular elements with resulting variability in viscosity. Indeed, the viscosity of blood has been shown to be an important determinant of PVR.[15]

Passive Control of Pulmonary Vascular Resistance

PVR can be modified passively in several ways. First, an increase in pulmonary arterial or pulmonary venous pressure causes PVR to fall (FIGURE 1-6A).

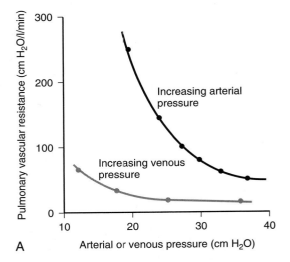

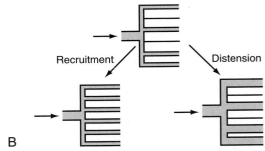

Figure 1-6. A. Effect of arterial and venous pressures on pulmonary vascular resistance. As arterial and venous pressures increase, there is a decrease in pulmonary vascular resistance. B. Recruitment and distention in the pulmonary vasculature, illustrating two likely mechanisms for the decrease in pulmonary vascular resistance seen as vascular pressure increases. (From West JB: *Respiratory physiology: The essentials,* 6th ed., Baltimore, 2000, Lippincott Williams and Wilkins.)

This observation was first described by Borst and colleagues[16] using a canine model in which they observed a decrease in PVR when either the pulmonary arterial or left atrial pressure was elevated. This is hypothesized to occur by two different mechanisms (FIGURE 1-6B). Increasing pulmonary vascular pressure opens portions of the pulmonary microcirculation previously closed, a process known as "recruitment." This is the primary mechanism for the fall in PVR when pulmonary vascular pressure is raised from low levels. At higher vascular pressures, further reductions in the PVR are accomplished primarily through distention of already opened resistance vessels and capillary segments. These two mechanisms can occur simultaneously. A concurrent increase in pulmonary artery pressures and reduction in PVR can be seen, for example, during exercise in normal adults.[17] With exercise, there is an increase in cardiac output, mPAP, and (to a lesser extent) PAOP, accompanied by a significant decrease in PVR (FIGURE 1-7).

Changes in lung volumes can also passively modify PVR by altering the caliber of extra-alveolar and alveolar vessels (FIGURE 1-8).[18] As discussed above, the radius of the extra-alveolar vessel can be affected by various forces. As the lung inflates, tethering of extra-alveolar vessels by the surrounding connective tissue and parenchyma results in an increase in vessel radius. This results in a decrease in vascular resistance. The smooth muscle and connective tissue of the extra-alveolar vessels, however, continuously oppose these tethering effects as volumes increase and result in increased vascular resistance at low lung volumes. The effect of lung volume on the resistance of intra-alveolar vessels is opposite that seen in extra-alveolar vessels. With increasing lung volume, there is a decrease in the intrapleural pressure and a resultant fall in pulmonary artery and venous pressures relative to alveolar pressure. Such a drop in arterial and venous pressures allows vessels to be compressed by the relatively greater alveolar pressures, thus causing their resistance to rise. In addition, stretching of alveolar walls occurs at higher lung volumes, further decreasing vessel caliber and increasing resistance.[19,20] At very low lung volumes, folding of the alveolar septum can occur, also resulting in a reduction of alveolar vessel

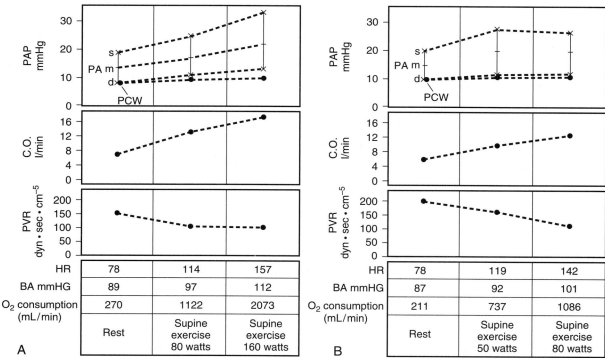

Figure 1-7. Decrease in pulmonary vascular resistance seen with exercise in humans. Pulmonary hemodynamics are shown during rest and exercise in normal man (**A**) and woman (**B**). *BA*, brachial artery pressure; *CO*, cardiac output; *PAP*, pulmonary arterial pressure; *s*, systolic pressure; *m*, mean pressure; *d*, diastolic pressure; *HR*, heart rate; *PCW*, pulmonary capillary wedge pressure; *PVR*, pulmonary vascular resistance. (From Fishman AP: Pulmonary circulation. In: Fishman AP, Fisher AB, editors: *Handbook of physiology, sec 3: The respiratory system, vol 1: Circulation and nonrespiratory functions*, Bethesda, 1985, American Physiological Society, pp 93-166.)

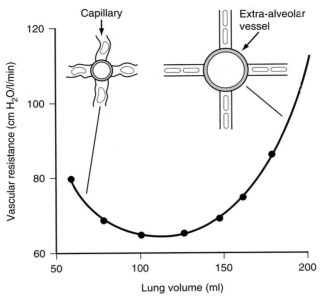

Figure 1-8. Effect of lung volume on pulmonary vascular resistance. At low lung volumes, resistance is elevated because extra-alveolar vessels are narrow. At high lung volumes, the alveolar vessels (capillaries) are stretched and their caliber is reduced, resulting in elevated resistance. (From West JB: *Respiratory physiology. The essentials,* 6th ed., Baltimore, 2000, Lippincott Williams and Wilkins.)

caliber and an increase in the resistance to blood flow. Therefore, because of the effects of lung volume on both extra-alveolar and alveolar blood vessels, the greatest increase in PVR occurs at extremes of lung volume.

A third mechanism by which PVR is passively controlled is gravity. As discussed, the contribution of alveolar pressure on PVR depends upon the lung zone. In the upright position, resistance to blood flow decreases passively from top to bottom of the lung due to the recruitment and distention of vessels associated with increasing hydrostatic pressure from gravity.[9] An exception to this rule occurs in the dependent zone (Zone 4) of the vertical lung, where pulmonary venous pressures are increased.[21] There PVR increases secondary to perivascular edema causing compression of the pulmonary vessels.

Active Control of Pulmonary Vascular Resistance

Hypoxic Pulmonary Vasoconstriction

A unique property of the pulmonary circulation is the vasoconstriction that occurs in response to hypoxia. First described by Von Euler and Liljestrand in 1946,[22] hypoxic pulmonary vasoconstriction (HPV) provides an autoregulatory mechanism by which blood flow is reduced to poorly

ventilated and oxygenated regions of the lung, and consequently increased in well-oxygenated lung units. The vasoconstriction induced by hypoxia is in stark contrast to the response of the systemic circulation, where arterial hypoxemia causes vasodilation. The pressor response to acute hypoxia occurs within a few breaths, peaking after about 3 minutes,[23] and may persist for hours or days depending upon the exposure and preparation used.[24,25] The strongest stimulus for HPV appears to be alveolar hypoxia, with a smaller contribution from mixed venous and bronchial artery oxygen tensions.[26] In humans, PVR increases by approximately 50 percent when the alveolar oxygen pressure (PO_2) falls below 50 mmHg.[27] Most segments of the pulmonary circulation, including the pulmonary veins, constrict to some degree in response to hypoxia. The major site of HPV however, is believed to be the small muscular precapillary arteries.[26] In contrast, the most proximal portions of the pulmonary artery dilate in response to hypoxia.[28,29] The central effector site of hypoxic pulmonary vasoconstriction is the smooth muscle cell of the pulmonary arteries, but this effect can be modified by endothelial and neurohumoral factors.

The exact mechanism by which hypoxia is sensed by the pulmonary vasculature remains incompletely understood, but one important component is a direct modulation of ion channel activity by hypoxia. One of the first systems in which this was described was the glomus cell of the carotid body, where chemosensory input regarding peripheral oxygen tension is provided to the respiratory neurons within the brainstem. Lopez-Barneo and colleagues[30] showed that hypoxia reduced K^+ current in these chemoreceptive cells of the carotid body. Electrophysiologic studies using whole-cell patch clamping of isolated pulmonary vascular smooth muscle cells also demonstrated that hypoxia inhibits K^+ currents and results in membrane potential depolarization.[31,32] In addition, this effect on K^+ current appears to be regionally specific, as membrane potential depolarization is seen predominantly in smooth muscle obtained from resistance vessels, but not conduit pulmonary artery segments.[29] The potassium channels involved are members of the voltage-gated (Kv) family, including the subtype Kv1.5.[33] HPV is severely impaired in genetically modified mice lacking the Kv1.5 potassium channel.[34]

HPV is also dependent upon the influx of calcium into the pulmonary smooth muscle cell. This has been demonstrated in the isolated rat lung, where the calcium antagonist verapamil inhibits HPV.[35] It is not clear whether Ca^{2+} channel activity is directly affected by hypoxia, secondarily by membrane depolarization due to hypoxia-induced K^+ channel closure, or by some soluble mediator released from a separate oxygen sensor. Similar to K^+ channels, the effects of hypoxia on L-type Ca^{2+} channel activity appear to be different in smooth muscle cells from resistance and conduit pulmonary vessels.[36] Whereas hypoxia inhibits L-type Ca^{2+} channel activity in main pulmonary arteries, it enhances Ca^{2+} activity in the resistance vessels.

A "redox theory" has been proposed by which hypoxia alters ion channel activity.[37] Under conditions of alveolar hypoxia, the production of oxidant mediators by the mitochondria of pulmonary artery smooth muscles cells is reduced. This results in the reduction of Kv channels, with their resultant closure and membrane depolarization. Nicotinamide adenine dinucleotide phosphate (NADPH) oxidase might similarly contribute to oxygen sensing within pulmonary smooth muscle cells. Under normoxic conditions NADPH oxidase produces oxygen free radicals. When oxygen levels decrease, however, the electron donors produced by NADPH oxidase are diminished, with resultant closure of Kv channels.

Several modulators of HPV have been described. Metabolic acidosis has been shown to enhance HPV[38,39] (FIGURE 1-9), whereas conflict-

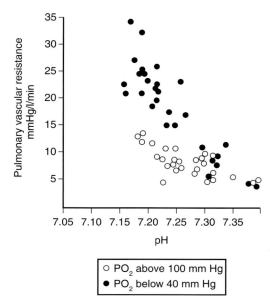

Figure 1-9. Response of pulmonary vascular resistance to changes in arterial pH at various oxygen tensions. Pulmonary vascular resistance increases with increasing acidemia. Note that hypoxemia appears to potentiate the effect of acidemia at any given pH. (From Rudolph AM, Yuan S: Response of the pulmonary vasculature to hypoxia and H^+ ion concentration changes. *J Clin Invest* 45:399-411, 1966.)

ing results have been reported regarding the effect of respiratory acidosis.[26,40] In contrast, respiratory alkalosis does modulate vascular tone to result in inhibition of HPV, likely through an increased release of prostacyclin.[41]

Nitric oxide (NO; also known also endothelium-derived relaxing factor) is synthesized and released by the pulmonary vascular endothelium during acute and chronic hypoxia. NO causes vasodilation and prevents excessive vasoconstriction.[42] Following its formation by endothelial nitric oxide synthase (eNOS), NO induces an increase in intracellular cyclic guanosine monophosphate (cGMP) within the pulmonary artery smooth muscle cell. This, in turn, results in a decrease in both calcium's entry into the cell and its release from intracellular stores, together producing vasodilation. Using a rat model of HPV, Zhao and colleagues[43] demonstrated that exposure to 10 percent O_2 for up to 2 days results in a greater than 50 percent reduction of pulmonary arterial pressure response to acute hypoxia. This reduction in the pulmonary artery response to acute hypoxia is blocked by the NOS inhibitor, N^G-monomethyl-L-arginine, suggesting that NO plays a role in modulating the effects of HPV. Using eNOS knock-out mice, Steudel and colleagues[44] showed that pulmonary hypertension in response to moderate hypoxia was more severe in eNOS-deficient mice than in wild-type controls, further supporting a role of NO in modulating HPV.

A more recently recognized second messenger in this system, carbon monoxide (CO), has been hypothesized to play a role in modulation of HPV. CO is produced in pulmonary artery smooth muscle cells by both constitutively expressed and inducible forms of heme oxygenase.[45] Levels of the inducible form, heme oxygenase-1, increase upon exposure to chronic hypoxia. CO causes pulmonary smooth muscle vasodilation similar to that caused by NO. Induction of heme oxygenase-1 with hypoxia and nickel chloride prevents HPV as well as pulmonary vascular remodeling in the rat.[46] Both heme oxygenases 1 and 2 are expressed in cultured human pulmonary artery, and exposure of these vessels to exogenous CO reduces pulmonary smooth muscle proliferation.[47]

Angiotensin II, a potent vascular vasoconstrictor, has been shown to augment HPV in a dose-dependent manner.[48] More recent studies have further substantiated a role for angiotensin II in the development of hypoxia-induced pulmonary vasoconstriction. In a rat model, the administration of captopril or the angiotensin II receptor antagonist, losartan, reduces the pulmonary remodeling and right ventricular hypertrophy associated with exposure to chronic hypoxia.[49]

The autonomic nervous system does not appear to play a role in HPV. Convincing evidence for this has been demonstrated in the isolated lung and autonomically isolated lung preparations,[26,50] as well as transplanted human lung.[51] In all preparations, sympathetic denervation, either by complete isolation or bilateral thoracic sympathectomy, did not prevent increases in PVR produced by alveolar hypoxia.

Humoral Regulators of Vascular Tone

The pulmonary circulation is a low-pressure system in most species. Under normoxic conditions, vasodilators have little effect on pulmonary vascular tone. This suggests a limited role for active basal control; however, several endogenous peptides and mediators can modulate pulmonary vascular tone in experimental systems (summarized in TABLE 1-1). The effect of these modulators on vascular tone, however, differs among animal species, strain, and gender. Their effects are also influenced by the experimental conditions employed, such as the presence or absence of endothelium, the dosage of a modulator applied, and the initial tone of the pulmonary vasculature at the time of its admin-istration. Thus, despite an observed influence on vascular tone under experimental conditions, the effect of a given modulator *in situ*, is less clear.

The pulmonary endothelium is the source of several modulators of vascular tone. In addition to its role in HPV described above, NO produced by vascular endothelial cells appears to be a major modulator of basal pulmonary vascular tone in humans.[52] Administration of the NO synthase inhibitor, N^G-monomethyl-L-arginine (L-NMMA), caused a 40 percent increase in PVR in normoxic healthy adults.[53] Deficiency of endothelial NO synthase is associated with mild pulmonary hypertension in mice, further suggesting that NO may participate in the low tone of the pulmonary circulation during normoxia.[54]

Endothelin-1 (ET-1) is another important modulator of pulmonary vascular tone produced by the endothelium. First described in 1988, ET-1 is the most abundant member of a family of 21 amino acid peptides.[55] ET-1 is expressed in multiple tissues, the highest levels being in the lung where it is produced by vascular endothelial, smooth muscle, airway epithelial, and a variety of other cell types. In addition to having mitogenic, fibrotic, and inflammatory effects, endothelin is among the most potent endogenous vasoconstrictor agents. Following conversion to its biologically active form, ET-1 can bind to either of two known endothelin receptors: ET_A or ET_B. The binding of endothelin to either ET_A or ET_B receptors on the surface of vascular smooth muscle cells results in potent vasoconstriction.[56,57] On endothelial cells, however, ET_B receptors mediate vasodilation by increasing the production of NO and prostacyclin.[58,59] ET_B receptors are also thought to be active in the clearance of circulating ET-1.[60] In normal volunteers under normoxic conditions, inhibition of ET-1 synthesis or blockade of its receptors results in a reduction in PVR, suggesting a role for ET-1 in the maintenance of normal basal vascular tone.[61] The relative expression of the endothelin receptors appears to vary according to vessel size and location within the pulmonary vasculature[62] and to be altered in some disease states,[63-65] which might influence the relative importance of their vasoconstricting and vasodilatory effects.

Prostacyclin (PGI_2), is another important modulator of pulmonary vascular tone produced by endothelial cells. A product of arachidonic acid metabolism, PGI_2 levels are increased in response to a number of stimuli. Shear stress on the pulmonary vascular endothelium is a potent stimulus for the release of PGI_2. Many vasoconstrictors such as hypoxia, angiotensin II, and ET-1 also

TABLE 1-1

Modulators of Pulmonary Vascular Tone

Modulator	Action
Acetylcholine	Variable
Angiotensin II	Vasoconstriction
Atrial natriuretic peptide	Variable
	Reduction of HPV
Brain natriuretic peptide	Reduction of HPV
Bradykinin	Vasodilation
	Reduction of HPV
Calcitonin gene-related peptide	Vasodilation
Endothelin	Vasodilation—low dose
	Vasoconstriction—high dose
Glucagon	Reduction in HPV
Histamine	Variable
Leukotrienes (LTC_4, LTD_4, LTE_4, LTB_4)	Vasoconstriction
Nitric oxide (EDRF)	Vasodilation
Prostaglandins	
PGI_2	Vasodilation
PGE_2	Vasodilation—low dose
	Vasoconstriction—high dose
$PGF_{2\alpha}$	Vasoconstriction
Serotonin	Vasoconstriction
Somatostatin	Increase in HPV
Substance P	Vasodilation
Thromboxane	Vasoconstriction
Vasopressin	Variable effect
	Reduction in HPV
Vasoactive intestinal peptide	Vasodilation

EDRF, *endothelium-derived relaxing factor;* HPV, *hypoxic pulmonary vasoconstriction;* LT, *leukotriene;* PG, *prostaglandin.*

can lead to increased levels of PGI_2. The mechanism for this is not clear but probably relates to the vasoconstriction produced by these endogenous modulators.[66,67]

The importance of PGI_2 in the modulation of vascular tone is supported by several observations. Transgenic mice that express excess prostacyclin synthase (an enzyme important to the production of PGI_2) are protected from the acute and chronic effects of hypoxia that would normally cause pulmonary hypertension.[68] Furthermore, in patients with severe pulmonary arterial hypertension, there is evidence for a reduction in the expression of PGI_2 synthase.[69] Administration of exogenous forms of prostacyclin is an important therapy for severe pulmonary arterial hypertension, by promoting significant vasodilation, vascular remodeling, and resultant improvements in hemodynamics, functional status, and survival.[70,71]

The complexity in control of pulmonary vascular tone is further illustrated by both the vasoconstricting and dilating effects of factors produced outside the pulmonary endothelium. In the kidney, renin converts liver-derived angiotensinogen into angiotensin I, which in turn is converted by its converting enzyme (ACE) to angiotensin II within the pulmonary vasculature. This peptide hormone, derived from products formed outside the lung, is a potent endogenous pulmonary vasoconstrictor and increases pulmonary vasoreactivity.[72] Binding of angiotensin II to its G-protein–coupled receptor activates protein kinase C and causes an increase in intracellular Ca^{2+} and smooth muscle contraction. Bradykinins released by inflammatory cells are also vasoactive molecules, predominantly causing vasodilation of the pulmonary vasculature.[73,74] In an isolated rat lung preparation, for example, bradykinin reduces hypoxic pulmonary vasoconstriction.[75] In fetal lamb lungs and in normal human volunteers, bradykinin causes vasodilation[73] and increased cardiac output.[74] Arginine vasopressin (AVP), a potent systemic vasoconstrictor produced by the neurohypophysis, has a variable affect on PVR. In the conscious dog, AVP causes pulmonary vasoconstriction[76] while in the rat it acts as a pulmonary vasodilator.[77] Infusion of AVP reduces the development of pulmonary hypertension in response to chronic hypoxia in rats.[78] Atrial natriuretic peptide, secreted by the cardiac atria, and brain natriuretic peptide, originally found in the brain but largely secreted by the cardiac ventricles, cause pulmonary artery relaxation and a reduction of HPV.[79,80] Secretion of these peptides during acute hypoxia may represent a mechanism to counteract the acute increase in afterload imposed upon the right ventricle by an elevated PVR.

Endogenous biogenic amines also appear to modulate pulmonary vascular tone. Indeed, acetylcholine was one of the first described pulmonary vasodilators used to attempt treatment of pulmonary hypertension in humans.[81] Its effects on the pulmonary circulation are likely mediated via the release of NO, and appear to depend on the concentration of acetylcholine administered.[82,83] Lower concentrations of acetylcholine cause vaso-dilation, while higher concentrations appear to cause vasoconstriction. Histamine, a major product released during mast cell degranulation, also has variable effects on pulmonary vascular tone, causing vasoconstriction in some animal models but vasodilation in others.[84-87] Serotonin released by activated platelets causes pulmonary vasoconstriction, notably in the presence of intravascular coagulation and thrombosis. In addition to its vasoconstriction properties, serotonin can promote pulmonary smooth muscle proliferation, suggesting a role in the pulmonary vascular remodeling observed with chronic pulmonary hypertension.[88,90] Norepinephrine, another biogenic amine, causes pulmonary vasoconstriction; however, its role in modulating pulmonary vascular tone has not been fully elucidated.

Although the pathophysiology and treatment of diseases characterized by elevations in PVR are discussed elsewhere, derangements in several of the factors discussed serve to emphasize their importance in the maintenance of normal vascular tone. Deficiencies in naturally occurring prostacyclin[69,91] or increases in the expression of endothelin-1,[65,92-95] for example, are associated with idiopathic and other forms of pulmonary arterial hypertension. The administration of prostacyclin analogues as noted above, or endothelin receptor antagonists, helps to restore PVR toward normal and thus improve hemodynamics and symptoms, as well as patient survival.[70,71] Such therapies aimed at altering pulmonary vascular tone are listed in TABLE 1-2. However, in addition to their positive effects, many of these same agents can acutely worsen oxygenation by increasing ventilation-perfusion mismatch by promoting vasodilation at sites where HPV should appropriately occur (for example, within atelectatic lung). This is further illustration of the importance of the many factors and systems that normally control local pulmonary vascular tone.

Neural Modulation of Pulmonary Vascular Tone

SYMPATHETIC INNERVATION. Vessels of the pulmonary and bronchial circulations are innervated by sympathetic nerves from cell bodies originating in the first five thoracic, the middle and inferior cervical, and the stellate ganglia.[96] Post-ganglionic fibers from these ganglia enter a complex array of plexuses that ultimately innervate the pulmonary vasculature and bronchial arteries. In animal models with an intact pulmonary vasculature, stimulation of the sympathetic nerves results in a frequency dependent increase in PVR and perfusion pressure.[97]

Four subtypes of adrenergic receptors have been identified in the pulmonary vasculature. Both β_1 and β_2 receptors mediate vasodilation in response to circulating catecholamines, as well as to the release of norepinephrine locally at nerve endings.[98,99] In contrast, α_1 and α_2 adrenergic receptors mediate vasoconstriction.[99,100] These effects can be inhibited by α-adrenergic blockade or chemical denervation by 6-hydroxydopamine.

The sympathetic nervous system may be important in maintaining basal pulmonary tone, primarily through its activation of α_1 adrenoreceptors.[101,102] Sympathetic nervous input may increase and bring about an increase in pulmonary vasoconstriction under pathophysiologic conditions such as systemic hypotension, pulmonary embolism, neurogenic pulmonary edema, or reperfusion injury.[102-106]

PARASYMPATHETIC INNERVATION. The pulmonary circulation also receives parasympathetic nervous system input, although it appears to have a less influential role on vascular tone than does the sympathetic system. Preganglionic parasympathetic nerve cell bodies are found in vagal nuclei within the brainstem and travel via the vagus nerve into the lungs. These nerve fibers then relay to postganglionic nerve cell bodies within the hila, from whence additional fibers proceed to innervate the pulmonary vasculature. The effect of acetylcholine release from parasympathetic nerve fibers depends upon the baseline tone of the pulmonary circulation. In the cat, acetylcholine produces vasoconstriction when applied under resting tone, but it causes vasodilation during conditions in which vascular tone is already elevated.[107] In humans, however, the predominant response to acetylcholine is vasodilation, regardless of initial tone.[108] This vasodilatory response to vagal

TABLE 1-2

Therapeutic Agents and Their Effects on Pulmonary Vascular Tone

Drug	Action	Mechanism
Angiotensin-converting enzyme inhibitor	Vasodilation	Increased PGI_2 synthesis
β-Sympathomimetic agents (isoproterenol, albuterol)	Vasodilation	β_2-Adrenergic receptor stimulation
Calcium channel blockers	Vasodilation	Decreased Ca^{2+} entry Decreased action of vasoconstrictors
Clonidine	Vasodilation	α_2-Adrenergic receptor stimulation
Cyclooxygenase inhibitor	Vasoconstriction	Inhibition of PGI_2 synthesis
Dopamine	Vasoconstriction	α_1-Adrenergic receptor stimulation
Endothelin receptor antagonists (ambrisentan, bosentan, sitaxsentan)	Vasodilation	ET_A and ET_B receptor inhibition
Ethanol	Vasodilation	? Membrane effect
Hydralazine	Vasodilation	Increased PGI_2 synthesis
Methylxanthines	Vasodilation	Increase in cAMP
Nitrates (nitroglycerin, nitroprusside)	Vasodilation	Increase in cAMP
Phentolamine	Vasodilation	α_1-Adrenergic receptor inhibition
Prostacyclin (epoprostenol, treprostinil, iloprost, beroprost)	Vasodilation	Increase in cAMP
Sildenafil	Vasodilation	Phosphodiesterase—Type 5 inhibitor

cAMP, *cyclic adenosine monophosphate*; ET, *endothelin*; PG, *prostaglandin*.

stimulation can be blocked by inhibition of NO,[109] suggesting that acetylcholine effects are dependent on NO release from the vascular endothelium.

Four types of muscarinic receptors are present in the pulmonary vasculature. The predominant subtypes are the M_1 and the M_3. M_3 muscarinic receptors mediate vasodilation,[110] whereas the M_1 receptor promotes vasoconstriction.[111-112] The predominance of any receptor subtype appears to vary among species, which is consistent with the variable response observed with the exogenous application of acetylcholine.

Parasympathetic activity does not appear to play a major role in the maintenance of basal pulmonary vascular tone, as blockade of cholinergic input does not significantly alter PVR or pulmonary arterial pressure.[113] Cholinergic input to the pulmonary circulation, however, does blunt HPV via carotid chemoreceptor feedback.[114] Using an anesthetized dog model, isolated carotid body stimulation increased blood flow in isolated hypoxic lung. This effect was blocked by vagotomy and atropine. Cholinergic input has also been implicated in the development of neurogenic pulmonary edema.[115] Using an *in vivo* guinea pig model and ^{125}I-labeled albumin as a marker of plasma extravasation, bilateral stimulation of the vagus nerve resulted in increased plasma leak in both parenchymal and tracheobronchial tissues.

NONADRENERGIC NONCHOLINERGIC NEURAL CONTROL. The nonadrenergic noncholinergic (NANC) nerves are modulators of the pulmonary circulation that are not inhibited by adrenergic or cholinergic blockade.[96] The response of the pulmonary circulation to NANC input can be either vasodilation or constriction. Several putative transmitters mediate the NANC neural response in the pulmonary circulation. Vasoactive intestinal peptide, calcitonin gene-related peptide, and tachykinins including substance P have each been shown to participate in mediating the NANC vasodilator response.[116-118] Each of these peptides appears to have a more potent vasodilator effect when pulmonary vascular tone is elevated.

Additional Functions of the Pulmonary Vasculature

The entire cardiac output passes through the pulmonary circulation. With its large surface area, the pulmonary endothelium is thus ideally placed to perform various metabolic and endocrine functions. In addition to the control of vasomotor tone as discussed above, substances produced by the pulmonary endothelium are active in various processes, such as leukocyte activation, platelet adhesion, cell growth and proliferation.

The pulmonary circulation is a major source of eicosanoids. These products of arachidonic acid include the prostaglandins, thromboxanes, leukotrienes, lipoxins, monohydroxyeicosatetraenoic acids, and epoxides. These eicosanoids are involved in an array of biologic functions, including determination of vascular permeability and tone, thrombosis, fibrinolysis, leukocyte activation, and cellular adhesion (as reviewed in Silverman ES, Gerritsen ME, Collins T).[119] The very low circulating serum levels of eicosanoids suggest that these substances act in an autocrine and paracrine manner. The predominant eicosanoids produced by the pulmonary circulation are prostacyclin (PGI_2) and prostaglandin E_2 (PGE_2),[120] both of which cause pulmonary vasodilation. The other metabolites of arachidonic acid, thromboxane and the leukotrienes, are pulmonary vasoconstrictors.

A number of factors increase eicosanoid synthesis by the pulmonary vascular endothelium. These include heparin, alcohol, hypoxia, increased sympathetic activity, nicotine, shear stress, and histamine. In addition to the synthesis of eicosanoids, the pulmonary vascular endothelium is the major site for their removal and inactivation. With the exception of PGI_2 and prostaglandins of the A series, most eicosanoids are removed by the lung.

The pulmonary circulation is also an important site for the regulation of circulating amino acids. This is accomplished primarily through their active transport. For example, L-arginine, a critical precursor in the production of NO, is actively transported by pulmonary vascular endothelial cells.

The pulmonary circulation removes adenosine and its derivatives from the circulation.[121,122] Adenosine, adenosine triphosphate (ATP), and adenosine diphosphate (ADP), are potent modulators of pulmonary of vasomotor tone.[123,124] Tight regulation of their activity within the lung is important so that these mediators do not reach the systemic circulation under normal conditions. The pulmonary vasculature removes the nucleotides by facilitated diffusion, as well as by nucleotidases localized to the endothelial membrane surface.[125]

The pulmonary circulation is remarkably selective in the breakdown of biogenic amines.[126,127] Serotonin is almost completely removed, whereas less than half of the norepinephrine presented is cleared by the pulmonary circulation during its first pass. This is in contrast to the other biogenic amines, including histamine, dopamine, and epinephrine, which pass freely through the pulmonary circulation without alteration.

The surface membrane of the pulmonary vascular endothelium is equipped with important enzymes active in the metabolism of various vasoactive peptides. One of the best studied and clinically important is angiotensin-converting enzyme (ACE).[128] ACE converts angiotensin I to angiotensin II, a potent vasoconstrictor and regulator of salt and water balance. ACE is also important for the breakdown of the vasodilator bradykinin. With its large surface area, the pulmonary circulation is the major site of angiotensin II production. Neutral endopeptidase is another important enzyme localized to the pulmonary endothelial surface. It contributes to the inactivation of vasoactive peptides including atrial natriuretic peptide, bradykinin, and the endothelins.[129]

The endothelium has fibrinolytic properties that help maintain a balance between procoagulant and anticoagulant activities. Endothelial cells synthesize and secrete both tissue plasminogen activator and urokinase plasminogen activator. In cultured human endothelial cells, tissue plasminogen activator enhances the enzymatic activity of the endothelial surface, allowing for enhanced fibrinolysis.[130,131]

Summary/Conclusions

The pulmonary circulation consists of several types of vessels that respond differently to changes in blood flow and pressure to optimize gas exchange while lung volume cyclically changes. Local control of pulmonary vascular tone is essential to the targeting ("matching") of blood perfusion to areas of high oxygen tension, and away from relatively hypoxic alveolar units. A complex host of mediators including peptides, hormones, and local metabolites interact to regulate vascular tone in a remarkably efficient manner. In addition to its active participation in its own regulation, the pulmonary vasculature serves important metabolic functions to regulate and catabolize hormones and peptides affecting other organ systems.

References

1. Hislop A, Reid L: Pulmonary arterial development during childhood: Branching pattern and structure. *Thorax* 28:129-135, 1973.
2. Howell JB, Permutt S, Proctor DF, et al: Effect of inflation of the lung on different parts of pulmonary vascular bed. *J Appl Physiol* 16:71-76, 1961.

3. Rosenzweig DY, Hughes JM, Glazier JB: Effects of transpulmonary and vascular pressures on pulmonary blood volume in isolated lung. *J Appl Physiol* 28:553-560, 1970.

4. Koyama S, Lamm WJ, Hildebrandt J, et al: Flow characteristics of open vessels in zone 1 rabbit lungs. *J Appl Physiol* 66:1817-1823, 1989.

5. Meyrick B, Reid L: Pulmonary hypertension. Anatomic and physiologic correlates. *Clin Chest Med* 4:199-217, 1983.

6. Gil J, Ciurea D: Functional structure of the pulmonary circulation. In: Peacock AJ, editor: *Pulmonary circulation: A handbook for clinicians*, London, 1996, Chapman and Hall Medical, pp 1-11.

7. Weibel ER: Design and morphometry of the pulmonary gas exchanger. In Crystal RG, West JB, Weibel ER, et al, editors: *The lung: Scientific foundations*, Philadelphia, 1997, Lippincott-Raven, pp 1147–1157.

8. Tsukimoto K, Mathieu-Costello O, Prediletto R, et al: Ultrastructural appearances of pulmonary capillaries at high transmural pressures. *J Appl Physiol* 71: 573-582, 1991.

9. West JB, Dollery CT, Naimark A: Distribution of blood flow in isolated lung; relation to vascular and alveolar pressures. *J Appl Physiol* 19:713-724, 1964.

10. Wiener F, Morkin E, Skalak R, et al: Wave propagation in the pulmonary circulation. *Circ Res* 19:834-850, 1966.

11. Hughes JM, Glazier JB, Maloney JE, et al: Effect of lung volume on the distribution of pulmonary blood flow in man. *Respir Physiol* 4:58-72, 1968.

12. Bhattacharya J, Staub NC: Direct measurement of microvascular pressures in the isolated perfused dog lung. *Science* 210:327-328, 1980.

13. Brody JS, Stemmler EJ, DuBois AB: Longitudinal distribution of vascular resistance in the pulmonary arteries, capillaries, and veins. *J Clin Invest* 47:783-799, 1968.

14. Swan HJ, Ganz W, Forrester J, et al: Catheterization of the heart in man with use of a flow-directed balloon-tipped catheter. *N Engl J Med* 283:447-451, 1970.

15. Murray JF, Karp RB, Nadel JA: Viscosity effects on pressure-flow relations and vascular resistance in dogs' lungs. *J Appl Physiol* 27:336-341, 1969.

16. Borst HG, McGregor M, Whittenberger JL, et al: Influence of pulmonary arterial and left atrial pressures on pulmonary vascular resistance. *Circ Res* 4:393-399, 1956.

17. Fishman AP: Handbook of physiology, Sec. 3: The respiratory system: Circulation and nonrespiratory functions. In: Fishman AP, Fishman AB, editors: *Pulmonary circulation, vol. 1*, Bethesda, 1985, American Physiological Society, pp 93-166.

18. Roos A, Thomas LJ, Jr., Nagel EL, et al: Pulmonary vascular resistance as determined by lung inflation and vascular pressures. *J Appl Physiol* 16:77-84, 1961.

19. Glazier JB, Hughes JM, Maloney JE, et al: Measurements of capillary dimensions and blood volume in rapidly frozen lungs. *J Appl Physiol* 26:65-76, 1969.

20. Mazzone RW, Durand CM, West JB: Electron microscopy of lung rapidly frozen under controlled physiological conditions. *J Appl Physiol* 45:325-333, 1978.

21. West JB, Dollery CT, Heard BE: Increased pulmonary vascular resistance in the dependent zone of the isolated dog lung caused by perivascular edema. *Circ Res* 17:191-206, 1965.

22. Von Euler US, Liljestrand G: Observations on the pulmonary arterial blood pressure in the cat. *Acta Physiol Scan* 12:301-320, 1946.

23. Malik AB, Kidd BS: Independent effects of changes in H^+ and CO_2 concentrations on hypoxic pulmonary vasoconstriction. *J Appl Physiol* 34:318-323, 1973.

24. Rubin LJ, Lazar JD: Nonadrenergic effects of isoproterenol in dogs with hypoxic pulmonary vasoconstriction. Possible role of prostaglandins. *J Clin Invest* 71:1366-1374, 1983.

25. Unger M, Atkins M, Briscoe WA, et al: Potentiation of pulmonary vasoconstrictor response with repeated intermittent hypoxia. *J Appl Physiol* 43:662-667, 1977.

26. Kato M, Staub NC: Response of small pulmonary arteries to unilobar hypoxia and hypercapnia. *Circ Res* 19:426-440, 1966.

27. Harris P, Heath, D: Influences of respiratory gases. In Harris P, Heath D, editors: *The human pulmonary circulation*, London, 1986, Churchill-Livingston, pp 456-483.

28. Zhao Y, Packer CS, Rhoades RA: Pulmonary vein contracts in response to hypoxia. *Am J Physiol* 265:L87-92, 1993.

29. Archer SL, Huang JM, Reeve HL, et al: Differential distribution of electrophysiologically distinct myocytes in conduit and resistance arteries determines their response to nitric oxide and hypoxia. *Circ Res* 78:431-442, 1996.

30. Lopez-Barneo J, Lopez-Lopez JR, Urena J, et al: Chemotransduction in the carotid body: K^+ current modulated by PO_2 in type I chemoreceptor cells. *Science* 241:580-582, 1988.

31. Post JM, Hume JR, Archer SL, et al: Direct role for potassium channel inhibition in hypoxic pulmonary vasoconstriction. *Am J Physiol* 262:C882-890, 1992.

32. Yuan XJ, Goldman WF, Tod ML, et al: Hypoxia reduces potassium currents in cultured rat

pulmonary but not mesenteric arterial myocytes. *Am J Physiol* 264:L116-123, 1993.

33. Archer SL, Souil E, Dinh-Xuan AT, et al: Molecular identification of the role of voltage-gated K⁺ channels, Kv1.5 and Kv2.1, in hypoxic pulmonary vasoconstriction and control of resting membrane potential in rat pulmonary artery myocytes. *J Clin Invest* 101:2319-2330, 1998.

34. Archer SL, London B, Hampl V, et al: Impairment of hypoxic pulmonary vasoconstriction in mice lacking the voltage-gated potassium channel Kv1.5. *FASEB J* 15:1801-1803, 2001.

35. McMurtry IF, Davidson AB, Reeves JT, et al: Inhibition of hypoxic pulmonary vasoconstriction by calcium antagonists in isolated rat lungs. *Circ Res* 38:99-104, 1976.

36. Franco-Obregon A, Lopez-Barneo J: Differential oxygen sensitivity of calcium channels in rabbit smooth muscle cells of conduit and resistance pulmonary arteries. *J Physiol* 491(Pt 2):511-518, 1996.

37. Archer S, Michelakis E: The mechanism(s) of hypoxic pulmonary vasoconstriction: Potassium channels, redox O_2 sensors, and controversies. *News Physiol Sci* 17:131-137, 2002.

38. Rudolph AM, Yuan S: Response of the pulmonary vasculature to hypoxia and H⁺ ion concentration changes. *J Clin Invest* 45:399-411, 1966.

39. Marshall C, Lindgren L, Marshall BE: Metabolic and respiratory hydrogen ion effects on hypoxic pulmonary vasoconstriction. *J Appl Physiol* 57:545-550, 1984.

40. Dumas M, Dumas JP, Rochette L, et al: Comparison of the effects of nicorandil, pinacidil and nitroglycerin on hypoxic and hypercapnic pulmonary vasoconstriction in the isolated perfused lung of rat. *Br J Pharmacol* 117:633-638, 1996.

41. Yamaguchi T, O'Brien RF, Hanson WL, et al: Prostacyclin contributes to inhibition of hypoxic pulmonary vasoconstriction by alkalosis. *Prostaglandins* 38:53-63, 1989.

42. Liu SF, Crawley DE, Barnes PJ, et al: Endothelium-derived relaxing factor inhibits hypoxic pulmonary vasoconstriction in rats. *Am Rev Respir Dis* 143:32-37, 1991.

43. Zhao L, Crawley DE, Hughes JM, et al: Endothelium-derived relaxing factor activity in rat lung during hypoxic pulmonary vascular remodeling. *J Appl Physiol* 74:1061-1065, 1993.

44. Steudel W, Scherrer-Crosbie M, Bloch KD, et al: Sustained pulmonary hypertension and right ventricular hypertrophy after chronic hypoxia in mice with congenital deficiency of nitric oxide synthase 3. *J Clin Invest* 101:2468-2477, 1998.

45. Morita T, Perrella MA, Lee ME, et al: Smooth muscle cell-derived carbon monoxide is a regulator of vascular cGMP. *Proc Natl Acad Sci U S A* 92:1475-1479, 1995.

46. Christou H, Morita T, Hsieh CM, et al: Prevention of hypoxia-induced pulmonary hypertension by enhancement of endogenous heme oxygenase-1 in the rat. *Circ Res* 86:1224-1229, 2000.

47. Stanford SJ, Walters MJ, Hislop AA, et al: Heme oxygenase is expressed in human pulmonary artery smooth muscle where carbon monoxide has an anti-proliferative role. *Eur J Pharmacol* 473:135-141, 2003.

48. Berkor S: Hypoxic pulmonary vasoconstriction in the rat. The necessary role of angiotensin II. *Circ Res* 35:256-261, 1974.

49. Morrell NW, Morris KG, Stenmark KR: Role of angiotensin-converting enzyme and angiotensin II in development of hypoxic pulmonary hypertension. *Am J Physiol* 269:H1186-1194, 1995.

50. Szidon JP, Flint JF: Significance of sympathetic innervation of pulmonary vessels in response to acute hypoxia. *J Appl Physiol* 43:65-71, 1977.

51. Robin ED, Theodore J, Burke CM, et al: Hypoxic pulmonary vasoconstriction persists in the human transplanted lung. *Clin Sci (Lond)* 72:283-287, 1987.

52. Ignarro LJ, Byrns RE, Buga GM, et al: Mechanisms of endothelium-dependent vascular smooth muscle relaxation elicited by bradykinin and VIP. *Am J Physiol* 253:H1074-1082, 1987.

53. Stamler JS, Loh E, Roddy MA, et al: Nitric oxide regulates basal systemic and pulmonary vascular resistance in healthy humans. *Circulation* 89:2035-2040, 1994.

54. Steudel W, Ichinose F, Huang PL, et al: Pulmonary vasoconstriction and hypertension in mice with targeted disruption of the endothelial nitric oxide synthase *(NOS3)* gene. *Circ Res* 81:34-41, 1997.

55. Yanagisawa M, Kurihara H, Kimura S, et al: A novel potent vasoconstrictor peptide produced by vascular endothelial cells. *Nature* 332:411-415, 1988.

56. Seo B, Oemar BS, Siebenmann R, et al: Both ETA and ETB receptors mediate contraction to endothelin-1 in human blood vessels. *Circulation* 89:1203-1208, 1994.

57. Pollock DM, Keith TL, Highsmith RF: Endothelin receptors and calcium signaling. *FASEB J* 9:1196-1204, 1995.

58. Hirata Y, Emori T, Eguchi S, et al: Endothelin receptor subtype B mediates synthesis of nitric oxide by cultured bovine endothelial cells. *J Clin Invest* 91:1367-1373, 1993.

59. Clozel M, Breu V, Gray GA, et al: In vivo pharmacology of Ro 46-2005, the first synthetic nonpeptide endothelin receptor antagonist: implications for endothelin physiology. *J Cardiovasc Pharmacol* 22(Suppl 8):S377-379, 1993.

60. Galie N, Manes A, Branzi A: The endothelin system in pulmonary arterial hypertension. *Cardiovasc Res* 61:227-237, 2004.

61. Johnson W, Nohria A, Garrett L, et al: Contribution of endothelin to pulmonary vascular tone under normoxic and hypoxic conditions. *Am J Physiol Heart Circ Physiol* 283:H568-575, 2002.

62. Davie N, Haleen SJ, Upton PD, et al: ET(A) and ET(B) receptors modulate the proliferation of human pulmonary artery smooth muscle cells. *Am J Respir Crit Care Med* 165:398-405, 2002.

63. de Lagausie P, de Buys-Roessingh A, Ferkdadji L, et al: Endothelin receptor expression in human lungs of newborns with congenital diaphragmatic hernia. *J Pathol* 205:112-118, 2005.

64. Bauer M, Wilkens H, Langer F, et al: Selective upregulation of endothelin B receptor gene expression in severe pulmonary hypertension. *Circulation* 105:1034-1036, 2002.

65. Abraham DJ, Vancheeswaran R, Dashwood MR, et al: Increased levels of endothelin-1 and differential endothelin type A and B receptor expression in scleroderma-associated fibrotic lung disease. *Am J Pathol* 151:831-841, 1997.

66. Voelkel NF, Gerber JG, McMurtry IF, et al: Release of vasodilator prostaglandin, PGI$_2$, from isolated rat lung during vasoconstriction. *Circ Res* 48:207-213, 1981.

67. Michiels C, Arnould T, Knott I, et al: Stimulation of prostaglandin synthesis by human endothelial cells exposed to hypoxia. *Am J Physiol* 264:C866-874, 1993.

68. Geraci MW, Gao B, Shepherd DC, et al: Pulmonary prostacyclin synthase overexpression in transgenic mice protects against development of hypoxic pulmonary hypertension. *J Clin Invest* 103:1509-1515, 1999.

69. Tuder RM, Cool CD, Geraci MW, et al: Prostacyclin synthase expression is decreased in lungs from patients with severe pulmonary hypertension. *Am J Respir Crit Care Med* 159:1925-1932, 1999.

70. Barst RJ, Rubin LJ, Long WA, et al.: A comparison of continuous intravenous epoprostenol (prostacyclin) with conventional therapy for primary pulmonary hypertension. The Primary Pulmonary Hypertension Study Group. *N Engl J Med* 334:296-302, 1996.

71. McLaughlin VV, Genthner DE, Panella MM, et al: Reduction in pulmonary vascular resistance with long-term epoprostenol (prostacyclin) therapy in primary pulmonary hypertension. *N Engl J Med* 338:273-277, 1998.

72. Goll HM, Nyhan DP, Geller HS, et al: Pulmonary vascular responses to angiotensin II and captopril in conscious dogs. *J Appl Physiol* 61:1552-1559, 1986.

73. Frantz E, Soifer SJ, Clyman RI, et al: Bradykinin produces pulmonary vasodilation in fetal lambs: role of prostaglandin production. *J Appl Physiol* 67:1512-1517, 1989.

74. Bönner G, Preis S, Schunk U, et al: Hemodynamic effects of bradykinin on systemic and pulmonary circulation in healthy and hypertensive humans. *J Cardiovasc Pharmacol* 15(Suppl 6):S46-56, 1990.

75. Archer SL, Rist K, Nelson DP, et al: Comparison of the hemodynamic effects of nitric oxide and endothelium-dependent vasodilators in intact lungs. *J Appl Physiol* 68:735-747, 1990.

76. Nyhan DP, Geller HS, Goll HM, et al: Pulmonary vasoactive effects of exogenous and endogenous AVP in conscious dogs. *Am J Physiol* 251:H1009-1016, 1986.

77. Walker BR, Haynes J, Jr., Wang HL, et al: Vasopressin-induced pulmonary vasodilation in rats. *Am J Physiol* 257:H415-422, 1989.

78. Jin HK, Yang RH, Chen YF, et al: Hemodynamic effects of arginine vasopressin in rats adapted to chronic hypoxia. *J Appl Physiol* 66:151-160, 1989.

79. Cigarini I, Adnot S, Chabrier PE, et al: Pulmonary vasodilator responses to atrial natriuretic factor and sodium nitroprusside. *J Appl Physiol* 67:2269-2275, 1989.

80. Hill NS, Klinger JR, Warburton RR, et al: Brain natriuretic peptide: possible role in the modulation of hypoxic pulmonary hypertension. *Am J Physiol* 266:L308-315, 1994.

81. Wood P: Pulmonary hypertension with special reference to the vasoconstrictive factor. *Br Heart J* 21:557, 1959.

82. Feddersen CO, Mathias MM, McMurtry IF, et al: Acetylcholine induces vasodilation and prostacyclin synthesis in rat lungs. *Prostaglandins* 31:973-987, 1986.

83. Barman SA, Senteno E, Smith S, et al: Acetylcholine's effect on vascular resistance and compliance in the pulmonary circulation. *J Appl Physiol* 67:1495-1503, 1989.

84. Ahmed T, Mirbahar KB, Oliver W, Jr., et al: Characterization of H1- and H2-receptor function in pulmonary and systemic circulations of sheep. *J Appl Physiol* 53:175-184, 1982.

85. Kadowitz PJ, Hyman AL: Pulmonary vascular responses to histamine in sheep. *Am J Physiol* 244:H423-428, 1983.

86. Rippe B, Allison RC, Parker JC, et al: Effects of histamine, serotonin, and norepinephrine on circulation of dog lungs. *J Appl Physiol* 57:223-232, 1984.

87. Shirai M, Sada K, Ninomiya I: Nonuniform effects of histamine on small pulmonary vessels in cats. *J Appl Physiol* 62:451-458, 1987.

88. Brody JS, Stemmler EJ: Differential reactivity in the pulmonary circulation. *J Clin Invest* 47:800-808, 1968.

89. Glazier JB, Murray JF: Sites of pulmonary vasomotor reactivity in the dog during alveolar hypoxia and serotonin and histamine infusion. *J Clin Invest* 50:2550-2558, 1971.

90. Lee SL, Wang WW, Lanzillo JJ, et al: Serotonin produces both hyperplasia and hypertrophy of bovine pulmonary artery smooth muscle cells in culture. *Am J Physiol* 266:L46-52, 1994.

91. Christman BW, McPherson CD, Newman JH, et al: An imbalance between the excretion of thromboxane and prostacyclin metabolites in pulmonary hypertension. *N Engl J Med* 327:70-75, 1992.

92. Giaid A, Yanagisawa M, Langleben D, et al: Expression of endothelin-1 in the lungs of patients with pulmonary hypertension. *N Engl J Med* 328:1732-1739, 1993.

93. Morelli S, Ferri C, Polettini E, et al: Plasma endothelin-1 levels, pulmonary hypertension, and lung fibrosis in patients with systemic sclerosis. *Am J Med* 99:255-260, 1995.

94. Rubens C, Ewert R, Halank M, et al: Big endothelin-1 and endothelin-1 plasma levels are correlated with the severity of primary pulmonary hypertension. *Chest* 120:1562-1569, 2001.

95. Yamakami T, Taguchi O, Gabazza EC, et al: Arterial endothelin-1 level in pulmonary emphysema and interstitial lung disease. Relation with pulmonary hypertension during exercise. *Eur Respir J* 10:2055-2060, 1997.

96. Liu SF, Barnes PJ: Neural control of pulmonary vascular tone. In: Crystal RG, West JB, editors: *The lung: Scientific foundations,* Philadelphia, 1997, Lippincott-Raven, pp 1457-1472.

97. Kadowitz PJ, Hyman AL: Effect of sympathetic nerve stimulation on pulmonary vascular resistance in the dog. *Circ Res* 32:221-227, 1973.

98. Boe J, Simonsson BG: Adrenergic receptors and sympathetic agents in isolated human pulmonary arteries. *Eur J Respir Dis* 61:195-202, 1980.

99. Hyman AL, Lippton HL, Kadowitz PJ: Analysis of pulmonary vascular responses in cats to sympathetic nerve stimulation under elevated tone conditions. Evidence that neuronally released norepinephrine acts on alpha 1-, alpha 2-, and beta 2-adrenoceptors. *Circ Res* 67:862-870, 1990.

100. Shebuski RJ, Fujita T, Ruffolo RR, Jr.: Evaluation of alpha-1 and alpha-2 adrenoceptor-mediated vasoconstriction in the in situ, autoperfused, pulmonary circulation of the anesthetized dog. *J Pharmacol Exp Ther* 238:217-223, 1986.

101. Duke HN, Stedford, RD: Pulmonary vasomotor responses to epinephrine and norepinephrine in the cat. Influence of the sympathetic nervous system. *Circ Res* 8:640-647, 1960.

102. Kabins SW, Fridman J, Kandelman M, et al: Effect of sympathectomy on pulmonary embolism-induced lung edema. *Am J Physiol* 202:687-689, 1962.

103. Malik AB: Mechanisms of neurogenic pulmonary edema. *Circ Res* 57:1-18, 1985.

104. Clougherty PW, Nyhan DP, Chen BB, et al: Autonomic nervous system pulmonary vasoregulation after hypoperfusion in conscious dogs. *Am J Physiol* 254:H976-983, 1988.

105. Sakakibara H, Hashiba Y, Taki K, et al: Effect of sympathetic nerve stimulation on lung vascular permeability in the rat. *Am Rev Respir Dis* 145:685-692, 1992.

106. Peterson WP, Trempy GA, Nishiwaki K, et al: Neurohumoral regulation of the pulmonary circulation during circulatory hypotension in conscious dogs. *J Appl Physiol* 75:1675-1682, 1993.

107. Hyman AL, Kadowitz PJ: Tone-dependent responses to acetylcholine in the feline pulmonary vascular bed. *J Appl Physiol* 64:2002-2009, 1988.

108. Greenberg B, Rhoden K, Barnes PJ: Endothelium-dependent relaxation of human pulmonary arteries. *Am J Physiol* 252:H434-438, 1987.

109. McMahon TJ, Hood JS, Kadowitz PJ: Pulmonary vasodilator response to vagal stimulation is blocked by N omega-nitro-L-arginine methyl ester in the cat. *Circ Res* 70:364-369, 1992.

110. McCormack DG, Mak JC, Minette P, et al: Muscarinic receptor subtypes mediating vasodilation in the pulmonary artery. *Eur J Pharmacol* 158:293-297, 1988.

111. el-Kashef HA, Hofman WF, Ehrhart IC, et al: Multiple muscarinic receptor subtypes in the canine pulmonary circulation. *J Appl Physiol* 71:2032-2043, 1991.

112. Altiere RJ, Travis DC, Roberts J, et al: Pharmacological characterization of muscarinic receptors mediating acetylcholine-induced contraction and relaxation in rabbit intrapulmonary arteries. *J Pharmacol Exp Ther* 270:269-276, 1994.

113. Murray PA, Lodato RF, Michael JR: Neural antagonists modulate pulmonary vascular pressure-flow plots in conscious dogs. *J Appl Physiol* 60:1900-1907, 1986.

114. Wilson LB, Levitzky MG: Chemoreflex blunting of hypoxic pulmonary vasoconstriction is vagally mediated. *J Appl Physiol* 66:782-791, 1989.

115. Liu S, Kuo HP, Sheppard MN, et al: Vagal stimulation induces increased pulmonary vascular permeability in guinea pig. *Am J Respir Crit Care Med* 149:744-750, 1994.

116. Hamasaki Y, Mojarad M, Said SI: Relaxant action of VIP on cat pulmonary artery: Comparison with

acetylcholine, isoproterenol, and PGE$_1$. *J Appl Physiol* 54:1607-1611, 1983.

117. McCormack DG, Mak JC, Coupe MO, et al: Calcitonin gene-related peptide vasodilation of human pulmonary vessels. *J Appl Physiol* 67:1265-1270, 1989.

118. McMahon TJ, Kadowitz PJ: Analysis of responses to substance P in the pulmonary vascular bed of the cat. *Am J Physiol* 264:H394-402, 1993.

119. Silverman ES, Gerritsen ME, Collins T: Metabolic functions of the pulmonary endothelium. In: Crystal RG, West JB, Weibel ER, et al: *The lung: Scientific foundations,* Philadelphia, 1997, Lippincott-Raven, pp 629-651.

120. Carley WW, Niedbala MJ, Gerritsen ME: Isolation, cultivation, and partial characterization of microvascular endothelium derived from human lung. *Am J Respir Cell Mol Biol* 7:620-630, 1992.

121. Pearson JD, Carleton JS, Hutchings A, et al: Uptake and metabolism of adenosine by pig aortic endothelial and smooth-muscle cells in culture. *Biochem J* 170:265-271, 1978.

122. Dieterle Y, Ody C, Ehrensberger A, et al: Metabolism and uptake of adenosine triphosphate and adenosine by porcine aortic and pulmonary endothelial cells and fibroblasts in culture. *Circ Res* 42:869-876, 1978.

123. Gaba SJ, Bourgouin-Karaouni D, Dujols P, et al: Effects of adenosine triphosphate on pulmonary circulation in chronic obstructive pulmonary disease. ATP: a pulmonary vasoregulator? *Am Rev Respir Dis* 134:1140-1144, 1986.

124. Steinhorn RH, Morin FC, 3rd, Van Wylen DG, et al: Endothelium-dependent relaxations to adenosine in juvenile rabbit pulmonary arteries and veins. *Am J Physiol* 266:H2001-2006, 1994.

125. Pearson JD, Carleton JS, Gordon JL: Metabolism of adenine nucleotides by ectoenzymes of vascular endothelial and smooth-muscle cells in culture. *Biochem J* 190:421-429, 1980.

126. Gaddum JH, Hebb CO, Silver A, et al: 5-Hydroxytryptamine; pharmacological action and destruction in perfused lungs. *Q J Exp Psychol* 38:255-262, 1953.

127. Fishman A, Pietra, G.G. Handling of bioactive materials by the lung. *New Engl J Med* 1974; 291:884-890.

128. Fanburg BL, Glazier JB. Conversion of angiotensin 1 to angiotensin 2 in the isolated perfused dog lung. *J Appl Physiol* 1973; 35:325-31.

129. de Nucci G, Thomas R, D'Orleans-Juste P, et al: Pressor effects of circulating endothelin are limited by its removal in the pulmonary circulation and by the release of prostacyclin and endothelium-derived relaxing factor. *Proc Natl Acad Sci U S A* 85:9797-9800, 1988.

130. Hajjar KA, Hamel NM, Harpel PC, et al: Binding of tissue plasminogen activator to cultured human endothelial cells. *J Clin Invest* 80:1712-1719, 1987.

131. Bevilacqua MP, Schleef RR, Gimbrone MA, Jr., et al: Regulation of the fibrinolytic system of cultured human vascular endothelium by interleukin 1. *J Clin Invest* 78:587-591, 1986.

Histopathology of Pulmonary Arterial Hypertension

Darren B. Taichman, MD, PhD,

Jennifer L. Snow, MD,

Giuseppe G. Pietra, MD

Histopathology of Pulmonary Arterial Hypertension

The pulmonary vasculature reacts to chronic elevations in pressure in a limited number of histologically recognizable patterns.[1,2] Accordingly, regardless of the clinical classification of pulmonary arterial hypertension (PAH), the histopathologic changes seen are qualitatively similar. Quantitative differences, however, can be noted in the distribution of these changes within individual portions of the vasculature, presumably reflecting differences in the pathogenesis of individual disorders. It remains important to acknowledge that neither the qualitative nor quantitative patterns observed in individual patients can be relied upon to indicate the etiology of the pulmonary hypertension. Indeed, both qualitative and quantitative differences in pathologic findings have been noted even among kindred patients with familial PAH.[3]

Structure of the Normal Pulmonary Vasculature

A description of the normal segments of the pulmonary circulation will aid in reviewing the histopathologic changes seen in patients with pulmonary hypertension.

As blood flows from the right ventricle to the left atrium it passes successively through large elastic pulmonary arteries, muscular pulmonary arteries, precapillary vessels, and subsequently the capillaries. It then travels via postcapillary venules and veins to the main pulmonary veins and into the left atrium. Elastic pulmonary arteries include the main pulmonary trunk and its intrapulmonary branches extending down to vessels approximately 1 mm in diameter (roughly at the junction of bronchi with bronchioli). These vessels are compliant conduits for blood flow composed of a multilayered latticework of elastic laminae separated by smooth muscle cells, fibroblasts, and proteoglycan matrix (FIGURE 2-1A). The relative dimensions and composition of each of these compartments of the arterial wall varies according to location. As the arteries decrease in size so does the number of elastic laminae, to the point that arteries 500-1000 μm in diameter are devoid of elastic tissue and have become entirely muscular. In these vessels, the innermost layer (intima) consists of a single layer of endothelial cells and its surrounding extracellular matrix (basement membrane). The medial layer contains circumferential rings of smooth muscle cells or other contractile cells such as myofibroblasts. The outermost adventitial layer is made of connective tissue matrix, fibroblasts, myofibroblasts, smooth muscle cells, and immune cells. Internal and external elastic laminae separate the medial from the intimal and adventitial layers, respectively (FIGURE 2-1B). Muscular arteries accompanying small airways outside the respiratory units are called "pre-acinar" vessels, while those within the respiratory units may be termed "intra-acinar" or "arterioles."

As vessels progress within the respiratory units toward the precapillary network, the muscular layer

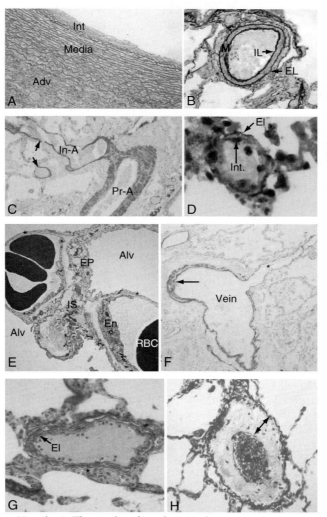

Figure 2-1. Normal Pulmonary Vessels. **A.** The media of an elastic pulmonary artery is composed of a latticework of coarse elastic laminae. A narrow strip of the intima *(Int)* overlying the media is visible. A normal adventitia *(Adv)* is also seen. **B.** Cross-section of a pre-acinar muscular pulmonary artery revealing a thin muscular media *(M)* bounded by internal *(IL)* and external *(EL)* elastic laminae. **C.** Branching off of an intra-acinar artery *(In-A)* from a pre-acinar artery *(Pr-A)*. The media of the vessels has been decorated with anti-smooth muscle actin antibody *(rust color)* to show the marked decrease in medial muscle as the caliber of the arteries decreases. The *arrows* point to a partial loss of the medial muscle in the vessel walls. **D.** Nonmuscular intra-acinar artery composed of intima *(Int)* and elastic lamina *(EL)*. **E.** Electron micrograph of an alveolar septum showing the subdivision of the interstitial space (IS) into thin (*) and thick zones by the eccentric course of the alveolar capillary. *RBC,* red blood cell; *EP,* Type 1 pneumocyte; *En,* endothelium; *Alv,* alveolar space. **F.** Intra-acinar venule (*) draining into an interlobular vein *(vein)*. Smooth muscle actin staining reveals the irregular distribution of the medial muscle in the venous wall *(arrow)*. **G.** Cross-section of an interlobular vein showing the single elastic lamina *(El)* separating the media from the adventitia. **H.** Cross-section of an interlobular vein showing age-related fibrous thickening of the intima *(double arrow)*. (Stains: **A, B, D, G,** and **H:** Verhoeff-van Gieson; **C** and **F:** Smooth muscle actin; **E:** Uranyl acetate-lead citrate.) (See Color Plate 1).

thins as the arterial diameter decreases. Although a continuous circumferential layer of muscle cells is present in larger vessels, in the smaller arteries the muscle fibers are spirally wound and gradually taper off until the nonmuscular precapillary arteries are reached (FIGURE 2-1C and FIGURE 2-2).[4] Thus, in cross-section, a precapillary artery can have a smooth muscle cell layer that normally is present only at part of its circumference; alternatively, it may appear entirely nonmuscular and composed of an intima separated from the adventitia by a single elastic lamina (FIGURE 2-1D). In conventional histological sections these arterioles are indistinguishable from postcapillary venules.

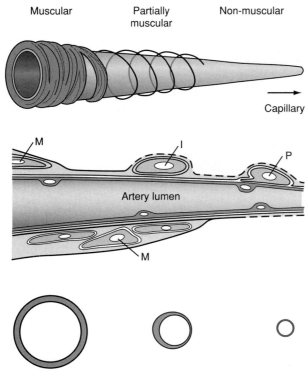

Muscular   Partially   Non-muscular
muscular

Capillary

M

I

P

Artery lumen

M

Figure 2-2. The muscular layer thins as the diameter of pulmonary arteries decreases. Initially a continuous layer of smooth muscle, the muscular coat eventually spirals as individual cells and surrounds only part of the circumference of small vessels. A cross-sectional schematic view is seen at the bottom. Proceeding distally, cells are initially typical of smooth muscle *(M)* and then of an intermediate type cell *(I)*; pericytes *(P)* are seen at the level of small precapillary arteries. (Reproduced with permission from DeMello DE, Reid LM: Prenatal and postnatal development of the pulmonary circulation. In: Haddad GG, Abman SH, Chernick V, editors: *Basic mechanisms of pediatric respiratory disease,* Hamilton, 2002, BC Decker, pp 77-101.)

The presence of precapillary and postcapillary segments within the pulmonary circulation is distinct from the arrangement of the systemic vascular bed. Changes within these vessels are important manifestations and causes of PAH. The normal, progressive thinning of the muscle that occurs in the precapillary arteries is of particular importance as distinct from the histopathologic changes seen in PAH, in which abnormal extension of muscularization is a prominent feature (see section titled "Constrictive Lesions" in this chapter).

Between the precapillary and postcapillary segments, the arterioles break up to form the alveolar capillary network. The alveolar capillaries are endothelial tubes lined by an endothelial monolayer whose basement membrane is enveloped by a wide-meshed network of pericytes. The alveolar capillaries course eccentrically within the alveolar septa, subdividing the interstitial space into thin and thick zones (FIGURE 2-1E). The thin zone is composed only of the fused endothelial and epithelial basement membranes, whereas the thick zone contains the nuclear region of the endothelial cell and the alveolar connective tissue. In the thick zone, within the collagen fibers and the proteoglycan matrix, are cellular elements such as pericytes, myofibroblasts, fibroblasts, mast cells, and immune, inflammatory, and peripatetic pluripotent cells. In the adult lung, only one capillary is present in cross-sections of the alveolar septa; therefore, the presence of a double layer of capillaries is an important histopathologic feature of the pulmonary microvasculopathy characteristic of pulmonary capillary hemangiomatosis, as will be discussed later.

Intra-acinar venules arise from the capillaries. As indicated previously, their structure is similar to that of the nonmuscular arterioles. They drain into larger veins located in the interlobular septa at the periphery of the acinus (FIGURE 2-1F) and are not related to the airways. Larger pulmonary veins within the interlobular septa have a well-developed media with smooth muscle cells, connective tissue matrix, and a distinct internal elastic lamina. The media blends gradually with the adventitia that is composed of connective tissue, smooth muscle cells, and elastic fibers (FIGURE 2-1G).

Histopathologic Features Common to All Forms of Pulmonary Hypertension

Pulmonary hypertension can occur in disease processes primarily isolated to the pulmonary vasculature itself, as in PAH, or in association with diseases in which the primary disturbance is one of respiratory function (e.g., chronic obstructive pulmonary disease) or of the left heart (e.g., mitral stenosis). Regardless, each of these causes of pulmonary hypertension can result in similar derangements at the elastic and muscular pulmonary vessels: atheromatous changes and dilation of large elastic pulmonary arteries, medial hypertrophy, and remodeling of muscular arteries. If pulmonary hypertension persists, right ventricular hypertrophy, dilation, and ultimately failure are common sequelae (FIGURE 2-3).

Medial hypertrophy is an abnormal increase in smooth muscle mass and occurs in the muscular

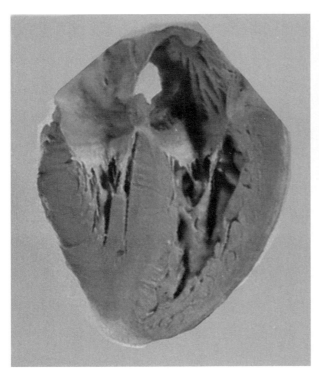

Figure 2-3. Right Ventricular Hypertrophy. Sagittal section of a patient with pulmonary hypertension and cor pulmonale with marked hypertrophy of the right ventricle. (Reproduced with permission from Pietra GG, Dessy E: Hypertensive pulmonary vasculopathies: Pathological findings. In: Lanzer P, Topol EJ, editors: *Panvascular medicine: Integrated clinical management,* New York, 2002, Springer Verlag, pp 1609-1618.)

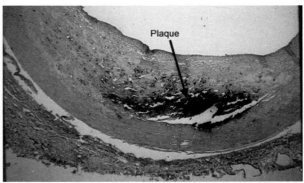

Figure 2-4. Low-power view of an elastic pulmonary artery from a patient with idiopathic pulmonary arterial hypertension showing a calcified atheromatous plaque. (Hematoxylin and eosin stain.) (See Color Plate 1).

and elastic arteries of all forms of pulmonary hypertension. Reduplication of the elastic laminae is another characteristic feature of the medial hypertrophy seen in pulmonary hypertension of multiple causes. Medial hypertrophy may be less obvious at elastic pulmonary arteries when significant arterial dilation occurs.[5] Significant arterial dilation, itself, can cause narrowing of adjacent airways and result in recurrent pneumonia, or it can compress the recurrent laryngeal nerve resulting in hoarseness (Ortner's sign). Localized medial hypertrophy and intimal thickening of muscular arteries can also develop as an isolated finding associated with tumors, interstitial lung diseases, or airway diseases in the absence of pulmonary hypertension.

Intimal atheromas confined to the elastic pulmonary arteries are additional features of all forms of pulmonary hypertension as are atherosclerotic changes in the systemic circulation with systemic hypertension (FIGURE 2-4). Atherosclerotic lesions

in the pulmonary circulation, however, tend to be shallow and nonobstructing.[5,6] Their presence should not be considered diagnostic of pulmonary hypertension, because atheromatous patches develop with aging in the nonhypertensive pulmonary circulation, particularly in the large elastic arteries at points of vessel branching.

Histopathologic Patterns in Pulmonary Arterial Hypertension

In addition to the histopathologic features common to all causes of pulmonary hypertension, each of the forms of PAH is associated with characteristic lesions involving both the pre-acinar and intra-acinar arteries. These include constrictive lesions at the vessel intima, remodeling of the media or adventitia, as well as complex lesions involving changes of the entire vessel wall.[1,7,8]

Constrictive Lesions
Medial hypertrophy is due to both an expansion in number (hyperplasia) and size (hypertrophy) of smooth muscle cells, as well as a change in their phenotype. It can involve the extension of smooth muscle cells into intra-acinar precapillary arteries that are normally only partially muscularized or nonmuscularized (FIGURE 2-5).[9] When marked thickening of the media occurs, presumably the result of long-standing elevations in pressure, the hypertrophied smooth muscle can undergo atrophy and be replaced by fibrous tissue (see FIGURE 2-5G). Atrophy can result in thinning of the media and dilation of the vessel lumen. When present, medial hypertrophy of the pre-acinar and intra-acinar vessels usually is accompanied by intimal thickening.

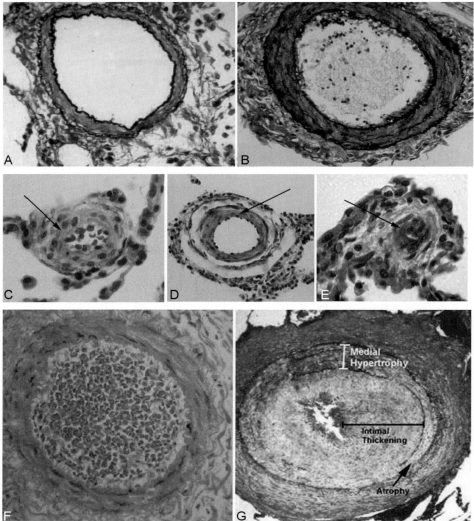

Figure 2-5. Medial Hypertrophy. As compared with a normal vessel (**A**), an increase in the medial smooth muscle is seen in the pulmonary artery of a patient with pulmonary hypertension (**B**). High-power photomicrographs showing extension of muscularization to involve small intra-acinar pulmonary arteries (**C, D, E,** *arrows*). Medial hypertrophy can occur as an isolated lesion (**F**) or in association with intimal fibrosis (**G**). Panel **G** shows a photomicrograph of a muscular pulmonary artery (approximately 20 microns) with marked nonlaminar concentric intimal thickening. Medial hypertrophy and segmental atrophy with partial destruction of the internal elastic lamina are seen. (Stains: **A, B, G**: Verhoeff-van Gieson; **C, D, E, F**: Hematoxylin and eosin.) (See Color Plate 2).

Intimal thickening can occur with or without associated hypertrophy or atrophy of the media. Three histopathologic patterns of intimal thickening are recognized: concentric laminar, eccentric, and concentric nonlaminar (FIGURE 2-6). Concentric laminar intimal thickening is a highly distinctive lesion composed of "onion skin-like" layers of fibroblasts, myofibroblasts, and smooth muscle cells. Acellular connective tissue can be seen, also. Although a characteristic feature of what was formerly conceptualized as "plexogenic arteriopathy," concentric laminar fibrosis in not unique to idiopathic ("primary") PAH and can be seen in other forms of PAH, such as that associated with systemic sclerosis or congenital heart disease with systemic-to-pulmonary shunt. In idiopathic PAH, concentric laminar fibrosis frequently is associated with atrophy of the medial layer.[7,10] Eccentric and concentric nonlaminar intimal thickenings are cushions of fibroblasts and connective tissue matrix. They can be localized to just one segment of the intima or can obliterate the entire lumen of the vessel. These

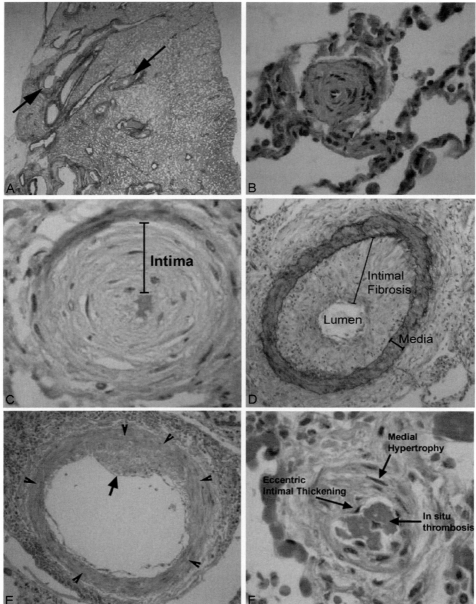

Figure 2-6. Intimal Thickening. **A.** Whole lung section from a patient with exposure to the appetite suppressant aminorex. Enlargement and thickening of the pulmonary arterial structures can be seen *(arrows)*. **B.** Concentric laminar intimal thickening in an intraacinar pulmonary artery of a patient with human immunodeficiency virus (HIV) infection. He did not meet criteria for a diagnosis of acquired immunodeficiency syndrome (AIDS) when pulmonary arterial hypertension was diagnosed. **C.** Pre-acinar pulmonary artery with marked concentric intimal thickening ("onion skinning") and resultant narrowing of the vessel lumen in a patient with systemic sclerosis and focal pulmonary fibrosis. This patient did not have pulmonary hypertension. The vascular lesions were localized to the areas of pulmonary fibrosis. **D** and **E.** Nonlaminar intimal thickening can be concentric (**D**) or eccentric (**E**, *arrow*) as seen in these pre-acinar muscular arteries. Medial hypertrophy is also seen *(arrow heads* and *label)*. **F.** High-power photomicrograph showing an intra-acinar pulmonary artery with eccentric nonlaminar intimal thickening, medial hypertrophy, and *in situ* thrombosis. (Stains: **A, D**: Verhoeff-Van Gieson; **B, C, E, F**: Hematoxylin and eosin.) (Reproduced with permission from Pietra GG: The pathology of primary pulmonary hypertension. In: Rubin LJ, Rich S, editors: *Primary pulmonary hypertension,* New York, 1997, Marcel Dekker, pp 19-61; Pietra GG, Capron F, Stewart S, et al: Pathologic assessment of vasculopathies in pulmonary hypertension. *J Am Coll Cardiol* 43(12 Suppl S):25S-32S, 2004.) (See Color Plate 3).

lesions may represent organization of thromboembolic material, but this cannot be proven on morphologic grounds and such an assumption should be discouraged. Indeed, such lesions can occur in the absence of any evidence of embolic disease. Adventitial thickening is difficult to define independently of alterations of the entire arterial wall. Thickening of the adventitia is found in persistent pulmonary hypertension of the newborn.[11,12]

Complex Lesions: Lesions Involving the Entire Vessel Wall

Plexiform lesions were once considered pathognomonic of idiopathic ("primary") PAH. Such lesions, however, can be seen in PAH of multiple types, as well as in non-PAH forms of pulmonary hypertension such as chronic thromboembolic disease.[13] They are nonetheless distinctive lesions and have been the focus of much attention in studies of the cellular and molecular pathogenesis of PAH.[14-17] Plexiform lesions consist of localized proliferations of endothelial cells, smooth muscle cells, myofibroblasts, and extracellular matrix (FIGURE 2-7). They can be found in precapillary and intra-acinar vessels, and are associated with aneurismal dilation of muscular vessels, typically near the vessel's branch origin from a larger parent vessel. The lumen of the parent artery often is narrowed or completely obliterated by intimal thickening proximal to the plexiform lesion, itself. The lumen of the plexiform lesion is replaced by a network of vascular channels lined by plump endothelial cells; fibrin thrombi and platelets are also frequently seen. Partial or total destruction of the media is associated with extension of the plexiform lesion into the surrounding adventitia.

Plexiform lesions were observed in 6 percent of 38 autopsies performed on patients in the National Institutes of Health Registry for the Characterization of Primary Pulmonary Hypertension.[2,18] These lesions occurred in less than 10 percent of muscular arteries seen. The frequency of plexiform lesions has varied significantly in reported series.[7,10,17-20] Although such variation no doubt reflects differences in the patients studied, the size of biopsy or autopsy material available, and the number of vessels assessed, it nonetheless emphasizes that the presence of plexiform lesions is neither sensitive for the presence of pulmonary hypertension or PAH, nor diagnosis-specific. Furthermore, plexiform lesions may be confused with recanalized thromboemboli ("colander-like" lesions) (see FIGURE 2-7E), which can also be found in patients with pulmonary hypertension.

Dilation lesions frequently are noted distal to plexiform lesions and are lined by thin-walled vessels (see FIGURE 2-7, F and G). Whether these lesions exist independently of plexiform lesions has been debated. These thin-walled vessels have been suggested as the site of rupture when pulmonary hemorrhage occurs in patients with PAH.[11] Arteritis with intimal and medial infiltration by acute and chronic inflammatory cells can be seen in association with complex lesions, but only rarely as a prominent, primary pathologic finding in patients with PAH (FIGURE 2-8). Arteritis can lead to necrosis of the vessel wall and scar formation involving the deposition of iron and calcium on degenerated elastic fibers ("ferruginization").

Pulmonary occlusive venopathy (POV) denotes occlusion of pulmonary veins of various sizes by fibrous tissue (FIGURE 2-9, A and B). Loosely organized and edematous fibrous tissue is felt to represent earlier stages of POV, while denser sclerotic fibrous tissue is seen at later stages. Intimal thickening is also seen, predominantly in smaller vessels and only rarely in larger pulmonary veins. This is distinct from the venous hyaline intimal thickening commonly seen in the lungs of elderly individuals (see FIGURE 2-1H), which is an isolated histological finding and not associated with the morphological evidence of chronic venous hypertension always present in POV. Multiple luminal channels may give the appearance of recanalized thrombus, and "arterialization" may be suggested by thickening of the media with the expansion of smooth muscle cells and elastic fibers. Large amounts of hemosiderin deposits within alveolar macrophages, Type 2 pneumocytes, and within the interstitium are also seen. Although the predominant pattern is one of venous involvement, medial hypertrophy of arterial (both large and precapillary) vessels are seen in approximately half of cases felt to primarily represent POV.[11,21,22]

Lymphatic dilation at the lung and pleura as well as alveolar congestion are additional prominent features of pulmonary occlusive venopathy, and shared by other causes of pulmonary venous hypertension such as left heart dysfunction. POV may be distinguished from other forms of venous hypertension by the presence of extensive fibrous tissue, and intimal and medial thickening mentioned above. Calcification of elastic fibers in the surrounding veins and alveoli are additional distinctive features of POV, which may be accompanied by a foreign body giant cell response. Interstitial lung disease (e.g., usual interstitial fibrosis) can be confused with POV because of the eventual fibrosis of interstitial

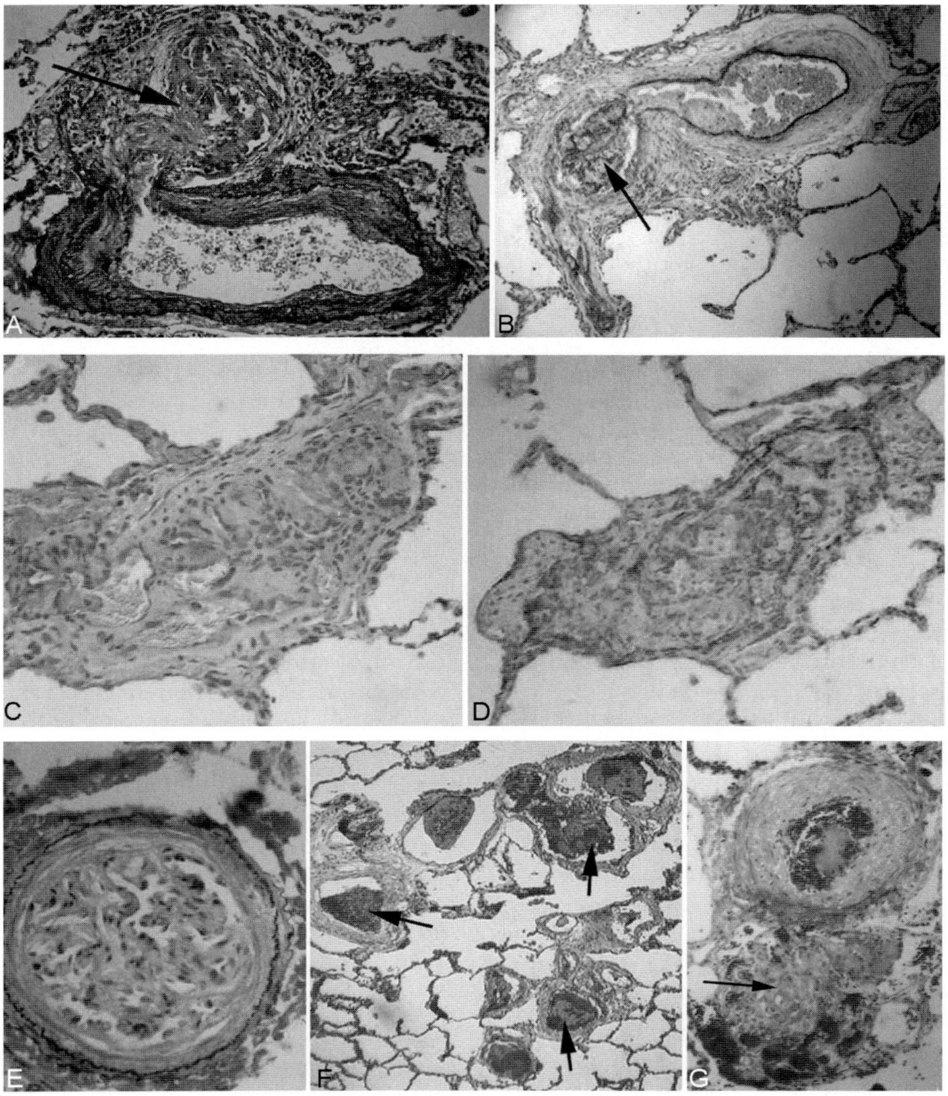

Figure 2-7. **A** and **B.** Plexiform lesions *(arrows)* often are located at the origin of a pulmonary artery at its branching point from a parent vessel. In (**A**), the vessel wall has been destroyed locally and is filled with small channels of blood and granulation tissue. Immunostaining for CD31 *(rust color)* reveals endothelial cells lining the parent vessel and within the plexiform lesion (**B**). **C** and **D.** Endothelial and smooth muscle cells within a plexiform lesion involving an intra-acinar pulmonary artery in a patient with idiopathic pulmonary arterial hypertension. Anti-factor VIII immunostaining *(rust color)* outlines endothelial cells (**C**) and anti-smooth muscle actin outlines smooth muscle cells (**D**) within the same plexiform lesion. **E.** A pre-acinar pulmonary artery displaying recanalized thrombus, giving rise to a "colander-like" lesion (often confused with plexiform lesions). **F.** Low-power photomicrograph showing dilation lesions *(arrows)* consisting of thin-walled sinusoidal channels within the alveolar-capillary network. These lesions usually are found distal to plexiform lesions and may result in hemoptysis if rupture occurs. **G.** Low-power photomicrograph showing a plexiform lesion *(arrow)* and dilation lesions in a patient with portopulmonary hypertension. (Stains: **A**: Verhoeff-Van Gieson; **F**, **G**: Hematoxylin and eosin.) (Reprinted with permission from [A] Pietra GG: The histopathology of primary pulmonary hypertension. In: Fishman AP, editor: *The pulmonary circulation: Normal and abnormal. Mechanisms, management, and the National Registry,* Philadelphia, 1990, University of Pennsylvania Press, pp 459-472; [F] Pietra GG, Capron F, Stewart S, et al: Pathologic assessment of vasculopathies in pulmonary hypertension. *J Am Coll Cardiol* 43[12 Suppl S]:25S-32S, 2004.) (See Color Plate 4).

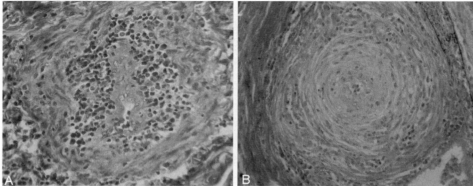

Figure 2-8. **A.** Medium-power photomicrograph of a pre-acinar pulmonary artery in a patient with pulmonary hypertension showing an inflammatory infiltrate in the vessel wall. (Hematoxylin and eosin stain.) **B.** A pre-acinar pulmonary artery with lymphocytic arteritis. (Verhoeff-Van Gieson stain). (Reproduced with permission from [B] Pietra GG, Capron F, Stewart S, et al: Pathologic assessment of vasculopathies in pulmonary hypertension. *J Am Coll Cardiol* 43[12 Suppl S]:25S-32S, 2004.) (See Color Plate 5).

edema that can be found predominantly within the lobular septa in cases of POV.

Pulmonary microvasculopathy (PM) is a rare finding marked by the proliferation of capillaries.[23] These angioproliferative lesions appear to invade the pulmonary vessels, interstitium and, rarely, the airways. These abnormal vessels extend into the walls of arteries and veins causing occlusion and can even extend beyond the vasculature[24-26] (see FIGURE 2-9, C and D). PM may thus be confused with an interstitial process but can be distinguished by the presence of numerous layers of small vessels containing many erythrocytes. PM also shares features with POV, as each may be accompanied by prominent hemosiderosis or medial hypertrophy of pulmonary arteries or both. Venous congestion can also cause confusion between PM and POV, the latter being distinguished by venous obliteration due to nonangiogenic fibrosis in contrast to the proliferating capillaries distinctive of pulmonary microvasculopathy.

The designation "pulmonary occlusive vasculopathy" corresponds to the predominant histological finding seen in the clinical diagnostic category of "pulmonary veno-occlusive disease."[27] Similarly, "pulmonary microvasculopathy" is a pathology term that describes findings that predominate in cases falling under the clinical diagnosis of "pulmonary capillary hemangiomatosis." Because of the overlap in histologic findings that can occur between these and other PAH diagnoses, it is preferable to adhere to descriptive pathology terms in describing tissue findings (see pathologic and clinical correlations below).

In Situ *Thrombosis*

In addition to constrictive and complex lesions, thrombosis of small vessels (both arterial and venous) is noted frequently in the absence of evidence to suggest an embolic source.[10,28,29] Platelet-fibrin thrombi with frequent recanalization can be found within precapillary and intra-acinar vessels, the vascular channels within plexiform lesions, and in association with the venous obstruction of POV (FIGURE 2-10).

Correlation of Pathologic and Clinical Parameters

In a study of 19 patients with idiopathic PAH who underwent lung biopsy close to the time of cardiac catheterization, the degree of medial thickening correlated with baseline hemodynamic measures. No histologic variables were predictive of response to the acute administration of vasodilators.[30] However, the degree of intimal thickening did correlate with clinical outcome, with greater intimal thickening associated with a more rapid clinical decline. Similar clinical-pathologic correlation studies have not been performed since multiple pharmacologic agents with long-term efficacy have become available for treatment of PAH. Furthermore, because tissue is now only rarely obtained in the antemortem evaluation of patients with pulmonary hypertension, such clinical-pathologic correlations have not been adopted into clinical management strategies.

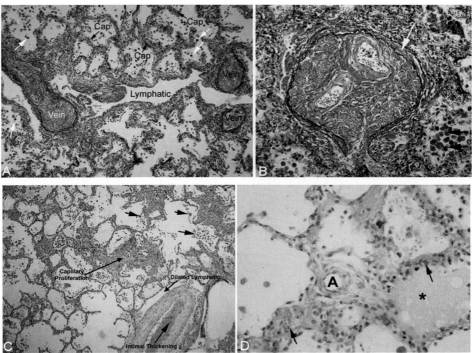

Figure 2-9. Pulmonary Obstructive Venopathy and Pulmonary Microvasculopathy. **A.** Low-power pho-tomicrograph showing near-total obstruction of pulmonary veins, lymphatic dilation, capil-lary congestion *(Cap, black arrows)*, and accumulation of hemosiderin-laden macrophages *(white arrows)* in pulmonary obstructive venopathy. (Verhoeff-Van Gieson stain.) **B.** High-power photomicrograph showing obstruction and recanalization of a pulmonary vein. Note also the arterialization characterized by medial muscle hypertrophy and the double elastic laminae *(white arrow)*. Hemosiderin-laden macrophages fill the alveolar spaces *(black arrows)*. This patient's clinical diagnosis was pulmonary veno-occlusive disease. (Verhoeff-Van Gieson stain.) **C.** Low-power photomicrograph showing pulmonary microvasculopathy, with patchy capillary proliferation and accumulation of hemosiderin-laden macrophages *(short arrows)* in the alveoli and interstitium. Intimal thickening within the artery as well as lymphatic dilation are seen. (Hematoxylin and eosin stain.) **D.** Low-power photomicrograph revealing the pres-ence of more than one capillary *(arrows)* in the widened alveolar septa, indicative of pulmonary microvasculopathy seen here in a patient with pulmonary capillary heman-giomatosis. Also seen is an intra-acinar artery *(A)* with medial hypertrophy. Note that in the normal adult lung, only one capillary is seen in cross-sections of the alveolar septa; a double layer of capillaries here is an important histopathologic feature of pulmonary microvascu-lopathy. (Hematoxylin and eosin stain.) (Reproduced with permission from [A] Pietra GG, Capron F, Stewart S, et al: Pathologic assessment of vasculopathies in pulmonary hyperten-sion. *J Am Coll Cardiol* 43[12 Suppl S]:25S-32S, 2004.) (See Color Plate 5).

As noted above, each of the histologic patterns of change described in patients with PAH can be found in the multiple clinical PAH diagnoses. In addition, significant variation in the patterns and frequency of lesions occurs among patients with the same clinical diagnosis.[3,18] Furthermore, obtain-ing lung tissue to clarify the diagnosis in patients with significant pulmonary hypertension is associ-ated with significant risk.[2,31] Thus, biopsy is reserved for cases where there is substantial doubt as to the etiology of dyspnea, or when establishing a diagnosis will impact planning treatment (even if

only to avoid needless risk associated with the use of therapies that will be ineffective), or when the diagnosis will provide important prognostic infor-mation to the patient.

For such instances in which a tissue diagnosis is sought to clarify treatment plans or assist in assess-ing prognosis, or when clinical-pathologic correla-tions are made at the time of autopsy, a uniform method of reporting the pathologic findings of PAH has been developed[11] (TABLE 2-1). Standardized reporting of pathologic findings should not only aid in interpreting the findings of biopsies taken in the

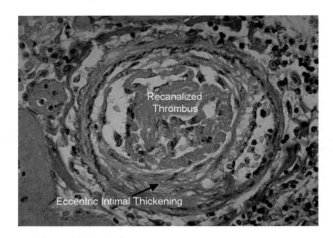

Figure 2-10. *In situ* thrombosis. Photomicrograph showing *in situ* thrombosis with organization and recanalization within a pre-acinar muscular artery with eccentric intimal thickening. (Verhoeff-Van Gieson stain.) (See Color Plate 6).

TABLE 2-1

Pathologic Classification of Pulmonary Vascular Lesions*

1. Pulmonary Arteriopathy (Pre-acinar and Intra-acinar Arteries)

Subsets

Pulmonary arteriopathy with isolated medial hypertrophy
Pulmonary arteriopathy with medial hypertrophy and intimal thickening (cellular, fibrotic)
Concentric laminar
Eccentric, concentric nonlaminar
Pulmonary arteriopathy with plexiform or dilation lesions or arteritis
Pulmonary arteriopathy with isolated arteritis

1a. As above but with coexisting venous-venular changes (cellular or fibrotic intimal thickening, muscularization)

The presence of the following changes should be noted:
Adventitial thickening; thrombotic lesions (fresh, organized, recanalized, colander lesion); necrotizing or lymphomonocytic arteritis; elastic artery changes (fibrotic or atheromatous intimal plaques, elastic laminae degeneration); bronchial vessel changes, ferruginous incrustation, calcifications, foreign body emboli, organized infarct perivascular lymphocytic infiltrates

2. Pulmonary Occlusive Venopathy (Veins of Various Size and Venules) With or Without Coexisting Arteriopathy

Histopathologic features:

Venous changes: Intimal thickening or obstruction (cellular, fibrotic); obstructive fibrous luminal septa (recanalization)
Adventitial thickening (fibrotic), muscularization, iron and calcium incrustation with foreign body reaction
Capillary changes: Dilated, congested capillaries, angioma-like lesions
Interstitial changes: Edema, fibrosis, hemosiderosis, lymphocytic infiltrates
Others: Dilated lymphatics, alveoli with hemosiderin-laden macrophages, Type 2 cell hyperplasia

3. Pulmonary Microvasculopathy With or Without Coexisting Arteriopathy or Venopathy

Histopathologic features:

Microvessel changes: Localized capillary proliferations within pulmonary interstitium, obstructive capillary proliferation in veins and venular walls
Venous-venular intimal fibrosis
Interstitial changes: Edema, fibrosis, hemosiderosis
Others: Dilated lymphatic vessels, alveoli with hemosiderin-laden macrophages, Type 2 cell hyperplasia

4. Unclassifiable**

---

*Nonvascular lung pathology needs to be listed as separate diagnosis.
**Atypical histopathologic features or inadequate sampling of blood vessels.
Reproduced with permission from Pietra GG, Capron F, Stewart S, et al: Pathologic assessment of vasculopathies in pulmonary hypertension. J Am Coll Cardiol 43(12 Suppl S):25S-32S, 2004.*

course of clinical care, it should also help to correlate pathologic with clinical, cellular, and molecular findings in studies of PAH pathogenesis and treatment.

References

1. Pietra GG: Histopathology of primary pulmonary hypertension. *Chest* 105(2 Suppl):2S-6S, 1994.
2. Pietra GG: The histopathology of primary pulmonary hypertension. In: Fishman AP, editor: *The pulmonary circulation: Normal and abnormal. Mechanisms, management, and the National Registry,* Philadelphia, 1990, University of Pennsylvania Press, pp 459-472.
3. Loyd JE, Atkinson JB, Pietra GG, et al: Heterogeneity of pathologic lesions in familial primary pulmonary hypertension. *Am Rev Respir Dis* 138:952-957, 1988.
4. DeMello DE, Reid LM: Prenatal and postnatal development of the pulmonary circulation. In: Haddad GG, Abman SH, Chernick V, editors: *Basic mechanisms of pediatric respiratory disease,* Hamilton, 2002, BC Decker, pp 77-101.
5. Edwards WD: The pathology of secondary pulmonary hypertension. In: Fishman AP, editor: *The pulmonary circulation: Normal and abnormal. Mechanisms, management, and the National Registry,* Philadelphia, 1990, University of Pennsylvania Press, pp 329-342.
6. Wissler RW, Vesselinovitch D: Atherogenesis in the pulmonary artery. In: Fishman AP, editor: *The pulmonary circulation: Normal and abnormal. Mechanisms, management, and the National Registry,* Philadelphia, 1990, University of Pennsylvania Press, pp 245-255.
7. Wagenvoort CA: Primary pulmonary hypertension: a pathologic study of the lung vessels in 156 clinically diagnosed cases. *Circulation* 42:1163-1184, 1970.
8. Wagenvoort CA, Wagenvoort N: Pulmonary vascular bed: Normal anatomy and responses to disease. In: Moser KM, editor: *Pulmonary vascular diseases: Lung biology in health and disease,* New York, 1979, Marcel Dekker, pp 100-109.
9. Heath D, Smith P, Gosney J: The pathology of the early and late stages of primary pulmonary hypertension. *Br Heart J* 58:204-213, 1987.
10. Bjornsson J, Edwards WD: Primary pulmonary hypertension: A histopathologic study of 80 cases. *Mayo Clin Proc* 60:16-25, 1985.
11. Pietra GG, Capron F, Stewart S, et al: Pathologic assessment of vasculopathies in pulmonary hypertension. *J Am Coll Cardiol* 43(12 Suppl S):25S-32S, 2004.
12. Chazova I, Loyd JE, Zhdanov VS, et al: Pulmonary artery adventitial changes and venous involvement in primary pulmonary hypertension. *Am J Pathol* 146:389-397, 1995.
13. Moser KM, Bloor CM: Pulmonary vascular lesions occurring in patients with chronic major vessel thromboembolic pulmonary hypertension. *Chest* 103:685-692, 1993.
14. Voelkel NF, Tuder RM, Weir EK: Pathophysiology of primary pulmonary hypertension: From physiology to molecular mechanisms. In: Rubin LJ, Rich S, editors: *Primary pulmonary hypertension,* New York, 1997, Marcel Dekker, pp 83-129.
15. Cool CD, Stewart JS, Werahera P, et al: Three-dimensional reconstruction of pulmonary arteries in plexiform pulmonary hypertension using cell-specific markers. Evidence for a dynamic and heterogeneous process of pulmonary endothelial cell growth. *Am J Pathol* 155:411-419, 1999.
16. Yeager ME, Halley GR, Golpon HA, et al: Microsatellite instability of endothelial cell growth and apoptosis genes within plexiform lesions in primary pulmonary hypertension. *Circ Res* 88:E2-E11, 2001.
17. Jamison BM, Michel RP: Different distribution of plexiform lesions in primary and secondary pulmonary hypertension. *Hum Pathol* 26:987-993, 1995.
18. Pietra GG, Edwards WD, Kay JM, et al: Histopathology of primary pulmonary hypertension. A qualitative and quantitative study of pulmonary blood vessels from 58 patients in the National Heart, Lung, and Blood Institute, Primary Pulmonary Hypertension Registry. *Circulation* 80:1198-1206, 1989.
19. Yi ES, Kim H, Ahn H, et al: Distribution of obstructive intimal lesions and their cellular phenotypes in chronic pulmonary hypertension. A morphometric and immunohistochemical study. *Am J Respir Crit Care Med* 162:1577-1586, 2000.
20. Pietra GG: The pathology of primary pulmonary hypertension. In: Rubin LJ, Rich S, editors: *Primary pulmonary hypertension,* New York, 1997, Marcel Dekker, pp 19-61.
21. Wagenvoort CA, Wagenvoort N: The pathology of pulmonary veno-occlusive disease. *Virchows Arch A Pathol Anat Histol* 364:69-79, 1974.
22. Mandel J, Mark EJ, Hales CA: Pulmonary veno-occlusive disease. *Am J Respir Crit Care Med* 162:1964-1973, 2000.
23. Wagenvoort CA, Beetstra A, Spijker J: Capillary haemangiomatosis of the lungs. *Histopathology* 2:401-406, 1978.
24. Havlik DM, Massie LW, Williams WL, et al: Pulmonary capillary hemangiomatosis-like foci. An

autopsy study of 8 cases. *Am J Clin Pathol* 113:655-662, 2000.

25. Erbersdobler A, Niendorf A: Multifocal distribution of pulmonary capillary haemangiomatosis. *Histopathology* 40:88-91, 2002.

26. Almagro P, Julia J, Sanjaume M, et al: Pulmonary capillary hemangiomatosis associated with primary pulmonary hypertension: report of 2 new cases and review of 35 cases from the literature. *Medicine* (Baltimore) 81:417-424, 2002.

27. Simonneau G, Galie N, Rubin LJ, et al: Clinical classification of pulmonary hypertension. *J Am Coll Cardiol* 43(12 Suppl S):5S-12S, 2004.

28. Cohen M, Fuster V, Edwards WD: Anticoagulation in the treatment of pulmonary hypertension. In: Fishman AP, editor: *The pulmonary circulation: Normal and abnormal. Mechanisms, management, and the National Registry.* Philadelphia, 1990, University of Pennsylvania Press, pp 501-510.

29. Fuster V, Steele PM, Edwards WD, et al: Primary pulmonary hypertension: natural history and the importance of thrombosis. *Circulation* 70:580-587, 1984.

30. Palevsky HI, Schloo BL, Pietra GG, et al: Primary pulmonary hypertension. Vascular structure, morphometry, and responsiveness to vasodilator agents. *Circulation* 80:1207-1221, 1989.

31. Wagenvoort CA: Lung biopsy specimens in the evaluation of pulmonary vascular disease. *Chest* 77:614-625, 1980.

32. Pietra GG, Dessy E: Hypertensive pulmonary vasculopathies: Pathological findings. In: Lanzer P, Topol EJ, editors: *Panvascular medicine: Integrated clinical management,* New York, 2002, Springer Verlag, pp 1609-1618.

Chapter 3

Pathobiologic Mechanisms of Pulmonary Arterial Hypertension

Jennifer L. Snow, MD,

Peter Lloyd Jones, PhD,

Darren B. Taichman, MD, PhD

Introduction

The development of pulmonary hypertension involves abnormal endothelial, platelet, and smooth muscle function. Alterations in ion channels, growth factors, and vasoactive proteins, as well as gene mutations, have been identified as contributors to these abnormalities. The host of cellular, molecular, histologic, and physiologic abnormalities associated with human pulmonary arterial hypertension (PAH), and the varying models that each reproduces some but not all of these derangements in experimental animals, suggest that no single etiologic factor is responsible. Rather, PAH likely can result from a number of abnormalities of pulmonary vascular cell function, initiated by one of a number of possible insults.

Furthermore, the propensity of such abnormalities to produce disease appears to be determined by both the intensity and duration of these derangements and an individual's predisposition to abnormal vascular responses. For example, the risk of developing PAH as a result of taking anorectic agents increases with the duration of exposure, yet not all patients develop disease even after years of exposure. Similarly, a minority of patients with either systemic sclerosis or human immunodeficiency virus (HIV) infection develop PAH. Patients' clinical courses can be strikingly different, with some responding well despite hemodynamically advanced disease at the initiation of

therapy, while others suffer inexorable decline despite initiating treatment when hemodynamic or functional changes are relatively mild. Thus, although it is tempting to assume that a "common final pathway" is operative in patients with different forms of PAH by the time the disease becomes clinically evident, such a view is certainly too simplistic.

In short, PAH results from one or more insults, in the setting of one or more genetic or other predisposing factors, that support a cascade of complex cellular and molecular changes in the pulmonary vasculature. These changes might not regress, either because the insult(s) is ongoing or because of a dysregulation of normal repair processes. This chapter will summarize some of the more important cellular and molecular processes that likely contribute to PAH.[1-6]

Cellular Derangements

The pathogenesis of PAH involves abnormal cellular proliferation, thrombosis, and alterations in the normal balance between vasoconstriction and vasodilation (FIGURE 3-1). Dysfunctional endothelial, platelet, smooth muscle, and perhaps other vascular cells each contribute to all three processes, mediated by a milieu of vasoactive products. It has not yet been possible to definitively differentiate initiating causes from secondary effects among the abnormalities

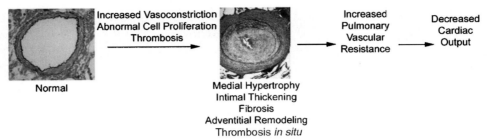

Figure 3-1. Schematic depiction of key pathobiologic processes involved in pulmonary arterial hypertension. Multiple factors contribute to abnormal vasoconstriction, cellular proliferation, and thrombosis. These changes result in an elevated resistance to the transit of blood through the pulmonary circulation and eventual right heart failure with impaired cardiac output. (Histologic images courtesy of G.G. Pietra, MD.) (See Color Plate 6).

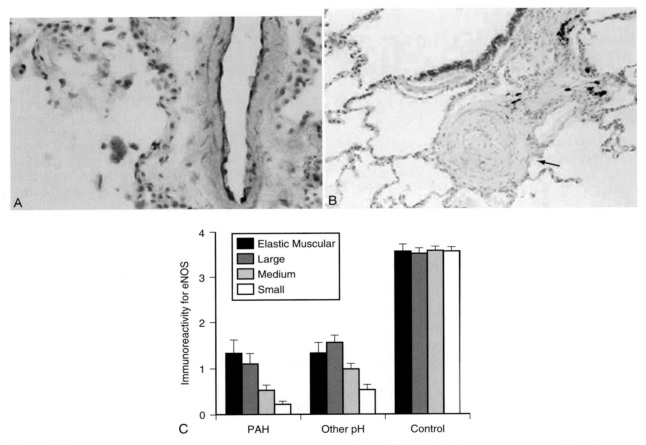

Figure 3-2. Decreased expression of endothelial nitric oxide synthase (eNOS) in the lungs of patients with pulmonary hypertension. Immunostaining (*rust color*) identifies eNOS on a muscular pulmonary artery from a normal (non–pulmonary hypertensive) lung (**A**). In the lung of a patient with pulmonary arterial hypertension (**B**), however, immunoreactivity for eNOS is seen on bronchial epithelial cells but not on an adjacent pulmonary artery (*arrow*), where intimal fibrosis and medial hypertrophy are found. Panel (**C**) shows a semi-quantitative assessment eNOS immunoreactivity on elastic and muscular pulmonary arteries from patients with pulmonary arterial hypertension (PAH) and non-PAH forms of pulmonary hypertension. For all vessel types and sizes, eNOS immunoreactivity was reduced as compared with that seen on vessels from normal (control) lungs. (Reproduced with permission from Giaid A, Saleh D: Reduced expression of endothelial nitric oxide synthase in the lungs of patients with pulmonary hypertension. *N Engl J Med* 333[4]:214-221, 1995.) (See Color Plate 6).

found in these cell types. Endothelial dysfunction, however, appears to be central to the initiation and propagation of the vascular derangements, regardless of whether it is the primary or secondary process.[7,8] Endothelial cells normally elaborate multiple vasoactive substances (such as nitric oxide and prostacyclin) with resulting vasodilatory and antiproliferative effects on vascular smooth muscle cells. In addition, the vascular endothelium normally maintains a relatively antithrombotic surface with an extremely slow rate of cellular turnover. Each of these normal homeostatic activities of the endothelium is disturbed in association with PAH.

Numerous morphologic changes indicating abnormal cell regulation are seen at all layers of the vessel wall. These include intimal thickening, medial hypertrophy, and thickening of the vessel adventitia (see Chapter 2). Ultrastructural changes at the endothelium include an increased rough endoplasmic reticulum, consistent with an elevated metabolic response. A neointima develops between the endothelial layer and internal elastic lamina and can include abnormally distributed myofibroblasts, macrophages, elastin, collagen, and other extracellular matrix (ECM) constituents. Within the internal elastic lamina itself, fragmentation of elastin by proteolytic enzymes and the accumulation of fibroblasts and myofibroblasts is seen. The normal distribution of cellular and ECM components of the media is also deranged, with hypertrophy of smooth muscle cells and their appearance within normally nonmuscularized vessels. Hyperplasia of fibroblasts, fibrosis, an increase in elastin and collagen, and neovascularization can all be seen within the vessel adventitia. In some vessels of patients with PAH, a characteristic plexiform lesion forms, consisting of abnormally proliferating endothelial cells and associated smooth muscle and ECM. In some such lesions a monoclonal expansion of endothelial cells has been demonstrated.[9,10] Finally, the vessel lumen, itself, frequently is obstructed by the formation of *in situ* thrombus.

These changes result in a thickened vessel wall with a markedly narrowed and, in some cases, completely obliterated lumen. These marked distortions along with abnormal vasoconstriction or deficiencies in vasodilation result in an elevated resistance to the transit of blood through the pulmonary circulation at rest and an inability to accommodate the augmented pulmonary blood flow required by exercise (see FIGURE 3-1). Some potential mechanisms underlying these changes are discussed below, with particular emphasis on how each may contribute to dysfunctional vasoconstriction, cellular proliferation, and thrombosis.

Molecular Derangements and Mechanisms

Nitric Oxide

Nitric oxide (NO) is a potent endogenous vasodilator active in the determination of resting vascular resistance. Within the vasculature, an endothelial isoform of NO synthase (eNOS) forms NO, which acts upon smooth muscle cells to increase cyclic guanosine monophosphate (cGMP) and produce vasodilation. Indeed, overexpression of eNOS in transgenic animals protects against hypoxia-induced pulmonary hypertension, whereas recombinant mice lacking eNOS develop severe pulmonary hypertension upon exposure to mild hypoxia.[11-13] Pulmonary hypertension induced by monocrotaline treatment of rats can be prevented, and indeed reversed, by the administration of endothelial progenitor cells that overexpress human eNOS.[14]

In addition to its role as a vasodilator, NO exerts anticoagulant effects by inhibiting the recruitment, adhesion, and aggregation of platelets. NO also inhibits proliferation of vascular smooth muscle cells and can promote their apoptosis. It modulates the growth of endothelial cells, protecting them from apoptosis at low concentrations while promoting cell death at higher concentrations.[15] Together, these vasodilatory, platelet, smooth muscle, and endothelial cell effects make NO central to vessel homeostasis.

eNOS messenger ribonucleic acid (mRNA) and protein expression by endothelial cells is markedly decreased in the lungs of patients with PAH as compared with normal lungs.[16] In an assessment of lung tissue from patients with pulmonary hypertension, the expression of eNOS was inversely correlated with total pulmonary resistance and the severity of the morphologic vascular changes. Intermediate levels were seen in patients with non-PAH forms of pulmonary hypertension (e.g., secondary to pulmonary fibrosis or congestive heart failure) (see FIGURE 3-2). However, another study, while similarly noting decreased eNOS expression on small pulmonary vessels, reported increased expression of eNOS within plexiform lesions.[17] Expression of eNOS by epithelial cells within the lung was unaffected by the presence of pulmonary hypertension.[16] It remains unclear whether altered expression of NO is a primary or secondary vascular abnormality in PAH and whether the discrepancies reported in expression within vascular lesions represent methodologic variables or context-specific differences in function.

Inhalation of NO to promote acute vasodilation is a common method of testing hemodynamic responsiveness at the time of patient evaluation,[18] whereas experience with its long-term use as a therapy has been limited, in part due to practical difficulties in administration.[19,20] Augmentation of endogenous NO production with L-arginine (the sole substrate for eNOS) also may promote vasodilation, although the results of small clinical trials of L-arginine therapy for PAH have been mixed.[21-23] Prolongation of NO activity by the inhibition of its degradation by phosphodiesterases has been successful in improving hemodynamics and capacity.[24,25,25b]

Prostacyclin

Prostacyclin (prostaglandin I2) is a product of endothelial cells with vasodilatory, anticoagulant, and growth modulatory properties. Its is decreased in patients with PAH. The importance of a deficiency in prostacyclin as either a primary or secondary process in the pathogenesis of PAH is underscored by the major impact its administration as therapy has on hemodynamics, exercise capacity, and patient survival. Synthesized primarily by the vascular endothelium, prostacyclin is a metabolite of arachidonic acid that activates adenylate cyclase to produce cyclic adenosine monophosphate (cAMP), which promotes vascular smooth muscle relaxation and vasodilation. Prostacyclin also inhibits platelet aggregation and reduces the proliferation of vascular smooth muscle cells. Overexpression of prostacyclin synthase in transgenic animals protects against hypoxia-induced pulmonary hypertension, while prostacyclin receptor–deficient mice develop severe pulmonary hypertension in response to hypoxia.

The expression of prostacyclin synthase is decreased within the pulmonary vasculature of patients with idiopathic as well as other forms of PAH, notably at small and medium-sized vessels, sites where the predominant histopathologic abnormalities typically are seen in PAH (see Chapter 2)

(FIGURE 3-3). As shown in FIGURE 3-4, the urinary excretion of prostacyclin metabolites is decreased in patients with PAH, and the relative excretion of vasoconstrictor metabolites (thromboxane) is increased. This relative deficiency in prostacyclin might contribute to the development of PAH by allowing unchecked vasoconstriction, platelet aggregation, and smooth muscle proliferation in response to other insults.[7]

Vasoactive Intestinal Peptide

Vasoactive intestinal peptide (VIP) is a neurotransmitter which has receptors that stimulate adenylate cyclase and the production of cAMP and cGMP. It is a powerful systemic and pulmonary vasodilator. VIP administration lowers pulmonary vascular resistance and pulmonary artery pressure in normal human volunteers, as well as in animals with monocrotaline-induced pulmonary hypertension. In addition, VIP is a potent inhibitor of both platelet activation and the proliferation of smooth muscle cells. One study demonstrated decreased immunoreactivity for VIP in the small blood vessels of lungs from patients with IPAH, while the density of VIP receptors was increased.[40] Also demonstrated was a dose-dependent decrease in the proliferation of pulmonary artery smooth muscle cells in vitro by VIP. Finally, in a series of eight patients with IPAH, inhalation of VIP resulted in an acute decrease in mean pulmonary arterial pressure and an increase in cardiac output. After 3 months of daily VIP treatments, pulmonary vascular resistance was decreased by approximately 50 percent, and 6-minute walk distance increased over baseline values.

Thromboxane

In addition to a deficiency in molecules that promote vasodilation, there is a relative excess of molecules that enhance vasoconstriction found in both experimental animal models and patients with PAH. Thromboxane is an arachidonic acid metabolite synthesized by endothelial cells and platelets. It produces vasoconstriction and platelet aggregation, and is a smooth muscle mitogen. In contrast to the decreased excretion of vasodilator (e.g., prostacyclin) metabolites in the urine of patients with pulmonary hypertension, increased thromboxane metabolites have been documented (see FIGURE 3-4).[33] In an initial trial of 10 patients

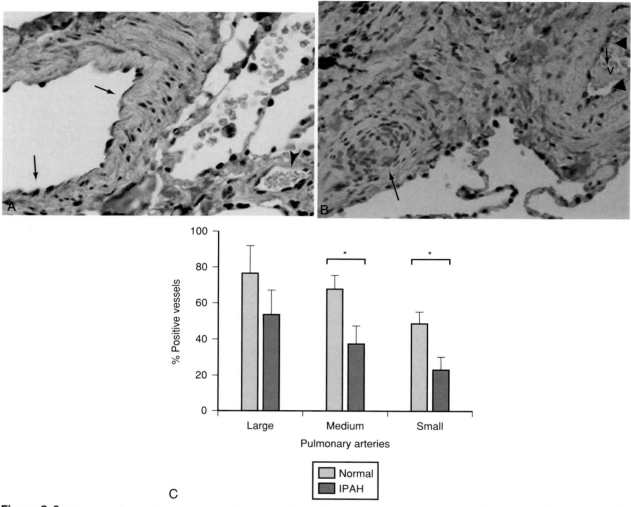

Figure 3-3. Decreased vascular expression of prostacyclin synthase in the lungs of patients with severe pulmonary arterial hypertension (PAH). Immunostaining *(rust color)* identifies the presence of prostacyclin synthase on the vessels of lung tissue from a patient without pulmonary hypertension *(arrows,* **A**). In a patient with idiopathic PAH (IPAH) (**B**), prostacyclin synthase expression is seen on histologically normal vessels *(V, arrowheads),* while absent on most endothelial cells within abnormal vessels, such as those within plexiform lesions *(arrow).* Although the frequency of large vessels expressing prostacyclin synthase was the same in lung tissue from patients with IPAH as compared with non–pulmonary hypertensive samples, there was a significant reduction on medium and small vessels from patients with IPAH (**C**; *P < .05). (Adapted with permission from Tuder RM, Cool CD, Geraci MW, et al: Prostacyclin synthase expression is decreased in lungs from patients with severe pulmonary hypertension. *Am J Respir Crit Care Med* 159[6]:1925-1932, 1999.) (See Color Plate 7).

with IPAH, the administration of a thromboxane inhibitor resulted in modest improvements in hemodynamics values. A larger randomized double-blinded placebo-controlled trial, however, was interrupted because of troubling leg pain in patients receiving the thromboxane inhibitor; at the time the trial was terminated there was no difference in the change in exercise tolerance or pulmonary hemodynamics between the groups receiving thromboxane inhibition and those receiving placebo.[41]

Endothelin

Endothelin-1 (ET-1) is the most abundant member of the endothelin peptides.[42] Found in numerous tissues, the highest level of ET-1 expression is in the

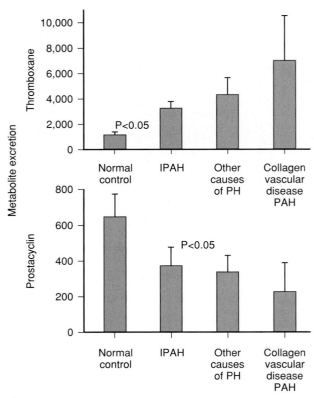

Figure 3-4. Altered levels of vasoconstrictor and vasodilator metabolites in patients with pulmonary arterial hypertension. Urinary expression of vasoconstrictor (thromboxane) metabolites are increased in patients with pulmonary hypertension of various types. In contrast, the excretion of vasodilator (prostacyclin) metabolites was decreased in these same patients. Vasoconstrictor or vasodilator excretion was similar to that of control subjects in patients with chronic obstructive pulmonary disease but without evidence of pulmonary hypertension (not shown). (Adapted with permission from Christman BW, McPherson CD, Newman JH, et al: An imbalance between the excretion of thromboxane and prostacyclin metabolites in pulmonary hypertension. *N Engl J Med* 327[2]: 70-75, 1992.)

lung where it is produced by vascular endothelial, smooth muscle, and airway epithelial cells. ET-1 is among the most potent endogenous vasoconstrictors known. Binding of ET-1 with either endothelin A (ET_A) or B (ET_B) receptors on the surface of smooth muscle cells results in potent vasoconstriction. Activation of ET_B receptors on vascular endothelial cells, by contrast, increases the production of NO, resulting in vasodilation. ET_B receptors are also thought to be important in endothelin cleaance. The net effect of such actions promoting vasoconstriction

or vasodilation may be site and context dependent. For example, the distribution of ET_A or ET_B receptors differs according to location in normal lung tissue, where ET_A receptors predominate on proximal arteries, with increasing density of ET_B receptors on smaller, distal vessels. Both receptors are more common in distal vessels in patients with IPAH as compared with patients with normal lungs[43] and some studies have suggested selective upregulation of ET_B receptors on smooth muscle cells that might augment vasoconstriction.[44]

In addition to being a potent vasoconstrictor, ET-1 may contribute to the development of pulmonary vascular disease as a smooth muscle mitogen and a profibrotic mediator. ET-1 promotes the proliferation of fibroblasts[45] and, in combination with other growth factors, the proliferation of cultured human vascular smooth muscle cells.[46] Biologically active endothelin isolated from bronchoalveolar lavage fluid of patients with systemic sclerosis induces the proliferation of cultured lung fibroblasts.[45] Finally, constitutive expression of endothelin-1 in recombinant mice results in pulmonary fibrosis,[47] an effect that does not necessarily lead to pulmonary hypertension. ET-1 has proinflammatory effects, causing the activation of monocytes and neutrophils and increasing their adhesion to endothelial cells when infused into rat venules. Platelet aggregation and damage to the endothelial lining are also seen following ET-1 infusion.[48] The activation of these multiple cell populations might, in turn, perpetuate the inflammatory response by their release of additional proinflammatory and prothrombotic mediators.

Endothelin has been implicated in the development of human PAH. In a group of 16 patients with idiopathic PAH (IPAH), a significant association was found between worsening pulmonary hemodynamics and increasing blood levels of endothelin in peripheral blood. Pulmonary vascular resistance rises while cardiac output and exercise capacity decline, each in association with rising peripheral blood levels of ET-1.[49] ET-1 is also elevated in the blood of patients with other forms of pulmonary hypertension. Among patients with either interstitial lung disease or chronic obstructive pulmonary disease (COPD), those with pulmonary hypertension (PH) tend to have higher arterial ET-1 levels than those without elevated pressures.[50] Further, the marked overexpression of ET-1 is evident in the lungs of patients with both idiopathic and secondary forms of pulmonary hypertension in which expression is increased on pulmonary arterial vessels and within plexiform lesions (FIGURE 3-5).[51]

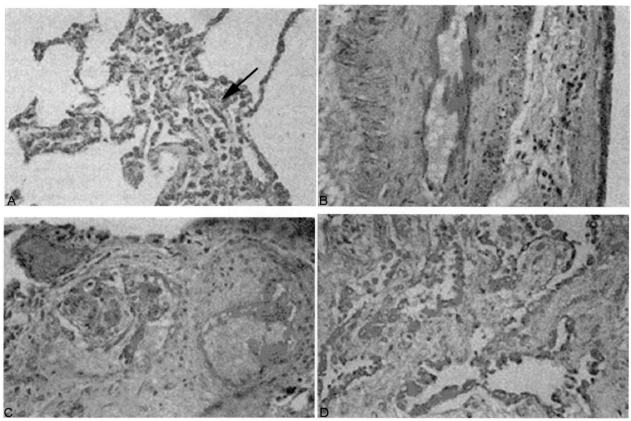

Figure 3-5. Increased expression of endothelin-1 in the lungs of patients with pulmonary hypertension. Immunostaining with an antibody to endothelin-1 decorates vascular endothelial cells in a normal (non–pulmonary hypertensive) lung (**A**, *rust color, arrow*). Markedly increased endothelin-1 expression is seen on pulmonary arteries of patients with idiopathic pulmonary arterial hypertension (**B** and **C**), including within plexiform lesions (**C**). Increased endothelin expression is also found in the lungs of patients with other forms of pulmonary hypertension, as well as on nonvascular cell populations such as on Type 2 alveolar pneumocytes (**D**). (Reproduced with permission from Giaid A, Yanagisawa M, Langleben D, et al: Expression of endothelin-1 in the lungs of patients with pulmonary hypertension. *N Engl J Med* 328[24]:1732-1739, 1993.) (See Color Plate 8).

The importance of endothelin in PAH is underscored by the ability of endothelin receptor antagonists to prevent and, in some cases, reverse pathologic changes in animal models of PH.[52,53] Most convincing of the importance of ET-1's in PAH (as either a primary or secondary effector) are the improvements seen in pulmonary hemodynamics and in exercise capacity with the use of oral endothelin receptor antagonists.[54-56]

Serotonin

Several observations suggest the importance of serotonin (5-HT) mediated vasoconstriction and smooth muscle cell proliferation in the development of pulmonary hypertension. Plasma 5-HT levels are elevated in patients with IPAH and remain so even after normalization of pulmonary hemodynamics with heart-lung transplantation, suggesting that the elevation in 5-HT seen with PAH is a primary and not a secondary process[57] (FIGURE 3-6). The anorexigens fenfluramine and aminorex have caused epidemics of PAH.[58,59] These agents increase plasma 5-HT levels by inducing the release of serotonin from platelets and interfering with its reuptake.[60] In addition to blood levels of 5-HT, expression of specific 5-HT receptor subtypes can be increased in patients with PAH and their activity potentiated by dexfenfluramine.[61,62]

A key regulator of 5-HT action is the serotonin transporter (5-HTT). 5-HTT is highly expressed in the lung, predominantly on pulmonary artery smooth muscle cells. Expression of 5-HTT is

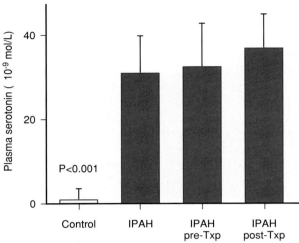

Figure 3-6. Elevated serotonin in the blood of patients with idiopathic pulmonary arterial hypertrophy (IPAH) before and after transplantation. Plasma serotonin levels are increased in patients with IPAH (n = 16) as compared with controls (n = 16), and remain elevated even after normalization of pulmonary hemodynamics following heart-lung transplantation (n = 6 for each patients with IPAH pretransplantation and posttransplantation). Bars show the mean ± standard error of plasma serotonin concentrations. (Adapted with permission from Herve P, Launay JM, Scrobohaci ML, et al: Increased plasma serotonin in primary pulmonary hypertension. *Am J Med* 99[3]:249-254, 1995.)

increased over normal on platelets and the pulmonary arteries of patients with IPAH. In addition, cultured smooth muscles cells isolated from patients with IPAH are more responsive to the mitogenic effects of serotonin than are cells from patients who don't have PAH.[63] Furthermore, overexpression of the *5-HTT* gene in recombinant mice results in worsened hypoxia-induced pulmonary hypertension,[64] whereas animals lacking the *5-HTT* gene are protected from hypoxia as well as from monocrotaline-induced disease.[65,66]

It has been suggested that polymorphisms in the *5-HTT* gene might alter susceptibility to pulmonary hypertension. An insertion in the gene's protomer region (L allele) increases *5-HTT* transcription as compared with the shorter (S) allele. In one study of 89 patients with IPAH, 65 percent were found to be homozygous for the L allele, as compared with 27 percent of controls[63]. An evaluation of 259 IPAH patients and 133 with associated forms of PAH, however, did not find an association with 5-HTTT alleles.[63b] An increased frequency of the LL genotype has also been reported in other forms of pulmonary hypertension.[67] Interestingly, while no difference in gene distribution (LL, LS, or SS) was found between controls and patients with pulmonary hypertension and COPD, the severity of the pulmonary hypertension in these patients was closely related to the presence of the LL genotype. Patients with COPD who are homozygous for the L allele had significantly higher mean pulmonary artery pressures and vascular resistance than those with either the LS or SS genotype.[68] These findings may suggest a mechanism for differences in the severity of pulmonary hypertension seen in patients with COPD not explained by the severity of airflow obstruction, because the forced expiratory volume in 1 second (FEV$_1$) was actually worse in the patients studied who had the LS and SS genotype.

Serotonin signaling might contribute to the pathogenesis of PAH through interaction with other pathways implicated in disease development. For example, 5-HT induces the transcription and secretion of S100A4/Mts1 (a member of the S100 family of calcium-binding proteins) by human pulmonary artery smooth muscle cells. Signaling events requiring the serotonin transporter are also necessary for the expression of S100A4/Mts1.[69] The expression of S100A4/Mts1 is markedly increased on pulmonary artery smooth muscle cells at the proliferative, occlusive lesions of the intima and adventitia found in patients with PAH, and the overexpression of this protein in transgenic animals results in the development of similar pathologic lesions.[70] S100A4/Mts1 may be involved in endothelial cell invasion and angiogenesis, both expected to be operative in the development of pulmonary hypertensive lesions. A further interaction of 5-HT signaling and other pathways operative in the development of PAH is through potassium channel activity. Inhibitors of potassium channels not only lead to vasoconstriction (as described below), they also cause the release of serotonin. Anorexigens which increase 5-HT levels can also inhibit potassium channels.[71] Thus, the intersection of multiple pathways, each of which is implicated in disease pathogenesis, might promote vasoconstriction and cellular proliferation.

Potassium Channels

The resting membrane potential of smooth muscle cells is established in large part by the efflux of potassium (K$^+$) through a family of voltage-gated K$^+$ (Kv) channels. These channels normally are inhibited by hypoxia, leading to an increase of intracellular K[+], membrane depolarization, and activation of calcium channels allowing for calcium accumulation and resultant smooth muscle cell contraction.[72] Whereas inhibition of Kv channels results in vasoconstriction, their activation promotes vasodilation. Expression of genes for members of the Kv family are downregulated in the lungs of patients with IPAH[73] and the Kv1.5 channel specifically on pulmonary artery smooth muscle cells.[74,75] Kv channel expression is also downregulated on the pulmonary artery smooth muscle cells from rats with hypoxia-induced experimental pulmonary hypertension (Kv1.5 and Kv2.1).[76,77] Pulmonary hypertension can be reversed in these animals by stimulating endogenous Kv channel expression with dichloroacetate[76] or increasing Kv1.5 expression by gene transfer.[78]

A potential role of Kv1.5 channels in PAH is further supported by their differential distribution within the pulmonary vasculature, being enriched in resistance vessels that in large part determine pulmonary vascular resistance.[79] Although it is not yet clear whether the changes in Kv channel activity in patients with IPAH are genetic or acquired, their potential role in disease is illustrated by their involvement in both harmful and beneficial pharmacologic effects. The anorexigens dexfenfluramine and aminorex inhibit smooth muscle Kv1.5 and Kv2.1 channels to cause pulmonary vasoconstriction.[80] The anorexigens can also block platelet Kv channels, resulting in the release of serotonin. In addition to inhibiting phosphodiesterase and elevating intracellular cGMP levels in smooth muscle, sildenafil may enhance Kv channel function to promote vasodilation.[76]

Abnormal Kv1.5 channel function might further contribute to the development of PAH by affecting apoptosis. Activation of potassium channels and the loss of intracellular potassium allows for a decrease in cell volume, an important step in apoptosis.[81] A decrease in the expression and function of Kv channels by pulmonary artery smooth muscle cells inhibits apoptosis-induced cell volume loss; resulting elevations in intracellular potassium further inhibits the function of caspases active in programmed cell death.[82] Thus, by inhibiting apoptosis, altered Kv function might enable unchecked smooth muscle cell proliferation in PAH.

Extracellular Matrix

The ECM traditionally has been associated with providing structural support and flexibility to cells within the pulmonary vasculature. Recent studies, however, have highlighted the importance of the ECM as a structure critical for pulmonary vascular homeostasis and one that is important in the development of PAH. Even under normal circumstances, the ECM is a dynamic entity that is constantly catabolized and renewed, and these processes are accelerated with the onset and progression of pulmonary vascular remodeling.[5,83] For example, the expression of one ECM component, tenascin-C (TN-C), is induced in a number of experimental and clinical forms of PAH regardless of etiology. Adult rats treated with the alkaloid toxin monocrotaline develop a fatal and irreversible form of PAH, characterized in part by the appearance of TN-C in the pulmonary vascular wall.[84,85] Similarly, neonatal swine subjected to increased pulmonary blood flow express high levels of TN-C on pulmonary artery smooth muscle cells.[86] Importantly, children with PAH secondary to a variety of congenital heart defects also show elevated levels of TN-C within their pulmonary arteries, including within plexiform lesions.[87] Recent studies indicate that TN-C is also expressed within remodeling pulmonary arteries of patients with idiopathic and sporadic forms of PAH underscored by mutations in bone morphogenetic protein receptor II (BMP-RII).[88]

At a functional level, TN-C promotes the proliferation and survival of pulmonary artery smooth muscle cells via its ability to cross-modulate the activity of important receptor tyrosine kinases, including epidermal growth factor (EGF) and fibroblast growth factor-2.[89] The importance of these findings is substantiated by the demonstration that antisense ablation of TN-C expression ameliorates monocrotaline-induced pulmonary vascular lesions,[90] and the inhibition of EGF receptor activity has similar effects.[91] Induction of TN-C transcription by endothelial, vascular smooth muscle, and fibroblast cells is regulated by the activation of extracellular signal-regulated protein kinase (ERK) 1/2 and mitogen-activated protein kinases (MAPK), as well as the binding of the paired-related homeobox gene transcription factor, Prx1. Of note, radiolabeled anti-TN-C antibodies are able to induce regression of human gliomas expressing high levels of stromal TN-C.[92,93] Whether similar treatments can be devised to modulate TN-C and its downstream effectors in patients with PAH awaits further investigation.

In Situ Thrombosis

Microvascular thrombosis is a frequent pathologic finding in many forms of PAH, occurring in the absence of evidence for a remote (embolic) source of clot.[94-97] Thrombosis may occur due to an imbalance of procoagulant and anticoagulant forces. The endothelial lining of vessels is normally an antithrombotic surface. In addition to a deficiency in antithrombotic activities already mentioned (e.g., decreased production of prostacyclin), the activation of procoagulant activity by endothelial cells is evident by abnormal von Willebrand factor activity, elevated plasma fibrinopeptide-A, and an increase in the half-life of fibrinogen[98,99] and plasminogen activator inhibitor type-1.[100] Decreased endothelial fibrinolytic activity is also seen in most patients with IPAH. Alterations in shear stress associated with elevated pressure or flow is one mechanism thought to activate these changes in the endothelium.

In addition to being influenced by endothelial cell activity, platelets themselves promote microvascular thrombus formation and likely influence endothelial and other vascular derangements in PAH by releasing vasoactive and mitogenic factors. Increased platelet activation in patients with PAH is indicated by elevated urinary levels of thromboxane metabolites.[33] Activated platelets also release vasoconstrictors such as serotonin, as well as growth factors that might promote cell proliferation and remodeling within the vessel walls (e.g., platelet-derived growth factor, transforming growth factor-β [TGF-β], and vascular endothelial growth factor [VEGF]).

Control of Cell Growth and Death: Bone Morphogenetic Protein Receptor II and Vascular Growth Factors

Germline mutations in the gene encoding the receptor BMP-RII have been identified in up to 60 percent of patients with familial PAH and in some patients with IPAH.[101-105] Mutations in this gene have been identified also in patients with PAH associated with anorexigens,[106] congenital heart disease,[107] and in a patient with pulmonary veno-occlusive disease.[108] The BMPs are members of the TGF-β superfamily of molecules, involved in diverse cell growth and differentiation processes in multiple systems. Mutations in another member of the TGFβ family, activin receptor-like kinase-1 (ALK-1), have been identified as conferring susceptibility of patients with hereditary hemorrhagic telangiectasia to developing PAH.[109,110] Upon engaging ligands, cell surface BMP receptors (type I and type II) normally form dimers, which then initiate activation of a series of intracellular mediators (Smads) and the translocation of a Smad complex to the cell nucleus.

Here the Smad complex binds deoxyribonucleic acid (DNA) sequences to regulate the transcription of target genes. The result can be activation of some genes and inhibition of others, and varies according to the BMP pathway and tissue involved. BMP signaling is essential to normal vascular development; animals lacking elements of the pathway die during early embryogenesis. In addition, BMP signaling functions in the maintenance of the normal adult pulmonary vasculature, likely by regulating the growth and apoptosis of both endothelial and smooth muscle cells. Loss of such regulation gives rise to pulmonary hypertension.[111]

Within the lung, BMPR-II is expressed primarily by the endothelium and, to a lesser extent, by smooth muscle cells. Expression is reduced in patients with various causes of PAH, most markedly so in those harboring mutations of the *BMP-RII* gene (FIGURE 3-7).[112] BMP function is also altered in PAH. Exposure of pulmonary artery smooth muscle cells isolated from normal lungs to varying BMPs results in inhibition of DNA synthesis and cell proliferation[113] as well as the induction of apoptosis.[114] These inhibitory effects, however, are suppressed in cells isolated from patients with PAH, despite the expression of BMP receptors by these cells. This altered response to BMP signaling appears to be relatively specific to smooth cells from smaller pulmonary vessels (approximately 1 to 2 mm, a location most often displaying proliferative, occlusive vascular pathology in IPAH). Whereas the proliferation of smooth muscle cells isolated from larger proximal vessels was inhibited normally, cells from distal, smaller pulmonary vessels failed to be suppressed by BMP signaling.[115]

BMP function may be inhibited by multiple mechanisms. Multiple mutations in *BMP-RII* have been identified that predict several mechanisms for impaired gene function, including premature truncation of the protein, incorrect protein trafficking, and perturbed ligand binding. Common to all of these mutants is ligand-independent activation of p38[MAPK] *in vitro*, potentially giving rise to enhanced proliferation signals.[5,116] Interference with BMP signaling can also occur in the absence of mutations known to promote the development of pulmonary hypertension. In patients with PAH of multiple types and without mutations of either *BMP-RII* or *ALK1*, Du and others have shown abnormally elevated expression of angiopoietin 1 and its ligand TIE2, molecules known to normally promote the maturation and stabilization of the developing vasculature. Elevations in these molecules correlated with the severity of PAH. A mechanistic link between elevations in angiopoietin and altered

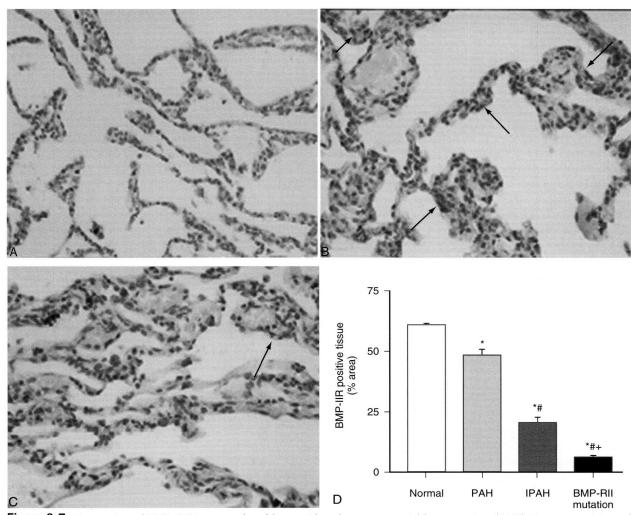

Figure 3-7. Expression of BMP-RII in normal and lung with pulmonary arterial hypertension (PAH). Immunostaining of lung tissue demonstrating the expression BMP-RII *(rust color)* in a control subject (**A**). Reduced expression is seen in the lung of patient with congenital heart disease–associated PAH (**B**) and markedly reduced in a patient with PAH and a mutation in the *BMP-RII* gene (**C**). The graph shows a semi-quantitative assessment of *BMP-RII* expression in normal lungs and those from patients with PAH associated with *BMP-RII* mutations, idiopathic (IPAH) and other forms of PAH. The reduction in staining in the tissue carrying *BMP-RII* was not due to a reduction in the number of endothelial cells, because no difference was seen upon staining with an endothelial cell marker (CD31, not shown). *P < .05 compared with control; #P < .05 compared with PAH; +P < .05 compared with IPAH. (Adapted with permission from Atkinson C, Stewart S, Upton PD, et al: Primary pulmonary hypertension is associated with reduced pulmonary vascular expression of type II bone morphogenetic protein receptor. *Circulation* 105[14]:1672-1678, 2002.) (See Color Plate 9).

BMP signaling was supported by the ability of angiopoietin to inhibit endothelial cell expression of a BMP receptor (BMP-R1A) required for normal BMP-RII signaling. A near absence of BMP-R1A expression was found in the lungs of these patients.[117] The mechanism by which angiopoietin becomes elevated in patients is not clear, and other experiments have shown a dramatic protective role of angiopoietin overexpression in an animal model of PAH induced by monocrotaline.[118]

Whether such discrepancies represent important differences between assessing human tissues as compared with an animal model is not yet clear.[119] Alternatively, the development of PAH likely requires multiple "hits"—including injury to the vascular endothelium and uncontrolled proliferation of smooth muscle cells.[1] Loss of BMP-RII function might not only allow for increased smooth muscle cell proliferation coupled with a loss of apoptosis, but might also affect endothelial cells by promoting their death via pro-apoptotic signaling.[1] In certain contexts, angiopoietin might serve to protect endothelial cells harmed by any of a number of injurious agents. In others, however, it may promote the development of PAH by altering BMP signaling as described above, or alternatively by increasing the production of serotonin (5-HT).[120]

VEGF is essential for normal vascular development, emphasized by the unique finding of embryonic lethality in animals lacking even a single *VEGF* allele.[121,122] VEGF is an endothelial cell mitogen that promotes vasculogenesis and angiogenesis in the developing embryo and at sites of injury or neoplasia in adults. The expression of VEGF and its receptor tyrosine kinase receptors are increased in the pulmonary vasculature of patients with PAH, particularly within plexiform lesions[9,123] in which its pro-angiogenic properties have been hypothesized to mediate disordered endothelial cell proliferation.[124] Increased VEGF expression in PAH, however, may also be a protective response to chronic hypoxia.[125] Blockade of VEGF receptor 2 in animals exposed to chronic hypoxia causes pulmonary endothelial cell death, occlusion of vessels by proliferating endothelial cells thought to be resistant to apoptosis, and severe pulmonary hypertension.[126] In another model, cell-based delivery of VEGF to the pulmonary vasculature protects animals from monocrotaline-induced PH.[127]

Several additional mechanisms by which the vascular endothelium might be damaged or proliferation induced in PAH have been proposed. Many of these same triggers might incite other dysfunctional endothelial responses (e.g., coagulation, vasoconstriction), lead to the exposure of subendothelial matrix, or alter the responses of other cells such as smooth muscle cells and platelets to promote further pathologic changes.[7] For example, inflammatory immune cytokine levels are elevated in patients with PAH,[128,129] and inflammatory infiltrates are seen in plexiform lesions.[130] Chemokine-dependent mechanisms lead to inflammatory cell recruitment in PAH.[129]

Cross-talk

The interaction of the multiple possible factors that contribute to PAH makes it difficult to determine primary from secondary events. It is unlikely that a single, common abnormality will be identified in all forms of PAH, or indeed even in all cases of a single form of the disease. An initiating trigger ("insult") might occur in a predisposed individual, setting off multiple abnormalities acting either simultaneously or sequentially that perpetuate the development of pulmonary hypertension.[1] Such predisposition might involve genetic abnormalities or another exposure (e.g., chronic hypoxia, infection, or toxin exposure). Unraveling these multiple and intersecting pathways has led to multiple forms of therapy and suggests additional pharmacologic interventions. Given that many of the simultaneously active paths that contribute to disease development and progression intersect or result in similar downstream events, it is perhaps not surprising that no single therapeutic approach is effective in all patients, and indeed none is as yet curative. Ultimately, like disease initiation and progression, cure will probably require a "multiple hit" approach.

References

1. Yuan JX, Rubin LJ: Pathogenesis of pulmonary arterial hypertension: The need for multiple hits. *Circulation* 111:534-538, 2005.
2. Newman JH, Fanburg BL, Archer SL, et al: Pulmonary arterial hypertension: Future directions: Report of a National Heart, Lung and Blood Institute/Office of Rare Diseases workshop. *Circulation* 109:2947-2952, 2004.
3. Archer S, Rich S: Primary pulmonary hypertension: A vascular biology and translational research "work in progress." *Circulation* 102:2781-2791, 2000.
4. Farber HW, Loscalzo J: Pulmonary arterial hypertension. *N Engl J Med* 351:1655-1665, 2004.
5. Humbert M, Morrell NW, Archer SL, et al: Cellular and molecular pathobiology of pulmonary arterial hypertension. *J Am Coll Cardiol* 43(12 Suppl S):13S-24S, 2004.
6. Mandegar M, Fung YC, Huang W, et al: Cellular and molecular mechanisms of pulmonary vascular remodeling: Role in the development of pulmonary hypertension. *Microvasc Res* 68:75-103, 2004.
7. Budhiraja R, Tuder RM, Hassoun PM: Endothelial dysfunction in pulmonary hypertension. *Circulation* 109:159-165, 2004.
8. Ghamra ZW, Dweik RA: Primary pulmonary hypertension: An overview of epidemiology and pathogenesis. *Cleve Clin J Med* 70(Suppl 1):S2-8, 2003.
9. Cool CD, Stewart JS, Werahera P, et al: Three-dimensional reconstruction of pulmonary arteries in plexiform pulmonary hypertension using cell-specific markers. Evidence for a dynamic and heterogeneous process of pulmonary endothelial cell growth. *Am J Pathol* 155:411-419, 1999.

10. Lee SD, Shroyer KR, Markham NE, et al: Monoclonal endothelial cell proliferation is present in primary but not secondary pulmonary hypertension. *J Clin Invest* 101:927-934, 1998.

11. Steudel W, Ichinose F, Huang PL, et al: Pulmonary vasoconstriction and hypertension in mice with targeted disruption of the endothelial nitric oxide synthase *(NOS3)* gene. *Circ Res* 81:34-41, 1997.

12. Ozaki M, Kawashima S, Yamashita T, et al: Reduced hypoxic pulmonary vascular remodeling by nitric oxide from the endothelium. *Hypertension* 37:322-327, 2001.

13. Fagan KA, Fouty BW, Tyler RC, et al: The pulmonary circulation of homozygous or heterozygous *eNOS*-null mice is hyperresponsive to mild hypoxia. *J Clin Invest* 103:291-299, 1999.

14. Zhao YD, Courtman DW, Deng Y, et al: Rescue of monocrotaline-induced pulmonary arterial hypertension using bone marrow-derived endothelial-like progenitor cells: Efficacy of combined cell and eNOS gene therapy in established disease. *Circ Res* 96:442-450, 2005.

15. Walford G, Loscalzo J: Nitric oxide in vascular biology. *J Thromb Haemost* 1:2112-2118, 2003.

16. Giaid A, Saleh D: Reduced expression of endothelial nitric oxide synthase in the lungs of patients with pulmonary hypertension. *N Engl J Med* 333:214-221, 1995.

17. Mason NA, Springall DR, Burke M, et al: High expression of endothelial nitric oxide synthase in plexiform lesions of pulmonary hypertension. *J Pathol* 185:313-318, 1998.

18. Sitbon O, Humbert M, Jagot JL, et al: Inhaled nitric oxide as a screening agent for safely identifying responders to oral calcium-channel blockers in primary pulmonary hypertension. *Eur Respir J* 12:265-270, 1998.

19. Ivy DD, Griebel JL, Kinsella JP, et al: Acute hemodynamic effects of pulsed delivery of low flow nasal nitric oxide in children with pulmonary hypertension. *J Pediatr* 133:453-456, 1998.

20. Channick RN, Newhart JW, Johnson FW, et al: Pulsed delivery of inhaled nitric oxide to patients with primary pulmonary hypertension: An ambulatory delivery system and initial clinical tests. *Chest* 109:1545-1549, 1996.

21. Mehta S, Stewart DJ, Langleben D, et al: Short-term pulmonary vasodilation with L-arginine in pulmonary hypertension. *Circulation* 92:1539-1545, 1995.

22. Baudouin SV, Bath P, Martin JF, et al: L-arginine infusion has no effect on systemic haemodynamics in normal volunteers, or systemic and pulmonary haemodynamics in patients with elevated pulmonary vascular resistance. *Br J Clin Pharmacol* 36:45-49, 1993.

23. Nagaya N, Uematsu M, Oya H, et al: Short-term oral administration of L-arginine improves hemodynamics and exercise capacity in patients with precapillary pulmonary hypertension. *Am J Respir Crit Care Med* 163:887-891, 2001.

24. Michelakis E, Tymchak W, Lien D, et al: Oral sildenafil is an effective and specific pulmonary vasodilator in patients with pulmonary arterial hypertension: Comparison with inhaled nitric oxide. *Circulation* 105:2398-2403, 2002.

25. Lepore JJ, Maroo A, Pereira NL, et al: Effect of sildenafil on the acute pulmonary vasodilator response to inhaled nitric oxide in adults with primary pulmonary hypertension. *Am J Cardiol* 90:677-680, 2002.

25b. Galie N, Ghofran, HA, Torbicki A, et al: Sildenafil citrate therapy for pulmonary arterial hypertension. *N Engl, J Med* 353:2148-2157, 2005.

26. Barst RJ, Rubin LJ, Long WA, et al: A comparison of continuous intravenous epoprostenol (prostacyclin) with conventional therapy for primary pulmonary hypertension. The Primary Pulmonary Hypertension Study Group. *N Engl J Med* 334:296-302, 1996.

27. McLaughlin VV, Genthner DE, Panella MM, et al: Reduction in pulmonary vascular resistance with long-term epoprostenol (prostacyclin) therapy in primary pulmonary hypertension. *N Engl J Med* 338:273-277, 1998.

28. McLaughlin VV, Shillington A, Rich S: Survival in primary pulmonary hypertension: The impact of epoprostenol therapy. *Circulation* 106:1477-1482, 2002.

29. Sitbon O, Humbert M, Nunes H, et al: Long-term intravenous epoprostenol infusion in primary pulmonary hypertension: Prognostic factors and survival. *J Am Coll Cardiol* 40:780-788, 2002.

30. Geraci MW, Gao B, Shepherd DC, et al: Pulmonary prostacyclin synthase overexpression in transgenic mice protects against development of hypoxic pulmonary hypertension. *J Clin Invest* 103:1509-1515, 1999.

31. Hoshikawa Y, Voelkel NF, Gesell TL, et al: Prostacyclin receptor-dependent modulation of pulmonary vascular remodeling. *Am J Respir Crit Care Med* 164:314-318, 2001.

32. Tuder RM, Cool CD, Geraci MW, et al: Prostacyclin synthase expression is decreased in lungs from patients with severe pulmonary hypertension. *Am J Respir Crit Care Med* 159:1925-1932, 1999.

33. Christman BW, McPherson CD, Newman JH, et al: An imbalance between the excretion of thromboxane and prostacyclin metabolites in pulmonary hypertension. *N Engl J Med* 327:70-75, 1992.

34. Gunaydin S, Imai Y, Takanashi Y, et al: The effects of vasoactive intestinal peptide on monocrotaline induced pulmonary hypertensive rabbits following

cardiopulmonary bypass: A comparative study with isoproterenol and nitroglycerine. *Cardiovasc Surg* 10:138-145, 2002.

35. Greenberg B, Rhoden K, Barnes PJ: Relaxant effects of vasoactive intestinal peptide and peptide histidine isoleucine in human and bovine pulmonary arteries. *Blood Vessels* 24:45-50, 1987.

36. Iwabuchi S, Ono S, Tanita T, et al: Vasoactive intestinal peptide causes nitric oxide-dependent pulmonary vasodilation in isolated rat lung. *Respiration* 64:54-58, 1997.

37. Soderman C, Eriksson LS, Juhlin-Dannfelt A, et al: Effect of vasoactive intestinal polypeptide (VIP) on pulmonary ventilation-perfusion relationships and central haemodynamics in healthy subjects. *Clin Physiol* 13:677-685, 1993.

38. Cox CP, Linden J, Said SI: VIP elevates platelet cyclic AMP (cAMP) levels and inhibits in vitro platelet activation induced by platelet-activating factor (PAF). *Peptides* 5:325-328, 1984.

39. Maruno K, Absood A, Said SI: VIP inhibits basal and histamine-stimulated proliferation of human airway smooth muscle cells. *Am J Physiol* 268:L1047-1051, 1995.

40. Petkov V, Mosgoeller W, Ziesche R, et al: Vasoactive intestinal peptide as a new drug for treatment of primary pulmonary hypertension. *J Clin Invest* 111:1339-1346, 2003.

41. Langleben D, Christman BW, Barst RJ, et al: Effects of the thromboxane synthetase inhibitor and receptor antagonist terbogrel in patients with primary pulmonary hypertension. *Am Heart J* 143:E4, 2002.

42. Fagan KA, McMurtry IF, Rodman DM: Role of endothelin-1 in lung disease. *Respir Res* 2:90-101, 2001.

43. Davie N, Haleen SJ, Upton PD, et al: ET(A) and ET(B) receptors modulate the proliferation of human pulmonary artery smooth muscle cells. *Am J Respir Crit Care Med* 165:398-405, 2002.

44. Kuc RE, Davenport AP: Endothelin-A receptors in human aorta and pulmonary arteries are downregulated in patients with cardiovascular disease: An adaptive response to increased levels of endothelin-1? *J Cardiovasc Pharmacol* 36(5 Suppl 1):S377-379, 2000.

45. Cambrey AD, Harrison NK, Dawes KE, et al: Increased levels of endothelin-1 in bronchoalveolar lavage fluid from patients with systemic sclerosis contribute to fibroblast mitogenic activity in vitro. *Am J Respir Cell Mol Biol* 11:439-445, 1994.

46. Yang Z, Krasnici N, Luscher TF: Endothelin-1 potentiates human smooth muscle cell growth to PDGF: Effects of ETA and ETB receptor blockade. *Circulation* 100:5-8, 1999.

47. Hocher B, Schwarz A, Fagan KA, et al: Pulmonary fibrosis and chronic lung inflammation in ET-1 transgenic mice. *Am J Respir Cell Mol Biol* 23:19-26, 2000.

48. Helset E, Lindal S, Olsen R, et al: Endothelin-1 causes sequential trapping of platelets and neutrophils in pulmonary microcirculation in rats. *Am J Physiol* 271:L538-546, 1996.

49. Rubens C, Ewert R, Halank M, et al: Big endothelin-1 and endothelin-1 plasma levels are correlated with the severity of primary pulmonary hypertension. *Chest* 120:1562-1569, 2001.

50. Yamakami T, Taguchi O, Gabazza EC, et al: Arterial endothelin-1 level in pulmonary emphysema and interstitial lung disease. Relation with pulmonary hypertension during exercise. *Eur Respir J* 10:2055-2060, 1997.

51. Giaid A, Yanagisawa M, Langleben D, et al: Expression of endothelin-1 in the lungs of patients with pulmonary hypertension. *N Engl J Med* 328:1732-1739, 1993.

52. Chen SJ, Chen YF, Meng QC, et al: Endothelin-receptor antagonist bosentan prevents and reverses hypoxic pulmonary hypertension in rats. *J Appl Physiol* 79:2122-2131, 1995.

53. Park SH, Saleh D, Giaid A, et al: Increased endothelin-1 in bleomycin-induced pulmonary fibrosis and the effect of an endothelin receptor antagonist. *Am J Respir Crit Care Med* 156:600-608, 1997.

54. Rubin LJ, Badesch DB, Barst RJ, et al: Bosentan therapy for pulmonary arterial hypertension. *N Engl J Med* 346:896-903, 2002.

55. Barst RJ, Rich S, Widlitz A, et al: Clinical efficacy of sitaxsentan, an endothelin-A receptor antagonist, in patients with pulmonary arterial hypertension: Open-label pilot study. *Chest* 121:1860-1868, 2002.

56. McLaughlin V, Sitbon O, Rubin LJ, et al: The effect of first-line Bosentan on survival of patients with primary pulmonary hypertension. *Am J Resp Crit Care Med* 167:A442, 2003.

57. Herve P, Launay JM, Scrobohaci ML, et al: Increased plasma serotonin in primary pulmonary hypertension. *Am J Med* 99:249-254, 1995.

58. Abenhaim L, Moride Y, Brenot F, et al: Appetite-suppressant drugs and the risk of primary pulmonary hypertension. International Primary Pulmonary Hypertension Study Group. *N Engl J Med* 335:609-616, 1996.

59. Rich S, Rubin L, Walker AM, et al: Anorexigens and pulmonary hypertension in the United States: Results from the surveillance of North American pulmonary hypertension. *Chest* 117:870-874, 2000.

60. Rothman RB, Ayestas MA, Dersch CM, et al: Aminorex, fenfluramine, and chlorphentermine are serotonin transporter substrates. Implications

for primary pulmonary hypertension. *Circulation* 100:869-875, 1999.

61. Eddahibi S, Adnot S, Frisdal E, et al: Dexfenfluramine-associated changes in 5-hydroxytryptamine transporter expression and development of hypoxic pulmonary hypertension in rats. *J Pharmacol Exp Ther* 297:148-154, 2001.

62. Launay JM, Herve P, Peoc'h K, et al: Function of the serotonin 5-hydroxytryptamine 2B receptor in pulmonary hypertension. *Nat Med* 8:1129-1135, 2002.

63. Eddahibi S, Humbert M, Fadel E, et al: Serotonin transporter overexpression is responsible for pulmonary artery smooth muscle hyperplasia in primary pulmonary hypertension. *J Clin Invest* 108:1141-1450, 2001.

63b. Machado RD, Koehler R, Glissmeyer E, et al: Genetic association of the serotonin transporter in pulmonary arterial hypertension. *Am J Resp Crit Care Med*, in press.

64. MacLean MR, Deuchar GA, Hicks MN, et al: Overexpression of the 5-hydroxytryptamine transporter gene: Effect on pulmonary hemodynamics and hypoxia-induced pulmonary hypertension. *Circulation* 109:2150-2155, 2004.

65. Eddahibi S, Hanoun N, Lanfumey L, et al: Attenuated hypoxic pulmonary hypertension in mice lacking the 5-hydroxytryptamine transporter gene. *J Clin Invest* 105:1555-1562, 2000.

66. Guignabert C, Raffestin B, Benferhat R, et al: Serotonin transporter inhibition prevents and reverses monocrotaline-induced pulmonary hypertension in rats. *Circulation* 111:2812-2819, 2005.

67. Marcos E, Fadel E, Sanchez O, et al: Serotonin-induced smooth muscle hyperplasia in various forms of human pulmonary hypertension. *Circ Res* 94:1263-1270, 2004.

68. Eddahibi S, Chaouat A, Morrell N, et al: Polymorphism of the serotonin transporter gene and pulmonary hypertension in chronic obstructive pulmonary disease. *Circulation* 108:1839-1844, 2003.

69. Lawrie A, Spiekerkoetter E, Martinez EC, et al: Interdependent serotonin transporter and receptor pathways regulate *S100A4/Mts1,* a gene associated with pulmonary vascular disease. *Circ Res* 97:227-235, 2005.

70. Greenway S, van Suylen RJ, Du Marchie Sarvaas G, et al: *S100A4/Mts1* produces murine pulmonary artery changes resembling plexogenic arteriopathy and is increased in human plexogenic arteriopathy. *Am J Pathol* 164:253-262, 2004.

71. Weir EK, Reeve HL, Johnson G, et al: A role for potassium channels in smooth muscle cells and platelets in the etiology of primary pulmonary hypertension. *Chest* 114(3 Suppl):200S-204S, 1998.

72. Post JM, Hume JR, Archer SL, et al: Direct role for potassium channel inhibition in hypoxic pulmonary vasoconstriction. *Am J Physiol* 262:C882-890, 1992.

73. Geraci MW, Moore M, Gesell T, et al: Gene expression patterns in the lungs of patients with primary pulmonary hypertension: A gene microarray analysis. *Circ Res* 88:555-562, 2001.

74. Yuan JX, Aldinger AM, Juhaszova M, et al: Dysfunctional voltage-gated K^+ channels in pulmonary artery smooth muscle cells of patients with primary pulmonary hypertension. *Circulation* 98:1400-1406, 1998.

75. Yuan XJ, Wang J, Juhaszova M, et al: Attenuated K^+ channel gene transcription in primary pulmonary hypertension. *Lancet* 351:726-727, 1998.

76. Michelakis ED, McMurtry MS, Wu XC, et al: Dichloroacetate, a metabolic modulator, prevents and reverses chronic hypoxic pulmonary hypertension in rats: Role of increased expression and activity of voltage-gated potassium channels. *Circulation* 105:244-250, 2002.

77. Platoshyn O, Yu Y, Golovina VA, et al: Chronic hypoxia decreases K(v) channel expression and function in pulmonary artery myocytes. *Am J Physiol Lung Cell Mol Physiol* 280:L801-812, 2001.

78. Pozeg ZI, Michelakis ED, McMurtry MS, et al: In vivo gene transfer of the O_2-sensitive potassium channel Kv1.5 reduces pulmonary hypertension and restores hypoxic pulmonary vasoconstriction in chronically hypoxic rats. *Circulation* 107:2037-2044, 2003.

79. Archer SL, Wu XC, Thebaud B, et al: Preferential expression and function of voltage-gated, O_2-sensitive K^+ channels in resistance pulmonary arteries explains regional heterogeneity in hypoxic pulmonary vasoconstriction: Ionic diversity in smooth muscle cells. *Circ Res* 95:308-318, 2004.

80. Weir EK, Reeve HL, Huang JM, et al: Anorexic agents aminorex, fenfluramine, and dexfenfluramine inhibit potassium current in rat pulmonary vascular smooth muscle and cause pulmonary vasoconstriction. *Circulation* 94:2216-2220, 1996.

81. Remillard CV, Yuan JX: Activation of K^+ channels: An essential pathway in programmed cell death. *Am J Physiol Lung Cell Mol Physiol* 286:L49-67, 2004.

82. Krick S, Platoshyn O, Sweeney M, et al: Activation of K^+ channels induces apoptosis in vascular smooth muscle cells. *Am J Physiol Cell Physiol* 280:C970-979, 2001.

83. Jeffery TK, Morrell NW: Molecular and cellular basis of pulmonary vascular remodeling in pulmonary hypertension. *Prog Cardiovasc Dis* 45:173-202, 2002.

84. Jones PL, Rabinovitch M: Tenascin-C is induced with progressive pulmonary vascular disease in rats and is functionally related to increased smooth

muscle cell proliferation. *Circ Res* 79:1131-1142, 1996.

85. Ivy DD, McMurtry IF, Colvin K, et al: Development of occlusive neointimal lesions in distal pulmonary arteries of endothelin B receptor-deficient rats: A new model of severe pulmonary arterial hypertension. *Circulation* 111:2988-2996, 2005.

86. Jones PL, Chapados R, Baldwin HS, et al: Altered hemodynamics controls matrix metalloproteinase activity and tenascin-C expression in neonatal pig lung. *Am J Physiol Lung Cell Mol Physiol* 282:L26-35, 2002.

87. Jones PL, Cowan KN, Rabinovitch M: Tenascin-C, proliferation and subendothelial fibronectin in progressive pulmonary vascular disease. *Am J Pathol* 150:1349-1360, 1997.

88. Ihida-Stansbury K, McKean DM, Gebb SA, et al: Paired-related homeobox gene *Prx1* is required for pulmonary vascular development. *Circ Res* 94:1507-1514, 2004.

89. Jones PL, Crack J, Rabinovitch M: Regulation of tenascin-C, a vascular smooth muscle cell survival factor that interacts with the alpha v beta 3 integrin to promote epidermal growth factor receptor phosphorylation and growth. *J Cell Biol* 139:279-293, 1997.

90. Cowan KN, Jones PL, Rabinovitch M: Elastase and matrix metalloproteinase inhibitors induce regression, and tenascin-C antisense prevents progression, of vascular disease. *J Clin Invest* 105:21-34, 2000.

91. Merklinger SL, Jones PL, Martinez EC, et al: Epidermal growth factor receptor blockade mediates smooth muscle cell apoptosis and improves survival in rats with pulmonary hypertension. *Circulation* 112:423-431, 2005.

92. Paganelli G, Grana C, Chinol M, et al: Antibody-guided three-step therapy for high grade glioma with yttrium-90 biotin. *Eur J Nucl Med* 26:348-357, 1999.

93. Riva P, Franceschi G, Frattarelli M, et al: [131]I radioconjugated antibodies for the locoregional radioimmunotherapy of high-grade malignant glioma—phase I and II study. *Acta Oncol* 38:351-359, 1999.

94. Bjornsson J, Edwards WD: Primary pulmonary hypertension: A histopathologic study of 80 cases. *Mayo Clin Proc* 60:16-25, 1985.

95. Cohen M, Fuster V, Edwards WD: Anticoagulation in the treatment of pulmonary hypertension. In: Fishman AP, editor: *The pulmonary circulation: Normal and abnormal. mechanisms, management, and the National Registry*, Philadelphia, 1990, University of Pennsylvania Press, pp 501-510.

96. Fuster V, Steele PM, Edwards WD, et al: Primary pulmonary hypertension: Natural history and the importance of thrombosis. *Circulation* 70:580-587, 1984.

97. Herve P, Humbert M, Sitbon O, et al: Pathobiology of pulmonary hypertension. The role of platelets and thrombosis. *Clin Chest Med* 22:451-458, 2001.

98. Geggel RL, Carvalho AC, Hoyer LW, et al: von Willebrand factor abnormalities in primary pulmonary hypertension. *Am Rev Respir Dis* 135:294-299, 1987.

99. Eisenberg PR, Lucore C, Kaufman L, et al: Fibrinopeptide A levels indicative of pulmonary vascular thrombosis in patients with primary pulmonary hypertension. *Circulation* 82:841-847, 1990.

100. Welsh CH, Hassell KL, Badesch DB, et al: Coagulation and fibrinolytic profiles in patients with severe pulmonary hypertension. *Chest* 110:710-717, 1996.

101. Deng Z, Morse JH, Slager SL, et al: Familial primary pulmonary hypertension (gene *PPH1*) is caused by mutations in the bone morphogenetic protein receptor-II gene. *Am J Hum Genet* 67:737-744, 2000.

102. Lane KB, Machado RD, Pauciulo MW, et al: Heterozygous germline mutations in *BMPR2*, encoding a TGF-β receptor, cause familial primary pulmonary hypertension. The International PPH Consortium. *Nat Genet* 26:81-84, 2000.

103. Thomson JR, Machado RD, Pauciulo MW, et al: Sporadic primary pulmonary hypertension is associated with germline mutations of the gene encoding BMPR-II, a receptor member of the TGF-β family. *J Med Genet* 37:741-745, 2000.

104. Newman JH, Wheeler L, Lane KB, et al: Mutation in the gene for bone morphogenetic protein receptor II as a cause of primary pulmonary hypertension in a large kindred. *N Engl J Med* 345:319-324, 2001.

105. Newman JH, Trembath RC, Morse JA, et al: Genetic basis of pulmonary arterial hypertension: Current understanding and future directions. *J Am Coll Cardiol* 43(12 Suppl S):33S-39S, 2004.

106. Humbert M, Deng Z, Simonneau G, et al: *BMPR2* germline mutations in pulmonary hypertension associated with fenfluramine derivatives. *Eur Respir J* 20:518-523, 2002.

107. Roberts KE, McElroy JJ, Wong WP, et al: *BMPR2* mutations in pulmonary arterial hypertension with congenital heart disease. *Eur Respir J* 24:371-374, 2004.

108. Runo JR, Vnencak-Jones CL, Prince M, et al: Pulmonary veno-occlusive disease caused by an inherited mutation in bone morphogenetic protein receptor II. *Am J Respir Crit Care Med* 167:889-894, 2003.

109. Trembath RC, Thomson JR, Machado RD, et al: Clinical and molecular genetic features of pulmonary hypertension in patients with hereditary

hemorrhagic telangiectasia. *N Engl J Med* 345:325-334, 2001.

110. Chaouat A, Coulet F, Favre C, et al: Endoglin germline mutation in a patient with hereditary haemorrhagic telangiectasia and dexfenfluramine associated pulmonary arterial hypertension. *Thorax* 59:446-448, 2004.

111. Stewart DJ: Bone morphogenetic protein receptor-2 and pulmonary arterial hypertension: Unraveling a riddle inside an enigma? *Circ Res* 96:1033-1035, 2005.

112. Atkinson C, Stewart S, Upton PD, et al: Primary pulmonary hypertension is associated with reduced pulmonary vascular expression of type II bone morphogenetic protein receptor. *Circulation* 105:1672-1678, 2002.

113. Morrell NW, Yang X, Upton PD, et al: Altered growth responses of pulmonary artery smooth muscle cells from patients with primary pulmonary hypertension to transforming growth factor-β(1) and bone morphogenetic proteins. *Circulation* 104: 790-795, 2001.

114. Zhang S, Fantozzi I, Tigno DD, et al: Bone morphogenetic proteins induce apoptosis in human pulmonary vascular smooth muscle cells. *Am J Physiol Lung Cell Mol Physiol* 285:L740-754, 2003.

115. Yang X, Long L, Southwood M, et al: Dysfunctional Smad signaling contributes to abnormal smooth muscle cell proliferation in familial pulmonary arterial hypertension. *Circ Res* 96:1053-1063, 2005.

116. Rudarakanchana N, Flanagan JA, Chen H, et al: Functional analysis of bone morphogenetic protein type II receptor mutations underlying primary pulmonary hypertension. *Hum Mol Genet* 11:1517-1525, 2002.

117. Du L, Sullivan CC, Chu D, et al: Signaling molecules in nonfamilial pulmonary hypertension. *N Engl J Med* 348:500-509, 2003.

118. Zhao YD, Campbell AI, Robb M, et al: Protective role of angiopoietin-1 in experimental pulmonary hypertension. *Circ Res* 92:984-991, 2003.

119. Rudge JS, Thurston G, Yancopoulos GD: Angiopoietin-1 and pulmonary hypertension: Cause or cure? *Circ Res* 92:947-949, 2003.

120. Sullivan CC, Du L, Chu D, et al: Induction of pulmonary hypertension by an angiopoietin 1/TIE2/serotonin pathway. *Proc Natl Acad Sci USA* 100:12331-12336, 2003.

121. Ferrara N, Carver-Moore K, Chen H, et al: Heterozygous embryonic lethality induced by targeted inactivation of the *VEGF* gene. *Nature* 380:439-442, 1996.

122. Carmeliet P, Ferreira V, Breier G, et al: Abnormal blood vessel development and lethality in embryos lacking a single *VEGF* allele. *Nature* 380:435-439, 1996.

123. Hirose S, Hosoda Y, Furuya S, et al: Expression of vascular endothelial growth factor and its receptors correlates closely with formation of the plexiform lesion in human pulmonary hypertension. *Pathol Int* 50:472-479, 2000.

124. Tuder RM, Chacon M, Alger L, et al: Expression of angiogenesis-related molecules in plexiform lesions in severe pulmonary hypertension: Evidence for a process of disordered angiogenesis. *J Pathol* 195:367-374, 2001.

125. Christou H, Yoshida A, Arthur V, et al: Increased vascular endothelial growth factor production in the lungs of rats with hypoxia-induced pulmonary hypertension. *Am J Respir Cell Mol Biol* 18:768-776, 1998.

126. Taraseviciene-Stewart L, Kasahara Y, Alger L, et al: Inhibition of the VEGF receptor 2 combined with chronic hypoxia causes cell death-dependent pulmonary endothelial cell proliferation and severe pulmonary hypertension. *FASEB J* 15:427-438, 2001.

127. Campbell AI, Zhao Y, Sandhu R, et al: Cell-based gene transfer of vascular endothelial growth factor attenuates monocrotaline-induced pulmonary hypertension. *Circulation* 104:2242-2248, 2001.

128. Humbert M, Monti G, Brenot F, et al: Increased interleukin-1 and interleukin-6 serum concentrations in severe primary pulmonary hypertension. *Am J Respir Crit Care Med* 151:1628-1631, 1995.

129. Dorfmuller P, Perros F, Balabanian K, et al: Inflammation in pulmonary arterial hypertension. *Eur Respir J* 22:358-363, 2003.

130. Tuder RM, Groves B, Badesch DB, et al: Exuberant endothelial cell growth and elements of inflammation are present in plexiform lesions of pulmonary hypertension. *Am J Pathol* 144:275-285, 1994.

4 Chapter

Genetics of Pulmonary Arterial Hypertension

C. Gregory Elliott, MD

Introduction

Recognition and understanding of the genetic basis of pulmonary arterial hypertension have evolved for more than 100 years.[1,2] The expansion of diagnostic techniques and clinical expertise has fueled this evolution. Early investigators had only the tools of clinical and pathologic examinations to study pulmonary hypertension.[1,3,4] In the modern era, these techniques are neither specific nor sufficient.[1,5] The introduction of right heart catheterization allowed direct measurement of pulmonary artery pressure and definition of "primary pulmonary hypertension," distinguished from secondary pulmonary hypertension by the absence of intrinsic heart or lung disease and the absence of mechanical obstruction in the pulmonary arteries (e.g., thromboemboli).[6,7] More recently, participants in major conferences have examined the definition and classification of pulmonary hypertension,[2,5,8] and the refined and improved definitions that have emerged have aided genetic investigations.

Historical Overview

Romberg first described pathologic changes characteristic of idiopathic pulmonary arterial hypertension in 1891.[1] Thirty-six years later Clarke described two sisters with right heart failure, but lung tissue was not available for examination, and specific diagnostic tests were not performed, leaving uncertainty as to the cause of their cor pulmonale.[3] In 1948, a large study hinted at an inherited basis for severe pulmonary hypertension, although exact diagnoses remained uncertain.[4]

In 1954, Dr. David Dresdale first recognized that a familial tendency might exist in patients with primary pulmonary hypertension (now referred to as "idiopathic pulmonary arterial hypertension").[9] Dr. Dresdale described a mother, her sister, and her son, all of whom displayed characteristic findings of primary pulmonary hypertension. A number of other physicians subsequently identified families affected by idiopathic pulmonary arterial hypertension.[10-23] These reports provided a foundation for Drs. Jim Loyd and John Newman, who contacted the patients or members of their families in order to identify new cases. In 1984 Loyd and colleagues reported analyses of nine families affected by primary pulmonary hypertension.[24] Striking findings included: a pattern of vertical transmission characteristic of autosomal dominant inheritance (FIGURE 4-1) as suggested by Melmon and Braunwald[14]; the occurrence of male-to-male transmission that excluded X-linkage of the gene; and varying expression of the disease among the families. Furthermore, it appeared that more women carried the gene, and that women who carried the gene were more likely to develop the disease. The age of disease onset varied considerably, and subsequent analysis indicated earlier onset of disease in successive generations.[25] This seminal work, accompanied by the banking of deoxyribonucleic acid (DNA), led to linkage studies using microsatellite markers.

By 1997, investigators including Morse and coworkers and Nichols and colleagues localized a marker for familial pulmonary arterial hypertension to chromosome 2q31-32 (FIGURE 4-2).[26] Three years later, two teams of investigators characterized mutations in the gene (BMPR2) that codes for bone morphogenetic protein receptor II (BMP-RII), a member of the transforming growth

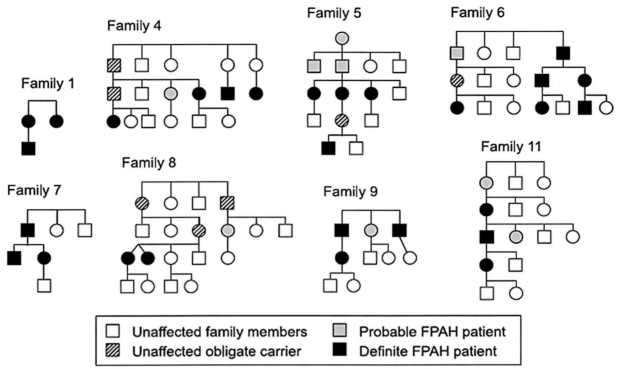

Figure 4-1. Pedigrees of families with familial primary pulmonary hypertension illustrate vertical transmission characteristic of the autosomal dominant pattern of inheritance. Note that unaffected obligate carriers in families 4, 5, 6, and 8 typify the incomplete penetrance of this inherited disease. (Reprinted with permission from Ref. 24)

factor-β (TGF-β) superfamily of receptors.[27,28] Shortly thereafter, *BMPR2* mutations were also identified in 13 of 50 patients diagnosed with sporadic (nonfamilial) pulmonary arterial hypertension.[29] This finding reinforced the concept that many patients with apparently sporadic idiopathic pulmonary arterial hypertension have an underlying genetic predisposition to this disorder.

In 1972, Dr. Erik Trell described individuals with both pulmonary arterial hypertension and hereditary hemorrhagic telangiectasia (HHT or Osler-Weber-Rendu disease).[30] Dr. Trell noted, "Apart from the associated hereditary hemorrhagic telangiectasia, the history of our patients and their family is reminiscent of so-called familial pulmonary arterial hypertension." More than 25 years later, Trembath and colleagues evaluated members of five kindred with HHT and identified ten cases of pulmonary arterial hypertension combined with telangiectasia. In 2001, Dr. Trembath reported that mutations in the gene that codes for another member of the TGF-β superfamily of cytokines, known as activin A receptor type II-like kinase-1 or activin receptor-like kinase-1 (ALK-1), predisposed patients

with classic HHT to develop pulmonary arterial hypertension.[31]

More recent investigations have suggested that pulmonary arterial hypertension is characterized by defects in the vascular signaling pathway involving angiopoietin-1 and its endothelial specific receptor, tunica intima endothelial kinase 2 (TIE2), proteins normally active in the recruitment of smooth muscle cells to developing vasculature.[32] These studies showed that the messenger ribonucleic acid (mRNA) and protein expression of angiopoietin-1, as well as the phosphorylation of TIE2, were strongly upregulated in the lungs of patients with a variety of forms of pulmonary hypertension not associated with known mutations of either *BMPR2* or *ALK1*. A near absence of *BMPR2* gene expression was seen in these patients with nonfamilial forms of pulmonary arterial hypertension. Furthermore, exposure to angiopoietin-1 was sufficient to inhibit the expression of *BMPR1A* by cultured human pulmonary artery endothelial cells, effectively blocking BMPR2 signaling. Thus, TGF-β molecular pathways appear to be pivotal in the pathogenesis of both familial and nonfamilial forms of pulmonary arterial hypertension.

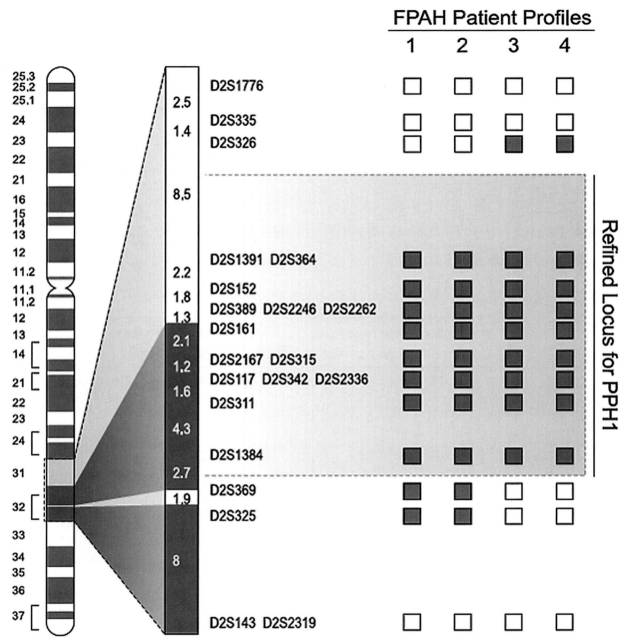

Figure 4-2. Investigators localized a gene responsible for familial pulmonary arterial hypertension (formerly familial primary pulmonary hypertension or PPH) to a critical region on chromosome 2. Linkage analyses identified recombinant events in six families bounded by the polymorphic sequenced tagged sites *(STS)* marked *D2S 326* and *D2S 369*. (From Nichols WC, Koller DL, Slovis B, et al: Localization of the gene for familial primary pulmonary hypertension to chromosome 2q31-32. *Nat Genet* 15(3):277-280, 1997.)

TGF-β Signaling

BMP-RII, ALK-1, and endoglin (ENG) are each cell surface, membrane-bound receptors of the TGF-β family. These receptors are involved in the control of a wide range of cellular processes, including cell growth, apoptosis, and cell type differentiation during development. Ligands for the TGF receptors include bone morphogenetic proteins, activins, inhibins, and TGF-β. Ligand binding by type II receptors (e.g., BMP-RII) causes heterodimerization and phosphorylation with a type I receptor. This, in turn, initiates the phosphorylation of specific intracellular signaling molecules (Smads). The Smads act as transcription factors to control nuclear gene expression. The resulting effects on gene expression and cellular activity can be both cell type and pathway specific.

Molecular Abnormalities

The gene responsible for familial pulmonary arterial hypertension is *BMPR2* (FIGURE 4-3).[27,28] This gene has 13 exons, more than 180,000 base pairs, and codes for 1,038 amino acids.[33] Intronic DNA constitutes more than 98 percent of the gene. The mature protein, the bone morphogenetic protein type II receptor, harbors four distinct functional domains. Exons 2 and 3 code for an extracellular binding ligand that spans amino acids 1-150. Exon 4 codes the transmembrane domain and spans amino acids 151-172. Exons 5 through 10 code for the serine-threonine kinase domain spanning amino acids 205-500, and exons 11 through 13 code for the cytoplasmic tail directing the assembly of amino acids 501-1038. Mutations have been found in all except exon 13. To date more than 140 *BMPR2* mutations have been identified in studies of patients in Europe and the United States,[34] Japan,[35,36] Israel,[37] India,[38] and China.[39] Most of these mutations occur in highly conserved, functionally important locations, suggesting that the mutations disrupt key protein actions such as ligand binding, kinase activity, or heterodimer formation.

Approximately one-half of patients with familial pulmonary arterial hypertension have *BMPR2* mutations identifiable by gene sequencing. Yet

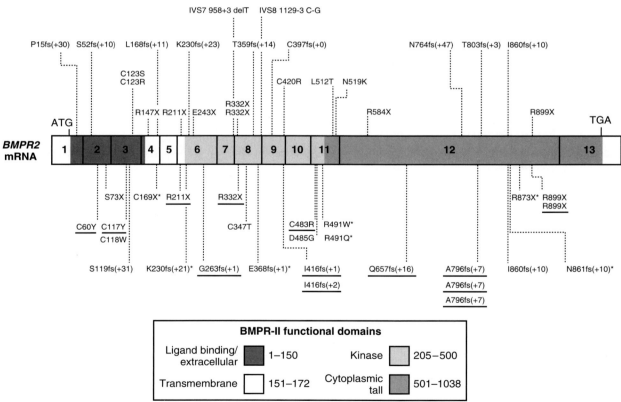

Figure 4-3. Complementary deoxyribonucleic acid (cDNA) structure of the gene that codes for bone morphogenetic protein receptor II, a transforming growth factor-β cell surface receptor. The gene has 13 exons (numbered *1-13* in this figure) and more than 100 Kb of intronic cDNA (not shown). The mutations were described by Machado, et al., 2001; Deng, et al. 2000; Thomson, et al. 2000; and Lane, et al. 2000. Since this report, scientists have characterized many more disease-causing mutations. A one-letter amino acid abbreviation and amino acid position number followed by the number of amino acids before the next stop codon (e.g., L 168 fs [+11]) identifies frame-shift mutations *(fs)*.(Reprinted with permission from Machado RD, Pauciulo MW, Thomson JR, et al: BMPR2 haploinsufficiency as the inherited molecular mechanism for primary pulmonary hypertension. *Am J Hum Genet* 68(1):92-102, 2001.)

undiscovered *BMPR2* mutations may exist within upstream regulatory regions, intronic sequences, or 3′ untranslated regions. Recently Cogan and others reported that 4 of 12 patients with familial pulmonary arterial hypertension have major rearrangements of *BMPR2* that were not detected by gene sequencing.[40] Using a ^{32}P-labeled *BMPR2* probe and Southern blot analysis of genomic DNA, they found unique bands suggestive of large *BMPR2* rearrangements. These data suggest that *BMPR2* mutations are the major cause of familial pulmonary arterial hypertension, although the existence of other causative genes has been proposed.[41]

A number of common *BMPR2* sequence variations have also been identified in exons 2, 3, 6, 8, and 12 (TABLE 4-1). However, these polymorphic variants are unlikely to cause pulmonary arterial hypertension, because they alter amino acids that are less well conserved in TGF-β receptors. Furthermore they occur in unaffected individuals. Nevertheless, the possibility remains that some of these *BMPR2* variants are associated with a very low penetrance of pulmonary arterial hypertension.

An association between additional genes that encode TGF-β cell surface receptors and pulmonary arterial hypertension has been identified (FIGURE 4-4).[31] *ALK1* and *ENG* mutations cause HHT (Rendu-Osler-Weber syndrome),[42,43] a syndrome characterized by a variety of vascular malformations.[44] Mucocutaneous telangiectasias are the most common lesions and consist of direct connections between arteries and veins (FIGURE 4-5, A and B). Arteriovenous malformations also may be found in the lung and brain. *ALK1* mutations cause diverse and sometimes overlapping vascular lesions, even within the same family (FIGURE 4-6).

Pulmonary arterial hypertension accompanying hereditary hemorrhagic telangiectasia has been recognized for decades, but mutations in *ALK1*[31,45,46] and perhaps *ENG*[47,48] as a molecular cause for pulmonary arterial hypertension were recognized only recently. The overlap of vascular dilations and vascular occlusions resulting in either low or high pulmonary vascular resistance suggests a dynamic interplay among signaling pathways that regulate vascular development and repair.

ALK1 is a gene located on chromosome 12 that has 10 exons and 1,512 base pairs. The gene codes for four functional domains. Exons 2, 3, and 4 code for extracellular ligand binding domains and a transmembrane domain. Exon 5 codes for the glycine-serine (GS) domain, and exons 6-10 code for the kinase domain. Investigators have identified multiple mutations located principally within exons 5 through 10 of *ALK1* (FIGURE 4-5C).[31,45,46] Most mutations represent missense changes located within the kinase domain and alter amino acids that are highly conserved across type I members of the TGF-β receptor family. None of these mutations has been found in control samples.[45] *ALK1* mutations mediate intracellular signaling through Smads 1, 5, and 8. Control of nuclear transcription factors by BMP-RI and BMP-RII complexes are also mediated by Smads 1, 5, and 8, raising the possibility that familial pulmonary arterial hypertension and pulmonary arterial hypertension related to HHT share a common pathogetic pathway.[49]

The TGF-β superfamily influences cell cycle behaviors including proliferation, apoptosis, adhesion, and migration.[50,51] The exact mechanism whereby mutations of *BMPR2* or *ALK1* result in

TABLE 4-1

cDNA Sequence Variations Identified Commonly in *BMPR2*

Location	Nucleotide Change	Amino Acid Change	Frequency	Reference
Exon 2	c.165 T > C	p.N55N	1.1%	35
Intron 3	c.420-43 delT	—	NK	52
Exon 6	c.672 G > T	p.E224D	NK	52
Exon 8	c.1107 A > G	p.E369E	NK	52
Exon 12	c.1937 C > G	p.A646G	0.5%	35
Exon 12	c.2379 A > C	p.T793T	2.1%	35
Exon 12	c.2539 A > G	p.Q844R	0.5%	35
Exon 12	c.2811 G > A	p.R937R	14%	35

cDNA, *complementary deoxyribonucleic acid; NK, not known.*
From Morisaki H, Nakanishi N, Kyotani S, et al: BMPR2 mutations found in Japanese patients with familial and sporadic primary pulmonary hypertension. Hum Mutat 23(6):632, 2004; Machado RD, Pauciulo MW, Thomson JR, et al: BMPR2 haploinsufficiency as the inherited molecular mechanism for primary pulmonary hypertension. Am J Hum Genet 68(1):92-102, 2001.

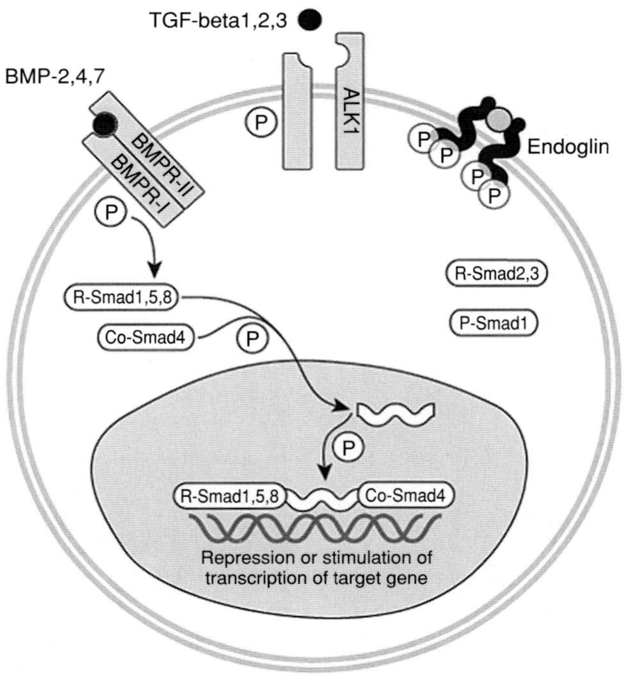

Figure 4-4. Molecular alterations of three members of the transforming growth factor-β (TGF-β) superfamily lead to some cases of pulmonary arterial hypertension. Bone morphogenetic protein receptor type II (BMP-RII) is a cell surface receptor situated immediately adjacent to the BMP-RI receptor. These two receptors bind in the presence of ligand. Once bound, BMP-RII phosphorylates the transmembrane region of BMP-RI, activating the kinase region. Activated BMP-RI phosphorylates receptor series of intracellular mediators (R-Smad), and this activates one or more cytoplasmic Smad proteins (Smad 1, Smad 5, and Smad 8). These activated Smads bind with Smad 4 and enter the nucleus, where they combine with nuclear binding factor before either repressing or stimulating the transcription of target genes. Activin receptor-like kinase-1 (ALK-1) also leads to phosphorylation of receptor Smad proteins (Smads 1, 5, and 8), and the potential exists for common effects of mutations that alter BMP-RII or ALK-1 upon downstream behavior of these pathways. The role and significance of endoglin (ENG), the third TGF-β cell surface receptor, is less certain.

pulmonary arterial hypertension remains undefined in spite of recent functional studies. These studies have shown a heterogeneous array of functional differences in the translated BMP-RII protein, reflecting a diversity of *BMPR2* mutations.[52] *BMPR2* missense mutations produce alterations of cysteine residues in the extracellular or kinase domains. These protein receptors appear unable to escape the cytoplasm to transduce BMP-mediated signaling pathways.[53] *BMPR2* mutations which alter the cytoplasmic tail of the BMP-RII appear to cause less efficient phosphorylation of the intracellular signal-transducing

molecule, Smad 5.[52] Similarly most *ALK1* mutant constructs appear to be retained within cell cytoplasm in the endoplasmic reticulum.[45]

Most of the *BMPR2* and *ALK1* mutations predict premature termination of the transcript with loss of function through the process of nonsense-mediated decay. Machado and co-workers and Harrison and colleagues have suggested that haploinsufficiency, the process whereby heterozygosity for a gene mutation leads to insufficient protein product for normal function, explains the development of pulmonary arterial hypertension in the presence of

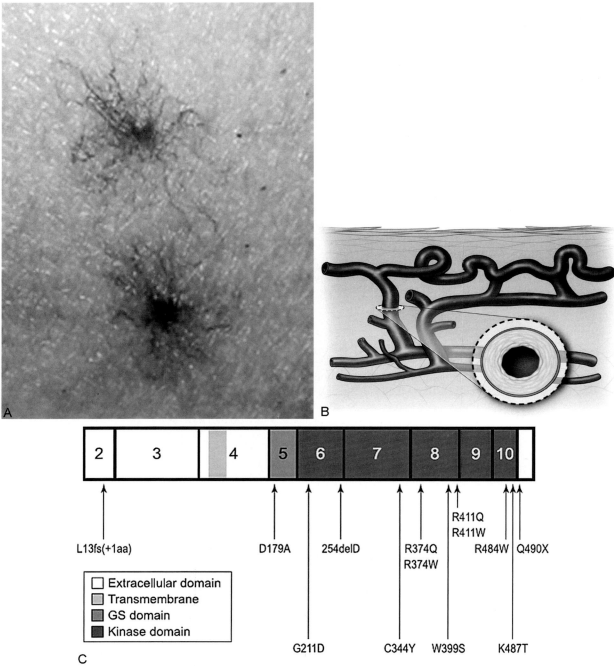

Figure 4-5. Mucocutaneous telangiectasias characterize hereditary hemorrhagic telangiectasia. Panel **A** illustrates typical lesions on the skin. Panel **B** demonstrates pathologic changes in the dermis. These changes include (1) dilation of post capillary venules with a vessel wall that has increased numbers of smooth muscle cells (**inset**); (2) direct communication between arterioles and venules without intervening capillaries. Patients with these lesions may have coexistent pulmonary arterial hypertension related to mutations in the gene that codes for activin receptor-like kinase-1. Panel **C** illustrates the complementary deoxyribonucleic acid (cDNA) structure of the gene that codes for the activin A receptor type II-like kinase-1 or activin receptor-like kinase-1 (ACVRL-1 or ALK-1). Investigators have detected multiple mutations, most located in the kinase domain, that are associated with pulmonary arterial hypertension accompanying hereditary hemorrhagic telangiectasia. (Panel B modified from: Guttmacher AE, Marchuk DA, White RI, Jr: Hereditary hemorrhagic telangiectasia. *N Engl J Med* 333(14):918-924, 1995, with permission; C, modified from Harrison RE, Flanagan JA, Sankelo M, et al: Molecular and functional analysis identifies ALK-1 as the predominant cause of pulmonary hypertension related to hereditary haemorrhagic telangiectasia. J Med Genet 40(12):865-871, 2003, with permission.)

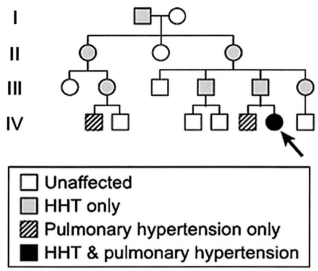

Figure 4-6. Pedigree of a family with hereditary hemorrhagic telangiectasia and pulmonary arterial hypertension. Seven members of this family demonstrated typical features of hereditary hemorrhagic telangiectasia, whereas two members had only features of pulmonary arterial hypertension. One member of the family had both telangiectasia and pulmonary arterial hypertension.

BMPR2 or *ALK1* mutation.[45,53] However, a dominant negative effect in which the altered gene product adversely affects cell function is also possible. Interestingly, *BMPR2* knockout mice die at gastrulation, whereas heterozygotes appear healthy.[54]

Serotonin and the Human Serotonin Transporter

Serotonin (5-hydroxytryptamine [5-HT]) may contribute to the pathogenesis of pulmonary arterial hypertension. Serotonin causes vasoconstriction and proliferation of pulmonary artery smooth muscle cells.[55] Excess circulating levels of serotonin are present in patients with idiopathic pulmonary arterial hypertension.[56] Investigators also have described excess serotonin levels in a patient with pulmonary arterial hypertension associated with familial platelet pool storage disease.[57] Furthermore, serotonin levels can be increased markedly when pulmonary arterial hypertension accompanies glycogen storage disease.[58] Serotonin receptors (5-HT 1B/D, 2A, and 2B) mediate vasoconstriction. However, the

mitogenic and co-mitogenic effects of serotonin require intracellular transfer of serotonin by the serotonin transporter (5-HT transporter [5-HTT]).[59,60]

A polymorphism in the promoter region of the human 5-HTT gene alters levels of serotonin transcription.[61] This polymorphism consists of two common alleles: the first codes for a 44 base pair deletion and is termed the short (S) allele; and the second codes for a 44 base pair insertion termed the long (L) allele. The L allele produces 2 to 3 times more serotonin transporter mRNA than the S allele. Homozygosity for the L allele occurs more often in patients with idiopathic pulmonary arterial hypertension (65 percent of such patients) as compared with controls (27 percent).[55]

In animal models, upregulation of 5-HT and 5-HTT occur with exposure to dexfenfluramine and in response to hypoxia.[62,63] Administration of the 5-HTT inhibitors fluoxetine or paroxetine decreases pulmonary artery smooth muscle cell proliferation and pulmonary artery pressure in rat models of pulmonary hypertension triggered by hypoxia.[60] 5-HTT inhibitors, however, have not been studied in human pulmonary arterial hypertension.

Factor V Leiden

Microscopic *in situ* thrombosis is a prominent pathologic finding in some patients with familial pulmonary arterial hypertension[64] and sporadic pulmonary arterial hypertension.[65] In a study of pathologic lesions, Dr. Jim Loyd identified organized thrombi in the small pulmonary arteries of all 23 patients with familial pulmonary arterial hypertension, although only a small minority of vessels contained thrombi.[64] These investigators suggested that coagulation at the endothelial surface might be an important pathogenetic mechanism.

An abnormal factor V (factor V Leiden) causes thrombosis and occurs relatively commonly in Caucasians.[66,67] A single point mutation in the factor V gene leads to an amino acid substitution, resulting in resistance to cleavage by activated protein C and thus promoting thrombosis. However, factor V Leiden is not found more commonly in patients with idiopathic pulmonary arterial hypertension than it is in healthy reference populations (TABLE 4-2).[68] In this study, only 1 of 42 patients with idiopathic pulmonary arterial hypertension demonstrated a factor V Leiden mutation, and none of 10 individuals with familial pulmonary arterial hypertension displayed a factor V Leiden mutation.

TABLE 4-2

Factor V Leiden Mutation Is Not Common in Idiopathic or Familial Pulmonary Arterial Hypertension

Study Population	n	Heterozygotes	Homozygotes	Allele Frequency (95% CI)
Europe	618	50	2	4.4 (3.3 -5.5)
USA	704	42	0	3.0 (2.2 -4.1)
IPAH	42	1	0	1.2 (0.0 -6.3)

IPAH, *idiopathic pulmonary arterial hypertension.*
From Elliott CG, Leppert MF, Alexander GJ, et al: Factor V Leiden is not common in patients diagnosed with primary pulmonary hypertension. Eur Respir J 12(5):1177-1180, 1998.

Genetic and Environmental Interaction

Several lines of evidence suggest that an environmental exposure (trigger) causes pulmonary arterial hypertension in a genetically susceptible individual. First, environmental exposure coupled with genetic susceptibility leads to a host of serious diseases (e.g., lung cancer, emphysema, melanoma). Second, the low level of penetrance in familial pulmonary arterial hypertension, and even lower penetrance in patients with sporadic pulmonary arterial hypertension and *BMPR2* mutations, suggests that additional factors, either genetic or environmental, are necessary to cause disease. Third, strong links exist between inflammation and pulmonary arterial hypertension.[69] Latent infection with human herpes virus-8[70] or human immunodeficiency virus,[71] exposure to anorexigens,[72] or as yet unrecognized environmental exposures may trigger the development of pulmonary arterial hypertension in genetically susceptible individuals. Yeager and others reported microsatellite instability, caused by insertion or deletion of complementary DNA (cDNA) base pairs during repair, in approximately one-half of all lung tissue specimens from patients with idiopathic pulmonary arterial hypertension.[73] These may represent somatic mutations acquired after an environmental insult.

Inheritance Pattern

Studies of familial pulmonary arterial hypertension have revealed an autosomal dominant pattern of inheritance.[24] Penetrance is incomplete as evidenced by skipped generations, although asymptomatic carriers of *BMPR2* mutations may have mild pulmonary hypertension detected by echocardiographic estimates of pulmonary artery pressure

during exercise.[74] Father-to-son transmission excludes X chromosome linkage.[24] A shorter lifespan is observed in successive generations of family members affected by pulmonary arterial hypertension (FIGURE 4-7).[25,75] This observation suggests genetic anticipation, a pattern of worsening of familial disease in subsequent generations, as has been observed in fragile X syndrome,[76,77] myotonic dystrophy,[78,79] and Friedreich ataxia.[80] Unlike the trinucleotide repeats observed in myotonic dystrophy, investigators have not found a molecular pattern to explain the phenomenon of genetic anticipation among patients with familial pulmonary arterial hypertension.

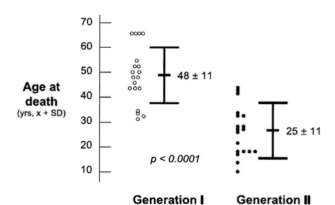

Figure 4-7. Studies of nine pedigrees yielded 19 pairs of individuals affected by familial pulmonary arterial hypertension. The age at death of patients found in the first generation (generation I) was significantly older than the age of death of the subsequent generation (generation II). Although this pattern suggests genetic anticipation caused by unstable nucleotide repeats, no repeats have been identified in patients with familial pulmonary arterial hypertension.

Epidemiologic Features

From 1981 through 1985, the National Institutes of Health sponsored a patient registry to characterize the clinical features and natural history of idiopathic pulmonary arterial hypertension.[7] This project identified 187 patients diagnosed with idiopathic pulmonary arterial hypertension. Twelve of these 187 patients (6 percent) had one or more immediate family members who were affected by idiopathic pulmonary arterial hypertension; the remaining 175 patients were said to have sporadic pulmonary arterial hypertension. Comparisons of patients with sporadic pulmonary arterial hypertension and those with familial disease showed no differences in age at diagnosis, hemodynamic abnormalities, or symptoms.

In 1995, investigators reported an epidemiologic study of Utah families diagnosed with idiopathic pulmonary arterial hypertension.[81] This study showed common ancestry for two apparently sporadic cases. The common ancestry in these cases was highly unlikely to be explained by chance alone. In 2001, Newman and colleagues reported extensive work linking apparently sporadic cases into a large family pedigree characterized by a single mutation in the gene that codes for BMP-RII.[82] These observations suggest that many patients with apparently sporadic idiopathic pulmonary arterial hypertension actually have a genetic predisposition to develop this condition. Some of these patients had developed *BMPR2* mutations spontaneously, because neither parent carries the mutation,[29] whereas others had a *BMPR2* mutation transmitted from a parent who never developed clinical disease (incomplete penetrance).[29] Misclassification of familial pulmonary arterial hypertension as sporadic pulmonary arterial hypertension likely reflects misdiagnosis, incomplete family histories, small family size, or low levels of disease expression among family members with a genetic predisposition to develop the disease (i.e., incomplete penetrance).

BMPR2 Mutations in Nonfamilial Forms of Pulmonary Arterial Hypertension

Idiopathic Pulmonary Arterial Hypertension

Studies of the hypothesis that many patients with apparently sporadic idiopathic pulmonary arterial hypertension have a genetic predisposition have yielded disparate results.[29,35,83-85] The first study

found *BMPR2* mutations in 13 of 50 patients (26 percent).[29] More recent reports suggest that the frequency of *BMPR2* mutations in sporadic pulmonary arterial hypertension is lower,[83-85] although one such study from Japan found that 12 of 30 patients harbored *BMPR2* mutations.[35] In spite of varying estimates of the frequency, the important point remains that any patient with apparently sporadic pulmonary arterial hypertension may have a predisposing *BMPR2* mutation.

Pulmonary Veno-occlusive Disease and Pulmonary Capillary Hemangiomatosis

Pathologic classification of the vasculopathies of pulmonary hypertension distinguishes changes occurring at the arterial and venous vessels.[86] Although changes within both can occur in each of the various clinical diagnoses associated with these histopathologic patterns, idiopathic and associated forms of pulmonary arterial hypertension are predominantly characterized by heterogeneous lesions, including medial and intimal proliferation in small muscular pulmonary arteries. The clinical entity pulmonary capillary hemangiomatosis, in contrast, is most notable for pulmonary microvasculopathy, characterized by a cytologically benign-appearing vascular proliferation of capillaries confined to the lung and causing pulmonary hypertension.[87] Pulmonary veno-occlusive disease is characterized by pulmonary occlusive venopathy involving a pronounced intimal and adventitial thickening of the pulmonary veins, with arterialization of veins greater than 50 μm in external diameter. The latter two conditions are extremely rare. There are no reports of *BMPR2* mutations in patients with pulmonary capillary hemangiomatosis, although one report of familial pulmonary capillary hemangiomatosis exists.[88] However, an example of pulmonary veno-occlusive disease associated with a frameshift mutation located in exon 1 of *BMPR2* (predicted to truncate BMP-RII) has been reported.[89]

Fenfluramine Derivatives

Some hypothesize that *BMPR2* mutations predispose people to develop pulmonary arterial hypertension after ingesting the anorectic drug fenfluramine or its derivatives. However, direct sequencing for *BMPR2* mutations in patients with pulmonary arterial hypertension related to fenfluramine ingestion has yielded few mutations.[90,91] Humbert reported *BMPR2* mutations in 3 of 33 (9 percent) of unrelated patients with pulmonary arterial hypertension after fenfluramine exposure,[90] and Scholand and colleagues found BMPR2 mutations in only 2 of 36 such patients.[91] One of these patients had a mother and two maternal uncles who were affected by idiopathic pulmonary arterial hypertension even though they had not been exposed to fenfluramine. Thus, it does not appear that BMPR2 mutations are the susceptibility factor that explains why only approximately 1 of every 10,000 individuals exposed to fenfluramine developed pulmonary arterial hypertension.

Congenital Heart Disease

The pivotal role of TGF-β receptors, including BMP-RII, in cellular growth and differentiation during embryogenesis engendered a search for mutations among patients with pulmonary arterial hypertension and congenital systemic-to-pulmonary shunts.[53,92,93] Roberts and others reported that 6 percent of 106 patients with congenital heart disease and pulmonary arterial hypertension had BMPR2 mutations.[94] Although BMPR2 mutations were found in three of four adults with complete atrioventricular canal defects, none was found in six children with the same defect.

Connective Tissue Diseases

Pulmonary arterial hypertension complicates a number of connective tissue diseases, especially limited scleroderma. However, only a small fraction of patients with connective tissue disease develop pulmonary arterial hypertension, again raising the question of genetic predisposition. BMPR2 mutations were not found in two small studies of patients with connective tissue diseases complicated by pulmonary arterial hypertension.[95,96]

Human Immunodeficiency Virus Infection

Pulmonary arterial hypertension complicates approximately 0.5 percent of human immunodeficiency virus infections.[97] Nunes and co-workers did not find BMPR2 mutations in 19 patients with human immunodeficiency virus infection and pulmonary arterial hypertension, suggesting that BMPR2 mutations do not foster susceptibility to the development of pulmonary arterial hypertension in those with human immunodeficiency virus infection.[98]

Portopulmonary Hypertension

Pulmonary arterial hypertension occurs in approximately 2-5 percent of patients with portal hypertension.[97] The frequency of BMPR2 mutations in this population, however, has not been reported.

Hereditary Hemorrhagic Telangiectasia

HHT is characterized by vascular dysplasias in visceral organs, mucous membranes, and skin.[44] Arteriovenous malformations can be found in the brain, lungs, liver, and the gastrointestinal tract. Similar lesions also occur on the lips, tongue, nasal mucosa, and fingertips. The inheritance pattern is autosomal dominant, and the disorder is caused by mutations in genes that code for TGF-β cell surface receptors, endoglin, and ALK-1. Eric Trell and others first recognized the association of HHT and pulmonary arterial hypertension.[30] Richard Trembath and colleagues subsequently identified mutations in the gene for ALK-1 as the molecular mechanism responsible for this uncommon combination.[31,45] Endoglin mutations have also been associated with pulmonary arterial hypertension related to HHT.[45-48]

Pulmonary Hypertension Related to Chronic Alveolar Hypoxia

Acute alveolar hypoxia is a potent stimulus for pulmonary arteriolar constriction, and chronic alveolar hypoxia stimulates pulmonary arterial smooth muscle proliferation and the development of chronic pulmonary hypertension.[99] Long-term oxygen therapy does little to reverse these changes once pulmonary hypertension is established when the patient has chronic parenchymal lung disease.[100] However, even severe pulmonary hypertension can be reversed to a large degree in chronic alveolar hypoventilation.

Genetic susceptibility may predispose to pulmonary hypertension induced by alveolar hypoxia. For example, native Tibetans, residing on the Himalayan plateau (3,600 meters above sea level) for many generations, have nearly normal pulmonary artery pressures,[101] whereas the Han Chinese, who moved to this region from lower elevations, develop pulmonary hypertension and cor pulmonale.[102] A susceptible subgroup of Kyrgyz residents (3,000 meters above sea level) develops pulmonary hypertension and right-sided heart failure.[103] Polymorphisms in the angiotensin-I-converting enzyme gene may contribute to differential susceptibility for the development of pulmonary hypertension triggered by alveolar hypoxia.[104,105]

Gene Testing

Clinical Laboratory Improvement Act (CLIA)-approved gene tests are available for a number of serious diseases such as cystic fibrosis and breast cancer.[106] CLIA-approved genetic testing for *BMPR2* is available at a few pulmonary hypertension centers. Genetic tests include full DNA sequencing, Southern blot, dye-binding high-resolution thermal denaturation, and reverse transcriptase–polymerase chain reaction (RT-PCR). Limited data suggest that full sequencing by a CLIA certified laboratory detects *BMPR2* cDNA sequence variations with high sensitivity and specificity. Dye-binding high-resolution thermal denaturation also appears to detect *BMPR2* cDNA sequence variations with high sensitivity and specificity,[107,108] although this technique usually is followed by direct sequencing of an exon region for precise identification of mutations.[109] RT-PCR–amplified mRNA products (i.e., cDNA) can be used to detect large gene rearrangements (i.e., exon deletions or duplications), as well as specific mutations detected by conventional sequencing. Sequence variations in exon 1 or 13 of *BMPR2* cannot be detected by RT-PCR. The Southern blot detects large gene rearrangements, but it does not identify specific cDNA sequence variations. Gene sequencing and Southern blot tests are used most widely, but other methods are under development.

Gene tests may be used to characterize an individual family member's risk of developing pulmonary arterial hypertension. Simply stated, a first-order relative who carries a disease-causing mutation of the *BMPR2* gene has approximately one chance in five of developing the disease. Of equal importance, a family member who does not carry a disease-causing *BMPR2* mutation has the same risk as others in the general population, about one chance in a million of developing this disease. Without testing, 1 chance in 10 is a reasonable estimate of the likelihood that a first-degree relative of a patient with known familial idiopathic pulmonary arterial hypertension will develop the disease. Professional genetic counseling is essential, both before and after genetic testing, because of the serious implications of the results.

Current guidelines call for gene testing of family members of patients with familial pulmonary arterial hypertension when the mutation is known and genetic counseling is available.[83,110]

Future Directions

Future work must answer a number of critical questions. First, why do some individuals with a *BMPR2* mutation develop pulmonary arterial hypertension, while other members of the same family, with the same mutation, never develop this devastating disease? The answer may reflect other modifying genes, or environmental triggers, or both. An important first step will be to perform genome-wide comparisons of affected and unaffected members of the same family, to identify mutations or polymorphisms that may explain these differences. Studies to explore molecular pathways that integrate *BMPR2* mutations with expression of the serotonin transporter gene may yield an explanation for incomplete penetrance and the intriguing predisposition of individuals with the LL genotype to develop pulmonary arterial hypertension. Other genes, such as nitric oxide synthase, angiotensin II, endothelin, vasoactive intestinal peptide, or carbamoylphosphate synthase, also need further study as possible modifiers of risk. Second, the genetic substrate that underlies pulmonary arterial hypertension complicating collagen vascular diseases, portal hypertension, human immunodeficiency virus infection, and congenital cardiovascular disorders characterized by systemic to pulmonary shunts must be identified.

The development of multiple classes of drugs to treat pulmonary arterial hypertension opens the door for future pharmacogenetic studies. Opportunities exist to describe polymorphisms that affect the response to specific drugs, or classes of drugs (e.g., endothelin receptor antagonists, phosphodiesterase-5 inhibitors), as well as to identify genetic predispositions to some of the rare, serious adverse reactions to drugs used to treat pulmonary arterial hypertension, such as liver toxicity related to endothelin receptor antagonists.

Rapid advances in understanding the genetics of pulmonary arterial hypertension provide real hope for the development of more effective methods to prevent or treat this disease. Early identification of individuals at high risk offers the prospect of early therapeutic intervention before pulmonary arterial hypertension progresses to irreversible pathologic changes. Similarly, identification of specific genetic abnormalities creates the opportunity for reprogramming cells to reverse the most basic pathobiologic abnormalities.

References

1. Romberge E: Uber Sklerose der Lungen Arterie. *Dtsch Arch Klin Med* 48:197-206, 1891.
2. Simonneau G, Galie N, Rubin LJ, et al: Clinical classification of pulmonary hypertension. *J Am Coll Cardiol* 43(12 Suppl S):5S-12S, 2004.
3. Clarke RC, Coombs CF, Favre C, et al: On certain abnormalities, congenital and acquired, of the pulmonary artery. *Quart J Med* 21:51-68, 1927.
4. Lange F: Die Essentielle Hypertonie der Lungenstrombahn und ir Familares Vorkhommen. *Dtsch Med Wochen* 73:322-326, 1948.
5. Barst RJ, McGoon M, Torbicki A, et al: Diagnosis and differential assessment of pulmonary arterial hypertension. *J Am Coll Cardiol* 43(12 Suppl S):40S-47S, 2004.
6. Dresdale DT, Schultz M, Michtom RJ: Primary pulmonary hypertension. I. Clinical and hemodynamic study. *Am J Med* 11:686-705, 1951.
7. Rich S, Dantzker DR, Ayres SM, et al: Primary pulmonary hypertension. A national prospective study. *Ann Intern Med* 107:216-223, 1987.
8. Rich S: Primary pulmonary hypertension: Executive summary from the world symposium. Available at: *http://www.who.int/ncd/cvd/pph.htm*, 1998.
9. Dresdale DT, Michtom RJ, Schultz M: Recent studies in primary pulmonary hypertension, including pharmacodynamic observations on pulmonary vascular resistance. *Bull N Y Acad Med* 30:195-207, 1954.
10. Schaffner F: Clinico-pathological conference. *Mt Sinai Hosp J* 25:470-494, 1958.
11. Husson GS, Wyatt TC: Primary pulmonary obliterative vascular disease in infants and young children. *Pediatrics* 23:493-506, 1959.
12. Sleeper JC, Orgain ES, McIntosh HD: Primary pulmonary hypertension. Review of clinical features and pathologic physiology with a report of pulmonary hemodynamics derived from repeated catheterization. *Circulation* 26:1358-1369, 1962.
13. Botteau GM, Kibranoff AJ: Primary pulmonary hypertension: Familial incidence. *Angiology* 14:260-264, 1963.
14. Melmon KL, Braunwald E: Familial pulmonary hypertension. *N Engl J Med* 269:770-775, 1963.
15. Rogge JD, Mishkin ME, Genovese PD: The familial occurrence of primary pulmonary hypertension. *Ann Intern Med* 65:672-684, 1966.
16. Kingdon HS, Cohen LS, Roberts WC, et al: Familial occurrence of primary pulmonary hypertension. *Arch Intern Med* 118:422-426, 1966.
17. Porter CM, Creech BJ, Billings FT, Jr: Primary pulmonary hypertension occurring in twins. *Arch Intern Med* 120:224-229, 1967.
18. Czarnecki SW, Rosenbaum HM, Wachtel HL: The occurrence of primary pulmonary hypertension in twins with a review of etiological considerations. *Am Heart J* 75:240-246, 1968.
19. Tsargaris TJ, Fikoff, G: Familial primary pulmonary hypertension. *Am Rev Respir Dis* 97:127-130, 1968.
20. Massoud H, Puckett W, Auerbach SH: Primary pulmonary hypertension: A study of the disease in four young siblings. *J Tenn Med Assoc* 63:299-305, 1970.
21. Inglesby TV, Singer JW, Gordon DS: Abnormal fibrinolysis in familial pulmonary hypertension. *Am J Med* 55:5-14, 1973.
22. Hendrix GH: Familial primary pulmonary hypertension. *South Med J* 67:981-983, 1974.
23. Tubbs RR, Levin RD, Shirey EK, et al: Fibrinolysis in familial pulmonary hypertension. *Am J Clin Pathol* 71:384-387, 1979.
24. Loyd JE, Primm RK, Newman JH: Familial primary pulmonary hypertension: Clinical patterns. *Am Rev Respir Dis* 129:194-197, 1984.
25. Loyd JE, Butler MG, Foroud TM, et al: Genetic anticipation and abnormal gender ratio at birth in familial primary pulmonary hypertension. *Am J Respir Crit Care Med* 152:93-97, 1995.
26. Nichols WC, Koller DL, Slovis B, et al: Localization of the gene for familial primary pulmonary hypertension to chromosome 2q31-32. *Nat Genet* 15:277-280, 1997.
27. Deng Z, Morse JH, Slager SL, et al: Familial primary pulmonary hypertension (gene *PPH1*) is caused by mutations in the bone morphogenetic protein receptor-II gene. *Am J Hum Genet* 67:737-744, 2000.
28. Lane KB, Machado RD, Pauciulo MW, et al: Heterozygous germline mutations in *BMPR2*, encoding a TGF-β receptor, cause familial primary pulmonary hypertension. The International PPH Consortium. *Nat Genet* 26:81-84, 2000.
29. Thomson JR, Machado RD, Pauciulo MW, et al: Sporadic primary pulmonary hypertension is associated with germline mutations of the gene encoding BMPR-II, a receptor member of the TGF-β family. *J Med Genet* 37:741-745, 2000.
30. Trell E, Johansson BW, Linell F, et al: Familial pulmonary hypertension and multiple abnormalities of large systemic arteries in Osler's disease. *Am J Med* 53:50-63, 1972.
31. Trembath RC, Thomson JR, Machado RD, et al: Clinical and molecular genetic features of pulmonary hypertension in patients with hereditary hemorrhagic telangiectasia. *N Engl J Med* 345:325-334, 2001.
32. Du L, Sullivan CC, Chu D, et al: Signaling molecules in nonfamilial pulmonary hypertension. *N Engl J Med* 348:500-509, 2003.
33. Liu F, Ventura F, Doody J, et al: Human type II receptor for bone morphogenic proteins (BMPs): Extension of the two-kinase receptor model to the BMPs. *Mol Cell Biol* 15:3479-3486, 1995.

34. Machado RD, Aldred MA, James V, et al: Mutations of the TGF-β type II receptor *BMPR2* in pulmonary arterial hypertension. *Hum Mutat,* 27:121-132, 2006.

35. Morisaki H, Nakanishi N, Kyotani S, et al: *BMPR2* mutations found in Japanese patients with familial and sporadic primary pulmonary hypertension. *Hum Mutat* 23:632, 2004.

36. Sugiyama S, Hirota H, Yoshida M, et al: Novel insertional mutation in the bone morphogenetic protein receptor type II associated with sporadic primary pulmonary hypertension. *Circ J* 68:592-594, 2004.

37. Cahn A, Meiner V, Leitersdorf E, et al: Identification of a novel mutation in the gene for bone morphogenetic protein receptor II in an Israeli patient with familial primary pulmonary hypertension. *Isr Med Assoc J* 6:156-159, 2004.

38. Rudarakanchana N, Flanagan JA, Chen H, et al: Functional analysis of bone morphogenetic protein type II receptor mutations underlying primary pulmonary hypertension. *Hum Mol Genet* 11:1517-1525, 2002.

39. Zhicheng J, Lihe L, Zhiyan H, et al: Bone morphogenetic protein receptor-II mutation Arg491Trp causes malignant phenotype of familial primary pulmonary hypertension. *Biochem Biophys Res Commun.* 315:1033-1038, 2004.

40. Cogan JD, Vnencak-Jones CL, Phillips JA, III, et al: Gross *BMPR2* gene rearrangements constitute a new cause for primary pulmonary hypertension. *Genet Med* 7:169-174, 2005.

41. Janssen B, Rindermann M, Barth U, et al: Linkage analysis in a large family with primary pulmonary hypertension: Genetic heterogeneity and a second primary pulmonary hypertension locus on 2q31-32. *Chest* 121(3 Suppl):54S-56S, 2002.

42. McAllister KA, Grogg KM, Johnson DW, et al: Endoglin, a TGF-β binding protein of endothelial cells, is the gene for hereditary haemorrhagic telangiectasia type 1. *Nat Genet* 8:345-351, 1994.

43. Johnson DW, Berg JN, Baldwin MA, et al: Mutations in the activin receptor-like kinase 1 gene in hereditary haemorrhagic telangiectasia type 2. *Nat Genet* 13:189-195, 1996.

44. Guttmacher AE, Marchuk DA, White RI, Jr: Hereditary hemorrhagic telangiectasia. *N Engl J Med* 333:918-924, 1995.

45. Harrison RE, Flanagan JA, Sankelo M, et al: Molecular and functional analysis identifies ALK-1 as the predominant cause of pulmonary hypertension related to hereditary haemorrhagic telangiectasia. *J Med Genet* 40:865-871, 2003.

46. Abdalla SA, Gallione CJ, Barst RJ, et al: Primary pulmonary hypertension in families with hereditary haemorrhagic telangiectasia. *Eur Respir J* 23:373-377, 2004.

47. Chaouat A, Coulet F, Favre C, et al: Endoglin germline mutation in a patient with hereditary haemorrhagic telangiectasia and dexfenfluramine-associated pulmonary arterial hypertension. *Thorax* 59:446-448, 2004.

48. Harrison RE, Berger R, Haworth SG, et al: Transforming growth factor-β receptor mutations and pulmonary arterial hypertension in childhood. *Circulation* 111:435-441, 2005.

49. Shi Y, Massague J: Mechanisms of TGF-β signaling from cell membrane to the nucleus. *Cell* 113:685-700, 2003.

50. Massague J, Wotton D: Transcriptional control by the TGF-β/Smad signaling system. *EMBO J* 19:1745-1754, 2000.

51. Blobe GC, Schiemann WP, Lodish HF: Role of transforming growth factor β in human disease. *N Engl J Med* 342:1350-1358, 2000.

52. Nishihara A, Watabe T, Imamura T, et al: Functional heterogeneity of bone morphogenetic protein receptor-II mutants found in patients with primary pulmonary hypertension. *Mol Biol Cell* 13:3055-3063, 2002.

53. Machado RD, Pauciulo MW, Thomson JR, et al: *BMPR2* haploinsufficiency as the inherited molecular mechanism for primary pulmonary hypertension. *Am J Hum Genet* 68:92-102, 2001.

54. Beppu H, Kawabata M, Hamamoto T, et al: BMP type II receptor is required for gastrulation and early development of mouse embryos. *Dev Biol* 221:249-258, 2000.

55. Eddahibi S, Humbert M, Fadel E, et al: Serotonin transporter overexpression is responsible for pulmonary artery smooth muscle hyperplasia in primary pulmonary hypertension. *J Clin Invest* 108:1141-1150, 2001.

56. Herve P, Launay JM, Scrobohaci ML, et al: Increased plasma serotonin in primary pulmonary hypertension. *Am J Med* 99:249-254, 1995.

57. Herve P, Drouet L, Dosquet C, et al: Primary pulmonary hypertension in a patient with a familial platelet storage pool disease: Role of serotonin. *Am J Med* 89:117-120, 1990.

58. Humbert M, Labrune P, Sitbon O, et al: Pulmonary arterial hypertension and type-I glycogen-storage disease: The serotonin hypothesis. *Eur Respir J* 20:59-65, 2002.

59. Lee SL, Wang WW, Moore BJ, et al: Dual effect of serotonin on growth of bovine pulmonary artery smooth muscle cells in culture. *Circ Res* 68:1362-1368, 1991.

60. Eddahibi S, Fabre V, Boni C, et al: Induction of serotonin transporter by hypoxia in pulmonary vascular smooth muscle cells. Relationship with the mitogenic action of serotonin. *Circ Res* 84:329-336, 1999.

61. Lesch KP, Wolozin BL, Estler HC, et al: Isolation of a cDNA encoding the human brain serotonin transporter. *J Neural Transm Gen Sect* 91:67-72, 1993.

62. Eddahibi S, Hanoun N, Lanfumey L, et al: Attenuated hypoxic pulmonary hypertension in mice lacking the 5-hydroxytryptamine transporter gene. *J Clin Invest* 105:1555-1562, 2000.

63. Welsh DJ, Harnett M, MacLean M, et al: Proliferation and signaling in fibroblasts: Role of 5-hydroxytryptamine 2A receptor and transporter. *Am J Respir Crit Care Med* 170:252-259, 2004.

64. Loyd JE, Atkinson JB, Pietra GG, et al: Heterogeneity of pathologic lesions in familial primary pulmonary hypertension. *Am Rev Respir Dis* 138:952-957, 1988.

65. Bjornsson J, Edwards WD: Primary pulmonary hypertension: A histopathologic study of 80 cases. *Mayo Clin Proc* 60:16-25, 1985.

66. Rees DC, Cox M, Clegg JB: World distribution of factor V Leiden. *Lancet* 346:1133-1134, 1995.

67. Ridker PM: Factor V Leiden and recurrent venous thromboembolism. *Thromb Haemost* 76:815-816, 1996.

68. Elliott CG, Leppert MF, Alexander GJ, et al: Factor V Leiden is not common in patients diagnosed with primary pulmonary hypertension. *Eur Respir J* 12:1177-1180, 1998.

69. Tuder RM, Voelkel NF: Pulmonary hypertension and inflammation. *J Lab Clin Med* 132:16-24, 1998.

70. Cool CD, Rai PR, Yeager ME, et al: Expression of human herpesvirus 8 in primary pulmonary hypertension. *N Engl J Med* 349:1113-1122, 2003.

71. Mette SA, Palevsky HI, Pietra GG, et al: Primary pulmonary hypertension in association with human immunodeficiency virus infection. A possible viral etiology for some forms of hypertensive pulmonary arteriopathy. *Am Rev Respir Dis* 145:1196-2000, 1992.

72. Abenhaim L, Moride Y, Brenot F, et al: Appetite-suppressant drugs and the risk of primary pulmonary hypertension. International Primary Pulmonary Hypertension Study Group. *N Engl J Med* 335: 609-616, 1996.

73. Yeager ME, Halley GR, Golpon HA, et al: Microsatellite instability of endothelial cell growth and apoptosis genes within plexiform lesions in primary pulmonary hypertension. *Circ Res* 88:E2-E11, 2001.

74. Grunig E, Janssen B, Mereles D, et al: Abnormal pulmonary artery pressure response in asymptomatic carriers of primary pulmonary hypertension gene. *Circulation* 102:1145-1150, 2000.

75. Alexander GJ, Elliott CG, Leppert MF, et al: Genetic anticipation is present in nine families with familial primary pulmonary hypertension. *Am J Respir Crit Care Med* 151:A723, 1995.

76. Fu YH, Kuhl DP, Pizzuti A, et al: Variation of the CGG repeat at the fragile X site results in genetic instability: Resolution of the Sherman paradox. *Cell* 67:1047-1058, 1991.

77. Verkerk AJ, Pieretti M, Sutcliffe JS, et al: Identification of a gene *(FMR-1)* containing a CGG repeat coincident with a breakpoint cluster region exhibiting length variation in fragile X syndrome. *Cell* 65:905-914, 1991.

78. Fu YH, Pizzuti A, Fenwick RG, Jr., et al: An unstable triplet repeat in a gene related to myotonic muscular dystrophy. *Science* 255:1256-1258, 1992.

79. Mahadevan M, Tsilfidis C, Sabourin L, et al: Myotonic dystrophy mutation: An unstable CTG repeat in the 3' untranslated region of the gene. *Science* 255:1253-1255, 1992.

80. Campuzano V, Montermini L, Molto MD, et al: Friedreich's ataxia: Autosomal recessive disease caused by an intronic GAA triplet repeat expansion. *Science* 271:1423-1427, 1996.

81. Elliott G, Alexander G, Leppert M, et al: Coancestry in apparently sporadic primary pulmonary hypertension. *Chest* 108:973-977, 1995.

82. Newman JH, Wheeler L, Lane KB, et al: Mutation in the gene for bone morphogenetic protein receptor II as a cause of primary pulmonary hypertension in a large kindred. *N Engl J Med* 345:319-324, 2001.

83. Newman JH, Trembath RC, Morse JA, et al: Genetic basis of pulmonary arterial hypertension: Current understanding and future directions. *J Am Coll Cardiol* 43(12 Suppl S):33S-39S, 2004.

84. Koehler R, Grunig E, Pauciulo MW, et al: Low frequency of *BMPR2* mutations in a German cohort of patients with sporadic idiopathic pulmonary arterial hypertension. *J Med Genet* 41:e127, 2004.

85. Grunig E, Koehler R, Miltenberger-Miltenyi G, et al: Primary pulmonary hypertension in children may have a different genetic background than in adults. *Pediatr Res* 56:571-578, 2004.

86. Pietra GG, Capron F, Stewart S, et al: Pathologic assessment of vasculopathies in pulmonary hypertension. *J Am Coll Cardiol* 43(12 Suppl S):25S-32S, 2004.

87. Wagenvoort CA, Beetstra A, Spijker J: Capillary haemangiomatosis of the lungs. *Histopathology* 2:401-406, 1978.

88. Langleben D, Heneghan JM, Batten AP, et al: Familial pulmonary capillary hemangiomatosis resulting in primary pulmonary hypertension. *Ann Intern Med* 109:106-109, 1988.

89. Runo JR, Vnencak-Jones CL, Prince M, et al: Pulmonary veno-occlusive disease caused by an inherited mutation in bone morphogenetic protein receptor II. *Am J Respir Crit Care Med* 167:889-894, 2003.

90. Humbert M, Deng Z, Simonneau G, et al: *BMPR2* germline mutations in pulmonary hypertension associated with fenfluramine derivatives. *Eur Respir J* 20:518-523, 2002.

91. Scholand MB, Singh NA, Leppert M, et al: *BMPR2* mutations are uncommon in North American patients with appetite suppressant associated pulmonary arterial hypertension. *Am J Respir Crit Care Med* 167:A167, 2003.

92. Schneider MD, Gaussin V, Lyons KM: Tempting fate: BMP signals for cardiac morphogenesis. *Cytokine Growth Factor Rev* 14:1-4, 2003.

93. Hogan BL: Bone morphogenetic proteins: Multifunctional regulators of vertebrate development. *Genes Dev* 10:1580-1594, 1996.

94. Roberts KE, McElroy JJ, Wong WP, et al: *BMPR2* mutations in pulmonary arterial hypertension with congenital heart disease. *Eur Respir J* 24:371-374, 2004.

95. Tew MB, Arnett FC, Reveille JD, et al: Mutations of bone morphogenetic protein receptor type II are not found in patients with pulmonary hypertension and underlying connective tissue diseases. *Arthritis Rheum* 46:2829-2830, 2002.

96. Morse J, Barst R, Horn E, et al: Pulmonary hypertension in scleroderma spectrum of disease: Lack of bone morphogenetic protein receptor 2 mutations. *J Rheumatol* 29:2379-2381, 2002.

97. Farber HW, Loscalzo J: Pulmonary arterial hypertension. *N Engl J Med* 351:1655-1665, 2004.

98. Nunes H, Humbert M, Sitbon O, et al: Prognostic factors for survival in human immunodeficiency virus-associated pulmonary arterial hypertension. *Am J Respir Crit Care Med* 167:1433-1439, 2003.

99. Meyrick B, Reid L: Hypoxia and incorporation of 3H-thymidine by cells of the rat pulmonary arteries and alveolar wall. *Am J Pathol* 96:51-70, 1979.

100. Timms RM, Khaja FU, Williams GW: Hemodynamic response to oxygen therapy in chronic obstructive pulmonary disease. *Ann Intern Med* 102:29-36, 1985.

101. Groves BM, Droma T, Sutton JR, et al: Minimal hypoxic pulmonary hypertension in normal Tibetans at 3,658 m. *J Appl Physiol* 74:312-318, 1993.

102. Niermeyer S, Yang P, Shanmina, et al: Arterial oxygen saturation in Tibetan and Han infants born in Lhasa, Tibet. *N Engl J Med* 333:1248-1252, 1995.

103. Aldashev AA, Sarybaev AS, Sydykov AS, et al: Characterization of high-altitude pulmonary hypertension in the Kyrgyz: Association with angiotensin-converting enzyme genotype. *Am J Respir Crit Care Med* 166:1396-1402, 2002.

104. Abraham WT, Raynolds MV, Gottschall B, et al: Importance of angiotensin-converting enzyme in pulmonary hypertension. *Cardiology* 86(Suppl 1): 9-15, 1995.

105. Kanazawa H, Otsuka T, Hirata K, et al: Association between the angiotensin-converting enzyme gene polymorphisms and tissue oxygenation during exercise in patients with COPD. *Chest* 121:697-701, 2002.

106. Burke W: Genetic testing. *N Engl J Med* 347:1867-1875, 2002.

107. Havlena G, Elliott CG, Carlquist J: Comprehensive variation scanning of the *BMPR2* gene using high resolution melting curve analysis. *Am J Respir Crit Care Proc* 169:A397, 2004.

108. Reed G, Wittwer CT: Sensitivity and specificity of single nucleotide polymorphism scanning by high-resolution melting analysis. *Clin Chem* 50:1748-1754, 2004.

109. Glissmeyer E, Havlena GT, Schmidt J, et al: *BMPR2* mutations identify patients with pulmonary arterial hypertension who are unlikely to demonstrate vasoreactivity. *Am J Respir Crit care Proc* 2:A192, 2005.

110. McGoon M, Gutterman D, Steen V, et al: Screening, early detection, and diagnosis of pulmonary arterial hypertension: ACCP evidence-based clinical practice guidelines. *Chest* 126(1 Suppl):14S-34S, 2004.

5 Chapter

Classification and Prognosis of Pulmonary Arterial Hypertension

Eliot B. Friedman, MD,

Harold I. Palevsky, MD,

Darren B. Taichman, MD, PhD

Introduction

What is now termed "idiopathic pulmonary arterial hypertension" (IPAH) was first described over 100 years ago, but during the past two decades intense basic and clinical investigations have led to major advances in therapy. Although IPAH is a rare disease, intensely focused epidemiologic studies have provided insight into both its natural history as well as the impact of current therapies on this and other forms of pulmonary hypertension (PH). This rapid pace of advances has prompted several recent changes in the classification of these diseases. Factors that previously predicted survival may no longer be as informative in an era of routinely employed effective therapies, while newly recognized prognostic factors have emerged. This chapter briefly outlines the evolution of the classification of PH and addresses risks and prognostic factors for pulmonary arterial hypertension (PAH). The prognosis of patients with PH associated with chronic respiratory diseases and hypoxemia is discussed in Chapter 10 and PAH in association with pregnancy in Chapter 17.

A Brief History of Classification

In 1891, Ernst von Romberg described the "Uber Sklerose der Lungen Arterie" (sclerosis of the pulmonary arteries) to explain abnormalities in the pulmonary blood vessels for which he was unable to uncover a cause.[1] In 1901, Abel Ayerza of Argentina used the term "cardiacos negros" for patients with a syndrome of PH and right ventricular failure. His colleagues subsequently referred to the disease as "Ayerza's disease" and believed it developed as a result of syphilitic pulmonary arteritis. This hypothesis prevailed until the 1940s, when Oscar Brenner reviewed 100 case reports of PH from the Massachusetts General Hospital. He examined the histopathologic lesions present in the muscular arteries and concluding that syphilis was not the cause.[2] The widespread introduction of cardiac catheterization during the 1950s initiated a new era when investigators could move beyond morphologic description and begin to study the disease in living patients from a physiologic perspective.

In 1951, David Dresdale and colleagues described a hypertensive vasculopathy of the pulmonary circulation. It involved vasoconstriction and an elevation in pulmonary arterial pressures that responded to the injection of the α-adrenergic antagonist vasodilator, tolazoline.[3] No cause could be found for the vasculopathy, and the term "primary pulmonary hypertension" (PPH) was coined. Cases of PH in which a demonstrable cause could be established were labeled "secondary" PH (e.g., PH secondary to left ventricular failure, chronic pulmonary diseases, hypoxemia, etc.).[4] Subsequently, Paul Wood employed a vasodilator that was eliminated within the pulmonary circulation (acetylcholine), thus allowing for a pulmonary-specific response when studying patients with PAH. Wood postulated that a "vasoconstrictive factor" was present and responsible for the disease.[2] In 1970, Wagenvoort and Wagenvoort described the extensive vascular injury and remodeling in a pathology series of 156 patients with PPH as "plexogenic pulmonary arteriopathy," believed to be pathognomonic of the disease.[5]

In the late 1960s and early 1970s, an epidemic of PAH in Australia, Switzerland, and West Germany was associated with the appetite suppressant drug, aminorex.[2] Prompted by this and related developments, the World Health Organization (WHO) sponsored an international working group that met in 1973 and proposed the first formal classification scheme of the disease. It was based primarily on histopathologic findings and included plexogenic pulmonary arteriopathy, thrombotic pulmonary arteriopathy, and pulmonary venous occlusive disease.[6] The working group also proposed that a multicenter collaborative study be conducted to better define the epidemiologic, clinical, and pathologic features of PPH (now termed IPAH).

In 1981, the National Institutes of Health (NIH) launched a multicenter prospective Registry for the Characterization of Primary Pulmonary Hypertension.[7] The registry enrolled 187 patients from 32 centers from 1981 to 1985. A hemodynamic definition of disease was adopted and except for minor modification has remained the standard used in practice and in clinical trials: PH is defined as a mean pulmonary arterial pressure (mPAP) of greater than 25 mmHg at rest or greater than 30 mmHg with exercise. A diagnostic evaluation for secondary causes of PH was standardized. The NIH registry was successful not only in furthering an understanding of PPH, but also in establishing an appropriate model to obtain epidemiologic, clinical, and pathologic information on a rare disease, and to foster continued cooperative investigation. As described by Dr. Alfred Fishman, the NIH registry "sharpened clinical and pathologic diagnostic criteria, provided a standardized format for data collection, led to the exploration and systematic evaluation of pulmonary vasodilators, promoted subsequent cooperative studies among the investigators at various centers, and promoted public awareness of the disease."[2]

In 1998, the Second World Symposium on Pulmonary Hypertension was held in Evian, France, at which the classification of PH as "primary" or "secondary" was abandoned.[8] The term "secondary" was problematic because of the heterogeneous nature of the conditions included. Many bore significant resemblance to PPH as diseases in which the pathogenesis appeared to directly involve the pulmonary vasculature. In addition, there were similarities in the clinical responses to therapy among PPH and certain "secondary" forms of PAH (e.g., PAH developing following the ingestion of appetite suppressant drugs or in patients with human immunodeficiency virus [HIV] infection). Thus, the 1998 Evian classification distinguished among conditions that directly affected the pulmonary vasculature (i.e., PAH) from those disorders in which the pulmonary circulation was affected by pulmonary venous hypertension (e.g., left heart ventricular or valvular disease) or by lung disease affecting respiratory function and structure. Although the term "secondary pulmonary hypertension" was abandoned, PPH was retained because of its familiarity.[9,10]

In 2003, a Third World Symposium on Pulmonary Arterial Hypertension convened in Venice, Italy, to address additional advances. These included the recognition that recently identified genetic factors responsible for familial cases of PAH appeared to be important in many sporadic, nonfamilial cases, as well. In addition, there was a growing awareness of overlap in histologic and certain clinical features in the disorders under the groupings of PAH and pulmonary veno-occlusive disease (classified as a form of pulmonary venous hypertension in the Evian nomenclature) and pulmonary capillary hemangiomatosis (included under a heterogenous group of disorders). The term "PPH" was abandoned in favor of "idiopathic" within the group of diseases known as "PAH," and both pulmonary veno-occlusive disease and pulmonary capillary hemangiomatosis were added to the same category (TABLE 5-1).[10] Maintained was the emphasis on distinguishing disorders under the grouping PAH from conditions involving PH caused by left-sided heart disease or respiratory function with resulting hypoxemia. Each successively adopted classification scheme has included a separate grouping of PH associated with chronic thromboembolic or other forms of pulmonary embolism (e.g., tumor cells or parasites).

Epidemiology of Pulmonary Arterial Hypertension

Risk Factors and Associated Conditions

The Second World Symposium on Pulmonary Arterial Hypertension also assessed the strength of data regarding risk factors for PAH. Factors

TABLE 5-1

Clinical Classification of Pulmonary Arterial Hypertension as adopted at the Third World Symposium on Pulmonary Arterial Hypertension (Venice, 2003) [4, 10]

Pulmonary Arterial Hypertension (PAH)
 Idiopathic (IPAH)
 Familial (FPAH)
 Associated with (APAH):
  Collagen vascular disease
  Congenital systemic-to-pulmonary shunts (large, small, repaired or nonrepaired)
  Portal hypertension
  HIV infection
  Drugs and toxins
  Other (glycogen storage disease, Gaucher disease, hereditary hemorrhagic telangiectasia, hemoglobinopathies, myeloproliferative disorders, splenectomy)
 Associated with significant venous or capillary involvement
  Pulmonary veno-occlusive disease
  Pulmonary capillary hemangiomatosis
Pulmonary venous hypertension
 Left-sided atrial or ventricular heart disease
 Left-sided valvular heart disease
Pulmonary hypertension associated with hypoxemia
 COPD
 Interstitial lung disease
 Sleep-disordered breathing
 Alveolar hypoventilation disorders
 Chronic exposure to high altitude
PH due to chronic thrombotic and/or embolic disease
 Thromboembolic obstruction of proximal pulmonary arteries
 Thromboembolic obstruction of distal pulmonary arteries
 Pulmonary embolism (tumor, parasites, foreign material)
Miscellaneous
 Sarcoidosis, histiocytosis X, lymphangiomatosis, compression of pulmonary vessels (adenopathy, tumor, fibrosing mediastinitis)

Reproduced with permission from [4, 10]

were categorized according to the strength of the evidence supporting their causal relationship or association with PAH. Some were categorized as "definite" risk factors or associations on the basis of controlled studies or clear-cut epidemics (e.g., a causal role of fenfluramine derivatives in anorexigen-induced PAH).[11,12] Others were termed "possible" risks or associations on the basis of fewer definitive data (e.g., case series). Intermediate levels of evidence were ranked accordingly (TABLE 5-2).

Idiopathic Pulmonary Arterial Hypertension

IPAH is a rare disease with an incidence estimated from 1 to 2 cases per million in industrialized countries.[11,13] The estimated incidence in a study from Israel was 1.4 new cases per million population per year; the estimated prevalence was 8 cases per million people.[14] IPAH affects young people, more commonly women. Among the 187 patients in the NIH registry, the mean age was 36.4 years, and age was similar for men and women (FIGURE 5-1).[7] Women outnumbered men, however, by a ratio of 1.7:1. Although generally a disease occurring in the third or fourth decade, IPAH can also emerge in elderly patients,[15] although the frequency is not well established. Only 9 percent of patients in the NIH registry were older than 60 years. The distribution of patients according to race and ethnicity in the NIH registry was similar to that of the general population, with 12.3 percent of patients described as African American and 2.3 percent described as Hispanic. Twelve cases (6 percent) were identified as familial PAH (defined by the presence of disease in a first-order blood relative).

A case series describing the experience from a PAH referral center in France between 1981 and 1992 included 173 patients and yielded very similar demographic characteristics as found in the

TABLE 5-2

Risk Factors for and Conditions Associated With the Development of Pulmonary Arterial Hypertension (as Assessed at the Second World Symposium on Pulmonary Arterial Hypertension, Evian, France, 1998)

A. Drugs and Toxins

1. Definite

Aminorex
Fenfluramine
Dexfenfluramine
Toxic rapeseed oil

2. Very Likely

Amphetamines
L-tryptophan

3. Possible

Meta-amphetamines
Cocaine
Chemotherapeutic agents

4. Unlikely

Antidepressants
Oral contraceptives
Estrogen therapy
Cigarette smoking

B. Demographic and Medical Conditions

1. Definite

Gender

2. Possible

Pregnancy
Systemic hypertension

3. Unlikely

Obesity

C. Diseases

1. Definite

HIV infection

2. Very Likely

Portal hypertension, liver disease
Collagen vascular diseases
Congenital systemic-pulmonary-cardiac shunts

3. Possible

Thyroid disorders

HIV, *human immunodeficiency virus.*
From Simonneau G, Galie N, Rubin LJ, et al: Clinical classification of pulmonary hypertension. J Am Coll Cardiol *43(12 Suppl S):5S-12S, 2004.*

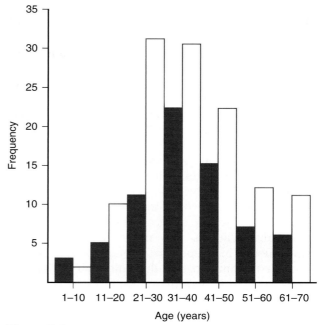

Figure 5-1. Distribution of patients with idiopathic pulmonary arterial hypertension entered into the National Institutes of Health Registry for the Characterization of Primary Pulmonary Hypertension. Patients entered into the registry were most often in their third and fourth decades of life, with a similar ratio of women to men (1.7:1) in all decades. *Open bars* represent women; *shaded bars* represent men. (Reproduced with permission from Rich S, Dantzker DR, Ayres SM, et al: Primary pulmonary hypertension. A national prospective study. *Ann Intern Med* 107(2):216-223, 1987.)

NIH registry,[16] as did a retrospective series from Japan involving 223 patients. In a retrospective series of 44 patients from Israel, the average age at onset was slightly higher (42.8 years), with a ratio of women to men of 3.4:1.[14] A prospective cohort of 61 patients from Mexico had a younger average age at onset (22.6 years) and a male-to-female ratio of 3:1.[17] Whether these discrepancies reflect true differences in the distribution of the disease across populations or were due to biases of enrollment in the individual studies remains unclear.

Clinical Findings at the Time of Diagnosis

The mean time from the onset of symptoms to diagnosis among patients in the NIH registry was 2.03 years, similar for men and women.[7] Dyspnea was the most common symptom when medical intervention was sought, occurring in 60 percent of patients. By the time patients were enrolled in the registry, fatigue was present in 73 percent of patients, chest pain in 47 percent, near syncope or syncope in 41 and 36 percent, respectively, edema in 37 percent, and palpitations in 33 percent. At the time of diagnosis, 75 percent of female patients and 64 percent of male patients were judged to have either class III or IV World Health Organization (WHO) functional class symptoms.

On physical examination, 93 percent of patients had an increased P_2 component of the second heart sound; right-sided third and fourth heart sounds were also common, as was a tricuspid regurgitant murmur. Cyanosis was reported in 20 percent and edema in 32 percent. Abnormal test results included prominence of the pulmonary artery on chest x-ray in 90 percent of cases; hilar vessels were enlarged in 98 percent and markings of peripheral vessels decreased in 51 percent. Most patients had signs of right ventricular strain on their electro-cardiograms (ECG). Among pulmonary function tests, the diffusing capacity for carbon monoxide was decreased in 69 percent of patients.

Initial hemodynamic testing found that the average mPAP was 60 + 18 mmHg and mean right atrial pressure (mRAP) was 9 + 6 mmHg. The mean cardiac index was 2.2 + 0.9 L/min/m². Hemodynamic values were similar for men and women. mPAP and mRAP were higher and cardiac index lower in patients with either WHO class III or IV symptoms. Similar hemodynamic variables were found in series of patients from France[16] and Israel[14]; however, mPAP was significantly higher (93 mmHg) in a cohort from Mexico, perhaps due to the high altitude at the study center.[17]

Prognosis of Idiopathic Pulmonary Arterial Hypertension

The prognosis of IPAH in the absence of effective therapy is very poor. In the NIH registry, the median survival of patients with IPAH was 2.8 years. The estimated rate of survival was 68 percent after 1 year, 48 percent after 3 years, and 34 percent after 5 years.[7] Other studies conducted in Mexico, Japan, and India show comparable survival rates for IPAH.[18] In one retrospective study of 120 patients with IPAH during the 1980s, only 21 percent survived 5 years; the cause of death was right ventricular failure in 63 percent of cases, pneumonia in 7 percent, and sudden death in 7

percent.[19] Fortunately, the introduction of effective therapies has improved survival significantly, as discussed below.

Factors Associated With Prognosis

Demographics

Age has not been established consistently as an independent predictor of survival in patients with IPAH, and increased mortality seen in elderly patients with PAH has been thought related to co-existing conditions.[20] In a retrospective cohort of 34 patients with IPAH evaluated between 1961 and 1981, some of whom were treated with warfarin but none with vasodilators, there was no relation between age at diagnosis and mean survival.[21] In contrast, older age at the time of disease onset was associated with a worsened survival in a cohort of 91 patients who were treated with epoprostenol.[22] No relationship between age and survival was seen in the patients in either the NIH registry or the series of patients from Israel,[14] whereas younger age was associated with a shorter length of survival in a series of 61 patients from India.[23] Published data are similarly inconsistent regarding the influence of the duration of symptoms before diagnosis on survival in IPAH.[14,24] Survival of men and women have been similar in several studies spanning periods both before and since the availability of effective therapies.[21,24-28] In one retrospective series of patients receiving standard therapies between 1994 and 2002, nonwhite race was identified as an independent poor prognostic factor, with patients who were of either African American or of Asian descent demonstrating an increased risk of death.[28]

Physical Examination

Few data support the use of physical examination findings to predict prognosis. In one retrospective study, Okada and others reported data on patients between 1980 and 1990 in Japan and found that those who died less than 1 year following initial cardiac catheterization had a faster heart rate than those who lived 1 year or more (93.6 versus 81.7 beats per minute, P = .007).[29] A prospective study of 60 patients with IPAH similarly found baseline heart rate to be related to mortality during an average follow-up of 24 months.[27] Other physical examination findings common among patients with significant PAH, such as an increased pulmonic component of the second heart sound, a right ventricular parasternal heave, right sided

S_3 gallop, or an S_4 gallop, have not been predictive of prognosis.

Functional Class

Functional status, as assessed by the WHO functional class (TABLE 5-3), is associated with survival in IPAH. Prognosis of patients with more advanced symptoms (WHO classes III and IV) has been worse than that of patients with less severe symptoms (classes I and II) in studies both before and since the introduction of effective therapies. In the NIH registry, the median survival of patients with either WHO class I or II symptoms was 58.6 months, as compared with 31.5 months for patients with class III and only 6 months with class IV symptoms.[7,24] Even with effective therapy such as epoprostenol, more advanced WHO functional class remains a significant risk factor for shorter length of survival.[14,22,26,30] For example, in a retrospective study of 162 patients treated with epoprostenol, those with baseline WHO class III symptoms had 3-year and 5-year survival rates of 81 and 79 percent, as compared with 47 and 27 percent, respectively, among patients with baseline WHO class IV symptoms.[25] Functional class remains an indicator of prognosis even after the institution of effective therapy, because patients with persistent class III or IV symptoms after several months of epoprostenol therapy have a significantly worse prognosis than those whose symptoms have improved to either class II or better.[25,26]

Electrocardiogram

The ECG can also be used as a prognostic marker in IPAH. In a prospective study of 51 patients with IPAH between 1992 and 1998, Bossone and colleagues found that ECG changes indicating abnormalities of the right ventricle were associated with a significantly increased risk of premature mortality. Management during the study period included epoprostenol, calcium channel antagonists, atrial septostomy, and lung transplantation. In particular, an increase in the amplitude of the P wave in lead II, a QR pattern in V_1, and right ventricular hypertrophy by WHO standards was each associated with shorter length of survival.[30]

Pulmonary Function Testing

Studies of the prognostic value of pulmonary function test findings have yielded inconsistent results. A decreased diffusing capacity for carbon monoxide was found to be predictive of a poorer outcome in patients with PAH associated with systemic sclerosis (SS)[22] but only weakly correlated with length of survival in some patients with IPAH.[24] The correlation has not been significant in other studies of patients with SS.[31] In a single study of patients with IPAH, a reduction in forced vital capacity was correlated with poorer survival.[17] Overall, pulmonary function testing currently is not helpful in predicting survival in patients with PAH.[18]

Exercise Testing

Exercise tolerance in patients with PAH is commonly evaluated with a 6-minute walk test (6MWT). Most patients, even those with right heart dysfunction or hypoxia, can complete this straightforward study in which the subject walks as far as possible on a flat surface for 6 minutes.[32,33] Protocols have varied, and certain studies have included some element of subject "encouragement," although most protocols prefer an "unencouraged" measurement.

TABLE 5-3

World Health Organization Functional Assessment Classification

Class I: Patients with PH but without resulting limitation of physical activity. Ordinary physical activity does not cause undue dyspnea or fatigue, chest pain, or near syncope.
Class II: Patients with PH resulting in slight limitation of physical activity. They are comfortable at rest. Ordinary physical activity causes undue dyspnea or fatigue, chest pain, or near syncope.
Class III: Patients with PH resulting in marked limitation of physical activity. They are comfortable at rest. Less than ordinary activity causes undue dyspnea or fatigue, chest pain, or near syncope.
Class IV: Patients with PH with inability to carry out any physical activity without symptoms. These patients manifest signs of right heart failure. Dyspnea and fatigue may even be present at rest. Discomfort is increased by any physical activity.

PH, *pulmonary hypertension.*
Adapted with permission from Rubin LJ: Diagnosis and management of pulmonary arterial hypertension: ACCP evidence-based clinical practice guidelines. Chest 126(1 Suppl):7S-10S, 2004.

6MWT distance correlates with maximal oxygen consumption ($\overset{\circ}{V}O_2$max) determined by full cardiopulmonary exercise testing in patients with PAH. In a study of 43 patients with IPAH who underwent pretreatment evaluations, the 6MWT distance was independently associated with survival. Most patients in this study were treated with epoprostenol or beraprost; a minority (n = 5) was intolerant of either treatment. Patients who were able to walk farther than 332 meters at baseline had a significantly longer survival after a mean follow-up of almost 2 years (FIGURE 5-2).[32]

Pretreatment 6MWT distance was also predictive of survival in a randomized trial of epoprostenol therapy for IPAH.[34] Although patients randomized to only "conventional" treatment had a lower baseline value, the 6MWT distance was an independent predictor of survival for the entire study population. All patients who died had a 6MWT distance of less than 150 meters. After a mean follow-up of 37 months in this cohort, the 6MWT distance remained an independent predictor of survival on univariate but not multivariate analysis.[35] In another study of 178 patients treated with continuous epoprostenol, a pretreatment 6MWT distance of less than 250 meters was associated with a worse prog-

nosis on univariate analysis. After 3 months of therapy, the absolute distance walked in the 6MWT was predictive of survival, although the change from the baseline value was not.[26]

In a cohort of 86 consecutive patients with IPAH, 70 were able to complete full cardiopulmonary exercise testing (CPET) with either a treadmill or cycle ergometer.[33] Most of these patients had WHO class III or IV symptoms, and treatments included calcium channel antagonists, anticoagulation, and oxygen; only two patients received iloprost. On multivariate analysis, a maximal oxygen consumption of greater than 10.4 ml/kg/min or an exercise peak systolic blood pressure greater than 120 mmHg were each associated with a better 1-year survival.

The fidelity of the 6MWT distance to discern changes may wane as exercise capacity improves (i.e., at greater distances). A recent analysis of data from a randomized controlled trial of sitaxsentan management for PAH demonstrated a "ceiling effect" such that patients with better baseline function (greater 6MWT distance) demonstrated less significant improvements in walk distance in response to therapy.[36] These findings may make the 6MWT distance less useful as an end point in clinical trials. A similar effect has not been evaluated in studies of the 6MWT distance as a prognostic indicator.

Echocardiography

Echocardiography is a widely available noninvasive test useful in screening for PH. Findings on echocardiogram are also useful in assessing prognosis in patients with IPAH. The presence and severity of a pericardial effusion are associated with an increased risk of death.[28,35,37,38] In a series of 26 patients treated with or without calcium channel antagonists during the 1980s, the severity of a pericardial effusion was independently associated with a shorter survival.[37] Follow-up of patients enrolled in a randomized trial of epoprostenol treatment[34] similarly revealed that a larger pericardial effusion was associated with an increased risk of death or lung transplantation after 1 year.[38] After a mean follow-up of 37 ± 15 months in 81 of these same patients, the hazard ratio of death or lung transplantation for patients with a pericardial effusion at baseline (versus no effusion) was 4.38 (95 percent confidence interval 1.41 – 13.67; p = 0.01)[35] Enlargement of the right atrium on echocardiogram was also associated with an increased risk of death.

An echocardiographic index of right ventricular function (also known at the "Tei index") measures the combined isovolumetric contraction and relaxation times divided by the right ventricular ejection time. A higher index signifies worsened right ventricular function and is associated with a poorer

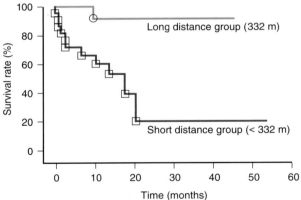

Figure 5-2. Survival in idiopathic pulmonary arterial hypertension according to 6-minute walk test distance. Kaplan-Meier survival curves according to the median value of distance walked in meters *(m)* during a 6-minute walk test. Patients unable to walk more than 332 meters had a lower survival (P < .001). (Reproduced with permission from Miyamoto S, Nagaya N, Satoh T, et al: Clinical correlates and prognostic significance of six-minute walk test in patients with primary pulmonary hypertension. Comparison with cardiopulmonary exercise testing. *Am J Respir Crit Care Med* 161(2 Pt 1):487-492, 2000.)

prognosis in IPAH. In a study of 53 patients treated with anticoagulation (in 79 percent), calcium channel antagonists (58 percent), or prostaglandins (26 percent), transplant-free survival after 5 years was only 4 percent among those with an elevated Doppler right ventricular index (>.83) as compared with 73% when the index was lower.[39]

Hemodynamic Measurements

The prognostic value of hemodynamic variables has been assessed in many descriptive and intervention studies of patients with IPAH. Despite isolated differences among studies, as a whole these studies have indicated that hemodynamic values reflecting right-sided heart failure are associated with a poorer prognosis. Thus, an increased mean right atrial pressure (mRAP) and a decreased cardiac index (CI) each portend a poorer prognosis in patients with IPAH. Although an increasing mean pulmonary artery pressure (mPAP) has been associated with a poorer prognosis in many studies, lower values have correlated with shorter survival in others— perhaps reflecting the natural history of right-sided heart failure in PAH. The mPAP initially rises progressively as vascular derangements worsen, but declines later as the right heart fails and is no longer able to generate increased pressures (FIGURE 5-3).

In the NIH registry, an increased mRAP, mPAP, and decreased CI were each associated with a higher risk of death and were incorporated into a regression equation used to determine the probability of survival[24] (FIGURE 5-4). In a subsequent study of 61 patients with IPAH during the same era and receiv-

ing similar treatments as patients in the NIH registry, the positive predictive value of the NIH equation was 87 percent after 1 year, 91 percent after 2 years, and 89 percent after 3 years.[17] Of the three

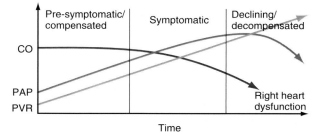

Figure 5-3. Hemodynamic changes with progression of pulmonary arterial hypertension. Schematic representation of the changes in cardiac output *(CO)*, mean pulmonary artery pressure *(PAP)* and pulmonary vascular resistance *(PVR)* in the absence of effective therapy. PVR rises progressively as the vascular derangements progress, eventually leading to the development of right heart dysfunction. PAPs initially rise as the right ventricle remains capable of generating the increased pressures required to maintain a given degree of cardiac output. Note, however, that with more advanced disease CO decreases and the PAP falls because the failing right ventricle is unable to generate increased pressures.

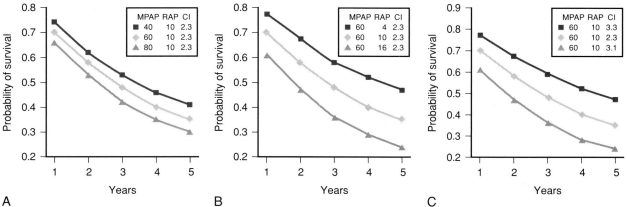

Figure 5-4. Probability of survival for patients with idiopathic pulmonary arterial hypertension according to the National Institutes of Health (NIH) Registry equation and before the availability of many current therapies. Differences in survival are shown as each mean pulmonary artery pressure *(MPAP)*, right atrial pressure *(MRAP)* and cardiac index *(CI)* are varied (in **A**, **B**, and **C**, respectively). The probability of survival is calculated according to the NIH registry equation[24] derived from patients enrolled between 1981 and 1985 and thus before the use of many currently approved therapies. (Reproduced with permission from McGoon MD: Prognosis and natural history. In: Rubin LJ, Rich S, editors: *Primary pulmonary hypertension,* New York, 1996, Marcel Dekker, pp 305-317.)

variables used in the NIH equation, mRAP has most consistently been a significant indicator of prognosis in other studies,[14,17,23,29] mPAP and CI less consistently so. Additional variables including resting heart rate, mixed venous oxygen saturation, and pulmonary vascular resistance have been identified as prognostic factors in other studies.[17,37,40]

Testing for acute pulmonary vasoreactivity to short-acting vasodilators is performed routinely during right heart catheterization as a means of identifying the few patients who are likely to respond to long-term treatment with oral calcium channel antagonists (see Chapter 7). A significant acute response, however, has significant prognostic information. What constitutes a significant hemodynamic response, however, has varied among studies. Rich and others used a reduction by at least 20 percent in both mPAP and PVR to identify 17 "responders" (from a group of 64 tested) who were subsequently treated with high doses of calcium channel antagonists. The 5-year survival for "responders" was 94 percent, as compared with 55 percent of "nonresponders" and 38 percent for patients from the NIH registry.[41] Although definitions of response have varied, a survival benefit has been similarly shown in additional studies treating responders with a calcium channel antagonist.[17,42,43]

The prognostic implication of acute vasoreactivity is less clear in patients treated with therapies other than calcium channel antagonists. Indeed, acutely responsive patients generally are treated with calcium channel antagonists because of the benefits discussed above. McLaughlin and coworkers have shown that the magnitudes of improvement in mPAP and CI following acute vasodilator administration at baseline were significantly correlated with improved survival among patients treated with long-term epoprostenol infusion.[25] No such correlation was reported at long-term follow-up of another cohort of patients treated with epoprostenol.[26] Although a significant survival benefit was observed for patients who were not acutely responsive in a randomized trial of epoprostenol, therapy was not randomized according to baseline vasoreactivity, so its prognostic importance could not be assessed.[34,44] In a retrospective analysis of 84 patients treated with calcium channel antagonists, prostanoids, bosentan, warfarin, or a combination, a lack of acute vasoreactivity at baseline was associated with a worse outcome for the whole cohort.[28]

Serum Markers

Blood levels of several proteins or metabolic products can be elevated in patients with PAH and have significant prognostic value. Serum uric acid (UA) levels are increased in hypoxemic states because of the degradation of adenosine nucleotides to their purine building blocks and UA. Serum UA is increased over normal in patients with IPAH,[45] and levels correlate with elevations in right atrial pressure.[46] Nagaya and colleagues followed 102 consecutive patients with PAH for a mean of 31 months from 1980 to 1998 and measured several potential prognostic serum markers. UA correlated with disease severity (as assessed by functional class and hemodynamics) and was an independent predictor of mortality.[45] Elevated plasma von Willebrand factor (vWF) levels were independently associated with survival in patients with IPAH and PAH associated with congenital heart disease.[47] Because vWF is a glycoprotein synthesized and stored in endothelial cells, its release is thought to reflect abnormal endothelial cell function in PAH. Increased plasma D-dimer levels are found in the blood of patients with IPAH, and the degree of elevation is associated with poorer prognosis.[48]

Troponin T (TnT), a serum marker specific for myocardial injury, has been studied in patients with PAH by Torbicki et al in a prospective follow-up of 56 patients (51 with IPAH and 5 with chronic thromboembolic disease). Fourteen percent of patients had elevated levels of TnT (>0.001 ng/ml) at the time of initial evaluation. Despite comparable hemodynamic variables, patients with an elevated TnT had a worse survival rate after 24 months than those with normal TnT levels (29 versus 81 percent). Even after controlling for differences in heart rate and 6MWT distance, an elevated TnT remained an independent risk factor for worse survival rates.[49]

Endothelin is a potent vasoconstrictor peptide with proinflammatory, fibrotic, and mitogenic properties operative in the pathogenesis of PAH. Increased serum endothelin levels correlate with elevations in right atrial pressure and depressions in oxyhemoglobin saturation.[50] Elevated endothelin levels also have functional significance. In one series of 16 consecutive patients, Rubens and others showed that elevated plasma endothelin levels correlated with hemodynamic indictors of disease severity as well as exercise capacity (6MWT distance).[51] Additional serum markers that are elevated in patients with PAH and correlate with hemodynamic measures include catecholamines and atrial natriuretic peptide (ANP).[50,52] Although certain of these hemodynamic values and exercise capacity have been shown to correlate with patient survival, none of the associated elevations in blood levels of endothelin, catecholamine, or ANP has been demonstrated unequivocally as an independent indicator of prognosis.

Levels of brain (B-type) natriuretic peptide (BNP) are associated with survival in PAH. Produced by myocardial cells in response to ventricular volume and pressure overload, BNP is a prognostic factor in left-sided heart failure.[53] Nagaya and colleagues demonstrated elevated levels of BNP in the blood of 60 consecutive patients with IPAH as compared with normal control subjects, and that levels before treatment correlated with WHO functional class and patient survival.[27] BNP levels decreased with improvements in hemodynamic parameters after 3 months of therapy (either epoprostenol or beraprost in most patients), and persistently elevated levels of BNP once again correlated with a poor prognosis. Patients with blood levels of BNP higher than 150 pg/ml before treatment or levels over 180 pg/ml following a mean of 3 months of therapy had a significantly lower survival rate (FIGURE 5-5).

In a retrospective study of 84 patients evaluated between 1994 and 2002 with a median follow-up of over 2 years, a low serum albumin level was associated with an increased risk of death. The association was independent of other measures of hepatic function or right atrial pressure, suggesting that the poorer survival seen with low serum albumin was not merely reflective of passive hepatic congestion and right-sided heart dysfunction.[28]

Changes in Prognosis With Therapy

Since the observational findings of the NIH registry and other cohort studies from the same period, advances in management have changed the prognosis of IPAH. Because of the dismal outcome expected in the absence of therapy, potential changes in survival rates resulting from new treatments frequently have been assessed by comparison with that predicted by the NIH registry equation. One randomized trial and several long-term series have demonstrated improved survival rates with the use of continuously infused epoprostenol. Barst and colleagues randomized 81 patients with IPAH to epoprostenol or conventional therapy in a 12-week trial. Of 41 epoprostenol-treated patients, 1 underwent lung transplantation, whereas 2 of the 40 conventional therapy patients received transplants and 8 died[34]. After long-term epoprostenol therapy in 162 patients, McLaughlin et al observed 1-year and 3-year survival rates were 88 and 62 percent, compared with rates of 59 and 35 percent predicted by the NIH registry equation.[25] Remarkably similar survival rates were observed by Sitbon et al in 178 epoprostenol treated patients after 1 and 3 years (85 and 63 percent, respectively); survival was 55 percent after 5 years of treatment. Here too, significant improvements over outcome predicted by the NIH registry equation were seen.[26] Kuhn and co-workers observed similar (although somewhat lower) survival with

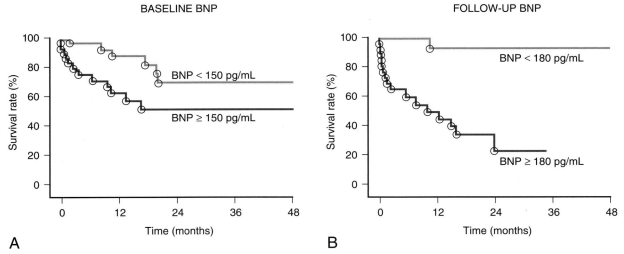

Figure 5-5. Poorer survival in patients with elevated blood levels of brain natriuretic peptide. Kaplan-Meier survival curves according to the median brain natriuretic peptide (BNP) value in patients with idiopathic pulmonary arterial hypertension before *(left)* or after a mean of 3 months of treatment *(right)*. P < .05 for comparison of survival between groups that had higher and lower BNP levels before treatment, and P < .0001 for comparison after treatment. (Reproduced with permission from Nagaya N, Nishikimi T, Uematsu M, et al: Plasma brain natriuretic peptide as a prognostic indicator in patients with primary pulmonary hypertension. *Circulation* 102(8): 865-870, 2000.)

improvement over predicted rates in a cohort of 91 patients.[22] The overall impact of epoprostenol on survival in IPAH has been summarized by McLaughlin and colleagues (FIGURE 5-6).[18]

Comparison with survival predicted by the NIH registry equation has also been used to assess the effect of therapy with the dual endothelin receptor antagonist bosentan. In 169 patients with IPAH who were treated with bosentan in the extension of randomized placebo-controlled trials, survival was 96 percent after 1 year and 89 percent after 2 years, compared with expected rates of 69 and 57 percent, respectively.[54] When patients from these same trials were compared with historical control patients treated with continuously infused epoprostenol, a noninferiority analysis demonstrated similar outcomes after 1 and 2 years.[55] In general, patients treated with epoprostenol in clinical trials and in current clinical practice have been sicker than those treated with oral agents. Prospective randomized trials directly comparing the efficacy of treatments have not been performed, thus limiting the conclusions that can be made regarding their relative impact on survival.

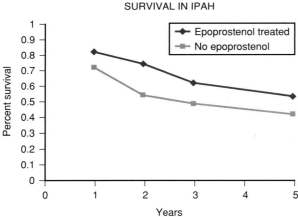

Figure 5-6. Effect of epoprostenol treatment on survival in patients with idiopathic pulmonary arterial hypertension. Estimated survival on the basis of patients treated with epoprostenol in three large series (total of 431 patients), as compared with survival in the absence of treatment predicted by the National Institutes of Health registry equation. (Reproduced with permission from McLaughlin VV, Presberg KW, Doyle RL, et al: Prognosis of pulmonary arterial hypertension: ACCP evidence-based clinical practice guidelines. *Chest* 126(1 Suppl): 78S-92S, 2004.)

The long-term prognosis is good for some patients with IPAH who demonstrate acute vasoreactivity when treated subsequently with calcium channel antagonists. A recent retrospective analysis of 557 patients with IPAH tested for acute vasoreactivity (defined as a fall in both mPAP and PVR of greater then 20 percent) found that survival rates were excellent among patients who were in WHO functional class I or II after at least 1 year of therapy with calcium channel antagonists. Thirty-seven of 38 (97 percent) of such long-term responders were alive after a mean follow-up of 7 years, as opposed to a 5-year survival of only 48 percent among the 32 patients who, despite demonstrating acute vasoreactivity at the time of initial testing, failed to achieve at least WHO functional class II for more than 1 year with calcium antagonist therapy.[43]

In situ thrombosis is seen frequently in patients with IPAH and other forms of PAH, and several nonrandomized studies have suggested that anticoagulation may improve survival. In a prospective nonrandomized trial demonstrating the benefit of calcium channel antagonists in acutely vasoreactive patients, warfarin use was associated with improved outcome, the effect being most significant in those without acute vasoreactivity.[41] Retrospective cohorts of patients with IPAH treated both before[19,41] and since[28] the introduction of currently available effective therapies, and in patients with PAH associated with anorectic agent use,[40] have all found the use of anticoagulants to be associated with a better outcome. Although diuretics and digoxin are used commonly to manage PAH, their effects on outcome have not been well studied.

The continued utility of the NIH registry equation in predicting survival has been questioned. Because this equation was derived from a data set reflecting survival in patients before the introduction of therapies now routinely used in PAH and which, as noted above, improve survival, it may no longer accurately predict survival in patients under the current standard of care. Kawut and co-workers evaluated the accuracy of the NIH registry equation to predict survival determined in a retrospective cohort of 84 patients followed at a single center between 1994 and 2002, during which time treatments included calcium channel antagonists, bosentan, prostanoids, and warfarin. They found that applying the registry equation to baseline values of patients in their cohort underestimated survival.[28] This observation has not been assessed in multicenter studies.

Cardiac Arrest

It is not surprising that the prognosis of patients with IPAH who have suffered cardiac arrest is dismal even when resuscitative efforts are initiated promptly. In a retrospective review of the records of over 3,000 patients, 132 episodes of attempted cardiopulmonary resuscitation following cardiac arrest were identified. Survival at 90 days following resuscitation was only 6 percent.[56]

Pulmonary Arterial Hypertension Associated With Other Conditions

Human Immunodeficiency Virus (HIV)
Infection with HIV is associated with an increased risk of developing PAH. The cumulative incidence of PAH in HIV-positive patients is estimated to be approximately 0.5 percent, significantly higher than in the general population. Among 74 HIV-positive patients with "cardiopulmonary complaints," echocardiographic evidence of PAH was found in 6 percent.[57] The annual incidence of PH in a large Swiss cohort of HIV-positive patients appears to be declining, with a peak of 0.24 percent in 1993 to 0.02 percent in 2001; this decline appears to correlate with the introduction of highly effective antiretroviral therapies.[58] The clinical manifestations and hemodynamic findings in PAH associated with HIV infection are similar to those of IPAH.[59] Survival also appears to be similar to that of IPAH.[59] Factors associated with a poorer outcome in patients with HIV-associated PAH include WHO class III or IV symptoms and a lower CD4 lymphocyte count (<212 cells/mm^3); mortality appears to be due to the PAH and right ventricular failure rather than other complications of HIV.[60] Indeed, survival in 19 HIV-positive patients with PAH followed for a mean of 1.3 years was much shorter than control HIV-positive patients without PAH (median survival 1.3 versus 2.6 years).[60b]

Systemic Sclerosis (SS)
The development of PAH in patients with the SS spectrum of disease (particularly the CREST variant [calcinosis, Raynaud's phenomenon, esophageal dysmotility, sclerodactyly, telangiectasia]) has been long recognized.[61] Stupi and colleagues reviewed records from 673 patients with SS who were treated between 1963 and 1983 at a single center and identified 331 with CREST. Of these, 59 patients had either proven or suspected PAH, of which 30 had isolated PAH (i.e., lacking evidence of interstitial lung disease); they estimated the prevalence of isolated PAH to be 9 percent of patients with CREST, and 13 percent of all patients with SS.[31] At another single center, a

retrospective review included 903 patients with SS and similarly estimated the cumulative prevalence of isolated pulmonary hypertension to be 13 percent.[62] In each of these studies, however, evaluations of possible PAH were made only when prompted by clinical suspicion, and PAH was defined by echocardiogram alone, with only a subset of cases confirmed as PAH by right heart catheterization. In both studies, patients with SS and isolated PAH had a greater risk of death than those with PH from other causes (e.g., interstitial lung or heart disease). In addition, survival of patients with SS and PAH is worse than those with IPAH, even with current therapies. As an example, in 91 consecutive patients treated with epoprostenol in one study, the risk of death was higher for patients with SS than for those with IPAH (hazard ratio 2.32).[22] Despite similar therapies including epoprostenol, calcium channel antagonists, and warfarin, Kawut and colleagues found the survival of 22 patients with SS to be shorter than of 33 with IPAH, even after adjusting for hemodynamic and demographic variables[63] (FIGURE 5-7).

Portal Hypertension
Patients with portal hypertension are at risk for PAH. The combination of conditions is referred to as "portopulmonary hypertension" (POPH).[64]

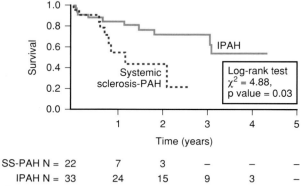

SS-PAH N =	22	7	3	–	–	–
IPAH N =	33	24	15	9	3	–

Figure 5-7. Survival in pulmonary arterial hypertension (PAH) associated with systemic sclerosis as compared with idiopathic PAH. Kaplan-Meier estimates of survival in patients with PAH associated with the systemic sclerosis spectrum of diseases *(SS-PAH)* and idiopathic PAH *(IPAH)*. (Reproduced with permission from Kawut SM, Taichman DB, Archer-Chicko CL, et al: Hemodynamics and survival in patients with pulmonary arterial hypertension related to systemic sclerosis. *Chest* 123(2):344-350, 2003.)

Neither the prevalence nor the incidence of this condition is well established. In a retrospective review of autopsy records from 1944 until 1981 at a single center, PAH was diagnosed in 0.73 percent of 1,241 patients with cirrhosis.[65] Prevalence estimates have been as high as 16 percent,[66] although typically in populations of patients with more advanced liver disease. In one series, for example, 8.5 percent of patients evaluated for liver transplantation had POPH.[67] The prognosis of patients with POPH without effective treatment is poor, with a mean survival of only 15 months in a retrospective series of 78 patients.[68] Survival with current therapies is also short compared with that of patients with IPAH. In one retrospective cohort of 13 patients with POPH and 33 with IPAH, survival estimates for those with POPH after 1 and 3 years were 85 and 38 percent as compared with 82 and 72 percent in patients with IPAH.[69] Mortality with liver transplantation is also increased in the presence of PAH, and management to decrease pressures may be required in order to permit transplantation to be attempted more safely[70-72] (see Chapter 9).

Anorexigens

In the 1960s, an epidemic of PAH in Australia, Switzerland, and West Germany occurred shortly after the appetite suppressant drug, aminorex fumarate, came into use.[73] Although only 2 percent of those exposed to the drug subsequently developed PAH, the relative risk compared with unexposed individuals was 52:1.[74] In the 1990s, cases of PAH were again noted in association with anorectic agent use (derivatives of fenfluramine),[75] prompting the establishment of the International Primary Pulmonary Hypertension Study Group in Europe to assess the incidence and risks of IPAH. Ninety-five patients were enrolled and anorectic agent use was clearly associated with an increased risk of developing PAH, especially when used for longer than 3 months (odds ratio, 23.8).[11] In the United States, the Surveillance of North American Pulmonary Hypertension study prospectively collected data on 579 patients with both idiopathic and other forms of PAH between 1996 and 1997. Fenfluramine use was associated strongly with the development of IPAH (odds ratio 7.5 with longer than 6 months use). A high prevalence of anorectic agent use in patients with other forms of PAH was also seen, suggesting these agents might also precipitate disease in the presence of other risks.[12]

Little is known regarding the prognosis of anorectic agent–associated PAH. With only anticoagulation therapy, survival was better among aminorex-exposed patients than patients with IPAH, although a benefit to anticoagulation was seen in both groups.[40] With additional therapies such as oral vasodilators and epoprostenol, however, survival in fenfluramine-exposed patients with PAH appear similar to that of patients with IPAH.[76] However, in a different study, when compared with IPAH patients matched according to treatment or for disease severity, survival at 1 and 5 years was poorer for those whose PAH was associated with fenfluramine use.[77]

Future Directions

During the past two decades, remarkable progress has been made as IPAH has been transformed from a routinely fatal disease, for which the only hope was lung transplantation, to one in which long-term survival is no longer rare, and progressively fewer organ transplantations are required. Following the demonstration of a survival benefit with continuously infused epoprostenol, the ethics of including long-term placebo arms in clinical trials have become increasingly problematic. As a growing number of effective drugs are becoming available, fewer treatment-naive patients are available for clinical trials. As a result, the relevance of comparing survival estimated on the basis of data from an era lacking effective management is questionable. Indeed, as noted previously, the NIH registry equation may no longer be sufficient for predicting survival given current standards of care and background therapies.[28] Future studies will involve comparisons of several effective management strategies, either alone or in combination.[78-80] Furthermore, studies focused on patients with non-IPAH forms of disease may reveal important differences in prognosis and in the appropriate approaches to care.[81,82]

It is possible that a growing understanding of the genetic underpinnings of PAH will lead to further revisions in classification. Currently, mutations in the gene encoding the bone morphogenetic protein receptor type II have been identified in approximately one-half of cases of familial PAH. In addition, primary genetic or secondary alterations in the function of this gene or signaling molecules with which it interacts are being recognized in sporadic, nonfamilial cases of PAH.[83-85] The penetrance of mutations appears to be low, and significant interactions among genetic and environmental factors likely influence disease activity. In addition, differences in gene expression patterns that might distinguish idiopathic from familial PAH are beginning to be recognized.[86,87] A better understanding of the gene mutations, differences in gene expression, and interactions with environmental or comorbid conditions that determine the clinical manifestations of PAH may make genetic-based classifications clinically appropriate and aid in the evaluation and assessment of management options.

References

1. Romberg E: Uber Sklerose der Lungen Arterie. *Dtsch Arch Klin Med* 48:197-206, 1891.

2. Fishman AP: A century of pulmonary hemodynamics. *Am J Respir Crit Care Med* 170:109-113, 2004.

3. Dresdale DT, Schultz M, Michtom RJ: Primary pulmonary hypertension. I. Clinical and hemodynamic study. *Am J Med* 11:686-705, 1951.

4. Rubin LJ: Diagnosis and management of pulmonary arterial hypertension: ACCP evidence-based clinical practice guidelines. *Chest* 126(1 Suppl):7S-10S, 2004.

5. Wagenvoort CA, Wagenvoort N: Primary pulmonary hypertension: a pathologic study of the lung vessels in 156 classically diagnosed cases. *Circulation* 42:1163-1184, 1970.

6. Moride Y, Abenhaim L, Xu J: Epidemiology of pulmonary hypertension in primary pulmonary hypertension. In: Rubin LJ, Rich S, editors: *Primary Pulmonary Hypertension*, 1997, pp 163-178.

7. Rich S, Dantzker DR, Ayres SM, et al: Primary pulmonary hypertension. A national prospective study. *Ann Intern Med* 107:216-223, 1987.

8. Rich S: Primary pulmonary hypertension: Executive Summary from the World Symposium, 1998.

9. Rubin LJ, Galie N: Pulmonary arterial hypertension: a look to the future. *J Am Coll Cardiol* 43(12 Suppl S):89S90S, 2004.

10. Simonneau G, Galie N, Rubin LJ, et al: Clinical classification of pulmonary hypertension. *J Am Coll Cardiol* 43(12 Suppl S):5S-12S, 2004.

11. Abenhaim L, Moride Y, Brenot F, et al: Appetite-suppressant drugs and the risk of primary pulmonary hypertension. International Primary Pulmonary Hypertension Study Group. *N Engl J Med* 335:609-616, 1996.

12. Rich S, Rubin L, Walker AM, et al: Anorexigens and pulmonary hypertension in the United States: Results from the surveillance of North American pulmonary hypertension. *Chest* 117:870-874, 2000.

13. Group IPPHS: The International Primary Pulmonary Hypertension Study. *Chest Supplement* 105:37S-41S, 1994.

14. Appelbaum L, Yigla M, Bendayan D, et al: Primary pulmonary hypertension in Israel: A national survey. *Chest* 119:1801-1806, 2001.

15. Braman SS, Eby E, Kuhn C, et al: Primary pulmonary hypertension in the elderly. *Arch Intern Med* 151:2433-2438, 1991.

16. Brenot F: Primary pulmonary hypertension: Case series from France. *Chest* 105:33S-36S, 1994.

17. Sandoval J, Bauerle O, Palomar A, et al: Survival in primary pulmonary hypertension. Validation of a prognostic equation. *Circulation* 89:1733-1744, 1994.

18. McLaughlin VV, Presberg KW, Doyle RL, et al: Prognosis of pulmonary arterial hypertension: ACCP evidence-based clinical practice guidelines. *Chest* 126(1 Suppl):78S-92S, 2004.

19. Fuster V, Steele PM, Edwards WD, et al: Primary pulmonary hypertension: Natural history and the importance of thrombosis. *Circulation* 70:580-587, 1984.

20. McGoon MD: Prognosis and natural history. In: Rubin LJ, Rich S, editors: *Primary pulmonary hypertension,* New York, 1996, Marcel Dekker, pp 305-317.

21. Rozkovec A, Montanes P, Oakley CM: Factors that influence the outcome of primary pulmonary hypertension. *Br Heart J* 55:449-458, 1986.

22. Kuhn KP, Byrne DW, Arbogast PG, et al: Outcome in 91 consecutive patients with pulmonary arterial hypertension receiving epoprostenol. *Am J Respir Crit Care Med* 167:580-586, 2003.

23. Rajasekhar D, Balakrishnan KG, Venkitachalam CG, et al: Primary pulmonary hypertension: Natural history and prognostic factors. *Indian Heart J* 46:165-170, 1994.

24. D'Alonzo GE, Barst RJ, Ayres SM, et al: Survival in patients with primary pulmonary hypertension. Results from a national prospective registry. *Ann Intern Med* 115:343-349, 1991.

25. McLaughlin VV, Shillington A, Rich S: Survival in primary pulmonary hypertension: The impact of epoprostenol therapy. *Circulation* 106:1477-1482, 2002.

26. Sitbon O, Humbert M, Nunes H, et al: Long-term intravenous epoprostenol infusion in primary pulmonary hypertension: Prognostic factors and survival. *J Am Coll Cardiol* 40:780-788, 2002.

27. Nagaya N, Nishikimi T, Uematsu M, et al: Plasma brain natriuretic peptide as a prognostic indicator in patients with primary pulmonary hypertension. *Circulation* 102:865-870, 2000.

28. Kawut SM, Horn EM, Berekashvili KK, et al: New predictors of outcome in idiopathic pulmonary arterial hypertension. *Am J Cardiol* 95:199-203, 2005.

29. Okada O, Tanabe N, Yasuda J, et al: Prediction of life expectancy in patients with primary pulmonary hypertension. A retrospective nationwide survey from 1980-1990. *Intern Med* 38:12-16, 1999.

30. Bossone E, Paciocco G, Iarussi D, et al: The prognostic role of the ECG in primary pulmonary hypertension. *Chest* 121:513-518, 2002.

31. Stupi AM, Steen VD, Owens GR, et al: Pulmonary hypertension in the CREST syndrome variant of systemic sclerosis. *Arthritis Rheum* 29:515-524, 1986.

32. Miyamoto S, Nagaya N, Satoh T, et al: Clinical correlates and prognostic significance of six-minute walk test in patients with primary pulmonary hypertension. Comparison with cardiopulmonary exercise testing. *Am J Respir Crit Care Med* 161:487-492, 2000.

33. Wensel R, Opitz CF, Anker SD, et al: Assessment of survival in patients with primary pulmonary hypertension: Importance of cardiopulmonary exercise testing. *Circulation* 106:319-324, 2002.

34. Barst RJ, Rubin LJ, Long WA, et al: A comparison of continuous intravenous epoprostenol (prostacyclin) with conventional therapy for primary pulmonary hypertension. The Primary Pulmonary Hypertension Study Group. *N Engl J Med* 334:296-302, 1996.

35. Raymond RJ, Hinderliter AL, Willis PW, et al: Echocardiographic predictors of adverse outcomes in primary pulmonary hypertension. *J Am Coll Cardiol* 39:1214-1219, 2002.

36. Frost AE, Langleben D, Oudiz R, et al: The 6-min walk test (6MW) as an efficacy endpoint in pulmonary arterial hypertension clinical trials: demonstration of a ceiling effect. *Vascul Pharmacol* 43:36-39, 2005.

37. Eysmann SB, Palevsky HI, Reichek N, et al: Two-dimensional and Doppler-echocardiographic and cardiac catheterization correlates of survival in primary pulmonary hypertension. *Circulation* 80:353-360, 1989.

38. Hinderliter AL, Willis PW, IV, Long W, et al: Frequency and prognostic significance of pericardial effusion in primary pulmonary hypertension. PPH Study Group. Primary pulmonary hypertension. *Am J Cardiol* 84:481-484, A10, 1999.

39. Yeo TC, Dujardin KS, Tei C, et al: Value of a Doppler-derived index combining systolic and diastolic time intervals in predicting outcome in primary pulmonary hypertension. *Am J Cardiol* 81:1157-1161, 1998.

40. Frank H, Mlczoch J, Huber K, et al: The effect of anticoagulant therapy in primary and anorectic drug-induced pulmonary hypertension. *Chest* 112:714-721, 1997.

41. Rich S, Kaufmann E, Levy PS: The effect of high doses of calcium-channel blockers on survival in primary pulmonary hypertension. *N Engl J Med* 327:76-81, 1992.

42. Raffy O, Azarian R, Brenot F, et al: Clinical significance of the pulmonary vasodilator response during short-term infusion of prostacyclin in primary pulmonary hypertension. *Circulation* 93:484-488, 1996.

43. Sitbon O, Humbert M, Jais X, et al: Long-term response to calcium channel blockers in idiopathic pulmonary arterial hypertension. *Circulation* 111:3105-3111, 2005.

44. Barst RJ, Rubin LJ, McGoon MD, et al: Survival in primary pulmonary hypertension with long-term continuous intravenous prostacyclin. *Ann Intern Med* 121:409-415, 1994.

45. Nagaya N, Uematsu M, Satoh T, et al: Serum uric acid levels correlate with the severity and the mortality of primary pulmonary hypertension. *Am J Respir Crit Care Med* 160:487-492, 1999.

46. Voelkel MA, Wynne KM, Badesch DB, et al: Hyperuricemia in severe pulmonary hypertension. *Chest* 117:19-24, 2000.

47. Lopes AA, Maeda NY, Goncalves RC, et al: Endothelial cell dysfunction correlates differentially with survival in primary and secondary pulmonary hypertension. *Am Heart J* 139:618-623, 2000.

48. Shitrit D, Bendayan D, Bar-Gil-Shitrit A, et al: Significance of a plasma D-dimer test in patients with primary pulmonary hypertension. *Chest* 122:1674-1678, 2002.

49. Torbicki A, Kurzyna M, Kuca P, et al: Detectable serum cardiac troponin T as a marker of poor prognosis among patients with chronic precapillary pulmonary hypertension. *Circulation* 108:844-848, 2003.

50. Nootens M, Kaufmann E, Rector T, et al: Neurohormonal activation in patients with right ventricular failure from pulmonary hypertension: Relation to hemodynamic variables and endothelin levels. *J Am Coll Cardiol* 26:1581-1585, 1995.

51. Rubens C, Ewert R, Halank M, et al: Big endothelin-1 and endothelin-1 plasma levels are correlated with the severity of primary pulmonary hypertension. *Chest* 120:1562-1569, 2001.

52. Nagaya N, Nishikimi T, Uematsu M, et al: Plasma brain natriuretic peptide as a prognostic indicator in patients with primary pulmonary hypertension. *J Cardiol* 37:110-111, 2001.

53. Omland T, Aakvaag A, Bonarjee VV, et al: Plasma brain natriuretic peptide as an indicator of left ventricular systolic function and long-term survival after acute myocardial infarction. Comparison with plasma atrial natriuretic peptide and N-terminal proatrial natriuretic peptide. *Circulation* 93:1963-1969, 1996.

54. McLaughlin V, Sitbon O, Rubin LJ, et al: Survival with first-line bosentan in patients with primary pulmonary hypertension. *EUR Resp J* 25:244-249, 2005.

55. Sitbon O, McLaughlin VV, Badesch DB, et al: Survival in patients with class III idiopathic pulmonary arterial hypertension treated with first-line oral bosentan compared with an historical cohort of patients started on IV epoprostenol. *Thorax* 60: 1025-1030, 2005.

56. Hoeper MM, Galie N, Murali S, et al: Outcome after cardiopulmonary resuscitation in patients with pulmonary arterial hypertension. *Am J Respir Crit Care Med* 165:341-344, 2002.

57. Speich R, Jenni R, Opravil M, et al: Primary pulmonary hypertension in HIV infection. *Chest* 100: 1268-1271, 1991.

58. Zuber JP, Calmy A, Evison JM, et al: Pulmonary arterial hypertension related to HIV infection: Improved hemodynamics and survival associated with antiretroviral therapy. *Clin Infect Dis* 38:1178-1185, 2004.

59. Petitpretz P, Brenot F, Azarian R, et al: Pulmonary hypertension in patients with human immuno-deficiency virus infection. Comparison with primary pulmonary hypertension. *Circulation* 89:2722-2727, 1994.

60. Nunes H, Humbert M, Sitbon O, et al: Prognostic factors for survival in human immunodeficiency virus–associated pulmonary arterial hypertension. *Am J Respir Crit Care Med* 167:1433-1439, 2003.

60b. Opravil M, Pechere M, Speich R, et al: HIV-associated primary pulmonary hypertension. A case control study. Swiss HIV cohort study. *Am J Resp Crit Care Med* 155:990-995, 1997.

61. Salerni R, Rodnan GP, Leon DF, et al: Pulmonary hypertension in the CREST syndrome variant of progressive systemic sclerosis (scleroderma). *Ann Intern Med* 86:394-399, 1977.

62. MacGregor AJ, Canavan R, Knight C, et al: Pulmonary hypertension in systemic sclerosis: Risk factors for progression and consequences for survival. *Rheumatology (Oxford)* 40:453-459, 2001.

63. Kawut SM, Taichman DB, Archer-Chicko CL, et al: Hemodynamics and survival in patients with pulmonary arterial hypertension related to systemic sclerosis. *Chest* 123:344-350, 2003.

64. Rodriguez-Roisin R, Krowka MJ, Herve P, et al: Pulmonary-Hepatic Vascular Disorders. *Eur Respir J* 24:861-880, 2004.

65. McDonnell PJ, Toye PA, Hutchins GM: Primary pulmonary hypertension and cirrhosis: Are they related? *Am Rev Respir Dis* 127:437-441, 1983.

66. Benjaminov FS, Prentice M, Sniderman KW, et al: Portopulmonary hypertension in decompensated cirrhosis with refractory ascites. *Gut* 52:1355-1362, 2003.

67. Ramsay MA, Simpson BR, Nguyen AT, et al: Severe pulmonary hypertension in liver transplant candidates. *Liver Transpl Surg* 3:494-500, 1997.

68. Robalino BD, Moodie DS: Association between primary pulmonary hypertension and portal hypertension: Analysis of its pathophysiology and clinical, laboratory and hemodynamic manifestations. *J Am Coll Cardiol* 17:492-498, 1991.

69. Kawut SM, Taichman DB, Ahya VN, et al: Hemodynamics and survival of patients with portopulmonary hypertension. *Liver Transpl* 11:1107-1111, 2005.

70. Krowka MJ, Mandell MS, Ramsay MA, et al: Hepatopulmonary syndrome and portopulmonary hypertension: A report of the multicenter liver transplant database. *Liver Transpl* 10:174-182, 2004.

71. Krowka MJ, Plevak DJ, Findlay JY, et al: Pulmonary hemodynamics and perioperative cardiopulmonary–related mortality in patients with portopulmonary hypertension undergoing liver transplantation. *Liver Transpl* 6:443-450, 2000.

72. Krowka MJ, Frantz RP, McGoon MD, et al: Improvement in pulmonary hemodynamics during intravenous epoprostenol (prostacyclin): A study of 15 patients with moderate to severe portopulmonary hypertension. *Hepatology* 30:641-648, 1999.

73. Gurtner HP: Aminorex pulmonary hypertension. In: A. P. Fisinman, editor: *The pulmonary circulation: Normal and abnormal,* Philadelphia, 1990, University of Pennsylvania Press, pp 397-411.

74. Brenot F: Risk factors for primary pulmonary hypertension. In: Rubin LJ, Rich S, editors: *Primary pulmonary hypertension,* New York, 1996, Marcel Dekker, pp 131-149.

75. Brenot F, Herve P, Petitpretz P, et al: Primary pulmonary hypertension and fenfluramine use. *Br Heart J* 70:537-541, 1993.

76. Simonneau G, Fartoukh M, Sitbon O, et al: Primary pulmonary hypertension associated with the use of fenfluramine derivatives. *Chest* 114(3 Suppl):195S-199S, 1998.

77. Rich S, Shillington A, McLaughlin V: Comparison of survival in patients with pulmonary hypertension associated with fenfluramine to patients with primary pulmonary hypertension. *Am J Cardiol* 92: 1366-1368, 2003.

78. Ghofrani HA, Rose F, Schermuly RT, et al: Oral sildenafil as long-term adjunct therapy to inhaled iloprost in severe pulmonary arterial hypertension. *J Am Coll Cardiol* 42:158-164, 2003.

79. Wilkins MR, Paul GA, Strange JW, et al: Sildenafil versus Endothelin Receptor Antagonist for Pulmonary

Hypertension (SERAPH) study. *Am J Respir Crit Care Med* 171:1292-1297, 2005.

80. Bhatia S, Frantz RP, Severson CJ, et al: Immediate and long-term hemodynamic and clinical effects of sildenafil in patients with pulmonary arterial hypertension receiving vasodilator therapy. *Mayo Clin Proc* 78:1207-1213, 2003.

81. Badesch DB, Tapson VF, McGoon MD, et al: Continuous intravenous epoprostenol for pulmonary hypertension due to the scleroderma spectrum of disease. A randomized, controlled trial. *Ann Intern Med* 132:425-434, 2000.

82. Sitbon O, Gressin V, Speich R, et al: Bosentan for the treatment of human immunodeficiency virus—associated pulmonary arterial hypertension. *Am J Respir Crit Care Med* 170:1212-1217, 2004.

83. Lane KB, Machado RD, Pauciulo MW, et al: Heterozygous germline mutations in *BMPR2*, encoding a TGF-β receptor, cause familial primary pulmonary hypertension. The International PPH Consortium. *Nat Genet* 26:81-84, 2000.

84. Thomson JR, Machado RD, Pauciulo MW, et al: Sporadic primary pulmonary hypertension is associated with germline mutations of the gene encoding BMPR-II, a receptor member of the TGF-β family. *J Med Genet* 37:741-745, 2000.

85. Du L, Sullivan CC, Chu D, et al: Signaling molecules in nonfamilial pulmonary hypertension. *N Engl J Med* 348:500-509, 2003.

86. Geraci MW, Moore M, Gesell T, et al: Gene expression patterns in the lungs of patients with primary pulmonary hypertension: A gene microarray analysis. *Circ Res* 88:555-562, 2001.

87. Bull TM, Coldren CD, Moore M, et al: Gene microarray analysis of peripheral blood cells in pulmonary arterial hypertension. *Am J Respir Crit Care Med* 170:911-919, 2004.

Chapter 6

Approach to the Patient With Pulmonary Hypertension

Jess Mandel, MD

When confronted with a patient who may have pulmonary hypertension, the clinician must ask and answer three questions:

- Is pulmonary hypertension present?
- What is the probable cause of pulmonary hypertension?
- What is the severity of pulmonary hypertension?

This chapter will review issues related to the diagnosis, evaluation, and screening of patients suspected of suffering from pulmonary hypertension.

Nomenclature

Several definitions of pulmonary hypertension have been proposed, but the most widely used is a mean pulmonary arterial pressure (mPAP) in excess of 25 mmHg at rest or 30 mmHg with exercise. The 2003 Venice Revised Clinical Classification of Pulmonary Hypertension divides the condition into five categories[1] (TABLE 6-1). Of these, pulmonary arterial hypertension (PAH) is in some ways the most critical to detect, because its management is uniquely focused upon medications to facilitate pulmonary vascular remodeling, rather than management of an underlying cause such as chronic obstructive pulmonary disease, ischemic cardiomyopathy, or obstructive sleep apnea.

Most of this chapter deals with the evaluation of undifferentiated pulmonary hypertension, although some issues are relevant only to the subset of patients with PAH. The reader must remain attentive to the manner in which these terms are employed.

Should Pulmonary Hypertension Be Suspected?

Pulmonary hypertension generally is suspected initially because of compatible patient history and physical examination findings, particularly when risk factors or conditions associated with pulmonary hypertension are present. However, because symptoms and signs can be nonspecific and overlap with other conditions that are far more common, a delay of 1 to 2 years is common between the development of symptoms and consideration of the proper diagnosis is not unusual.[2,3]

Patient History

In the United States National Institutes of Health cohort of 187 patients with idiopathic pulmonary arterial hypertension (IPAH, formerly called primary pulmonary hypertension) assembled during the mid-1980s, dyspnea was the most common initial complaint. It was noted in 60 percent of patients on initial presentation, and dyspnea was present in 98 percent by the time they were enrolled in the study by a participating center. Fatigue was the initial complaint in 19 percent and was present in 73 percent of patients at the time of study enrollment. Other common symptoms included chest pain, syncope or near syncope, lower extremity edema, and palpitations.[2] Syncope is considered a particularly worrisome historical element in patients with PAH, and evaluation should be expedited if syncope has been documented.

The pathophysiology of symptoms such as fatigue and exertional syncope is believed to relate to an impaired ability of the chronically pulmonary hypertensive heart to adequately augment cardiac

TABLE 6-1

Causes and Classification of Pulmonary Hypertension

1. Pulmonary Arterial Hypertension (PAH)
  1.1. Idiopathic (IPAH)
  1.2. Familial (FPAH)
  1.3. Associated with (APAH):
    1.3.1. Collagen vascular disease
    1.3.2. Congenital systemic-to-pulmonary shunts
    1.3.3. Portal hypertension
    1.3.4. HIV infection
    1.3.5. Drugs and toxins
    1.3.6. Other (thyroid disorders, glycogen storage disease, Gaucher disease, hereditary hemorrhagic telangiectasia, hemoglobinopathies, myeloproliferative disorders, splenectomy)
  1.4. Associated with significant venous or capillary involvement
    1.4.1. Pulmonary veno-occlusive disease (PVOD)
    1.4.2. Pulmonary capillary hemangiomatosis (PCH)
  1.5. Persistent pulmonary hypertension of the newborn
2. Pulmonary hypertension with left-sided heart disease
  2.1. Left-sided atrial or ventricular heart disease
  2.2. Left-sided valvular heart disease
3. Pulmonary hypertension associated with lung diseases or hypoxemia
  3.1. Chronic obstructive pulmonary disease
  3.2. Interstitial lung disease
  3.3. Sleep-disordered breathing
  3.4. Alveolar hypoventilation disorders
  3.5. Long-term exposure to high altitude
  3.6. Developmental abnormalities
4. Pulmonary hypertension due to chronic thrombotic or embolic disease or both
  4.1. Thromboembolic obstruction of proximal pulmonary arteries
  4.2. Thromboembolic obstruction of distal pulmonary arteries
  4.3. Nonthrombotic pulmonary embolism (tumor, parasites, foreign material)
5. Miscellaneous (sarcoidosis, histiocytosis X, lymphangiomatosis, compression of pulmonary vessels [adenopathy, tumor, fibrosing mediastinitis])

HIV, *human immunodeficiency virus.*
Adapted from Rubin LJ: Diagnosis and management of pulmonary arterial hypertension: ACCP evidence-based clinical practice guidelines.
Chest 126:7S-10S, 2004.

output during exertion, as well as from hypoxemia caused by suboptimal ventilation-perfusion matching. The normal plasticity of the pulmonary vascular bed is lost and, as a result, the normal mechanisms of accommodating an increased cardiac output and optimizing ventilation-perfusion matching via recruitment and distention of pulmonary vessels operates poorly. Arterial hypoxemia and an inadequate cardiac output with exertion due to underfilling of the left ventricle and ventricular interdependence ultimately result in tissue hypoxia.[4,5]

Chest pain may have characteristics of typical (Heberden) angina or may be atypical in nature. Several mechanisms historically have been proposed to explain its development, including pulmonary artery stretching and global right ventricular ischemia.[6-8] More recently, a number of patients with chest pain in the context of longstanding pulmonary hypertension (generally due to congenital systemic-to-pulmonary shunts or IPAH) have developed myocardial ischemia due to extrinsic compression of the left main coronary artery by an enlarged pulmonary artery.[9,10] Production of cardiac ischemia by this mechanism appears unlikely when the pulmonary artery diameter is less than 40 mm and when the ratio of the main pulmonary artery and aortic diameters is less than 1.21.[11] Stenting of the compressed area of the left main coronary artery has been accomplished successfully in some cases.[12,13]

Less commonly, patients with pulmonary hypertension may develop symptoms of cough, hemoptysis, or hoarseness, the last of which can be caused by compression of the left recurrent laryngeal nerve by an enlarged pulmonary artery. This hoarseness is referred to as "Ortner syndrome," although Ortner's original description involved a patient with mitral stenosis in whom impingement on the nerve by an enlarged left atrium may have been responsible, and the term is also applied to cardiovocal hoarseness caused by aortic aneurysm or dissection.[14,15]

Historical elements should also be sought which are consistent with conditions or exposures that are associated with pulmonary hypertension. Examples include a history of Raynaud phenomenon, that may be associated with autoimmune conditions; a history of witnessed nocturnal apneas and excessive daytime somnolence that may be associated with obstructive sleep apnea; liver disease; a family history of IPAH, or a history of cocaine, amphetamine, or anorectic drug use.

A thorough family history should be obtained. Patients should be questioned specifically about the presence in family members of pulmonary hypertension, autoimmune diseases, and thrombophilia, and deaths attributed to "heart disease" should be scrutinized to try to determine if undiagnosed PAH was present.

Physical Findings

The physical examination remains an important aspect of the evaluation of a patient in whom pulmonary hypertension is being considered. Characteristic physical findings become more pronounced as the disease progresses.

The most common cardiac abnormality is an accentuated intensity of the pulmonic component of the second heart sound, which was noted in more than 90 percent of patients in the NIH registry.[2] This finding presumably occurs because an increased force of pulmonic valve closure results from elevated pulmonary arterial pressures. Other cardiac auscultatory findings that may be present include narrow splitting of the second heart sound (although this will not occur if a right ventricular conduction delay has developed), an early systolic click as a result of resistance to pulmonic valve opening, a midsystolic ejection murmur caused by turbulent flow across the pulmonic valve, a holosystolic tricuspid regurgitant murmur, a diastolic pulmonary insufficiency murmur, or a right ventricular S_3 or S_4 gallop.[2,16,17] Right-sided murmurs generally are augmented with inspiration.

Palpation may reveal a left parasternal heave or a subxiphoid thrust. Jugular venous distention with prominent a and v waves may be observed, and peripheral edema is commonly seen. Pulsatile

hepatomegaly and ascites are particularly common when tricuspid regurgitation is pronounced.

Careful attention also should be paid to clues on physical examination that may suggest a specific cause of pulmonary hypertension. Examples include hyperresonance and hyperinflation of the thorax suggestive of chronic obstructive pulmonary disease, kyphoscoliosis characteristic of chest wall disease, redundancy of oropharyngeal soft tissues consistent with obstructive sleep apnea, skin changes or arthritis suggestive of autoimmune disease, or digital clubbing indicative of pneumoconiosis, congenital heart disease, or pulmonary veno-occlusive disease.[18]

Basic Diagnostic Tests

Laboratory tests are generally insensitive and nonspecific for confirming the diagnosis of pulmonary hypertension. However, such tests may have utility in the diagnosis of conditions with which pulmonary hypertension is associated. As examples, a strongly positive antinuclear antibody titer may point toward connective tissue disease; abnormal serum alanine and aspartate aminotransferase concentrations may suggest liver disease; and positive serology for human immunodeficiency virus (HIV) is diagnostic for HIV infection.

More recently, the potential diagnostic role of brain natriuretic peptide (BNP) for PAH has been examined. Although initially identified in brain tissue, BNP is also produced by the heart and stimulates natriuresis via several distinct mechanisms.[19,20] Plasma BNP concentrations are elevated in patients with PAH and may correlate with functional status, but are nonspecific; elevations in BNP are likewise seen in patients with left-sided heart failure or following acute coronary syndromes.[21-24] Thus, BNP is generally of limited utility in the initial evaluation of a patient with possible pulmonary hypertension.

Electrocardiography (ECG) frequently shows changes consistent with right ventricular hypertrophy and right atrial enlargement when pulmonary hypertension is present, but it does not have sufficient sensitivity or specificity to serve as a screening test for pulmonary hypertension.[16] As an example, in one series of 61 patients with PAH associated with collagen vascular disease, 13 percent demonstrated normal ECG findings despite an average mPAP of 47 mmHg during cardiac catheterization.[25] Furthermore, no significant correlation between hemodynamic parameters and ECG features such as P wave amplitude in lead II, frontal QRS ratio, QRS duration, R/S ratio in leads

I or V_6, or an inverted T wave in lead V_4 could be demonstrated. Other series have found similar results. In the 187 patients in the NIH registry, right ventricular hypertrophy was absent in 13 percent of patients, and right axis deviation was not present in 21 percent[2] (FIGURE 6-1).

Despite its shortcomings, an ECG generally is recommended for patients in whom pulmonary hypertension is suspected.[16] Abnormalities suggestive of congenital abnormalities or rhythm disturbances may be appreciated, and some data suggest that electrocardiographic evidence of right ventricular or right atrial enlargement connote a worse prognosis in patients with IPAH.[26-28]

Similarly, a chest radiograph generally is obtained when pulmonary hypertension is suspected, although its utility appears greater in detecting parenchymal lung disease, chest wall disease, or pulmonary venous congestion that may be associated with pulmonary hypertension, rather than pulmonary hypertension per se.[16,29,30] Radiographic findings consistent with pulmonary hypertension include enlarged hilar and main pulmonary arterial contours associated with attenuation of peripheral vascular shadows (known as "pruning"), and right ventricular enlargement appreciated as expansion of the chamber border into the retrosternal clear space on the lateral projection.[31]

The exact sensitivity and specificity of conventional chest radiographs for PAH is not entirely clear. In the NIH IPAH registry, 6 percent of patients had normal chest film findings, while 90 percent demonstrated prominence of the main pulmonary arteries, 80 percent showed enlarged hilar vessels, 74 percent displayed right ventricular hypertrophy, and 51 percent displayed decreased peripheral vascularity.[2]

An infrequently used radiologic index of pulmonary hypertension is obtained by measuring the horizontal distances from the midline to the first divisions of the right and left pulmonary arteries, then dividing the sum of these distances by the maximum transverse diameter of the thorax on a posteroanterior chest radiograph obtained by standard techniques. In one series of patients with cardiovascular disease and pulmonary hypertension, an index value above 0.38 correctly identified 111 of 150 patients with hemodynamic abnormalities, although the index value correlated poorly with the magnitude of disease.[32] However, this radiologic index is insufficiently validated to be adopted as a screening test.

Although computed tomography (CT) imaging is not obtained routinely when pulmonary hypertension is suspected, CT may reveal enlargement of central pulmonary arteries, right ventricular hypertrophy, and diminished caliber of peripheral pulmonary vessels when pulmonary hypertension is present[33] (FIGURE 6-2). Several series have examined the predictive power of main pulmonary artery diameter for pulmonary hypertension. One study of 32 patients with cardiopulmonary disease and 26 age-matched and sex-matched controls found that a main pulmonary artery diameter greater than 28.6 mm

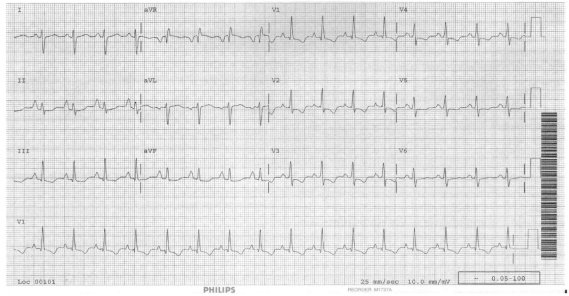

Figure 6-1. Right Ventricular Hypertrophy. Electrocardiogram from a 30-year-old woman with idiopathic pulmonary arterial hypertension shows right axis deviation, right atrial enlargement, and right ventricular hypertrophy with strain. (Courtesy of Donald D. Brown, M.D.).

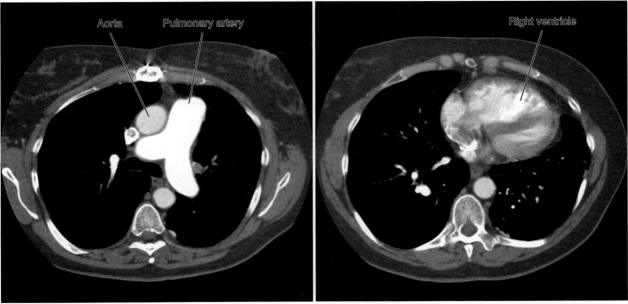

Figure 6-2. Computed Tomographic Findings of Pulmonary Hypertension. Contrast computed tomography of the chest in a patient with severe pulmonary arterial hypertension showing enlargement of the contrast-filled main pulmonary artery, which is larger in diameter than the adjacent ascending aorta (**A**); and enlargement of the right ventricle (**B**).

identified patients with pulmonary hypertension (defined as mPAP >18 mmHg) with a sensitivity of 69 percent and a specificity of 100 percent.[34] A different series of 36 patients with pulmonary hypertension due to parenchymal lung disease and 9 controls determined that the sensitivity and specificity of a main pulmonary artery diameter greater than 29 mm was 87 and 89 percent, respectively, for detecting an mPAP higher than 20 mmHg.[35] A segmental artery-to-bronchus ratio greater than 1.0 in three or four separate lobes appeared to be a more specific finding among these patients.

The ratio of main pulmonary artery and aortic diameters on axial imaging has also been examined. One report of 50 patients with pulmonary and cardiovascular disease found that a ratio of main pulmonary artery to aortic diameter greater than 1 on CT was 70 percent sensitive and 92 percent specific for an mPAP over 20 mmHg.[36] The literature regarding vascular diameters obtained by magnetic resonance imaging (MRI) is less robust, but one study of 12 patients with IPAH and 8 controls found that the ratio of main pulmonary artery to aortic diameter obtained by MRI was significantly elevated among patients with IPAH.[33,37] Of note, the mean ratio among control patients in this study was 1.3, emphasizing the need for separately derived CT and MRI normative values for this purpose.

CT and MRI can provide can provide a wealth of information, such as the appearance of the lung parenchyma, the presence or absence of central venous obstruction, and estimation of right ventricular mass. Nonetheless, these studies need not be obtained in all patients in whom pulmonary hypertension is suspected, but should instead be reserved to answer the specific clinical questions to which they are suited.

Is Pulmonary Hypertension Present?

If pulmonary hypertension is suspected on the basis of some combination of risk factors, symptoms, physical examination findings, electrocardiogram, and imaging studies, the focus of the evaluation turns to determining whether pulmonary hypertension is indeed present. Echocardiography and cardiac catheterization are the most important diagnostic modalities employed at this stage of the evaluation.

Echocardiography

Echocardiographic detection of pulmonary hypertension is based upon documentation of characteristic architectural changes by two-dimensional echocardiography, as well as elevated pulmonary artery pressures on color Doppler imaging[38] (TABLES 6-2 and 6-3). Two-dimensional echocardiography typically includes parasternal long-axis

TABLE 6-2

Echocardiographic and Color Doppler Features in Patients With Pulmonary Arterial Hypertension

Variables	Right Heart	Left Heart
M-mode Diminished or absent atrial wave of the pulmonary valve Mid-systolic closure or notching of the pulmonary valve		
2D Echocardiography	RV hypertrophy RV dilation RV abnormal systolic function RV pressure overload pattern of IVS Right atrial dilation Dilated pulmonary artery Interatrial septum bows right to left	Reduced LV end-diastolic volume Reduced LV end-systolic volume LV ejection fraction within normal limits Increased IVS thickness IVS-to-posterior wall thickness ratio >1
Color Doppler Imaging	Tricuspid regurgitation Pulmonary insufficiency Elevated PASP RVOT AT <0.1 sec	E/A ratio <1

E/A, ratio between early peak transmitral flow velocity and late peak systolic; IVS, intraventricular septum; LV, left ventricular; PASP, pulmonary artery systolic pressure; RV, right ventricular; RVOT AT, Right ventricular outflow tract acceleration time.
From Bossone E, Bodini B, Mazza E, et al: Pulmonary arterial hypertension. The key role of echocardiography. Chest 127:1836-1843, 2005.

TABLE 6-3

Noninvasive Estimation of Pulmonary Arterial Pressures From Echocardiographic Parameters

Pulmonary Arterial Systolic Pressure (PASP)

PASP = 4 × (peak tricuspid regurgitant velocity)^2 + right atrial pressure

Mean Pulmonary Arterial Pressure (mPAP)

mPAP = 79 − 0.45 × (right ventricular outflow tract acceleration time)
mPAP = 4 × (peak pulmonic regurgitant velocity)^2

Pulmonary End-diastolic Pressure (PEDP)

PEDP = 4 × (end-diastolic pulmonic regurgitant velocity)^2 + right atrial pressure

From Bossone E, Bodini B, Mazza E, et al: Pulmonary arterial hypertension. The key role of echocardiography. Chest 127:1836-1843, 2005.

and short-axis views at the mitral valve and papillary muscle levels, apical four-chamber, two-chamber, and three-chamber views, and subcostal views. Common morphologic abnormalities observed in patients with pulmonary hypertension include right ventricular dilation or hypertrophy or both (wall thickness >5 mm), right atrial enlargement, dilation of the pulmonary artery, and thickening, flattening, or bowing of the interventricular septum[39,40] (FIGURE 6-3). Left ventricular end-systolic and end-diastolic volumes may also be reduced, a ratio of interventricular septum to posterior wall thickness greater than 1.0 may be seen, and a pericardial effusion may be present.[41] In one series of 51 consecutive patients with known or suspected IPAH, right ventricular dilation was

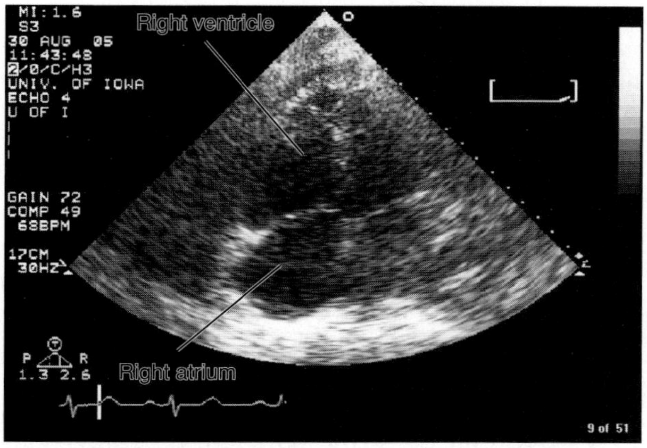

Figure 6-3. Severe Pulmonary Hypertension. Apical four-chamber echocardiographic view shows profound right atrial and right ventricular enlargement in a 74-year-old woman with chronic thromboembolic pulmonary hypertension. Her pulmonary arterial systolic pressure was estimated at 103 mmHg by echocardiography and was measured at 98 mmHg at cardiac catheterization. (Courtesy of Paul Lindower, MD.)

the most common two-dimensional feature, and was present in 98 percent of individuals.[42]

Color Doppler echocardiography assesses blood flow based on changes in the ultrasonographic signal due to the movement of erythrocytes relative to the transducer. The technique is useful in documenting the tricuspid regurgitation and pulmonic insufficiency that may be seen with pulmonary hypertension. Tricuspid regurgitation, present in up to 95 percent of patients, permits estimation of pulmonary artery systolic pressure (which is assumed to be equal to right ventricular systolic pressure [RVSP]) via the simplified Bernoulli equation:

$$RVSP = 4v^2 + \text{right atrial pressure}$$

in which v is the velocity of the tricuspid jet in meters per second.[16,43-45] Peak tricuspid regurgitant jet velocity generally is obtained from a spectral profile acquired in the parasternal long-axis view, parasternal short-axis view, or apical four-chamber view. It is critical that the intercept angle between the ultrasound beam and the direction of blood flow approaches zero for this technique to be accurate. A value for right atrial pressure is obtained either by measurement of jugular venous pressure on physical examination, by addition of a standardized value of 10-14 mmHg, or by observing the inferior vena cava for collapse to less than 50 percent of its initial diameter with inspiration.[46]

Failure of the inferior vena cava to collapse during inspiration implies an elevated right atrial pressure, generally assumed to be 10 mmHg or higher.

Right ventricular outflow tract acceleration time can also be obtained, usually from the parasternal short-axis view at the aortic valve level, where the pulsed wave Doppler sample volume is situated in the center of the right ventricular outflow tract immediately proximal to the pulmonic valve. A right ventricular outflow tract acceleration time less than 100 milliseconds is consistent with pulmonary hypertension.[47]

Finally, shunting across a patent foramen ovale may be noted, because right atrial pressures frequently exceed left atrial pressures for at least part of the cardiac cycle.[39] An experienced echocardiographer may be required to differentiate a patent foramen ovale from an atrial septal defect in this situation.

The accuracy of echocardiographic estimates of pulmonary artery pressures has been compared with hemodynamic values obtained during catheterization in a number of studies. In general, strong correlation coefficients have been reported, and several series have described a mean difference in pulmonary artery systolic pressures obtained by echocardiography and catheterization of less than 3 mmHg.[42-44,48,49] However, such results have not been universal. One study of 10 patients predominantly with IPAH found that echocardiography systematically underestimated pulmonary artery systolic pressure by more than 20 mmHg, and a different study of 81 patients with IPAH found that invasive measurement of pulmonary artery pressures exceeded echocardiographic estimates by more than 20 mmHg in 31 percent of patients.[50,51] In contrast, one study of 25 pregnant patients found that 32 percent of women in whom echocardiography suggested pulmonary hypertension displayed normal pulmonary artery pressures on subsequent catheterization.[52]

Cardiac Catheterization

Although echocardiography is an appropriate test for the noninvasive characterization of pulmonary hypertension, its accuracy is sufficiently variable that it should be considered an estimate, rather than a measurement, of pulmonary artery pressure. Cardiac catheterization remains necessary to definitively establish or exclude the diagnosis of pulmonary hypertension, determine if left atrial hypertension is present, exclude significant left-to-right intracardiac shunts by means of oximetric sampling, and enable assessment of pulmonary vasoreactivity in response to short-acting vasodilating agents. Pulmonary hypertension is considered present if an mPAP greater than 25 mmHg at rest or greater than 30 mmHg with exertion is noted. Pulmonary venous hypertension is excluded if a pulmonary capillary wedge pressure or left ventricular end-diastolic pressure (in the absense of mitral valve disease) of less than 15 mmHg and a pulmonary vascular resistance of more than 3 Wood units are documented.[17]

The specifics of cardiac catheterization are discussed elsewhere.[53] It is generally agreed that the safety and reliability of cardiac catheterization are maximized when consistency of personnel, equipment, and methodology are employed. Pressure measurements in the right side of the heart usually are obtained via femoral or internal jugular vein approaches. Zeroing of the system should be at the lateral mid-chest level, in order to correspond to the most anterior area of the left ventricular blood pool.[54] Right-sided pressures usually are obtained with a balloon-tipped flotation catheter with a uniform dynamic response of greater than 20 Hz. Pressure measurements are recorded in the central veins, right atrium, right ventricle, and pulmonary capillary wedge positions. If waveforms are questionable for assessing a wedged position, oximetric analysis of blood drawn from the distal port and comparison with a simultaneously obtained arterial sample may be required. If an elevated pulmonary capillary wedge pressure is noted, direct measurement of left ventricular end-diastolic pressure (LVEDP) should be considered, because the pulmonary capillary wedge pressure may overestimate LVEDP when there is pulmonary hypertension, volume overload, or chronic obstructive lung disease, and LVEDP is more accurate measurement of left ventricular preload. Exercise via arm or bicycle ergometry can be attempted to record changes in pulmonary artery pressure with exertion, but exercise introduces difficulties in the quality of measurements obtained, as well as with normative values.[55]

Cardiac output generally should be calculated according to both thermodilution and Fick methods. The Fick method tends to be more reliable in low cardiac output states, or when there is severe tricuspid regurgitation, pulmonic insufficiency, or a left-to-right shunt.

In addition to measurement of intravascular pressures and cardiac output, serial blood samples from the vena cava, right atrium, right ventricle, and pulmonary artery should be analyzed by oximetry to exclude a left-to-right shunt. In general, shunts smaller than 20 percent of pulmonary blood flow are not detectable. A left-to-right shunt is suggested by a step-up of 9 percent in hemoglobin oxygen saturation between superior vena cava and right atrium, 5 percent between right atrium and right ventricle, or 3 percent between right ventricle and pulmonary artery.[56,57]

Finally, if PAH is confirmed during catheterization, the response to short-acting pulmonary vasodilator agents should be assessed. The agents most commonly used for this diagnostic purpose are inhaled nitric oxide, usually administered at 10-80 ppm in conjunction with high-flow supplemental oxygen; intravenous epoprostenol, usually infused at a rate of 2 ng/kg/minute initially and then titrated upward in 2 ng/kg/minute increments to a maximum of 10 mg/kg/min; or intravenous adenosine, usually begun at 50 mcg/kg/minute and titrated upward to a maximum dosage of 300–500 mcg/kg/minute.[58-61] If no pulmonary vasoreactivity can be documented, the patient is not a candidate for therapy with a calcium channel antagonist. In general, fewer than 10 percent of patients with PAH demonstrate vasoreactivity[62] (see Chapter 7).

Longer acting pulmonary vasodilators, such as dihydropyridine calcium channel antagonists, should not be employed for assessing pulmonary vasoreactivity, because fatalities have occurred in this situation.[63] Pulmonary vasodilators should not be employed if pulmonary veno-occlusive disease is suspected (e.g., when pulmonary hypertension is accompanied by pulmonary septal thickening or Kerley B lines and a normal pulmonary capillary wedge pressure), because acute pulmonary edema may ensue.[18,64,65]

Regardless of the short-acting agent employed, a significant positive response is defined as an acute decrease in mPAP of 10 mmHg or more to reach an mPAP of less than 40 mmHg with an increased or unchanged cardiac output.[17] The relatively few patients in whom acute pulmonary vasoreactivity is documented generally respond to treatment with oral calcium channel antagonists and have a much better prognosis than those in whom pulmonary vasoreactivity is absent.[66] If short-acting pulmonary vasodilators are not tolerated or fail to produce a significant positive response, the likelihood that the patient will respond to oral calcium channel antagonists is very small, and their use should not be attempted.[67]

What is the Etiology of Pulmonary Hypertension?

When pulmonary hypertension is suspected on the basis of clinical findings, and documented by catheterization or highly suggestive echocardiographic data, the clinician must then attempt to determine the etiology of pulmonary hypertension so that prognosis can be determined and therapy maximized. An organized, thorough approach is required (FIGURE 6-4):

- The history and physical examination should be reexamined for clues to the presence of conditions associated with pulmonary hypertension, such as connective tissue disorders, liver disease, HIV infection, or structural lung disease.

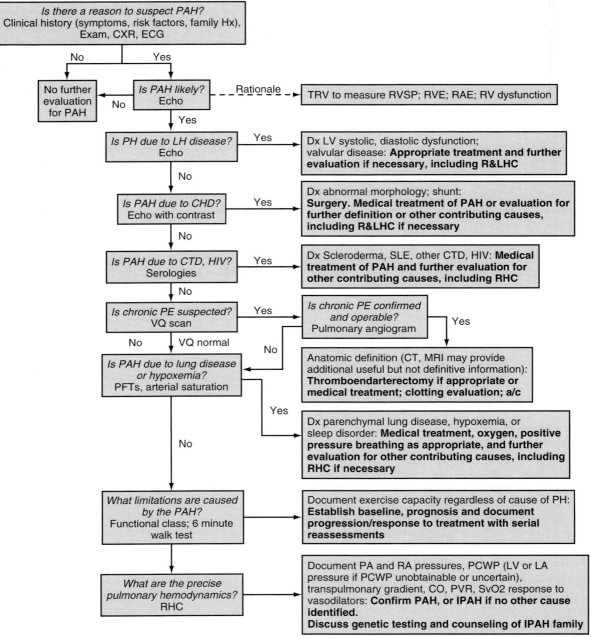

Figure 6-4. Evaluation of Suspected Pulmonary Arterial Hypertension. *a/c,* anticoagulation; *CHD,* congenital heart disease; *CO,* cardiac output; *CTD,* connective tissue disease; *Dx,* diagnosis; *Echo,* echocardiography; *Hx,* history; *LA,* left atrial; *LH,* left heart; *LV,* left ventricular; *PCWP,* pulmonary capillary wedge pressure; *PE,* pulmonary embolism; *PFT,* pulmonary function test; *PVR,* pulmonary vascular resistance; *RAE,* right atrial enlargement; *RHC,* right heart catheterization; *R&LHC,* right and left heart catheterization; *RV,* right ventricular; *RVE,* right ventricular enlargement; *SvO₂,* mixed venous oxygen saturation *TRV,* peak velocity of tricuspid regurgitant jet. (From McGoon M, Gutterman D, Steen V, et al: Screening, early detection, and diagnosis of pulmonary arterial hypertension. ACCP evidence-based clinical practice guidelines. *Chest* 126:14S-34S, 2004.)

- Serologic examination for antinuclear antibodies (ANA) should be perfomed as presumptive evidence of an autoimmune process. An ANA titer greater than 1:80 generally is considered significant, and may prompt additional clinical or serologic evaluation to properly classify autoimmune syndromes associated with PAH.[68,69]
- Serologic examination for HIV-1 and HIV-2 should be obtained, because pulmonary hypertension is a well-described complication of HIV infection.[70,71] Because indeterminate enzyme-linked immunosorbent assay results may occur in those with autoimmune conditions, confirmatory Western blot analysis is mandatory.
- Liver function tests should be obtained, including measurements of serum aminotransferases, bilirubin, and γ-glutamyl transpeptidase as screening tests for liver disease, because pulmonary hypertension may develop in association with portal hypertension.[72] Further evaluation, including liver imaging, may be necessary if portal hypertension is strongly suspected. In some situations, liver biopsy is required to differentiate passive liver congestion from primary liver pathology in patients with newly diagnosed pulmonary hypertension.
- Spirometry and measurement of lung volumes and diffusing capacity should be performed to exclude chronic lung conditions, such as chronic obstructive pulmonary disease, interstitial lung disease, chest wall disease, or neuromuscular disease, as potential causes.[73,74]
- Overnight oximetry should be performed as a screening test for obstructive sleep apnea in patients in whom there is not a high pretest suspicion for the diagnosis. A negative study result makes the presence of sleep apnea unlikely, whereas a positive test result requires polysomnography for confirmation and titration of positive pressure therapy.[75] If a high suspicion of obstructive sleep apnea is present, it is generally prudent to proceed directly to polysomnographic evaluation.[76]
- Ventilation-perfusion ($\dot{V}/\dot{Q}$) lung scintigraphy is the modality of choice for excluding the diagnosis of chronic thromboembolic pulmonary hypertension, and will generally display at least one segmental or larger defect when that condition is present.[77] Overall, the sensitivity of ($\dot{V}/\dot{Q}$) scintigraphy for detecting chronic thromboembolism in patients with pulmonary hypertension is estimated at between 90 and 100 percent, while specificity is estimated in excess of 94 percent.[78-80] ($\dot{V}/\dot{Q}$) scintigraphy does not predict the degree and extent of vascular obstruction with precision,

and conventional angiography should be obtained in cases in which perfusion scintigraphy results are abnormal in order to precisely characterize the features, degree, and location of vascular defects, and to assess surgical accessibility.[16,81,82] The roles of CT and MRI in excluding chronic thromboembolic disease are less well established, and these studies should not be relied upon.[16,83]

- Other blood tests, such as renal function tests, thyroid studies, and uric acid levels, may be obtained, although the strengths of association between pulmonary hypertension and end-stage renal disease, thyroid abnormalities, and hyperuricemia are not entirely clear.[84-87]
- In unusual cases, lung biopsy is required to confirm the diagnosis or clarify the cause of pulmonary hypertension. Transbronchial biopsy generally is contraindicated because of an increased risk of hemorrhage, and thoracoscopic lung biopsy carries significant risks primarily related to the anesthesia required for the procedure. Surgical lung biopsy usually is reserved for situations in which the definitive diagnosis of a condition such as pulmonary veno-occlusive disease, pulmonary capillary hemangiomatosis, interstitial lung disease, or active pulmonary vasculitis would substantially alter therapy.[17]
- Right heart catheterization is recommended to exclude a systemic-to-pulmonary shunt, and also to define precisely the hemodynamic severity of pulmonary hypertension and its response to pulmonary vasodilators.

What is the Severity of Pulmonary Hypertension?

After the etiology of pulmonary hypertension has been established, it is important to then stratify the severity of pulmonary hypertension, so that appropriate prognostic information can be communicated and difficult therapeutic decisions (e.g., consideration of lung transplantation or enrollment in a clinical trial) can be undertaken optimally. In addition, accurate baseline data regarding disease severity is essential for objectively determining the benefit of therapeutic interventions. Although many prognostic variables have been described, the severity of pulmonary hypertension (particularly PAH) generally is assessed on the basis of several interrelated parameters, including hemodynamic measurements, functional measurements or indices, changes in right ventricular geometry or performance, and other markers with a bearing on survival.[16,88]

Direct measurement of pulmonary arterial pressures and cardiac performance during cardiac catheterization remains an important means of grading the severity of pulmonary hypertension. In addition, right atrial pressure, mixed venous oxygen saturation, and pulmonary vascular resistance can be measured easily. In the era before effective therapies, a prognostic formula was derived from the NIH IPAH cohort that incorporated a given patient's mPAP, mean right atrial pressure, and cardiac index.[89] This formula is less useful in predicting the course of patients receiving therapy in the current era.[88]

Originally published in 1928 as a classification and prognostic schema of patients with cardiac disease, the New York Heart Association (NYHA) classification has a long history of use in categorizing the severity of disease in patients with pulmonary hypertension. The 1998 World Symposium on Primary Pulmonary Hypertension in Evian, France, published a modified form of this classification, which commonly is referred to as the WHO classification (see below)[90] (TABLE 6-4). Although its prognostic value is inexact, numerous studies have demonstrated the association of NYHA or WHO class III or IV with higher mortality in both treated and untreated patients with IPAH. The classification is used routinely in characterizing the severity of disease among patients with pulmonary hypertension from other causes, although its prognostic power in these populations has been less well studied.[88]

In recent years, the 6-minute walk test (6MWT) has found increasing use both as a measure of disease severity among patients with pulmonary hypertension and a metric of response to therapeutic intervention. The test evolved from a 12-minute running test originally developed as a measure of fitness among healthy young men, to a 12-minute walking test for assessing disability among patients with chronic airflow obstruction, to the current 6MWT that is used as an assessment tool for patients with a variety of cardiopulmonary conditions.[91-94] Although some differences in the technique for obtaining a 6MWT have been described, patients generally are taken to a premeasured, unobstructed 100-foot hallway and instructed to walk at their own pace, stop to rest if needed, and cover as much distance as possible in the 6 minutes provided. The examiner may or may not be scripted to encourage a patient during the test. Patients generally are excluded from the test if they regularly use a cane or walker, have a resting oxygen saturation of less than 90 percent, a resting heart rate less than 50 or more than 110 beats per minute, chest pain within the previous month, or have experienced a myocardial infarction, coronary angioplasty, or bypass grafting within the

TABLE 6-4

New York Heart Association and World Health Organization Functional Classification

Class	New York Heart Association	World Health Association
I	Patients with cardiac disease but without resulting limitation of physical activity. Ordinary physical activity does not cause undue fatigue, palpitation, dyspnea, or anginal pain.	Patients with pulmonary hypertension but without resulting limitation of physical activity. Ordinary physical activity does not cause undue dyspnea or fatigue, chest pain, or near syncope.
II	Patients with cardiac disease resulting in slight limitation of physical activity. They are comfortable at rest. Ordinary physical activity results in fatigue, palpitation, dyspnea, or anginal pain.	Patients with pulmonary hypertension resulting in slight limitation of physical activity. These patients are comfortable at rest, but ordinary physical activity causes undue dyspnea or fatigue, chest pain, or near syncope.
III	Patients with cardiac disease resulting in marked limitation of physical activity. They are comfortable at rest. Less than ordinary physical activity results in fatigue, palpitation, dyspnea, or anginal pain.	Patients with pulmonary hypertension resulting in marked limitation of physical activity. These patients are comfortable at rest, but less than ordinary physical activity causes undue dyspnea or fatigue, chest pain, or near syncope.
IV	Patients with cardiac disease resulting in inability to carry on any physical activity without discomfort. Symptoms of cardiac insufficiency or of the anginal syndrome may be present even at rest. If any physical activity is undertaken, discomfort is increased.	Patients with pulmonary hypertension resulting in inability to perform any physical activity without symptoms. These patients manifest signs of right-sided heart failure. Dyspnea or fatigue or both may be present at rest, and discomfort is increased by any physical activity.

preceding 3 months. Data correlating 6MWT with survival and thus with disease severity have been mixed in patients with IPAH, but the measurement is being used increasingly to stratify the severity of PAH among patients undergoing enrollment in clinical trials.[88]

Several echocardiographic parameters can provide prognostic information and assess disease severity, including right atrial size and the presence of a pericardial effusion in patients with IPAH.[95,96] In addition, investigators have reported the prognostic utility in IPAH patients of the Doppler right ventricular index or "Tei index," consisting of the sum of isovolumic contraction time and the isovolumic relaxation time, divided by ejection time.[97,98] Of note, echocardiographic estimates of pulmonary artery systolic pressure have not had good statistical predictive power and, overall, the use of echocardiographic variables alone is not widespread for the purpose of characterizing the severity of pulmonary hypertension.

Similarly, a number of groups have investigated the use of serum biomarkers for stratifying the disease severity. Associations between survival and serum concentrations of BNP, uric acid, and von Willebrand factor antigen have been described, but none is used commonly to classify disease severity.[84,99,100]

In short, despite the availability of numerous potential markers for disease severity, measurements of functional status (NYHA or WHO functional classification and 6MWT) remain the most widely employed metrics of disease severity, while hemodynamic values such as right atrial pressure, pulmonary artery pressures, and measures of cardiac performance obtained during catheterization play an adjunctive role. With the proliferation of new therapeutic strategies in the management of PAH, these metrics require continued close scrutiny, because they will be applied increasingly to patients who are managed in ways different from the reference population in which their utility was demonstrated.

Screening

The role of screening for pulmonary hypertension in asymptomatic but higher risk individuals remains controversial. In general, screening for any condition is recommended only when the test is relatively safe and inexpensive, when true positive results are not decisively outnumbered by false positive results and, most importantly, when early detection of a disease at a presymptomatic phase enables interventions that have been demonstrated definitively to improve outcome. Although all of these conditions have not been fulfilled unequivocally for the practice of screening asymptomatic persons for pulmonary hypertension, some authors have recommended the echocardiographic screening of individuals with the following risk factors:[17]

- Known genetic risk factor for PAH
- A first-degree relative with PAH
- Diagnosed scleroderma spectrum illness
- Systemic-to-pulmonary shunts due to congenital cardiac disease
- Portal hypertension, in patients undergoing evaluation for orthotopic liver transplantation

However, there is not universal consensus regarding these patients, and there is even less consensus regarding screening in other populations, such as those with sickle cell disease or related hemoglobinopathies.[101]

The most spirited debate has centered on patients with the scleroderma spectrum of illnesses. Several studies have demonstrated that the fraction of such patients with echocardiographically detected pulmonary hypertension (not always defined by the same criteria) ranges between 13 and 61 percent.[102-105] However, the utility of screening is limited, because a relatively small number of patients with PAH detected in this manner demonstrate progression of disease over several years of follow-up, particularly in the absence of interstitial lung disease.[104,105] Furthermore, the cut point values must be set high when echocardiography or diffusing capacity of carbon monoxide is used for screening purposes to avoid generating a prohibitive number of false positive results. Consequently, these tests do not provide accurate reliable information when assessing patients for mild to moderate PAH during presymptomatic phases.[106]

Despite these caveats and the lack of clear evidence that presymptomatic detection of PAH improves outcome in those with the scleroderma spectrum of diseases, the practice of screening these patients is becoming more common, with screening commonly performed at yearly intervals.[16,17,107] The wisdom, or lack of wisdom, of this practice will likely become apparent over the next decade, as the natural history of pulmonary vascular disease among asymptomatic, at-risk individuals with rheumatologic diseases becomes better defined, and data accrue regarding the long-term safety and efficacy of early pharmacologic therapy of PAH in this population.

References

1. Simonneau G, Galie N, Rubin L, et al: Clinical classification of pulmonary hypertension. *J Am Coll Cardiol* 43:5S-12S, 2004.

2. Rich S, Dantzker D, Ayres S, et al: Primary pulmonary hypertension. A national prospective study. *Ann Intern Med* 107:216-223 1987.

3. Yung G, Rubin L: Approach to pulmonary hypertension. *Curr Rheumatol Rep* 2:517-523, 2000.

4. Lucas C: Fluid mechanics of the pulmonary circulation. *Crit Rev Biomed Eng* 10:317-393, 1984.

5. Vizza C, Lynch J, Ochoa L, et al: Right and left ventricular dysfunction in patients with severe pulmonary disease. *Chest* 113:576-583, 1998.

6. Viar W, Harrison T: Chest pain in association with pulmonary hypertension: Its similarity to the pain due to coronary disease. *Circulation* 5:1-11, 1952.

7. Ross R: Right ventricular hypertension as a cause of precordial pain. *Am Heart J* 61:134-135, 1961.

8. Morrison D, Klein C, Walsh C: Relief of right ventricular angina and increased exercise capacity with long-term oxygen therapy. *Chest* 100:534-539, 1991.

9. Schaffer A, Bonaccorsi B, Tchertkoff V: Compressibility of the coronary artery by pulmonary artery distension. *Am J Cardiol* 12:406-407, 1961.

10. Kawut S, Silvestry F, Ferrari V, et al: Extrinsic compression of the left main coronary artery by the pulmonary artery in patients with long-standing pulmonary hypertension. *Am J Cardiol* 83:984-986, 1999.

11. Mesquita S, Castro C, Ikari N, et al: Likelihood of left main coronary artery compression based on pulmonary trunk diameter in patients with pulmonary hypertension. *Am J Med* 116:369-374, 2004.

12. Rich S, McLaughlin V, O'Neill W: Stenting to reverse left ventricular ischemia due to left main coronary artery compression in primary pulmonary hypertension. *Chest* 120:1412-1415, 2001.

13. Gomez Varela S, Montes Orbe PM, Alcibar Villa J, et al: [Stenting in primary pulmonary hypertension with compression of the left main coronary artery.] *Rev Esp Cardiol* 57:695-698, 2004.

14. Ortner N: Recurrenslahmung bei Mitralstenose. *Wein Klin Wochenschr* 10:753-755, 1897.

15. Sengupta A, Dubey S, Chaudhuri D, et al: Ortner's syndrome revisited. *J Laryngol Otol* 112:377-379, 1998.

16. McGoon M, Gutterman D, Steen V, et al: Screening, early detection, and diagnosis of pulmonary arterial hypertension. ACCP evidence-based clinical practice guidelines. *Chest* 126:14S-34S, 2004.

17. Barst R, McGoon M, Torbicki A, et al: Diagnosis and differential assessment of pulmonary arterial hypertension. *J Am Coll Cardiol* 43:40S-47S, 2004.

18. Holcomb BJ, Loyd J, Ely E, et al: Pulmonary veno-occlusive disease: a case series and new observations. *Chest* 118:1671-1679, 2000.

19. Levin E, Gardner D, Samson W: Natriuretic peptides. *N Engl J Med* 339:321-328, 1998.

20. Davidson N, Struthers A: Brain natriuretic peptide. *J Hypertens* 12:329-336, 1994.

21. Nagaya N, Nishikimi T, Okano Y, et al: Plasma brain natriuretic peptide levels increase in proportion to the extent of right ventricular dysfunction in pulmonary hypertension. *J Am Coll Cardiol* 31:202-208, 1998.

22. Leuchte H, Neurohr C, Baumgartner R, et al: Brain natriuretic peptide and exercise capacity in lung fibrosis and pulmonary hypertension. *Am J Respir Crit Care Med* 170:360-365, 2004.

23. McDonagh T, Robb S, Murdoch D, et al: Biochemical detection of left-ventricular systolic dysfunction. *Lancet* 351:9-13, 1997.

24. de Lemos J, Morrow D, Bentley J, et al: The prognostic value of B-type natriuretic peptide in patients with acute coronary syndromes. *N Engl J Med* 345:1014-1021, 2001.

25. Ahearn G, Tapson V, Rebeiz A, et al: Electrocardiography to define clinical status in primary pulmonary hypertension and pulmonary arterial hypertension secondary to collagen vascular disease. *Chest* 122:524-527, 2002.

26. Bossone E, Paciocco G, Iarussi D, et al: The prognostic role of the ECG in primary pulmonary hypertension. *Chest* 121:513-518, 2002.

27. Kanemoto N: Electrocardiogram in primary pulmonary hypertension—with special reference to prognosis. *Tokai J Exp Clim Med* 12:173-179, 1987.

28. Kanemoto N: Electrocardiogram in primary pulmonary hypertension. *Eur Respir J* 12:181-193, 1981.

29. Gehlbach B, Geppert E: The pulmonary manifestations of left heart failure. *Chest* 125:669-682, 2004.

30. Sanders C: The radiographic diagnosis of emphysema. *Radiol Clin North Am* 29:1019-1030, 1991.

31. Walcott G, Burchell H, Brown AJ: Primary pulmonary hypertension. *Am J Med* 49:70-79, 1970.

32. Lupi E, Dumont C, Tejada V, et al: A radiologic index of pulmonary arterial hypertension. *Chest* 68:28-31, 1975.

33. Frazier A, Galvin J, Franks T, et al: From the archives of the AFIP: Pulmonary vasculature: Hypertension and infarction. *Radiographics* 20:491-524, 2000.

34. Kuriyama K, Gamsu G, Stern R, et al: CT-determined pulmonary artery diameters in predicting pulmonary hypertension. *Invest Radiol* 19:16-22, 1984.

35. Tan R, Kuzo R, Goodman L, et al: Utility of CT scan evaluation for predicting pulmonary hypertension in patients with parenchymal lung disease. *Chest* 113:1250-1256, 1998.

36. Ng C, Wells A, Padley S: A CT sign of chronic pulmonary arterial hypertension: The ratio of main pulmonary artery to aortic diameter. *J Thorac Imaging* 14:270-278, 1999.

37. Murray T, Boxt L, Katz J, et al: Estimation of pulmonary artery pressure in patients with primary pulmonary hypertension by quantitative analysis of magnetic resonance images. *J Thorac Imaging* 9:198-204, 1994.

38. Bossone E, Bodini B, Mazza E, et al: Pulmonary arterial hypertension. The key role of echocardiography. *Chest* 127:1836-1843, 2005.

39. Bossone E, Chessa M, Butera G, et al: Echocardiographic assessment of overt or latent unexplained pulmonary hypertension. *Can J Cardiol* 19:544-548, 2003.

40. Schnittger I, Gordon E, Fitzgerald P, et al: Standardized intracardiac measurements of two-dimensional echocardiography. *J Am Coll Cardiol* 2:934-938, 1983.

41. Hinderlater A, Willis PT, Long W, et al: Frequency and prognostic significance of pericardial effusion in primary pulmonary hypertension. PPH study group. Primary pulmonary hypertension. *Am J Cardiol* 84:481-484, 1999.

42. Bossone E, Duong-Wagner T, Paciocco G, et al: Echocardiographic features of primary pulmonary hypertension. *J Am Soc Echocardiogr* 12:655-662, 1999.

43. Yock P, Popp R: Noninvasive estimation of right ventricular systolic pressure by Doppler ultrasound in patients with tricuspid regurgitation. *Circulation* 70:657-662, 1984.

44. Currie P, Seward J, Chan K, et al: Continuous wave Doppler determination of right ventricular pressure: A simultaneous Doppler-catheterization study in 127 patients. *J Am Coll Cardiol* 6:750-756, 1985.

45. Borgesson D, Seward J, Miller FJ, et al: Frequency of Doppler measurable pulmonary artery pressures. *J Am Soc Echocardiogr* 9:832-837, 1996.

46. Ommen S, Nishimura R, Hurrell D, et al: Assessment of right atrial pressure with 2-dimensional and Doppler echocardiography: A simultaneous catheterization and echocardiographic study. *Mayo Clin Proc* 75:24-29, 2000.

47. Niederle P, Starek A, Jezek V, et al: Doppler echocardiography in the diagnosis of pulmonary hypertension. *Cor Vasa* 30:272-280, 1988.

48. Naeije R, Torbicki A: More on the noninvasive estimation of right ventricular systolic pressure by Doppler ultrasound in patients with tricuspid regurgitation. *Eur Respir J* 8:14445-14449, 1995.

49. Kim W, Krowka M, Plevak D, et al: Accuracy of Doppler echocardiography in the assessment of pulmonary hypertension in liver transplant candidates. *Liver Transpl* 6:453-458, 2000.

50. Hinderlater A, Willis P, Barst R, et al: Effects of long-term infusion of prostacyclin (epoprostenol) on echocardiographic measures of right ventricular structure and function in primary pulmonary hypertension. *Circulation* 95:1479-1486, 1997.

51. Brecker S, Gibbs J, Fox K, et al: Comparison of Doppler derived haemodynamic variables and simultaneous high fidelity pressure measurements in severe pulmonary hypertension. *Br Heart J* 72:384-389, 1994.

52. Penning S, Robinson K, Major C, et al: A comparison of echocardiography and pulmonary artery catheterization for evaluation of pulmonary artery pressures in pregnant patients with suspected pulmonary hypertension. *Am J Obstet Gynecol* 184:1568-1570, 2001.

53. Baim DS, Grossman W: *Grossman's Cardiac Catheterization, Angiography, and Intervention,* 6th ed, 2000, New York: Lippincott, Williams & Wilkins.

54. Courtois M, Fattal P, Kovacs SJ, et al: Anatomically and physiologically based reference level for measurement of intracardiac pressures. *Circulation* 92:1994-2000, 1995.

55. Chemla D, Castelain V, Herve P, et al: Haemodynamic evaluation of pulmonary hypertension. *Eur Respir J* 20:1314-1331, 2002.

56. Fuster V, Alexander R, O'Rourke R, et al: *Hurst's the heart,* 11th ed, 2004, New York: McGraw-Hill.

57. Freed M, Miettinen O, Nadas A: Oximetric detection of intracardiac left-to-right shunts. *Br Heart J* 42:690-694, 1979.

58. Morgan J, McCormack D, Griffiths M, et al: Adenosine as a vasodilator in primary pulmonary hypertension. *Circulation* 84:1145-1149, 1991.

59. Krasuski R, Warner J, Wang A, et al: Inhaled nitric oxide selectively dilates pulmonary vasculature in adult patients with pulmonary hypertension, irrespective of etiology. *J Am Coll Cardiol* 36:2204-2211, 2000.

60. Rubin L, Groves B, Reeves J, et al: Prostacyclin-induced acute pulmonary vasoreactivity in primary pulmonary hypertension. *Circulation* 66:334-338, 1982.

61. Sitbon O, Brenot F, Denjean A, et al: Inhaled nitric oxide as a screening vasodilator agent in primary pulmonary hypertension. A dose-response study and comparison with prostacyclin. *Am J Respir Crit Care Med* 151:384-389, 1995.

62. Sitbon O, Humbert M, Jais X, et al: Long-term response to calcium channel blockers in idiopathic pulmonary arterial hypertension. *Circulation* 111:3105-3111, 2005.

63. Partanen J, Nieminem M, Luomanmaki K: Death in a patient with primary pulmonary hypertension after 20 mg of nifedipine. *N Engl J Med* 329:812-813, 1993.

64. Palmer S, Robinson L, Wang A, et al: Massive pulmonary edema and death after prostacyclin infusion in a patient with pulmonary veno-occlusive disease. *Chest* 113:237-240, 1998.

65. Mandel J, Mark E, Hales C: Pulmonary veno-occlusive disease. *Am J Respir Crit Care Med* 162:1964-1973, 2000.

66. Rich S, Kaufmann E, Levy P: The effect of high doses of calcium-channel blockers on survival in primary pulmonary hypertension. *N Engl J Med* 327:76-81, 1992.

67. Runo J, Loyd J: Primary pulmonary hypertension. *Lancet* 361:1533-1544, 2003.

68. Yanai-Landau H, Amital H, Bar-Dayan Y, et al: Autoimmune aspects of primary pulmonary hypertension. *Pathobiology* 63:71-75, 1995.

69. Rich S, Kieras K, Hart K, et al: Antinuclear antibodies in primary pulmonary hypertension. *J Am Coll Cardiol* 8:1307-1311, 1986.

70. Pellicelli A, D'Ambrosio C, Vizza C, et al: HIV-related pulmonary hypertension. From pathogenesis to clinical aspects. *Acta Cardiol* 59:323-530, 2004.

71. Burkhart K, Farber H: HIV-associated pulmonary hypertension: Diagnosis and treatment. *Adv Cardiol* 40:197-207, 2003.

72. Budhiraja R, Hassoun P: Portopulmonary hypertension. A tale of two circulations. *Chest* 123:562-576, 2003.

73. Barbera J, Peinado V, Santos S: Pulmonary hypertension in chronic obstructive pulmonary disease. *Eur Respir J* 21:892-905, 2003.

74. Shapiro S: Management of pulmonary hypertension resulting from interstitial lung disease. *Curr Opin Pulm Med* 9:426-430, 2003.

75. Series F, Marc I, Cormier Y, et al: Utility of nocturnal home oximetry for case finding in patients with suspected sleep apnea hypopnea syndrome. *Ann Intern Med* 119:449-453, 1993.

76. Atwood CJ, McCrory D, Garcia J, et al: Pulmonary artery hypertension and sleep-disordered breathing: ACCP evidence-based clinical practice guidelines. *Chest* 126:72S-77S, 2004.

77. Fedullo P, Auger W, Kerr K, et al: Chronic thromboembolic pulmonary hypertension. *N Engl J Med* 345:1465-1472, 2001.

78. Worsley D, Palevsky H, Alavi A: Ventilation-perfusion lung scanning in the evaluation of pulmonary hypertension. *J Nucl Med* 35:793-796, 1994.

79. Bergin C, Hauschildt J, Rios G, et al: Accuracy of MR angiography compared with radionuclide scanning in identifying the cause of pulmonary arterial hypertension. *Am J Roentgenol* 168:1549-1555, 1997.

80. D'Alonzo G, Bower J, Dantzker D: Differentiation of patients with primary and thromboembolic pulmonary hypertension. *Chest* 85:457-461, 1984.

81. Ryan K, Fedullo P, Davis G, et al: Perfusion scan findings understate the severity of angiographic and hemodynamic compromise in chronic thromboembolic pulmonary hypertension. *Chest* 93:1180-1185, 1988.

82. Azarian R, Wartski M, Collignon M, et al: Lung perfusion scans and hemodynamics in acute and chronic pulmonary embolism. *J Nucl Med* 38:980-983, 1997.

83. Ley C, Kauczor H, Heussel C, et al: Value of contrast-enhanced MR angiography and helical CT angiography in chronic thromboembolic pulmonary hypertension. *Eur Radiol* 13:2365-2371, 2003.

84. Nagaya N, Uematsu M, Satoh T, et al: Serum uric acid levels correlate with the severity and the mortality of primary pulmonary hypertension. *Am J Respir Crit Care Med* 160:487-492, 1999.

85. Lozano H, Sharma C: Reversible pulmonary hypertension, tricuspid regurgitation and right sided heart failure associated with hyperthyroidism. Case report and review of the literature. *Cardiol Rev* 12:299-305, 2004.

86. Curnock A, Dweik R, Higgins B, et al: High prevalence of hypothyroidism in patients with primary pulmonary hypertension. *Am J Med Sci* 318:289-292, 1999.

87. Yigla M, Nakhoul F, Sabag A, et al: Pulmonary hypertension in patients with end-stage renal disease. *Chest* 123:1577-1582, 2003.

88. McLaughlin V, Presberg K, Doyle R, et al: Prognosis of pulmonary arterial hypertension: ACCP evidence-based clinical practice guidelines. *Chest* 126:78S-92S, 2004.

89. D'Alonzo G, Barst R, Ayers S, et al: Survival in patients with primary pulmonary hypertension. Results from a national prospective registry. *Ann Intern Med* 115:343-349, 1991.

90. Executive Summary, World Symposium on Primary Pulmonary Hypertension, Evian, France, 6-10 September, 1998, World Health Organization.

91. Cooper K: A means of assessing maximal oxygen intake. Correlation between field and treadmill testing. *JAMA* 203:201-204, 1968.

92. McGavin C, Gupta S, McHardy G: Twelve-minute walking test for assessing disability in chronic bronchitis. *Br Med J* 1:822-823, 1976.

93. Butland R, Pang J, Gross E, et al: Two-, six-, and 12-minute walking tests in respiratory disease. *Br Med J* 284:1607-1608, 1982.

94. Enright P, McBurnie M, Bittner V, et al: The 6-min walk test: A quick measure of functional status in elderly adults. *Chest* 123:387-398, 2003.

95. Eysmann S, Palevsky H, Reichek N, et al: Two-dimensional and Doppler-echocardiographic and cardiac catheterization correlates of survival in primary pulmonary hypertension. *Circulation* 80:353-360, 1989.

96. Raymond R, Hinderliter A, Willis P, et al: Echocardiographic predictors of adverse outcomes in primary pulmonary hypertension. *J Am Coll Cardiol* 39:1214-1219, 2002.

97. Yeo T, Dujardin K, Tei C, et al: Value of a Doppler-derived index combining systolic and diastolic time intervals in predicting outcome in primary pulmonary hypertension. *Am J Cardiol* 81:1157-1161, 1998.

98. Tei C, Dujardin K, Hodge D, et al: Doppler echocardiographic index for assessment of global right ventricular function. *J Am Soc Echocardiogr* 9:838-847, 1996.

99. Nagaya N, Nishikimi T, Uematsu M, et al: Plasma brain natriuretic peptide as a prognostic indicator in patients with primary pulmonary hypertension. *Circulation* 102:865-870, 2000.

100. Lopes A, Maeda N, Concalves R, et al: Endothelial cell dysfunction correlates differentially with survival in primary and secondary pulmonary hypertension. *Am Heart J* 139:618-623, 2000.

101. Ataga K, Sood N, De Gent G, et al: Pulmonary hypertension in sickle cell disease. *Am J Med* 117:665-669, 2004.

102. Battle R, Davitt M, Cooper S, et al: Prevalence of pulmonary hypertension in limited and diffuse scleroderma. *Chest* 110:1515-1519, 1996.

103. Yamane K, Ihn H, Asano Y, et al: Clinical and laboratory features of scleroderma patients with pulmonary hypertension. *Rheumatology (Oxford)* 39:1269-1271, 2000.

104. MacGregor A, Canavan R, Knight C, et al: Pulmonary hypertension in systemic sclerosis: risk factors for progression and consequences for survival. *Rheumatology (Oxford)* 40:453-459, 2001.

105. Hesselstrand R, Ekman R, Eskilsson J, et al: Screening for pulmonary hypertension in systemic sclerosis: The longitudinal development of tricuspid gradient in 227 consecutive patients, 1992-2001. *Rheumatology (Oxford)* 44:366–371, 2005.

106. Mukerjee D, St George D, Knight C, et al: Echocardiography and pulmonary function as screening tests for pulmonary arterial hypertension in systemic sclerosis. *Rheumatology (Oxford)* 43:461-466, 2004.

107. Korn J: Clinical manifestations and evaluation of scleroderma lung disease. In: Rose B, editor: *UpToDate*, vol 12.3. Wellesley, MA, 2004, UpToDate.

Chapter 7

Treatment for Pulmonary Arterial Hypertension

Jess Mandel, MD

Despite significant advances in management over the past two decades, pulmonary arterial hypertension (PAH) remains an incurable and potentially deadly disease that is difficult to manage adequately.[1,2] Nonetheless, significant progress has occurred in the therapeutic approach to PAH, particularly for idiopathic pulmonary arterial hypertension (IPAH), during the past 15 years. This chapter will focus on the therapeutic approach to patients with IPAH. Many of these therapeutic principles are also applied to PAH from other causes, although in the absence of extensive experience or well-controlled data, such extrapolation should be undertaken with extreme care.

Basic Management

For most of the twentieth century, therapy for IPAH relied almost entirely upon oxygen, cardiac glycosides, anticoagulants, and diuretics, and was minimally efficacious.[3,4] Nonetheless, all of these therapies remain part of the basic therapeutic regimen of patients with IPAH, despite a paucity of high-grade evidence in favor of their effectiveness.[1]

Oxygen

Hypoxemia, particularly with exertion, is common among patients with PAH. It may result from a combination of mechanisms such as poor ventilation-perfusion matching, an inability to normally recruit and distend pulmonary capillaries with exercise, impairment of cardiac performance resulting in desaturation of venous blood, and right-to-left shunting via a patent foramen ovale. Although long-term oxygen therapy is documented to delay mortality in patients with chronic obstructive pulmonary disease (COPD), data on the utility of long-term, low-flow oxygen therapy in patients with PAH are sparse. Nonetheless, oxygen prescription is recommended in patients with PAH, using the same parameters as in patients with COPD accompanied by evidence of cor pulmonale: titration to maintain an oxygen saturation over 90 percent with rest and exertion for 24 hours per day.[5,6] This goal may be particularly difficult to achieve when hypoxemia is caused by shunt physiology. Care must be taken to ensure patients' access to portable equipment that will have the smallest negative impact upon their mobility.

Anticoagulation

Anticoagulation has been prescribed in PAH for many decades, yet its benefit has never been documented in appropriate prospective randomized trials. Rather, anticoagulation is justified on the basis of postmortem studies that have described *in situ* or embolic thrombosis in the small vessels of a substantial number of patients with IPAH[7,8] and observational, nonrandomized studies that have suggested a survival benefit for IPAH patients treated with anticoagulation.[7,9,10] As an example, one study of 64 patients with IPAH who were treated with calcium channel antagonists found 3-year survival to be significantly improved if warfarin was also employed (47 versus 31 percent).[10] Registry data from a different group suggested that patients with PAH associated with anorectic drug use benefited from earlier, rather than delayed, warfarin initiation.[9]

In addition, anticoagulation is justified in part because of the increased prevalence of risk factors for venous thromboembolism among patients with PAH, such as heart failure and relative immobility. Pulmonary emboli tend to be poorly tolerated in this population because of diminished cardiopulmonary reserve.[1]

Based upon this circumstantial evidence of efficacy, most clinicians recommend initiation of warfarin titrated to an International Normalized Ratio of approximately 1.5 to 2.5 in patients with IPAH, provided that contraindications are not present.[1,5] However, there is a lack of unanimity regarding the threshold pulmonary artery pressures at which anticoagulation should be initiated, or whether this therapy should be applied strictly to patients with IPAH or generalized to other forms of PAH as well. There are no compelling data to suggest a routine role for heparin, antiplatelet agents, or other anticoagulants in preference to warfarin, or to suggest that a combination of anticoagulants is superior to warfarin alone. A potential role for aspiration is being investigated in ongoing trials.

Cardiac Glycosides

Various forms of digitalis have been used in medical practice for centuries, yet the ideal manner in which to employ these agents for pulmonary hypertension remains controversial. Long-term, prospective, randomized trials have not been performed in patients with PAH. However, one study examined hemodynamics in 17 patients with IPAH and symptomatic heart failure immediately before and 2 hours after the intravenous administration of 1.0 mg of digoxin. Investigators noted a significant increase in cardiac output (from 3.49 to 3.81 L/min), a significant fall in plasma norepinephrine concentrations, and a significant increase in the plasma concentration of atrial natriuretic peptide.[11] These data, in conjunction with the observation that a low cardiac output is a poor prognostic indicator, persuade a number of clinicians to routinely initiate digoxin in patients with PAH if symptomatic right ventricular failure is present. Nonetheless, given the limited clinical data on the issue, a firm recommendation regarding the use of long-term digoxin in PAH cannot be made confidently.

Diuretics

The obvious clinical utility of diuretic therapy in patients with symptomatic right heart failure is such that few rigorous data have been collected regarding their optimal acute and long-term use. Volume overload in pulmonary hypertension exacerbates elevations of central venous pressure, hepatic and abdominal congestion, ascites, and peripheral edema. Dyspnea can worsen because diaphragmatic excursion is limited, and ventricular septal displacement limits left ventricular performance.

Diuretic therapy should be individualized based upon symptoms and signs of hypervolemia, including weight gain. Education and limitation of dietary salt intake are of paramount importance. Loop diuretics are generally the agents of first choice, and are administered with appropriate electrolyte repletion and care to avoid iatrogenic hypovolemia. Furosemide remains the most widely used initial agent, although the more dependable bioavailability of torsemide may offer advantages in some patients.[12] In more diuretic-refractory cases, a loop diuretic may need to be combined with a potassium-sparing or thiazide diuretic. Patients do not require diuretic therapy if heart failure has not developed.

Contraception

Pregnancy is discouraged among patients with significant pulmonary hypertension because of increased maternal and fetal risks related to the disease, the teratogenicity of medications such as warfarin and endothelin receptor antagonists, and the potential for shortened maternal life expectancy (see Chapter 17).[13,14] Although successful pregnancies have been reported in patients with IPAH and other conditions, most practitioners strongly recommend effective contraception in women of childbearing potential. Surgical sterilization of the male partner is the safest and most effective method of contraception for the woman with pulmonary hypertension, although barrier methods and hormonal methods and are also used widely, provided no contraindications such as venous thromboembolism are present. Of note, the effectiveness of hormonal contraceptives may be diminished by certain medications for PAH, such as bosentan.[15]

Physical Activity

Although vigorous exercise to exhaustion is hazardous to the individual with significant pulmonary hypertension, patients need to remain as active as their condition reasonably permits in order to avoid deconditioning.[1] Patients should engage in activities of daily living and mild aerobic exercise such as walking. Supplemental oxygen should be employed to avoid oxyhemoglobin desaturation, and patients should be counseled to pace exercise so as to avoid dizziness, syncope, or severe dyspnea. Evaluation and monitoring by an experienced physical therapist is recommended before physical activity is increased substantially. Indeed, enrollment in a pulmonary or cardiac rehabilitation program may help to improve exercise tolerance by providing emotional encouragement, patient confidence in the safety of exercise, and teaching of coping mechanisms to manage troubling symptoms.

Calcium Channel Antagonists

After scientists in the mid-twentieth century hypothesized that IPAH was related to excessive vasoconstriction, a number of vasodilator agents were employed to treat patients with this condition, including acetylcholine, tolazoline, phentolamine, hydralazine, diazoxide, isoproterenol, and calcium channel antagonists.[16,17] None of these medications proved consistently successful in altering the symptoms or the course of the disease.

Calcium channel antagonists, such as nifedipine and diltiazem, became the vasodilator medications of choice after the description of 64 patients treated with high doses of these drugs. Seventeen patients demonstrated acute decreases in pulmonary arterial pressures and pulmonary vascular resistance in response to acute drug administration during a monitored hemodynamic trial. Significant sustained improvements in hemodynamics and longer survival were seen in this group with long-term administration of calcium antagonists, better than the response of the 47 patients who did not respond acutely to such medications[10] (FIGURES 7-1, 7-2, and 7-3).

However, only 5–10 percent of patients with IPAH respond to calcium channel antagonists. Intensive care unit admission is required for oral vasodilator testing, and deaths can occur during the acute administration of these medications. Thus, safer methods of predicting calcium channel antagonist response were sought.[18–20] It became apparent that testing for calcium channel antagonist responsiveness could be performed more safely by means of a two-step process:

- Initial testing for pulmonary vasoreactivity with short-acting pulmonary vasodilators
- Follow-up testing only of responders with orally administered calcium channel antagonists.

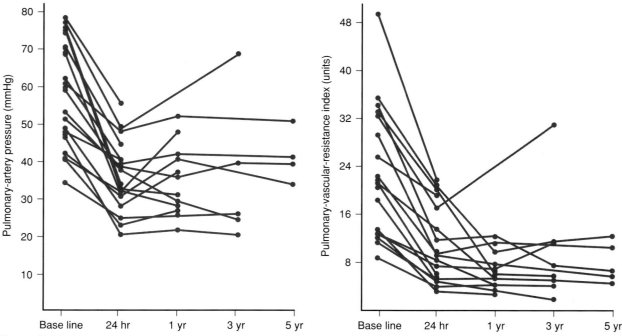

Figure 7-1. Mean Pulmonary Artery Pressure and Pulmonary Vascular Resistance Index in the Patients Who Had Favorable Responses to Calcium Channel Antagonists. Values shown were measured at baseline, after the initial assessment of the effectiveness of the drug, and then periodically for up to 5 years. (From Rich S, Kaufmann E, Levy P: The effect of high doses of calcium-channel blockers on survival in primary pulmonary hypertension. *N Engl J Med* 327:76–81, 1992.)

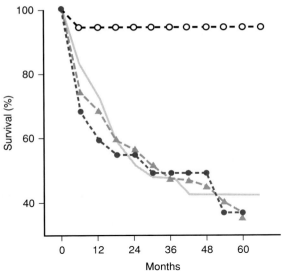

Figure 7-2. Kaplan-Meier estimates of survival among patients who responded to treatment *(open circles)*, those who did not respond *(solid line)*, patients enrolled in the National Institutes of Health (NIH) registry who were treated at the University of Illinois *(solid circles)*, and the NIH registry cohort *(triangles)*. The percentages were calculated every 6 months for 5-{1/2} years. The rate of survival was significantly better in the patients who responded (P = .003) than in the other groups. (From Rich S, Kaufmann E, Levy P: The effect of high doses of calcium-channel blockers on survival in primary pulmonary hypertension. *N Engl J Med* 327:76–81, 1992.)

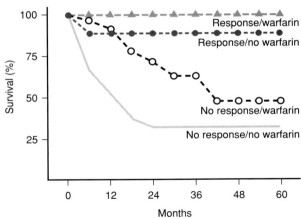

Figure 7-3. Kaplan-Meier estimates of survival, according to the presence or absence of a response to calcium channel blockers and to the use of concurrent therapy with warfarin. Overall survival was significantly improved by warfarin therapy (P = .025). (From Rich S, Kaufmann E, Levy P: The effect of high doses of calcium-channel blockers on survival in primary pulmonary hypertension. *N Engl J Med* 327:76–81, 1992.)

Testing for Acute Pulmonary Vasoreactivity

Based upon their high pulmonary vasodilatory activities and their short half-lives, inhaled nitric oxide, intravenous epoprostenol, intravenous adenosine, or inhaled epoprostenol or iloprost are the agents currently used to assess acute pulmonary vasoreactivity, defined as a fall in mean pulmonary arterial pressure of at least 10 mmHg to a final value of 40 mmHg, without a fall in cardiac output.[5] Only one short-acting vasodilator needs to be employed to test for pulmonary vasoreactivity, and there is no established benefit to trying multiple agents in a single patient.

- Inhaled nitric oxide offers the advantage of a half-life of 15-30 seconds and production of pulmonary vasodilation with minimal systemic effects. It is generally administered at a dosage of 10-80 ppm for a duration of 5-10 minutes.[21,22]
- Intravenous adenosine has a half-life of 5-10 seconds and can decrease both pulmonary and systemic vascular resistance, as well as produce coronary vasodilation. For testing of pulmonary vasoreactivity, adenosine generally is administered at an initial rate of 50 mcg/kg/min, and increased by 20-50 mcg/kg/minute increments every 2 minutes until hemodynamic targets are met; dosage-limiting symptoms such as hypotension, severe chest pain, severe dyspnea, or dysrhythmias develop; or a maximum dosage of 350-500 mcg/kg/min is reached.[23]
- Intravenous epoprostenol has a serum half-life of approximately 3-6 minutes, and like adenosine has effects on both the pulmonary and systemic vascular beds. Acute vasoreactivity testing generally is performed with a starting dosage of 1.0-2.5 ng/kg/min, which is increased by 2.0-2.5 ng/kg/min increments every 5-10 minutes until hemodynamic targets are met; dosage-limiting symptoms such as nausea, emesis, or systemic hypotension develop; or a maximum dosage of 10 ng/kg/min is reached.[24]
- There is less experience with inhaled iloprost or inhaled epoprostenol for vasodilator testing, but they appear to have reasonably specific effects on the pulmonary vasculature and to produce acute hemodynamic changes that are similar those achieved with intravenous epoprostenol.[25,26] In this setting, iloprost can be delivered as a single inhaled dose of 10-18 mcg.

Follow-up Testing of Responders

If a patient does not respond to a short-acting pulmonary vasodilator agent, the chance of producing a sustained positive response with a calcium channel antagonist is very small, and no further testing or calcium channel antagonist therapy is advised. Thus, calcium channel antagonists should not be used to manage PAH in the absence of demonstrated acute pulmonary vasoreactivity.[5]

However, if a patient displays a positive acute response to a short-acting pulmonary vasodilator agent, then the pulmonary artery catheter should be left in place, and the patient should be transferred to an intensive care unit setting for testing the safety and effectiveness of oral calcium channel antagonists. After baseline hemodynamic values are recorded, the patient should receive 20 mg of oral nifedipine (or 60 mg of oral diltiazem if tachycardia is present) each hour until there is a fall in mean pulmonary arterial pressure of at least 10 mmHg, to a final value of 40 mmHg without a fall in cardiac output, dosage-limiting symptoms develop, or a total of 8 hourly doses have been administered. If hemodynamic targets are achieved, the cumulative dose should be administered every 8 hours on a long-term basis, or a long-acting preparation can be used to deliver the same cumulative daily dosage. In general, the target long-term dosage of calcium channel antagonists should be achieved after slowly titrating upward over several weeks to minimize adverse effects. High dosages of calcium channel antagonists generally are required to treat PAH in responsive patients; in some series, up to 240 mg/day of nifedipine or 900 mg/day of diltiazem have been prescribed.[10,27] Systemic hypotension and peripheral edema may limit tolerance of these agents.

Of note, the benefits of calcium channel antagonists have not been documented in large randomized trials. Although one study documented an impressive improvement in survival among responders to calcium channel antagonists, the comparison group was nonresponders, rather than responders in whom calcium channel antagonists were withheld.[10] Because the presence of pulmonary vasoreactivity connotes a better prognosis, this choice of comparison group may impute more benefit to the intervention than is truly the case.[28]

All in all, relatively few patients benefit from sustained treatment with a calcium channel antagonist. Because of the risks of dysrhythmia, hypotension, progression of cor pulmonale, and worsened hypoxemia when these drugs are employed, consultation with an experienced PAH referral center is recommended before they are employed in this setting.

Prostacyclin Derivatives (Prostanoids)

Prostacyclin initially was described in 1976, and shortly thereafter it received attention as a potentially important molecule in both the development and the therapy of PAH.[29] A product of arachidonic acid metabolism, prostacyclin produces relaxation in both pulmonary and systemic vascular smooth muscle cells and inhibits vascular smooth muscle proliferation and platelet aggregation; at least some of these properties result from stimulation of the intracellular production of cyclic adenosine monophosphate (cAMP).[30] Decreased release of endogenous prostacyclin has been documented in patients with pulmonary hypertension from a variety of causes, suggesting that this phenomenon may be a consequence, rather than a fundamental cause, of the condition.[31] Nonetheless, administration of prostacyclin (epoprostenol sodium) and the synthetic prostaglandin analogs treprostinil and iloprost form a cornerstone of therapy for PAH.

Epoprostenol (Prostacyclin)

Prostacyclin is administered pharmacologically as epoprostenol sodium (Flolan). The drug cannot be used orally and has a short half-life (<6 minutes for a single intravenous dose, and 15 minutes as a continuous intravenous infusion); this necessitates delivery of the medication as a continuous infusion via a long-term, tunneled intravenous catheter. In addition, it is unstable at room temperature and thus requires cooling until infusion.

Epoprostenol is begun at a low dosage (1-4 ng/kg/min) and titrated upward in 1-2 ng/kg/min increments at a rate that is dependent upon patient response and side effects. Most patients reach a plateau dosage between 20 and 40 ng/kg/min, at which point further increase in dosage may produce additional adverse effects without additional benefit, although dosage must be individualized. Common side effects, most of which are dosage related, include hypotension, headache, flushing, masticatory jaw pain, nausea, diarrhea, leg pain, and rash. Long-term overdosage may produce high-output cardiac failure.[32] Patients are at risk for catheter-related infections and thrombosis, and interruption of the infusion may cause clinical deterioration within 30 minutes. For this reason, proper training of the patient and a second individual in mixing and administering the drug is essential, and patients should always have a spare functional pump and additional reconstituted drug available. Ongoing assessment of functional status and repeat cardiac catheterizations every 6-12 months may be required to optimize dosing, which may be titrated to a goal cardiac index of 2.5 to 4.0 L/min/meter[2].[33]

The first successful long-term use of continuous intravenous epoprostenol to treat a patient with severe IPAH was reported in 1984.[34] Several uncontrolled trials subsequently reported positive hemodynamic and functional outcomes among epoprostenol-treated patients, but it was not until 1996 that a randomized, open-label trial was reported in which functional and survival advantages were documented.[35] In this 12-week trial, 81 patients with IPAH were randomized to receive conventional therapy (including anticoagulants, oral vasodilators, diuretics, cardiac glycosides, and supplemental oxygen) or conventional therapy plus epoprostenol (approximately 5.0 ng/kg/min at initiation, and 9.0 ng/kg/min at the end of the study). Statistically significant differences between treatment groups were noted after 12 weeks in mortality

(20 versus zero percent), 6-minute walk distance (+31 meters versus –29 meters), quality of life, and in several hemodynamic indices (TABLE 7-1; FIGURE 7-4). Serious complications of epoprostenol management included four episodes of catheter-related sepsis and one of paradoxical embolism. Largely on the basis of this trial, the United States Food and Drug Administration (FDA) approved continuous intravenous epoprostenol for IPAH management in late 1995.

Subsequently, it has been well documented that acute improvements following the initiation of epoprostenol in patients with IPAH are generally sustained for several years or longer.[36] Perhaps even more significant has been that the absence of an acute hemodynamic response to epoprostenol or other acute vasodilating agents does not preclude improvement in function and hemodynamics with long-term infusion.[37] This observation suggests that epoprostenol exerts an effect that produces advantageous remodeling of the pulmonary vasculature in addition to its vasodilating properties.

Because of success in managing IPAH with epoprostenol, the drug has also been used to treat patients with PAH from other causes. One randomized controlled trial of 111 patients with PAH accompanying the scleroderma spectrum of

TABLE 7-1

Short-term Hemodynamic Effects of Epoprostenol at the Maximal Tolerated Dosage During Short-term Dosage Ranging*

Variable	Change From Baseline		95% Confidence Interval[†]
	Epoprostenol (n = 41)	Conventional Therapy (n = 40)	
Mean pulmonary artery pressure (mmHg)	–2.4 ± 1.1	–1.4 ± 1.3	–4.4 to 2.4
Mean right atrial pressure (mmHg)	–0.2 ± 0.4	–1.3 ± 0.6	–0.3 to 2.5
Mean systemic artery pressure (mmHg)	–13.6 ± 1.5	–11.9 ± 1.2	–5.5 to 2.2
Mean pulmonary capillary wedge pressure (mmHg)	–1.5 ± 0.9	–1.0 ± 0.8	–2.0 to 2.9
Cardiac index (L/min/m²)	–0.9 ± 0.1	–0.5 ± 0.2	0 to 0.8
Heart rate (beats/min)	–6.8 ± 1.2	–6.1 ± 1.9	–3.7 to 5.1
Systemic arterial oxygen saturation (%)	–0.6 ± 0.7	–1.3 ± 1.0	–4.2 to 0.5
Mixed venous oxygen saturation (%)	–5.8 ± 1.4	–8.9 ± 1.3	–7.0 to 0.9
Stroke volume (mL/beat)	–14.8 ± 2.7	–5.8 ± 3.0	1.1 to 17.0
Pulmonary vascular resistance (mmHg/L/min)	–5.5 ± 0.8	–3.9 ± 0.8	–4.0 to 0.7
Systemic vascular resistance (mmHg/L/min)	–10.5 ± 0.9	–7.3 ± 0.9	–5.7 to –0.6

*Plus-minus values are mean (±SE) changes from baseline. The maximal tolerated dosages were 9.2 ± 0.5 ng per kilogram per minute in the epoprostenol group and 7.6 ± 0.5 nh per kilogram per minute in the conventional therapy group.
[†]95 Percent confidence intervals are for the differences in mean changes between treatment groups. A confidence interval that does not contain zero indicates statistical significance.
SE, standard error.
From Barst R, Rubin L, Long W, et al: A comparison of continuous intravenous epoprostenol (prostacyclin) with conventional therapy for primary pulmonary hypertension. The Primary Pulmonary Hypertension Study Group. N Engl J Med 334:296–302, 1996.

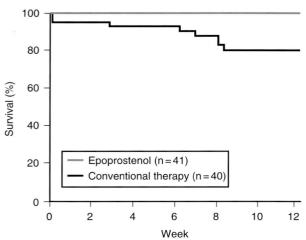

Figure 7-4. Survival Among the 41 Patients Treated With Epoprostenol and the 40 Patients Receiving Conventional Therapy. Data on patients who underwent transplantation during the 12-week study were censored at the time of transplantation. Estimates were made by the Kaplan-Meier product-limit method. The two-sided P value from the log-rank test was .003. Survival analysis with data on patients receiving transplants not censored at transplantation resulted in the same level of significance (two-sided P = .003 by the log-rank test). (From Barst R, Rubin L, Long W, et al: A comparison of continuous intravenous epoprostenol (prostacyclin) with conventional therapy for primary pulmonary hypertension. The Primary Pulmonary Hypertension Study Group. *N Engl J Med* 334: 296-302, 1996.)

connective tissue disease (in the absence of significant interstitial lung disease) documented an improvement in NYHA functional class in 38% of patients receiving epoprostenol, versus no improvement among patients treated with conventional therapy alone; likewise, the change in 6-minute walk distance after 12 weeks was significantly greater in the epoprostenol group (+46 versus –48 meters). No difference in mortality after 12 weeks was demonstrated.[38] Although randomized controlled trials have not been performed in other types of PAH, case reports and case series have suggested that epoprostenol is efficacious for PAH associated with other conditions, including systemic lupus erythematosus, human immunodeficiency virus infection, anorectic drug use, cocaine or amphetamine use, congenital heart disease, portal hypertension, chronic thromboembolic disease, and scleroderma with associated interstitial lung disease.[39-45]

Of note, epoprostenol should be used with great care in patients with pulmonary veno-occlusive disease or pulmonary capillary hemangiomatosis, because life-threatening pulmonary edema may ensue.[46,47] This complication may result from dilation of pulmonary arterioles in lungs with relatively fixed venous changes, producing an increase in transcapillary hydrostatic pressure and consequent pulmonary edema.

Patients with pulmonary venous hypertension from left-sided heart failure have also fared poorly with epoprostenol. The drug was associated with increased mortality (despite improvements in hemodynamic parameters) among patients who had NYHA class IIIB to IV symptoms caused by left ventricular failure and who were randomized to treatment with epoprostenol.[48]

With the demonstration of the efficacy of epoprostenol for PAH, the therapy of pulmonary hypertension entered a new era. A condition that previously was refractory to treatment now could be managed in many cases, although not cured. Initially regarded a bridge to lung transplantation, epoprostenol therapy quickly was recognized as a viable long-term alternative to transplantation, and changed the treatment paradigm from one of vasodilation alone to one of vascular remodeling. Because of epoprostenol and subsequent therapies, PAH has become the only major indication for lung transplantation for which there has been a dramatic decrease in demand for the procedure.[49] Despite its cost, side effects, and inconvenient delivery system, epoprostenol remains an attractive therapeutic option because of its established efficacy and the extensive clinical experience with its use.

Treprostinil

Treprostinil (Remodulin) is an analog of prostacyclin with a longer half-life (approximately 3 hours), near-neutral pH, and greater stability at room temperature. The chemical properties of treprostinil permit continuous subcutaneous administration, thereby eliminating the need for and complications of long-term intravenous access. The medication may be particularly advantageous among patients with recurrent episodes of line sepsis; in contrast to the life-threatening nature of line sepsis, infectious complications of subcutaneous catheters are frequently minor and treatable with catheter repositioning, or oral antibiotics, or both. More recently, treprostinil has received FDA approval for use via the intravenous route, and inhaled and oral formulations of the drug are under investigation.

A randomized, placebo-controlled, double-blind, 12-week trial of 470 patients with IPAH or PAH associated with connective tissue disease or congenital systemic-to-pulmonary shunts examined the risks and benefits of subcutaneous treprostinil.[50] Patients were enrolled in 40 centers in North America, Europe, Israel, and Australia and were randomized to receive standard therapy (oral vasodilators, anticoagulants, and diuretics, with or without digitalis) and either subcutaneous treprostinil or vehicle placebo. Compared with placebo, a modest but statistically significant median improvement in 6-minute walk distance of 16 meters was noted with subcutaneous treprostinil, as were small but statistically significant improvements in mean pulmonary artery pressure, pulmonary vascular resistance, and cardiac index.

However, significant adverse effects were also noted, most notably infusion site pain, which occurred in 85 percent of patients receiving treprostinil versus 27 percent in the placebo group. Prostanoid side effects, such as jaw pain, diarrhea, and flushing, were also observed. There is no uniformly effective treatment for infusion site pain; some patients find relief with cold packs or topical anesthetics, while others cannot obtain acceptable palliation of symptoms even with oral nonsteroidal antiinflammatory agents or opiates.

Intravenous treprostinil was approved by the FDA in 2004 and offers several advantages over epoprostenol. First, its stability at room temperature obviates the need to apply cooling packs to the infusion pump. Second, the drug is supplied in prefilled syringes, so that sterile mixing is not required. Third, its longer half-life theoretically suggests that short interruptions in intravenous administration should be better tolerated than is the case with epoprostenol. Studies of the efficacy of intravenous treprostinil are relatively few, but they suggest that similar short-term hemodynamic effects as are achieved with epoprostenol.[51] Fewer data are available comparing the benefits of long-term treprostinil and epoprostenol administration. In general, an intravenous dose of epoprostenol requires multiplication by a factor of 1.1 to 1.5 to obtain an equivalent intravenous dose of treprostinil.

More recently, inhaled treprostinil is undergoing investigation. Preliminary experiments suggest that the drug may be effective with only four inhalations per day, employing briefer inhalation times than iloprost (see below).[52] High-quality controlled trials of inhaled treprostinil for pulmonary hypertension have not yet been performed. Trials of oral treprostinil are even more preliminary.[53]

Iloprost

Iloprost (Ilomedin, Ventavis) is another synthetic analog of prostacyclin. Like prostacyclin and treprostinil, it dilates pulmonary and systemic vascular beds and decreases platelet aggregation. Its plasma half-life is approximately 12-25 minutes, which is longer than that of epoprostenol but significantly shorter than that of treprostinil.[54] The drug has been used in intravenous form to manage pulmonary and systemic vasculopathies, but currently it is employed more widely in its inhaled form to manage PAH.

Intravenous iloprost has been used for over a decade in patients with PAH, primarily when the cause is idiopathic or related to connective tissue diseases.[55,56] Although large-scale therapeutic equivalency trials have not been performed with intravenous iloprost and intravenous epoprostenol, small trials have suggested similar hemodynamic effects can be achieved with intravenous infusion of either drug.[55,57] Because intravenous iloprost has also been used to manage digital ulcers, a number of rheumatologists prefer it over epoprostenol when an intravenous prostanoid is required for the treatment of PAH associated with the scleroderma spectrum of diseases.[58] Intravenous iloprost is approved for use in a number of European countries and elsewhere, but not in the United States.

In contrast, inhaled iloprost was approved for use in the United States in December 2004 and is also widely available worldwide. Several delivery devices have been studied (e.g., the Ilo-Neb, Ventstream, and HaloLite systems), and similar responses can be obtained from each if calibrated to a standard delivered dose.[59] Systems require an inhalation time of approximately 10 minutes; inhalations are performed roughly every 2 hours while awake for a minimum of 6 and a maximum of 9 inhalations per 24-hour period.

Even with multiple doses of inhaled iloprost, pulmonary vasodilation is achieved for only a small portion of each 24-hour period. As an example, one study of five vasoreactive ambulatory patients using an implantable right ventricular pressure monitor found a mean effective treatment time of 49 minutes after the initiation of each treatment. A regimen of 5-6 daily inhalations (given no more frequently than every 4 hours) was used and resulted in pulmonary vasodilation being achieved only during 13 percent of each 24-hour period.[60]

Uncontrolled trials showed conflicting reports of efficacy. One uncontrolled trial of 19 severely ill patients (including 12 with IPAH and 3 with PAH associated with connective tissue diseases) reported a 6-minute walk distance improvement of 148 meters after 3 months of treatment.[61] A different observational trial of 12 severely ill patients, most with IPAH, found that none manifested improvement in hemodynamics or exercise tolerance after a mean treatment time of 10 months.[62]

A multicenter, randomized, placebo-controlled trial was organized to help resolve these conflicting results.[63] A total of 203 patients in WHO classes III and IV, primarily with IPAH, chronic thromboembolic pulmonary hypertension, or PAH associated with connective tissue diseases were randomized to receive placebo or 2.5-5.0 mcg of iloprost inhaled 6-9 times daily while awake. At the conclusion of the 12-week study, 6-minute walk distance measured after iloprost inhalation improved by an average of 36 meters over the placebo group. The proportion of patients who had an increase of at least 10 percent in their 6-minute walk distances was not significantly different between the placebo and control groups, and preinhalation hemodynamic measurements were largely unchanged after 12 weeks in the iloprost group. Overall, iloprost was well tolerated, with only jaw pain, cough, and syncope occurring more significantly than in the placebo group. Syncope was not associated with clinical deterioration, and its pathophysiology in this situation is not well understood. Systemic hypotension has developed upon initiation of inhaled iloprost, and for that reason the initial two doses should be administered in an observed setting.

Inhaled iloprost has entered widespread use in the United States relatively recently. Many questions about its true sustained efficacy and it optimal role in the treatment of PAH will likely be answered during the next several years as worldwide experience with this therapy continues to accrue.

Beraprost

Beraprost (Berasil, Dorner, Procylin) is an orally active prostacyclin analogue that is absorbed rapidly and has an elimination half-life of approximately 40 minutes.[64] Two major randomized trials have examined its safety and efficacy.

One study randomized 130 patients with WHO class II and III symptoms of PAH (primarily with IPAH, congenital systemic-to-pulmonary shunts, and portal hypertension) to receive placebo or the maximally tolerated dose of beraprost (median 80 mcg 4 times per day).[65] At the end of the 12-week study period, mean 6-minute walk distance in the beraprost group was 25 meters longer than in the

placebo group. No significant changes in hemodynamics or WHO functional class were observed. Adverse effects such as headache, flushing, jaw pain, leg pain, diarrhea, and nausea were far more common in the beraprost group, although they tended to improve after the first 6 weeks of therapy.

A second trial randomized 116 patients with PAH due to IPAH, connective tissue diseases, or congenital systemic-to-pulmonary shunts and with WHO class II and III functional status to treatment with beraprost or placebo for 12 months.[66] Some improvements over placebo in 6-minute walk distance and disease progression were observed among beraprost-treated patients during the first 6 months of therapy, but these were not sustained at months 9 and 12. Adverse effects were noted in a high proportion of both beraprost and placebo patients, but headache, jaw pain, vasodilation, diarrhea, and asthenia were significantly more common among patients receiving beraprost.

Because of its lack of sustained proven benefit and frequent adverse reactions, beraprost has not found widespread use outside of Japan for PAH management.

Endothelin Antagonists

The endothelins are a family of peptides that are secreted by endothelial cells and have important vasoconstrictor, proliferative, and regulatory effects on vascular smooth muscle and endothelial cells within the pulmonary circulation.[67] Of the multiple molecules identified in the family, endothelin-1 (ET-1) is the predominant isoform, and it is approximately 100-fold more powerful as a vasoconstrictor than norepinephrine.

Pre-pro ET-1 is synthesized within endothelial cells, then cleaved to big ET-1 by an endopeptidase. Big ET-1 is subsequently processed to the 21 amino acid sequence of ET-1 by any of several enzymes, including at least two types of endothelin-converting enzymes, at least two distinct chymases, and other metallo-proteases[68] (FIGURE 7-5). ET-1 is secreted both into the lumen and abluminally toward vascular smooth muscle cells. Endothelin A (ET$_A$) receptors are found primarily on vascular smooth muscle cells, where they stimulate vasoconstriction (via G-protein-induced phospholipase C activation) and cellular proliferation.[69] ET$_B$ receptors are also found on vascular smooth muscle cells and have similar effects, but the receptors are additionally present on endothelial cells where they are important for clearance of ET-1 and play a

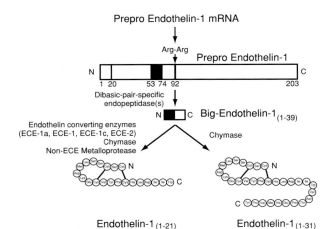

Figure 7-5. Biosynthesis of Endothelin (ET)-1$_{1-21}$ and ET-1$_{1-31}$ Peptides. Pre-pro ET-1 messenger ribonucleic acid is translated into prepro-ET-1 protein, a 203-amino acid peptide, which is cleaved by furin convertase to the 38-amino acid precursor, big ET-1$_{1-38}$. Big ET$_A$ is processed into ET-1$_{1-21}$ by endothelin-converting enzyme(s) (ECE[s]), mast cell and smooth muscle cell chymases, and non-ECE metalloprotease *(left)*. By a novel pathway involving mast cell chymase 31-amino acid, ET-1$_{1-31}$ is formed *(right)*. (Modified from Yanagisawa M, Kurihara H, Kimura S, et al: A novel potent vasoconstrictor peptide produced by vascular endothelial cells. *Nature* 332:411–415, 1988; and Luscher T, Barton M: Endothelins and endothelin receptor antagonists. Therapeutic considerations for a novel class of cardiovascular drugs. *Circulation* 102:2434–2440, 2000.)

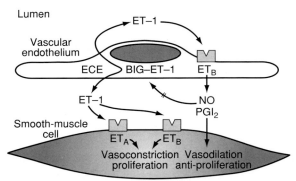

ET–1 = endothelin–1, BIG–ET–1 = proendothelin–1, ECE = endothelin–converting enzyme, NO = nitric oxide, PGI$_2$ = prostacyclin

Figure 7-6. Endothelin System in Vascular Tissue. (From Dupuis J: Endothelin-receptor antagonists in pulmonary hypertension. *Lancet* 358: 1113–1114, 2001.)

counter-regulatory role: stimulation of endothelial ET$_B$ receptors increases endothelial production of nitric oxide and prostacyclin (with vasodilatory and antiproliferative effects) and suppresses cellular production of big ET-1[70] (FIGURE 7-6).

ET-1 levels are elevated in pulmonary hypertension from a variety of causes, suggesting that endothelial dysfunction (probably related to both increased ET-1 production and decreased uptake by endothelial ET$_B$ receptors) occurs as a consequence, rather than an underlying cause, of the syndrome.[71] Nonetheless, the endothelin system likely plays an important role in disease propagation and acceleration and therefore has become an important therapeutic target. Both nonselective and ET$_A$ receptor-selective agents have been developed. Although theoretic advantages have been proposed for both classes of agents, compelling clinical differences have not been demonstrated among the various agents in the endothelin receptor antagonist class.[72]

Bosentan

Bosentan (Tracleer) is considered a nonspecific ET-1 receptor antagonist, because it has only minimally higher affinity for the ET$_A$ receptor.[73] It is administered orally twice daily; after an initial oral dosage of 62.5 mg twice per day for 4 weeks, the dosage is increased to 125 mg twice per day. Two double-blind, randomized, placebo-controlled studies have demonstrated the efficacy of the drug versus placebo. In the first, 32 patients with IPAH or PAH associated with scleroderma were assigned to bosentan or placebo groups with the primary end point of a change in 6-minute walk distance.[74] At the conclusion of the 12-week study, the bosentan group had a mean improvement of 76 meters versus the placebo group, and improvements in hemodynamics and Borg dyspnea index were observed. The second trial employed a similar design but randomized a total of 213 patients with IPAH or PAH associated with connective tissue disease (almost all with WHO class III functional symptoms) to placebo or one of two dosages of bosentan for a period of 16 weeks.[75] A statistically significant 6-minute walk distance difference of 44 meters was observed between the bosentan groups and the placebo group (FIGURE 7-7). Subsequent observations have suggested that among those who benefit from bosentan, the benefit is largely

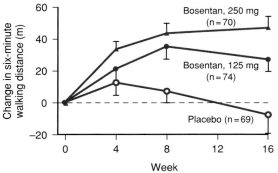

Figure 7-7. Mean (±SE) Change in 6-Minute Walking Distance From Baseline to Week 16 in the Placebo and Bosentan Groups. P < .01 for the comparison between the 125-mg dose of bosentan and placebo, and P < .001 for the comparison between the 250-mg dose and placebo by the Mann-Whitney U test. There was no significant difference between the two bosentan groups (P = .16 by the Mann-Whitney U test). (From Rubin L, Badesch D, Barst R, et al: Bosentan therapy for pulmonary arterial hypertension. *N Engl J Med* 346: 896–903, 2002.)

maintained after a year or more of treatment.[76] Although an effect of bosentan upon survival has not been demonstrated directly, comparison of bosentan-treated patients with the historical control group of the NIH cohort of IPAH patients from the 1980s suggests that bosentan may positively impact the mortality of the disease.[77] Nonetheless, a high-grade, sustained response to bosentan is not universal.

Bosentan is absolutely contraindicated in pregnancy (FDA category X) because of its potent teratogenicity. Women of childbearing age who are candidates for therapy must document negative pregnancy tests at initiation and monthly thereafter, and ideally they should use two methods of contraception (of which at least one is nonhormonal). Other safety concerns have focused on hepatotoxicity, given that an approximately 9 percent excess of transaminase elevation to more than 3 times the upper limit of normal has been noted in patients taking bosentan in pooled clinical trials.[73] For this reason, liver function tests must be obtained monthly for as long as patients remain on the drug, and the medication must be discontinued if elevations greater than 5 times the upper limits of normal are observed. The drug has been reintroduced successfully in a number of cases, but this should be undertaken cautiously only if the benefits of therapy clearly outweigh the risks.

Other adverse effects observed with bosentan have included worsened fluid retention and anemia early in therapy, headache, and nasopharyngeal irritation. The drug should not be used concomitantly with glyburide or cyclosporine, and because of its metabolism by the cytochrome P-450 system (CYP2C8/9 and 3A4), it has numerous potential drug interactions.

Sitaxsentan

Sitaxsentan (Thelin) is an orally active ET-1 receptor antagonist that binds approximately 6,500 times as avidly to ET_A as to ET_B receptors, and has a half-life of 5-7 hours that permits once-daily dosing.[78] One study randomized 178 patients with IPAH, or PAH associated with connective tissue disorders or congenital systemic-to-pulmonary shunts, to receive placebo or 100 mg or 300 mg daily of sitaxsentan.[79] Most patients were WHO functional class II or III, and the primary end point of the study was change in peak oxygen uptake after 12 weeks of therapy. Patients in the 300 mg/day group demonstrated a statistically significant improvement in peak oxygen uptake of 3.1 percent, compared with those taking placebo. Both sitaxsentan groups demonstrated an improvement in 6-minute walk distance of approximately 35 meters greater than those in the placebo group at the conclusion of the study, and showed improvements in mean pulmonary artery pressure, cardiac index, and pulmonary vascular resistance (FIGURE 7-8). Long-term experience with sitaxsentan is limited, but small studies suggest that most patients who improve on the drug experience benefit for 1 year or longer.[80]

Adverse effects of sitaxsentan are similar to those of bosentan: the medication is a potent teratogen which is absolutely contraindicated in pregnancy, and monthly monitoring of transaminases is recommended because of the risk of drug-induced hepatitis.[81] Headache, peripheral edema, nausea, nasal congestion, and dizziness can occur. The drug is also metabolized via the cytochrome P-450 CYP2C9 enzyme system, and thus has multiple drug interactions, including potentiation of the effects of warfarin.[79]

Ambrisentan

Ambrisentan is an orally active ET-1 receptor antagonist with preferential binding to the ET_A receptor, although its relative avidity for the

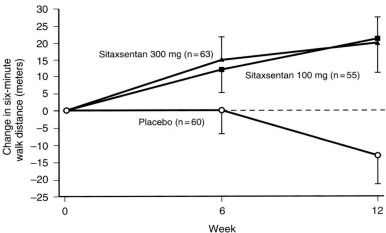

Figure 7-8. Mean (±SE) Change in 6-Minute Walk Distance From Baseline to Week 12 in Placebo and Sitaxsentan Groups. Pair-wise (versus placebo) P values are from analysis of covariance including baseline response in the model and are adjusted for multiple comparisons using Dunnett's method. P values less than .01 for the comparison between each sitaxsentan dose (100 mg and 300 mg) and placebo. (From Barst R, Langleben D, Frost A, et al: Sitaxsentan therapy for pulmonary arterial hypertension. *Am J Respir Crit Care Med* 169:441–447, 2004.)

ET_A receptor is less pronounced than that of sitaxsentan.[82] It entered clinical trials later than the other two endothelin receptor antagonists, so fewer clinical data are available regarding its efficacy. Open-label studies have suggested similar efficacy and adverse effects as are seen in other members of the class, but randomized trials have not yet been published.[83] The drug is not metabolized via the cytochrome P-450 system and thus has fewer drug interactions than bosentan or sitaxsentan.

Phosphodiesterase Inhibitors

Nitric oxide released from endothelial cells plays an important role in dilating the pulmonary vascular bed and is a significant antiproliferative stimulus to pulmonary vascular smooth muscle.[84,85] An important signal transduction pathway for nitric oxide within pulmonary vascular smooth muscle cells is the activation of guanylate cyclase, which catalyzes the formation of cyclic guanosine monophosphate (cGMP), and in turn leads to changes in myosin light chain kinase and cellular calcium pumps that facilitate relaxation. cGMP is inactivated by a number of phosphodiesterases, the most important and most cGMP-specific of

which is phosphodiesterase 5 (PDE5).[86] Thus, inhibition of PDE5 can produce pulmonary vasodilation and remodeling. Of note, PDE5 is strongly expressed in the vascular smooth muscle cells of the genitals and the retina, as well as the lung.

Sildenafil

Sildenafil (Viagra, Revatio) was developed as a treatment for erectile dysfunction because of its potency as a PDE5 inhibitor. Case reports and case series describing its potential efficacy in the management of PAH and persistent pulmonary hypertension of the newborn proliferated around the turn of the millennium.[87-89]

The SUPER-1 trial randomized 278 patients to placebo or treatment with 20 mg, 40 mg, or 80 mg of sildenafil 3 times daily[89b]. Most patients had IPAH or PAH associated with connective tissue disease, and most had WHO class II or III function. At the conclusion of the 12-week study, 6-minute walk distance improved by a mean of 45 meters in the sildenafil groups over those in the placebo group, and no significant differences were demonstrated among the different dosing regimens. More recent studies suggest that patients with IPAH who are treated with sildenafil experience longer survival than did historical controls in the NIH registry from the 1980s.[90] Headache, flushing, and epistaxis have been the most common adverse effects of PAH management. Systemic hypotension may result if the drug is taken concomitantly with nitrates.

Large comparison trials between sildenafil and endothelin receptor antagonists have not been performed, but preliminary data suggest that sildenafil does not represent inferior management. One study randomized 26 WHO functional class III patients with IPAH or PAH associated with connective tissue disease to receive therapy with bosentan or sildenafil in a double-blinded fashion for 16 weeks.[91] At the conclusion of the study, there were no significant differences among the groups by intention to treat analysis, although sildenafil patients who completed the protocol had significantly higher 6-minute walk distances and Kansas City Cardiomyopathy quality of life scores.

Although data on sildenafil are relatively preliminary, the drug shows significant promise for the management of PAH. Sildenafil was approved by the FDA for PAH management in mid-2005. There are far fewer data for the use of other PDE5 inhibitors, such as vardenafil and tadalafil, for this indication, and their use is not recommended until their efficacy and safety have been comparably demonstrated in patients with PAH.[92]

Combination Therapy

Whereas PAH was essentially an untreatable disease in most patients until the mid-1990s, the proliferation of effective therapies now permits combination therapy. Unfortunately, the relative rarity of PAH has made the conduct of large trials of combination therapy challenging. Combination therapy varies widely among centers, and there are few data to guide decision making.

Parenteral Prostanoid Plus Endothelin Receptor Antagonist

The best-studied combination regimen is intravenous epoprostenol plus oral bosentan. One study randomized 33 patients with PAH (predominantly IPAH) to begin using open-label epoprostenol and to receive also either bosentan or placebo.[93] Both groups demonstrated improvements in 6-minute walk distance and hemodynamics after 16 weeks, but no significant benefit to the additional bosentan

was detected. Of note, the power of the study was limited, and combination therapy appeared safe provided that standard monitoring protocols for endothelin receptor antagonist-related toxicity were employed.

Parenteral Prostanoid Plus PDE5 Inhibitor

Several uncontrolled series have reported improvements in patients treated with continuous infusion epoprostenol or treprostinil when sildenafil was added to their regimens.[94,95,95b] Randomized controlled trials are in progress to test the safety and efficacy of this combination more thoroughly.

Inhaled or Oral Prostanoid Plus Endothelin Receptor Antagonist

Very little has been published regarding the combination of a nonparenteral prostanoid with an endothelin receptor antagonist.[96,97] One series of 20 patients with IPAH who were stable on inhaled iloprost or oral beraprost suggested that the addition of bosentan improved maximal oxygen consumption after 3 months of combination therapy.[97] More recently, a trial randomized 67 patients stable on bosentan to add inhaled placebo or iloprost for 12 weeks.[97b] At the conclusion of the trial, patients randomized to bosentan plus iloprost displayed a statistically significant improvement of 30 meters on 6 minute walk distance versus patients receiving bosentan plus placebo.

Inhaled Prostanoid Plus PDE5 Inhibitor

The combination of inhaled iloprost plus oral sildenafil has been described to reduce acutely pulmonary artery pressures more effectively than iloprost alone.[98] In addition, the combination results in a longer period of vasodilation than iloprost alone, and the area under the curve for reduction in pulmonary vascular resistance is greater than that of the sum of iloprost and sildenafil monotherapy.[99] A case series reported that the addition of sildenafil to 14 patients whose condition was deteriorating on treatment with inhaled iloprost alone produced hemodynamic improvement in all subjects and reversed their clinical deterioration.[100] Despite these promising initial results, rigorous prospective randomized trials have not yet been performed to clarify the exact role this combination of therapies should play in the care of patients with PAH.

Endothelin Receptor Antagonist Plus PDE5 Inhibitor

The prospect of a combination of an endothelin receptor antagonist and a PDE5 inhibitor is very appealing, because both medications are active when taken orally and are relatively well tolerated. One series reported the course of 9 patients with IPAH whose condition had initially improved on bosentan but subsequently declined.[101] Three months after the addition of sildenafil, mean 6-minute walk distance improved by over 100 meters, and maximal oxygen uptake was likewise enhanced.

Combination of an endothelin receptor antagonist and a PDE5 inhibitor may have pharmacokinetic implications. When bosentan and sildenafil are combined, higher levels of bosentan and lower levels of sildenafil result than when either is taken alone.[102] However, the clinical significance of these changes on the efficacy and safety of both drugs is unclear.[103,104] The magnitude of pharmacokinetic interactions between sildenafil and either sitaxsentan or ambrisentan appears less significant.[105]

Miscellaneous Agents

A number of medications are in early stages of development for PAH management, or have shown promise in limited case reports or series. Because none of these has yet demonstrated benefit in rigorous prospective randomized trials, their routine use cannot be recommended at present.

Inhaled Nitric Oxide

Endogenous nitric oxide plays an important role in regulating pulmonary vascular tone and cellular proliferation. Inhaled nitric oxide frequently is used as a diagnostic agent to determine whether pulmonary vasoreactivity is present, as a short-term therapy in the perioperative setting, or when persistent pulmonary hypertension of the newborn occurs.[106] In contrast, inhaled nitric oxide has not been well studied as a long-term therapy for PAH, with only rare case reports and case series appearing in print.[107-109]

L-Arginine

Because L-arginine is the precursor for the formation of nitric oxide in the pulmonary endothelium, a potential therapeutic role for L-arginine has been hypothesized. Several reports have noted hemodynamic improvements following infusion of L-arginine.[110] One study randomized 19 patients with pulmonary hypertension (most with IPAH or chronic thromboembolic pulmonary hypertension) to receive either oral L-arginine supplementation or placebo.[111] Sixty minutes after administration, patients receiving L-arginine had significant reductions in pulmonary vascular resistance and systemic vascular resistance. After 1 week of supplementation, patients receiving L-arginine demonstrated a significant improvement in peak oxygen uptake, in contrast to patients receiving placebo.

HMG-CoA Reductase Inhibitors (Statins)

3-Hydroxy-3-methylglutaryl-coenzyme A (HMG-CoA) reductase inhibitors, also known as statins, play an important role in the management of hypercholesterolemia. They also appear to have direct effects on the vasculature, exerting antiproliferative stimuli and facilitating endothelial production of nitric oxide.[112,113] Simvastatin has been effective in animal models of PAH, but human experience is limited.[114] One open-label study of 16 patients with pulmonary hypertension found that the addition of simvastatin to their regimen was well tolerated, and that two patients demonstrated improvements in pulmonary vascular resistance without prostanoid therapy.[115] In contrast, a different small study found no deterioration following the withdrawal of atorvastatin from patients receiving bosentan and sildenafil.[103] Additional human trials of statins in PAH are ongoing.

Angiotensin Antagonists

Because of the important role that angiotensin II plays in the pathobiology of vascular remodeling, angiotensin-converting enzyme inhibitors or angiotensin receptor antagonists have been considered as potential therapeutic agents in PAH.[116,117] However, their use frequently is complicated by systemic hypotension, and none of these agents has demonstrated a clinically meaningful impact on PAH.

Vasoactive Intestinal Peptide

Vasoactive intestinal peptide (VIP) is a 28-amino acid peptide hormone that is synthesized in pancreatic islet cells and influences water and electrolyte trafficking in the gastrointestinal tract. It also is a systemic and pulmonary vasodilator and inhibits platelet activation and vascular smooth muscle proliferation. Decreased serum and lung tissue VIP levels have been seen in patients with PAH. One group treated eight patients with IPAH with VIP inhalation 4 times daily; after 3 months, significant decreases in pulmonary artery pressure and pulmonary vascular resistance and increases in cardiac output and mixed venous oxygen saturation were noted. Few adverse effects were reported.[118]

Surgical Therapies: Lung Transplantation, Pulmonary Thromboendarterectomy, and Atrial Septostomy

Issues pertaining to lung transplantation and pulmonary thromboendarterectomy are discussed elsewhere in this volume (see Chapters 8, 13). Atrial septostomy, in which a communication is established between the atria with the intention of creating a right-to-left shunt and reducing the load on the right side of the heart, has been employed in cases of unremitting right-sided heart failure.[119-122] The procedure appears to be associated with an immediate mortality of around 13 percent, although hemodynamic benefits that are sustained for 2 years or more have also been documented.[123] The high procedural mortality of atrial septostomy coupled with the availability of multiple effective medications for PAH has rendered the procedure rarely indicated.

Conclusions

In less than a decade, PAH has evolved from a condition in which few patients could be treated successfully, to one in which a multitude of generally effective medications from a variety of classes are available. There is, however, an absence of head-to-head medication trials, a paucity of data on combination therapies, and a lack of clinical information by which to determine whether a "front-loaded" strategy of initial multiple agents is superior to a "stepped therapy" approach by which therapy progresses to parenteral agents or multiple agents only if deterioration occurs[124]. Thus, it is not possible to offer a single algorithm by which all patients with PAH should be treated. Nonetheless, several recommendations can be made:

- All patients should be evaluated for treatment with oxygen and diuretics, and counseling regarding exercise and pregnancy should be undertaken. We favor the use of warfarin and digoxin unless contraindications are present.
- Right heart catheterization with a short-acting vasodilator challenge should be performed to identify patients who are candidates for calcium channel antagonist therapy unless contraindications are present. Because of their low cost and established safety profiles, calcium channel antagonists should be employed in hemodynamically reactive patients.
- Patients with less severe disease who are not vasoreactive generally should be treated with an endothelin receptor antagonist, sildenafil, or both; inhaled and parenteral prostanoids should be reserved for patients whose disease progresses despite oral therapies, or who are severely ill at initial evaluation.
- Atrial septostomy or lung transplantation should be undertaken only in patients whose medical management is unequivocally failing.

References

1. Humbert M, Sitbon O, Simonneau G: Treatment of pulmonary hypertension. *N Engl J Med* 351:1425–1436, 2004.
2. McLaughlin V, Presberg K, Doyle R, et al: Prognosis of pulmonary arterial hypertension: ACCP evidence-based clinical practice guidelines. *Chest* 126:78S-92S, 2004.
3. Dresdale D, Schultz M, Michtom R: Primary pulmonary hypertension. I. Clinical and hemodynamic study. *Am J Med* 11:686–705, 1951.
4. Walcott G, Burchell H, Brown AJ: Primary pulmonary hypertension. *Am J Med* 49:70–79, 1970.
5. Badesch D, Abman S, Ahearn G, et al: Medical therapy for pulmonary arterial hypertension. ACCP evidence-based clinical practice guidelines. *Chest* 126:35S-62S, 2004.
6. Tarpy S, Celli B: Long-term oxygen therapy. *N Engl J Med* 333:710–714, 1995.
7. Fuster V, Steele P, Edwards W, et al: Primary pulmonary hypertension: Natural history and the importance of thrombosis. *Circulation* 70:580–587, 1984.
8. Bjornsson J, Edwards W: Primary pulmonary hypertension: A histopathologic study of 80 cases. *Mayo Clin Proc* 60:16–25, 1995.
9. Frank H, Mlczoch J, Huber K, et al: The effect of anticoagulant therapy in primary and anorectic drug-induced pulmonary hypertension. *Chest* 112:714–721, 1997.

10. Rich S, Kaufmann E, Levy P: The effect of high doses of calcium-channel blockers on survival in primary pulmonary hypertension. *N Engl J Med* 327:76–81, 1992.

11. Rich S, Seidlitz M, Dodin E, et al: The short-term effects of digoxin in patients with right ventricular dysfunction from pulmonary hypertension. *Chest* 1998:787–792, 1998.

12. Murray M, Deer M, Ferguson J, et al: Open label randomized trial of torsemide compared with furosemide therapy for patients with heart failure. *Am J Med* 111:513–520, 2001.

13. Weiss B, Hess O: Pulmonary vascular disease and pregnancy: Current controversies, management strategies, and perspectives. *Eur Heart J* 21:104–115, 2000.

14. McCaffrey R, Dunn L: Primary pulmonary hypertension in pregnancy. *Obstet Gynecol Surv* 19:567–591, 1964.

15. Taichman D, Palevsky H: Treatment of pulmonary arterial hypertension with the endothelin receptor antagonist bosentan. *Clin Pulm Med* 12:121–127, 2005.

16. Wood P: Primary pulmonary hypertension, with special reference to vasoconstrictive factors. *Br Heart J* 20:557–565, 1958.

17. Fishman A, Pietra G: Primary pulmonary hypertension. *Ann Rev Med* 31:421–431, 1980.

18. Weir E, Rubin L, Ayers S, et al: The acute administration of vasodilators in primary pulmonary hypertension. Experience from the National Institutes of Health Registry on Primary Pulmonary Hypertension. *Am Rev Respir Dis* 140:1623–1630, 1989.

19. Partanen J, Nieminen M, Luomanmaki K: Death in a patient with primary pulmonary hypertension after 20 mg of nifedipine. *N Engl J Med* 329:812, 1993.

20. Sitbon O, Humbert M, Ioos V, et al: Who benefits from long-term calcium channel blocker (CCB) therapy in primary pulmonary hypertension (PPH)? *Am J Respir Crit Care Med* 167:A440, 2003 (abstract).

21. Ricciardi M, Knight B, Martinez F, et al: Inhaled nitric oxide in primary pulmonary hypertension. A safe and effective agent for predicting a response to nifedipine. *J Am Coll Cardiol* 32:1068–1073, 1998.

22. Sitbon O, Humbert M, Jagot J, et al: Inhaled nitric oxide as a screening agent for safely identifying responders to oral calcium-channel blockers in primary pulmonary hypertension. *Eur Respir J* 12:263–264, 1998.

23. Schrader B, Inbar S, Kaufmann L, et al: Comparison of the effects of adenosine and nifedipine in pulmonary hypertension. *J Am Coll Cardiol* 19:1060–1064, 1992.

24. Sitbon O, Brenot F, Denjean A, et al: Inhaled nitric oxide as a screening vasodilator agent in primary pulmonary hypertension. A dose-response study and comparison with prostacyclin. *Am J Respir Crit Care Med* 151:384–389, 1995.

25. Olschewski H, Walmrath D, Schermuly R, et al: Aerosolized prostacyclin and iloprost in severe pulmonary hypertension. *Ann Intern Med* 124:820–824, 1996.

26. Opitz C, Wensel R, Bettmann M, et al: Assessment of the vasodilator response in primary pulmonary hypertension. Comparing prostacyclin and iloprost administered by either infusion or inhalation. *Eur Heart J* 24:356–365, 2003.

27. Rich S, Kaufmann E: High-dose titration of calcium channel blocking agents for primary pulmonary hypertension: guidelines for short-term drug testing. *J Am Coll Cardiol* 18:1323–1327, 1991.

28. Raffy O, Azarian R, Brenot F, et al: Clinical significance of the pulmonary vasodilator response during short-term infusion of prostacyclin in primary pulmonary hypertension. *Circulation* 93:484–488, 1996.

29. Moncada S, Gryglewski R, Bunting S, et al: An enzyme isolated from arteries that transforms prostaglandin endoperoxidases to an unstable substance that inhibits platelet aggregation. *Nature* 263:663–665, 1976.

30. Clapp L, Finney P, Turcato S, et al: Differential effects of stable prostacyclin analogs on smooth muscle proliferation and cyclic AMP generation in human pulmonary artery. *Am J Respir Crit Care Med* 26:194–201, 2002.

31. Christman B, McPherson C, Newman J, et al: An imbalance between the excretion of thromboxane and prostacyclin metabolites in pulmonary hypertension. *N Engl J Med* 327:70–75, 1992.

32. Rich S, McLaughlin V: The effects of chronic prostacyclin therapy on cardiac output and symptoms in primary pulmonary hypertension. *J Am Coll Cardiol* 34:1184–1187, 1999.

33. McLaughlin V, Rich S: Pulmonary hypertension. *Curr Probl Cardiol* 29:575–634, 2004.

34. Higenbottam T, Wheeldon D, Wells F, et al: Long-term treatment of primary pulmonary hypertension with continuous intravenous epoprostenol (prostacyclin). *Lancet* 1:1046–1047, 1984.

35. Barst R, Rubin L, Long W, et al: A comparison of continuous intravenous epoprostenol (prostacyclin) with conventional therapy for primary pulmonary hypertension. The Primary Pulmonary Hypertension Study Group. *N Engl J Med* 334:296–302, 1996.

36. McLaughlin V, Shillington A, Rich S: Survival in pulmonary hypertension. The impact of epoprostenol therapy. *Circulation* 106:1477–1482, 2002.

37. McLaughlin V, Genthner D, Panella M, et al: Reduction in pulmonary vascular resistance with long-term epoprostenol (prostacyclin) therapy in primary pulmonary hypertension. *N Engl J Med* 338:273–277, 1998.

38. Badesch D, Tapson V, McGoon M, et al: Continuous intravenous epoprostenol for pulmonary hypertension due to the scleroderma spectrum of disease. A randomized, controlled trial. *Ann Intern Med* 132:425–434, 2000.

39. Simonneau G, Fartoukh M, Sitbon O, et al: Primary pulmonary hypertension associated with the use of fenfluramine derivatives. *Chest* 114:195S–199S, 1998.

40. Robbins I, Gaine S, Schilz R, et al: Epoprostenol for treatment of pulmonary hypertension in patients with systemic lupus erythematosus. *Chest* 117:14–18, 2000.

41. Aguilar R, Farber H: Epoprostenol (prostacyclin) therapy in HIV-associated pulmonary hypertension. *Am J Respir Crit Care Med* 162:1846–1850, 2000.

42. Kuo P, Johnson L, Plotkin J, et al: Continuous intravenous infusion of epoprostenol for the treatment of portopulmonary hypertension. *Transplantation* 63:604–606, 1997.

43. Rosenzweig E, Kerstein D, Barst R: Long-term prostacyclin for pulmonary hypertension associated with congenital heart defects. *Circulation* 99:1858–1865, 1999.

44. McLaughlin V, Genthner D, Panella M, et al: Compassionate use of continuous prostacyclin in the management of secondary pulmonary hypertension: A case series. *Ann Intern Med* 130:740–743, 1999.

45. Strange C, Bolster M, Mazur J, et al: Hemodynamic effects of epoprostenol in patients with systemic sclerosis and pulmonary hypertension. *Chest* 118:1077–1082, 2000.

46. Mandel J, Mark E, Hales C: Pulmonary veno-occlusive disease. *Am J Respir Crit Care Med* 162:1964–1973, 2000.

47. Almagro P, Julia J, Sanjaume M, et al: Pulmonary capillary hemangiomatosis associated with primary pulmonary hypertension: Report of 2 new cases and review of 35 cases from the literature. *Medicine (Baltimore)* 81:417–424, 2002.

48. Califf R, Adams K, McKenna W, et al: A randomized controlled trial of epoprostenol therapy for severe congestive heart failure: The Flolan International Randomized Survival Trial (FIRST). *Am Heart J* 134:44–54, 1997.

49. Lang G, Klepetko W: Lung transplantation for end-stage primary pulmonary hypertension. *Ann Transplant* 9:25–32, 2004.

50. Simonneau G, Barst R, Galie N, et al: Continuous subcutaneous infusion of treprostinil, a prostacyclin analogue, in patients with pulmonary arterial hypertension. A double-blind, randomized, placebo-controlled trial. *Am J Respir Crit Care Med* 165: 800–804, 2002.

51. McLaughlin V, Gaine S, Barst R, et al: Efficacy and safety of treprostinil: An epoprostenol analog for primary pulmonary hypertension. *J Cardiovasc Pharmacol* 41:293–299, 2003.

52. Voswinckel R, Enke E, Kreckel A, et al: Pharmacologic testing with inhaled treprostinil for pulmonary hypertension and nine month treatment experience. *Proc Am Thorac Soc* 2:A199, 2005 (abstract).

53. Mottola D, Laliberte K, Phares K, et al: Pharmacokinetics and safety of treprostinil diethanolamine (UT-15C), a novel salt of treprostinil for oral delivery. *Proc Am Thorac Soc* 2:A197, 2005 (abstract).

54. Scott J, Higenbottam T, Wallwork J: The acute effect of the synthetic prostacyclin analog iloprost in primary pulmonary hypertension. *Br J Clin Pharmacol* 6:231–234, 1990.

55. Higenbottam T, Butt A, McMahon A, et al: Long-term intravenous prostaglandin (epoprostenol or iloprost) for treatment of severe pulmonary hypertension. *Heart* 80:151–155, 1998.

56. de la Mata J, Gomez-Sanchez M, Aranzana M, et al: Long-term iloprost infusion therapy for severe pulmonary hypertension in patients with connective tissue diseases. *Arthritis Rheum* 37:1528–1533, 1994.

57. Higenbottam T, Butt A, Dihn-Xuan A, et al: Treatment of pulmonary hypertension with the continuous infusion of a prostacyclin analog, iloprost. *Heart* 79:175–179, 1998.

58. Bettoni L, Geri A, Airo P, et al: Systemic sclerosis therapy with iloprost: A prospective observational study of 30 patients treated for a median of 3 years. *Clin Rheumatol* 21:244–250, 2002.

59. Olschewski H, Rohde B, Behr J, et al: Pharmacodynamics and pharmacokinetics of inhaled iloprost, aerosolized by three different devices, in severe pulmonary hypertension. *Chest* 124:1294, 2003.

60. Fruhwald F, Kjellstrom B, Perthold W, et al: Continuous hemodynamic monitoring in pulmonary hypertensive patients treated with inhaled iloprost. *Chest* 124:351–359, 2003.

61. Olschewski H, Ghofrani H, Schmehl T, et al: Inhaled iloprost to treat severe pulmonary hypertension. An uncontrolled trial. *Ann Intern Med* 132:435–443, 2000.

62. Machherndl S, Kneussl M, Baumgartner H, et al: Long-term treatment of pulmonary hypertension with aerosolized iloprost. *Eur Respir J* 17:8–13, 2001.

63. Olschewski H, Simonneau G, Galie N, et al: Inhaled iloprost for severe pulmonary hypertension. *N Engl J Med* 347:322–329, 2002.

64. Okano Y, Yoshioko T, Shimouchi A, et al: Orally active prostacyclin analogue in primary pulmonary hypertension. *Lancet* 349:1365, 1997.

65. Galie N, Humbert M, Vachiery J, et al: Effects of beraprost sodium, an oral prostacyclin analogue, in patients with pulmonary arterial hypertension: A randomized, double-blind, placebo-controlled trial. *J Am Coll Cardiol* 39:1496–1502, 2002.

66. Barst R, McGoon M, McLaughlin V, et al: Beraprost therapy for pulmonary arterial hypertension. *J Am Coll Cardiol* 41:2119, 2003.

67. Yanagisawa M, Kurihara H, Kimura S, et al: A novel potent vasoconstrictor peptide produced by vascular endothelial cells. *Nature* 332:411–415, 1988.

68. Luscher T, Barton M: Endothelins and endothelin receptor antagonists. Therapeutic considerations for a novel class of cardiovascular drugs. *Circulation* 102:2434–2440, 2000.

69. Takuwa Y, Kasuya Y, Takuwa N, et al: Endothelin receptor is coupled to phospholipase C via a pertussis toxin-insensitive guanine nucleotide-binding regulatory protein in vascular smooth muscle cells. *J Clin Invest* 85:653–658, 1990.

70. Dupuis J: Endothelin-receptor antagonists in pulmonary hypertension. *Lancet* 358:1113–1114, 2001.

71. Giaid A, Yanagisawa M, Langleben D, et al: Expression of endothelin-1 in the lungs of patients with pulmonary hypertension. *N Engl J Med* 328:1732–1739, 1993.

72. Wilkins M: Selective or nonselective endothelin receptor blockade in pulmonary arterial hypertension. *Am J Respir Crit Care Med* 169:433–436, 2004 (editorial).

73. Channick R, Sitbon O, Barst R, et al: Endothelin receptor antagonists in pulmonary arterial hypertension. *J Am Coll Cardiol* 43:62S-67S, 2004.

74. Channick R, Simonneau G, Sitbon O, et al: Effects of the dual endothelin-receptor antagonist bosentan in patients with pulmonary hypertension: A randomised placebo-controlled study. *Lancet* 358:1119–1123, 2001.

75. Rubin L, Badesch D, Barst R, et al: Bosentan therapy for pulmonary arterial hypertension. *N Engl J Med* 346:896–903, 2002.

76. Sitbon O, Badesch D, Channick R, et al: Effects of the dual endothelin receptor antagonist bosentan in patients with pulmonary arterial hypertension: A 1-year follow-up study. *Chest* 124:247–254, 2003.

77. McLaughlin V, Sitbon O, Badesch D, et al: Survival with first-line bosentan in patients with primary pulmonary hypertension. *Eur Respir J* 25:244–249, 2005.

78. Wu C, Chan M, Stavros F, et al: Discovery of TBC11251, a potent, long-acting, orally active endothelin receptor-A selective antagonist. *J Med Chem* 40:1690–1697, 1997.

79. Barst R, Langleben D, Frost A, et al: Sitaxsentan therapy for pulmonary arterial hypertension. *Am J Respir Crit Care Med* 169:441–447, 2004.

80. Langleben D, Hirsch A, Shalit E, et al: Sustained symptomatic, functional, and hemodynamic benefit with the selective endothelin-A receptor antagonist, sitaxsentan, in patients with pulmonary arterial hypertension. *Chest* 126:1377–1381, 2004.

81. Barst R, Rich S, Widlitz A, et al: Clinical efficacy of sitaxsentan, an endothelin-A receptor antagonist, in patients with pulmonary arterial hypertension. *Chest* 121:1860–1868, 2002.

82. Billman G: Ambrisentan (Myogen). *Curr Opin Investig Drugs* 3:1483–1486, 2002.

83. Galie N, Keogh A, Frost A, et al: Ambrisentan long-term safety and efficacy in pulmonary arterial hypertension—one year follow-up, American Thoracic Society International Conference, San Diego, CA, May 20–25 2005 (abstract).

84. Palmer R, Ferrige A, Moncada S: Nitric oxide release accounts for the biological activity of endothelium-derived relaxing factor. *Nature* 327:524–526, 1987.

85. Olschewski H, Olschewski A, Rose F, et al: Physiologic basis for the treatment of pulmonary hypertension. *J Lab Clin Med* 138:287–297, 2001.

86. Rabe K, Tenor H, Dent G, et al: Identification of PDE isoenzymes in human pulmonary artery and effect of selective PDE inhibitors. *Am J Physiol* 266:L536–543, 1994.

87. Prasad S, Wilkinson J, Gatzoulis M: Sildenafil in primary pulmonary hypertension. *N Engl J Med* 343:1342, 2000 (letter).

88. Michelakis E, Tymchak W, Lien D, et al: Oral sildenafil is an effective and specific pulmonary vasodilator in patients with pulmonary arterial hypertension: Comparison with inhaled nitric oxide. *Circulation* 105:2398–2403, 2002.

89. Kumar S: Indian doctor in protest after using Viagra to save "blue babies." *Br Med J* 325:181, 2002.

89b. Galie N, Ghofrani HA, Torbicki A, et al: Sildenafil citrate therapy for pulmonary arterial hypertension. *N Engl J Med* 353:2148–2157, 2005.

90. Galie N, Burgess G, Parpia T, et al: Effects of sildenafil on 1-year survival of patients with idiopathic pulmonary arterial hypertension (PAH), American Thoracic Society International Conference, San Diego, CA, May 20–25 2005 (abstract).

91. Wilkins M, Paul G, Strange J, et al: Sildenafil versus endothelin receptor antagonist for pulmonary hypertension (SERAPH) study. *Am J Respir Crit Care Med* 171:1292–1297, 2005.

92. Ghofrani H, Voswinckel R, Reichenberger F, et al: Differences in hemodynamic and oxygenation

responses to three different phosphodiesterase-5 inhibitors in patients with pulmonary arterial hypertension: A randomized prospective study. *J Am Coll Cardiol* 44:1488–1496, 2004.

93. Humbert M, Barst R, Robbins I, et al: Combination of bosentan with epoprostenol in pulmonary arterial hypertension: BREATHE-2. *Eur Respir J* 24:353–359, 2004.

94. Kataoka M, Satoh T, Manabe T, et al: Oral sildenafil improves primary pulmonary hypertension refractory to epoprostenol. *Circ J* 69:461–465, 2005.

95. Stiebellehner L, Petkov V, Vonbank K, et al: Long-term treatment with oral sildenafil in addition to continuous IV epoprostenol in patients with pulmonary arterial hypertension. *Chest* 123: 1293–1295, 2003.

95b. Gomberg-Maitland M, McLaughlin V, Gulati M, Rich S. Efficacy and safety of sildenafil added to treprostinil in pulmonary hypertension. *Am J Cardiol* 96:1334–1336, 2005.

96. Beghetti M, Nicod L, Barazzone-Argiroffo C, et al: New combined treatments avoided transplantation in a child with severe pulmonary hypertension. *Heart* 90:154, 2004.

97. Hoeper M, Taha N, Bekjarova A, et al: Bosentan treatment in patients with primary pulmonary hypertension receiving nonparenteral prostanoids. *Eur Respir J* 22:330–334, 2003.

97b. McLaughlin VV, Oudiz R, Frost A et al: A randomized, double-blind, placebo controlled study of iloprost inhalation as add-on therapy to bosentan in pulmonary arterial hypertension. American College of Chest Physicians Annual Meeting, Montreal, Canada, October 29—November 3, 2005 (abstract).

98. Wilkens H, Guth A, Konig J, et al: Effect of inhaled iloprost plus oral sildenafil in patients with primary pulmonary hypertension. *Circulation* 104:1218–1222, 2001.

99. Ghofrani H, Wiedemann R, Rose F, et al: Combination therapy with oral sildenafil and inhaled iloprost for severe pulmonary hypertension. *Ann Intern Med* 136:515–522, 2002.

100. Ghofrani H, Rose F, Schermuly R, et al: Oral sildenafil as long-term adjunct therapy to inhaled iloprost in severe pulmonary arterial hypertension. *J Am Coll Cardiol* 42:158–164, 2003.

101. Hoeper M, Faulenbach C, Golpon H, et al: Combination therapy with bosentan and sildenafil in idiopathic pulmonary arterial hypertension. *Eur Respir J* 24:1007–1010, 2004.

102. Wittke B, Burgess G, Ng T, et al: Mutual pharmacokinetic interactions between steady-state bosentan and sildenafil, American Thoracic Society International Conference, San Diego, CA, 2005 (abstract).

103. Gomberg-Maitland M, McLaughlin V, Gulati M: Efficacy and safety of sildenafil and atorvastatin added to bosentan therapy for pulmonary arterial hypertension, American Thoracic Society International Conference, San Diego, CA, May 20–25 2005 (abstract).

104. Hoeper M, Kiely D, Carlsen J, et al: Safety profile of pulmonary arterial hypertension patients treated with bosentan and sildenafil: Results from a European surveillance program, American Thoracic Society International Conference, San Diego, CA, May 20–25 2005.

105. Coyne T, Garces P, Kramer W: No clinical interaction between sitaxsentan and sildenafil, American Thoracic Society International Conference, San Diego, CA, May 20-25 2005.

106. Ichinose F, Roberts JJ, Zapol W: Inhaled nitric oxide. A selective pulmonary vasodilator. Current uses and therapeutic potential. *Circulation* 109:3106–3111, 2004.

107. Snell G, Salamonsen R, Bergin P, et al: Inhaled nitric oxide used as a bridge to heart-lung transplantation in a patient with end-stage pulmonary hypertension. *Am J Respir Crit Care Med* 151:1263–1266, 1995.

108. Channick R, Newhart J, Johnson F, et al: Pulsed delivery of inhaled nitric oxide to patients with primary pulmonary hypertension. An ambulatory delivery system and initial clinical tests. *Chest* 109:1545–1549, 1996.

109. Koh E, Niimura J, Nakamura T, et al: Long-term inhalation of nitric oxide for a patient with primary pulmonary hypertension. *Jpn Circ J* 62:940–942, 1998.

110. Mehta S, Stewart D, Langleben D, et al: Short-term pulmonary vasodilation with L-arginine in pulmonary hypertension. *Circulation* 92:1539–1545, 1995.

111. Nagaya N, Uematsu M, Oya H, et al: Short-term oral administration of L-arginine improves hemodynamic and exercise capacity in patients with precapillary pulmonary hypertension. *Am J Respir Crit Care Med* 163:887–891, 2001.

112. Kureishi Y, Luo Z, Shiojima I, et al: The HMG-CoA reductase inhibitor simvastatin activates the protein kinase Akt and promotes angiogenesis in normocholesterolemic animals. *Nat Med* 6:1004–1010, 2000.

113. Laufs U, Liao J: Direct vascular effects of HMG-CoA reductase inhibitors. *Trends Cardiovasc Med* 10:143–148, 2000.

114. Nishimura T, Vaszar L, Faul J, et al: Simvastatin rescues rats from fatal pulmonary hypertension by inducing apoptosis of neointimal smooth muscle cells. *Circulation* 108:1640–1645, 2003.

115. Kao P: Simvastatin treatment of pulmonary hypertension. An observational case series. *Chest* 127:1446–1452, 2005.

116. Morrell N, Upton P, Higham M, et al: Angiotensin II stimulates proliferation of human pulmonary

artery smooth muscle cells via the AT1 receptor. *Chest* 114(1 Suppl):90S-91S, 1998.

117. Jeffery T, Wanstall J: Pulmonary vascular remodeling: a target for therapeutic intervention in pulmonary hypertension. *Pharmacol Ther* 92:1–20, 2001.

118. Petkov V, Mosgoeller W, Ziesche R, et al: Vasoactive intestinal peptide as a new drug for treatment of primary pulmonary hypertension. *J Clin Invest* 111:1339–1346, 2003.

119. Sandoval J, Gaspar J, Pulido T, et al: Graded balloon dilation atrial septostomy in severe primary pulmonary hypertension. A therapeutic alternative for patients nonresponsive to vasodilator treatment. *J Am Coll Cardiol* 32:297–304, 1998.

120. Nihill M, O'Laughlin M, Millins C: Effects of atrial septostomy in patients with terminal cor pulmonale due to pulmonary vascular disease. *Cathet Cardiovasc Diagn* 24:166–172, 1991.

121. Kerstein D, Levy P, Hsu D, et al: Blade balloon atrial septostomy in patients with severe primary pulmonary hypertension. *Circulation* 91:2028–2035, 1995.

122. Kothari S, Yusuf A, Juneja R, et al: Graded balloon atrial septostomy in severe pulmonary hypertension. *Indian Heart J* 54:164–169, 2002.

123. Doyle R, McCrory D, Channick R, et al: Surgical treatments/interventions for pulmonary arterial hypertension. ACCP evidence-based clinical practice guidelines. *Chest* 126:63S-71S, 2004.

124. Hoeper MM, Markevych E, Spickerkoetter, et al: Goal-oriented treatment and combination therapy for pulmonary arterial hypertension. *Eur Respir J* 26:858–863, 2005.

Chapter 8

Lung Transplantation for Pulmonary Arterial Hypertension

Vivek N. Ahya, MD,

Jeffrey S. Sager, MD, MSCE,

Robert M. Kotloff, MD

Lung transplantation is an accepted therapeutic option for select patients with end-stage lung disease of diverse causes, including pulmonary arterial hypertension. For patients with severe functional impairment and limited life expectancy, lung transplantation offers the possibility of a markedly improved quality of life and, in some cases, longer survival. Although the introduction of potent immunosuppressive agents and surgical advances has propelled the field forward and made intermediate-term survival an achievable goal, the lung transplant recipient remains susceptible to multiple complications that threaten the quality and duration of life.[1] The 2004 International Society for Heart and Lung Transplantation (ISHLT) Registry reported actuarial survival rates of 74 percent after 1 year, 47 percent after 5 years, and 24 percent after 10 years for all lung transplant recipients who received their new organs between January 1990 and June 2002. Patients with idiopathic pulmonary arterial hypertension (IPAH; formerly termed "primary pulmonary hypertension") had somewhat poorer short-term survival but displayed similar outcomes 5 years after transplantation.[2] These sobering statistics justify the use of lung transplantation only as the final option for the treatment of appropriate patients with pulmonary arterial hypertension.

The first successful heart-lung transplant procedure was performed in 1981 in a patient with IPAH.[3] Since this initial report, pulmonary arterial hypertension has been an important indication for heart-lung, double lung, and single lung transplan-

tation. In the last decade, however, new therapeutic agents such as calcium channel blockers, prostacyclin analogues and, more recently, endothelial receptor antagonists and phosphodiesterase-5 inhibitors have provided safer alternatives to transplantation. Consequently, transplantation generally is reserved for patients not responsive to or unable to tolerate medical therapy. Although it accounted for 10 percent of all transplants performed in 1990, IPAH is currently the indication for only 4 percent of all those performed, a testament to the significant impact of these medical alternatives.[4]

Transplant Center Referral

A seminal study published in 1991 that analyzed data from a large national patient registry reported a median survival of 2.8 years for patients with IPAH. Patients with poor functional status, World Health Organization (WHO) functional class III or IV, and cor pulmonale had the highest risk for death.[5] The exceedingly poor prognosis documented in this study led to the recommendation that patients with IPAH be referred to transplant centers early in the course of their disease, particularly in the United States where waiting times exceeding 18–24 months were commonplace.[6] The subsequent development of effective medical therapy has favorably impacted the natural history of IPAH and has influenced referral practices for transplantation. The most extensively studied agent is intravenous epoprostenol (prostacyclin, Flolan), whose administration has been demonstrated to result in sustained intermediate and long-term improvement in hemodynamic and functional parameters as well as in improved survival.[7-9] At one active transplant center, improvement in functional status associated with initiation of intravenous epoprostenol permitted transplant listing to be deferred in 70 percent of patients.[10] However, it is clear that not all patients respond to vasodilator therapy and among those that do, the response may not be sustained. Mortality among treated patients remains considerable, with approximately one-third of patients dying within 3 years after treatment is initiated.[9,11,12] Patients who are the most debilitated at the initiation of therapy (WHO functional class IV) have a poorer long-term survival. Further, the persistence of more significant functional impairment (WHO class III or IV) following at least 3 months of therapy conferred a particularly poor prognosis. Thus, referral for lung transplantation is appropriate for those patients with WHO class III or IV functional status, who do not demonstrate significant hemodynamic and functional improvement within 3 months of initiating vasodilator treatment or have progression after initial improvement with treatment. Concerns that such patients may not survive the long waiting times to transplantation were addressed by a new lung allocation policy in the United States in May 2005. It prioritizes patients on the basis of net transplant benefit and medical urgency rather than simply on time accrued on the waiting list.

There are no clear guidelines regarding the appropriate timing of referral for patients with other ("secondary") forms of pulmonary arterial hypertension. Survival rates vary among the different disease processes, and decisions about transplantation must be individualized.

Eisenmenger syndrome represents a unique condition that may require either lung transplantation with concurrent correction of the cardiac abnormality or heart-lung transplantation. It is characterized by pulmonary arterial hypertension and elevated pulmonary vascular resistance with right-to-left shunting of blood, usually through an intracardiac defect.[13] Overall, patients with Eisenmenger syndrome represent a heterogeneous group with a better prognosis when compared with patients who have IPAH. One study comparing the survival of patients with severe pulmonary arterial hypertension awaiting transplantation showed that although there was a trend toward higher pulmonary arterial pressures in the group with Eisenmenger syndrome, these patients had significantly better 1-year and 3-year survival (97 percent and 77 percent versus 77 percent and 35 percent, respectively).[14] Interestingly, lower right atrial pressures and greater cardiac indices were documented in the patients with Eisenmenger syndrome, suggesting that the right-to-left shunt may exert a protective effect by decompressing the right ventricle and allowing it to adapt more slowly.[15] Thus, it is not surprising that elevated right atrial pressure, right ventricular dilation and dysfunction, and reduced cardiac index have been associated with increased mortality in those with Eisenmenger syndrome.[16,17] Other factors that may also be associated with shorter survival include poor WHO functional class, younger age, and supraventricular dysrhythmias that require medical therapy.[18] Patients with these characteristics should be considered for earlier referral for lung or heart-lung transplant evaluation.

Selection Criteria

The numerous complications associated with transplantation necessitate that stringent selection criteria be applied to potential candidates to increase the likelihood of a successful outcome. Because of the limited supply of donor organs, a concerted effort must be made to avoid selecting poor candidates simply because of the desperate nature of their situations.[1] The ideal transplant recipient should have advanced lung disease without evidence of extrapulmonary organ damage that may jeopardize the success of transplantation (TABLE 8-1).

Patients should be ambulatory and free of clinically significant cardiac, renal, or hepatic impairment. Isolated right-sided heart dysfunction secondary to severe pulmonary arterial hypertension is not a contraindication to lung transplantation, because dramatic post-transplant reduction in right ventricular afterload permits rapid recovery of right ventricular function.[19] Patients with complex congenital heart disease not amenable to surgical repair, however, require combined heart-lung transplantation.

Other contraindications include severe malnutrition or morbid obesity, active or recent cancer with the exception of basal cell or squamous cell skin cancer, severe psychiatric illness, noncompliance with medical therapy, recent cigarette smoking, acute critical illness, and infection with human immunodeficiency virus.[1] Hepatitis C infection is not universally accepted as an absolute contraindication, and some centers will proceed

TABLE 8-1

Guidelines for the Selection of Lung Transplantation Candidates

Indications

Advanced obstructive, fibrotic, or pulmonary vascular disease with a high risk of death within 2 to 3 years
Lack of success or availability of alternative therapies
Severe functional limitation, but preserved ability to walk
Age of 55 years or less for candidates for heart-lung transplantation, age of 60 years or less for candidates for bilateral lung transplantation, and age of 65 years or less for candidates for single lung transplantation

Absolute Contraindications

Severe extrapulmonary organ dysfunction, including renal insufficiency with a creatinine clearance below 50 ml/min, hepatic dysfunction with coagulopathy or portal hypertension, and left ventricular dysfunction or severe coronary artery disease (consider heart-lung transplantation)
Acute, critical illness
Active cancer or recent history of cancer with substantial likelihood of recurrence (except for basal cell and squamous cell carcinoma of the skin)
Active extrapulmonary infection (including infection with human immunodeficiency virus; hepatitis B, indicated by the presence of hepatitis B surface antigen; and hepatitis C with evidence of liver disease on biopsy)
Severe psychiatric illness, noncompliance with therapy, and drug or alcohol dependence
Active or recent (preceding 3 to 6 months) cigarette smoking
Severe malnutrition (<70 percent of ideal body weight) or marked obesity (>130 percent of ideal body weight)
Inability to walk, with poor rehabilitation potential

Relative Contraindications

Chronic medical conditions that are poorly controlled or associated with target-organ damage
Daily requirements for more than 20 mg of prednisone (or equivalent)
Mechanical ventilation (excluding noninvasive ventilation)
Extensive pleural thickening from prior thoracic surgery or infection
Active collagen vascular disease
Preoperative colonization of the airways with pan-resistant bacteria (in patients with cystic fibrosis)

Reproduced with permission from Arcasoy SM, Kotloff RM: Lung transplantation. N Engl J Med 340:1081–1091, 1999; and adopted from Maurer JR, Frost AE, Estenne M, et al: International guidelines for the selection of lung transplant candidates. The International Society for Heart and Lung Transplantation, the American Thoracic Society, the American Society of Transplant Physicians, the European Respiratory Society. J Heart Lung Transplant 17:703–709, 1998.

with transplantation as long as there is neither histologic evidence of significant fibrosis or cirrhosis nor clinical evidence of significant hepatic dysfunction. This policy, however, does not suggest that hepatitis C infection is benign, but rather reflects the belief that complications of hepatitis C infection may not impact short-term and intermediate-term outcomes after transplantation.[20]

Patients with pulmonary arterial hypertension in addition to underlying scleroderma pose additional problems related to the frequent presence of esophageal dysmotility and gastroesophageal reflux disease. Data suggesting that silent aspiration of gastric contents may lead to accelerated graft dysfunction following transplantation have prompted exclusion at most centers of patients with scleroderma who have significant esophageal involvement.[21]

In recognition of the somewhat poorer outcomes among older patients and the rigors of more extensive surgical procedures, age limits have been adopted by most transplant centers: 55 years for candidates for heart-lung transplantation, and 65 years for candidates for single and bilateral lung transplantation.[2,22]

Organ Allocation

Donor lungs are scarce in comparison with the number of patients in need. Previously, donor lungs were allocated based upon the time accrued by the recipient on the lung transplantation waiting list. Recognizing that such a system may disadvantage sicker patients with more advanced or rapidly progressive disease, the United Network for Organ Sharing (UNOS) implemented a revised lung allocation system in May 2005.[23] This new system has two major goals: (1) to reduce the number of deaths on the lung transplant waiting list and (2) to increase the benefit for candidates who receive a lung transplant. Under the new system, a "lung allocation score" is assigned to each transplant candidate. This score is calculated using clinical variables predictive of 1-year survival with a transplant and variables predictive of survival without transplantation. A higher allocation score reflects a greater margin between the respective survival calculations (and thus a greater expected benefit in survival as a result of transplantation). Factors included in calculating the lung allocation score include:

- Diagnosis
- Age
- Body mass index
- New York Heart Association functional class
- 6-Minute walk distance
- Forced vital capacity (% predicted)
- Need for supplemental oxygen
- Continuous mechanical ventilation
- Diabetes mellitus
- Serum creatinine levels
- Pulmonary artery pressures
- Pulmonary capillary wedge mean pressure

These variables are not applied uniformly, because their significance may vary among disease groups. For example, because all patients with IPAH listed for transplant have elevated pulmonary artery pressures, this variable does not give one the ability to discriminate between patients who are at higher versus lower risk for death. For additional information on how the lung allocation score is calculated, the reader is referred to the UNOS web site (*http://www.unos.org/resources/professionalresources. asp?index=8; accessed February 2006*).

It is not yet clear how this allocation system will impact the availability or success of lung transplantation for patients with pulmonary arterial hypertension. Of concern is that the lung allocation score calculates probability of transplant benefit by using 1-year survival statistics. Survival of patients with pulmonary arterial hypertension has been noted previously to be poorer than that of other groups, but equivalent after 5 years.[2] Thus, the allocation score calculations may underestimate the benefit of transplantation for patients with pulmonary arterial hypertension and negatively

impact their assigned priority on the waiting list. Additionally, the revised system does not consider factors generally accepted as indicating a poorer prognosis in pulmonary arterial hypertension (e.g., hemoptysis and syncope).[24] UNOS plans to update periodically the allocation algorithm to address such concerns so that the new system indeed optimizes utilization of the limited number of donor lungs.

Procedure Options

Three transplant options exist for patients with pulmonary hypertension: single lung transplantation, bilateral lung transplantation, and combined heart-lung transplantation. The choice of which procedure to perform varies significantly among transplant centers.[25] Right ventricular dysfunction associated with severe pulmonary arterial hypertension led to initial recommendations supporting heart-lung transplantation as the procedure of choice. However, because isolated right ventricular dysfunction can recover dramatically following reduction of afterload by lung transplantation and because thoracic organs are in severely short supply, heart-lung transplantation in North America is reserved for patients with complex and surgically irreparable congenital heart disease[19,26–28] (FIGURE 8-1).

Both single and bilateral lung transplantation have been performed successfully in patients with severe pulmonary arterial hypertension. Bilateral transplantation is strongly preferred for this patient population by the vast majority of centers in the United States.[29] This preference is fueled by concerns that following single lung transplantation, nearly the entire cardiac output will flow to the freshly implanted allograft (where vascular resistance is lower), potentially magnifying the degree of reperfusion edema that is encountered and compromising graft function. Indeed, one study of patients with pulmonary arterial hypertension reported the development of significant graft edema in 82 percent of patients following single lung transplantation compared with 59 percent following bilateral procedures.[27] This study and several others demonstrated superior functional outcomes and survival after bilateral lung transplantation.[27,30,31] In contrast, advocates of single lung transplantation argue that this is a shorter and more straightforward procedure and, consequently, both ischemic and cardiopulmonary bypass times can be reduced. In support

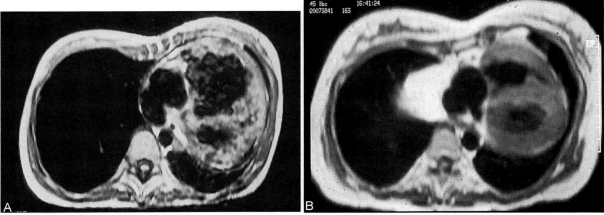

Figure 8-1. Cardiac magnetic resonance imaging obtained prior to lung transplantation (**A**) shows evidence of severe right ventricular dilation with resultant left ventricular restriction. Several months following lung transplantation, (**B**) right ventricular afterload has improved, with normalization of pulmonary artery pressures leading to remodeling of the right ventricle and normalization of left ventricular morphology. (Courtesy of Larry Kaiser, MD.)

of single lung transplantation, several single-center studies have reported outcomes similar to those achieved with the more extensive bilateral procedure.[32,33] Even more compelling, the 2004 ISHLT International Registry reported no difference in survival rates between single and bilateral lung transplant recipients with underlying IPAH, although this must be interpreted with caution because it is not clear that the groups were comparable with respect to disease severity before transplantation, and assignment to a specific procedure was not randomized.[2]

In the final analysis, heart-lung, single lung, and bilateral lung transplantation have all been employed successfully in the management of pulmonary hypertension. Each is characterized by unique advantages and disadvantages, and no single procedure has proven clearly superior. Until future studies clarify this controversy, the availability of donor organs, severity of the recipient's illness, and institutional practices will remain the primary factors in determining the surgical procedure for a particular patient.

Outcomes

One-year survival following lung transplantation for IPAH is approximately 65 percent, significantly lower than that associated with transplantation in other patient populations, such as those with emphysema or cystic fibrosis.[2] Perioperative mortality is particularly high and is related to surgical

complexity, the requirement for cardiopulmonary bypass and consequent risk of bleeding, increased incidence of hemodynamic instability due in part to underlying cardiac impairment, and early graft dysfunction.[19] Five-year survival, however, is 45 percent, a figure comparable with those of other disease groups.[2]

Post-transplantation improvements in hemodynamic parameters and functional status are critical to achieving lung transplantation's principal goal: improvement in quality of life. For patients with pulmonary vascular disease, both single lung and bilateral lung transplantation result in immediate and sustained improvements in pulmonary vascular resistance and pulmonary arterial pressure.[33] This is accompanied by an immediate increase in cardiac output and more gradual remodeling of the right ventricle, with a decrease in ventricular wall thickness.[28,32,34]

Most patients who undergo lung transplantation have sufficient improvement in exercise capacity within 1 year of the procedure to permit resumption of an active lifestyle. As a reflection of this, over 80 percent of lung recipients report no limitations to activity, and less than 4 percent require total assistance.[2] Survivors have also reported long-term improvements in functional status. Objective measures of exercise capacity confirm these findings. Studies comparing results of cardiopulmonary exercise testing (CPET) before and after single, bilateral, and heart-lung transplantation for various disease groups, including pulmonary vascular disease, have shown dramatic improvement in exercise tolerance after transplantation. Significant increases in peak oxygen uptake (arV>O_2max), O_2 pulse, and work capacity have been reported consistently. Peak exercise capacity, however, although considerably enhanced, remains suboptimal when compared with that of normal volunteers. CPET measurements typically show a reduced anaerobic threshold and $\dot{V}O_2$max despite the absence of significant cardiac or ventilatory limitations.[35–39] These findings suggest that abnormal peripheral oxygen utilization at the level of the skeletal muscle, possibly resulting from calcineurin inhibitor-induced impairment in mitochondrial function, may contribute to peak exercise limitations.[40–43]

Specific data comparing quality of life before and after lung transplantation for pulmonary arterial hypertension are lacking. However, quality of life surveys assessing physical, social, and psychologic functioning in the general lung transplant population reveal significant short-term and intermediate-term improvements in quality of life. Long-term quality of life benefit is more variable and depends on the presence and number of comorbidities and, in particular, on the degree to which graft function is compromised by chronic rejection.[44–47]

Complications

Lung transplantation, although offering a vital therapeutic option for select patients, is associated with numerous complications that threaten the quality and duration of the recipient's life. These complications may be technical, mediated by allograft-specific immune response, or consequences of global immunosuppression.

Primary Graft Dysfunction

The most common early post-transplant complication is pulmonary edema. Mild, transient edema is a nearly universal feature of the freshly transplanted lung allograft. It is presumed to be a consequence of ischemia-reperfusion injury and attendant increase in microvascular permeability, although surgical trauma and lymphatic disruption may also be important contributing factors.[48] In 12–22 percent of cases, injury is sufficiently severe to cause a form of acute respiratory distress syndrome termed "primary graft dysfunction" (PGD).[49,50] Risk factors for PGD have been identified preliminarily in one single-center study and include donor female sex, donor African American

ethnicity, donor age (less than 21 or more than 45 years), and a recipient diagnosis of IPAH.[49] Other studies have reported an association between prolonged graft ischemic time and PGD, but this has not been observed uniformly.[51] The diagnosis of PGD is based upon the development of widespread radiographic infiltrates and markedly impaired oxygenation within 72 hours of transplantation (FIGURE 8-2), and exclusion of other causes of early graft dysfunction such as volume overload, pneumonia, hyperacute rejection, atelectasis, and pulmonary venous outflow obstruction. Histopathologic examination of lung tissue from patients with PGD reveals a prevailing pattern of diffuse alveolar damage.[52]

Treatment typically is supportive, relying primarily on lung-protective mechanical ventilation strategies. Rarely, extracorporeal life support is required in cases of severe respiratory failure or hemodynamic instability.[53,54] Prophylactic use of nitric oxide for all recipients at the time of implantation does not appear to reduce the incidence of PGD. It is not yet clear if selective administration of nitric oxide to a high-risk population, such as patients with pulmonary hypertension, will improve their outcome.[55] With an in-hospital mortality rate of 42–60 percent, PGD is the leading cause of perioperative deaths among transplant recipients.[48,56] Recovery among survivors is often protracted and incomplete, although attainment of

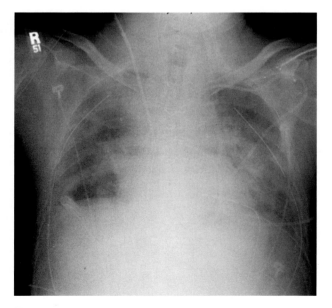

Figure 8-2. Chest radiograph obtained 24 hours after bilateral lung transplantation for pulmonary hypertension reveals diffuse interstitial and alveolar infiltrates consistent with the diagnosis of primary graft dysfunction.

normal lung function and exercise tolerance is possible. Results of emergent retransplantation in this situation have been poor.[57]

Anastomotic Complications

Major dehiscence of the bronchial anastomosis was once a leading cause of perioperative mortality, but refinements in surgical technique, tissue preservation, and immunosuppression have reduced the risk to a negligible level. Focal dehiscence, incidentally detected on bronchoscopy or heralded by a spontaneous pneumothorax, is still encountered in 1–6 percent of patients.[58–60] Tube thoracostomy may be required for evacuation of pneumothoraces, but focal dehiscence usually heals without surgical intervention.

The most common form of airway complication is anastomotic narrowing, with a reported frequency of 12–24 percent in contemporary series.[58,61] Narrowing of the anastomosis can result from ischemia-induced stricture or bronchomalacia, or from excessive granulation tissue. Independent of the mechanism, anastomotic narrowing typically develops within several weeks of transplantation. Clues to its presence include focal wheezing on the involved side, recurrent bouts of pneumonia or purulent bronchitis, and suboptimal pulmonary function studies demonstrating airway obstruction. Diagnosis is based on direct bronchoscopic visualization. Techniques commonly employed to reverse anastomotic narrowing include balloon dilation, electrocautery, or laser debridement of excessive granulation tissue, followed by endobronchial stent placement.[58]

Acute Rejection

Lung transplant recipients are at considerable risk for pulmonary injury mediated by alloreactive T-lymphocytes. This form of injury, termed "acute rejection," occurs in 55–75 percent of transplant recipients within the first year after transplantation, despite continuous administration of immunosuppressive agents.[62,63] Factors that influence the likelihood of acute rejection remain poorly defined. The degree of human leukocyte antigen disparity between the donor and recipient has been inconsistently identified as a risk factor.[64,65]

Symptoms of acute rejection are nonspecific and include malaise, low-grade fever, dyspnea, and cough. Radiographic infiltrates, a decline in oxygen saturation at rest or with exercise, and an abrupt fall of greater than 10 percent in spirometric values are important clues to the possibility of acute rejection, although respiratory infections may present a similar clinical picture.[1] The gold standard for the diagnosis of acute rejection remains transbronchial biopsy. The histopathologic hallmark of acute rejection is perivascular lymphocytic infiltrates that, in more severe cases, spill over into the adjacent interstitium and alveolar spaces. These findings may be associated with lymphocytic involvement of the bronchi and bronchioles[66] (FIGURE 8-3).

Conventional management of acute rejection consists of a 3-day pulse of high-dose intravenous methylprednisolone. In most cases, this results in rapid improvement in symptoms, pulmonary function, and radiographic abnormalities, although up to 44 percent of patients with moderate acute rejection have histopathologic evidence of persistent rejection and may require additional intensified treatment with immunosuppressive agents.[67]

Chronic Rejection

Chronic rejection, in the form of bronchiolitis obliterans, develops in up to two-thirds of lung transplant recipients and represents the major impediment to long-term graft and patient survival.[68–70] Bronchiolitis obliterans is a fibroproliferative process characterized by submucosal inflammation and fibrosis of the bronchiolar walls, ultimately leading to complete obliteration of the airway lumen. The functional consequence of this process is progressive and irreversible airflow obstruction. Because the characteristic histology of chronic rejection is difficult to demonstrate by transbronchial lung biopsy, a clinical surrogate for its presence based on the magnitude of decline in forced expiratory volume in 1 second (FEV1), termed "bronchiolitis obliterans syndrome" (BOS), has been created to more easily identify these patients.[71]

Acute rejection, particularly when recurrent or severe, and lymphocytic bronchiolitis have been identified consistently as major risk factors for development of BOS, supporting the view that BOS is a consequence of alloimmune injury.[68–70,72–74] Nonimmune factors may also be important in initiating or perpetuating injury but have been substantiated more variably. These factors include cytomegalovirus and other respiratory viral infections, a synergistic interaction between older donor age and prolonged ischemic times, and gastroesophageal reflux with occult aspiration.[71,74]

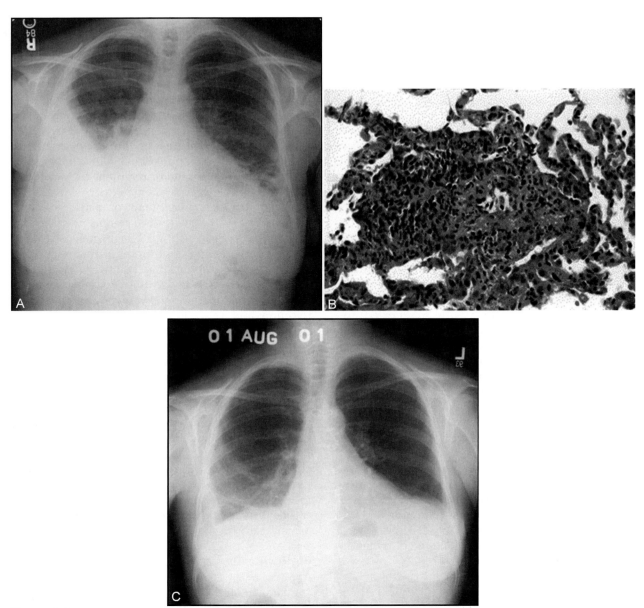

Figure 8-3. Chest radiograph (**A**) obtained several weeks after bilateral lung transplantation demonstrates increasing peri-ihilar and interstitial infiltrates, as well a new pleural effusions. Subsequent transbronchial biopsy (**B**) reveals near-circumferential perivascular mononuclear cell infiltrates that extend into the interstitium. These findings indicate moderate (A3) acute rejection. Subsequent treatment with high-dose intravenous methylprednisolone (Solu-Medrol) led to rapid radiographic resolution of the infiltrates (**C**).

The incidence of BOS is greatest within the first 2 years, but the risk remains considerable and steady beyond this point.[72] The onset of BOS typically is insidious but may be abrupt in more aggressive cases. Dyspnea, cough, and recurrent bouts of purulent tracheobronchitis, with recovery of *Pseudomonas aeruginosa* from sputum cultures, are highly characteristic features. Although chest radiographic findings are usually unremarkable, high-resolution computed tomography of the chest reveals air trapping on expiratory images in most patients and evidence of bronchiectasis in some.[75–77] Progressive airflow obstruction is the rule, although the pace of decline is highly variable and the course may be interrupted by periods of functional stability. The prognosis is generally poor, with a 40 percent mortality rate within two years of onset.[78] Patients with the onset of BOS within the first 3 years experience a more rapid decline in lung function and higher mortality during that time.[79]

A myriad of immunosuppressive modalities have been employed in the management of BOS, including pharmacologic agents, antilymphocyte antibodies, photopheresis, and total lymphoid irradiation, but consensus is lacking on the optimal approach.[78,80–84] At best, immunosuppressive measures appear to slow the rate of decline rather than to arrest or reverse the process. The only definitive treatment is retransplantation, but this strategy remains highly controversial in the context of a scarce donor organ pool.[85]

Infectious Complications

Infection is a constant threat to the lung transplant recipient and is an important cause of both early and late mortality. Infection rates appear to be higher than those encountered in other solid organ transplant populations, likely related to the higher levels of immunosuppression and the unique exposure of the lung allograft to the external environment.[86] The scope of this topic, unfortunately, is sufficiently broad to allow only a superficial discussion. The reader is referred to two reviews for a more in-depth discussion of infectious complications.[48,87]

Bacterial infections of the lower respiratory tract predominate and have a bimodal distribution. During the early period after transplantation, bacterial pneumonia is common, with an incidence rate of 16 percent in one 2002 series.[88] In addition to the immunocompromised state of the recipient, other factors that predispose to early bacterial pneumonia include the need for prolonged mechanical ventilation, blunted cough due to postoperative pain and lung denervation, disruption of lymphatics, and ischemic injury to the bronchial mucosa with resultant impairment of mucociliary clearance.[1] Passive transfer of occult pneumonia initially acquired by the donor is also a concern, although interestingly, the presence of organisms on Gram stain of donor bronchial washings is not predictive of subsequent pneumonia in the recipient.[88] Bacterial infections re-emerge as important late complications after transplant in the form of purulent bronchitis, bronchiectasis, and pneumonia among patients who develop chronic rejection. Gram-negative pathogens, especially *Pseudomonas aeruginosa*, are isolated most frequently in association with both early and late infectious events.[89,90]

Cytomegalovirus is the most common viral pathogen encountered during the post-transplant period. Although antiviral therapy has dramatically reduced direct mortality from cytomegalovirus infection, this virus continues to cause frequent, troubling infections, is associated with an increased risk of bacterial and fungal superinfections, and has been implicated as a risk factor for chronic rejection.[91,92] Recent studies suggest that other respiratory viral pathogens such as respiratory syncytial virus, parainfluenza virus, and adenovirus may also be associated with progressive graft dysfunction and chronic rejection.[93]

Although a number of opportunistic and endemic fungal pathogens cause pulmonary infections in lung transplant recipients, *Aspergillus* species are by far the most frequent and lethal pathogens encountered. Approximately 5 percent of lung recipients develop *Aspergillus* infections of the airway.[94] The devitalized cartilage and foreign suture material of the fresh bronchial anastomosis create a favorable environment for localized fungal infection at the anastomotic site. A more diffuse ulcerative tracheobronchitis occasionally is seen following severe ischemic injury to the bronchial mucosa.[95] *Aspergillus* infections of the airway typically occur during the first 6 months following transplantation and usually respond to appropriate antifungal therapy, although progression to invasive pneumonia or fatal erosion into an adjacent pulmonary artery rarely have been reported.[94,96,97]

Invasive aspergillosis is the most serious and devastating form of *Aspergillus* infection. An overall incidence rate of 5 percent has been calculated from pooled studies.[86] Most cases occur within the first post-transplant year. Despite management with antifungal agents, the mortality rate approaches 60 percent.[94]

Other Complications

In addition to infections, immunosuppression also increases the risk of neoplastic complications. As an example, post-transplant lymphoproliferative disorder refers to a spectrum of abnormal B-cell proliferative responses ranging from benign polyclonal hyperplasia to malignant lymphomas, and is seen in 2 to 8 percent of the lung transplant population.[98–100] Epstein-Barr virus has been identified as a potent stimulus for B-cell proliferation, which proceeds in an unchecked fashion because of muted cytotoxic T-cell responses in the immunosuppressed host.[101]

Long-term use of immunosuppressive agents may also contribute to other medical problems such as osteoporosis, renal insufficiency, hypertension, hypercholesterolemia, gastroparesis, and reflux disease.[86] The physician caring for the lung recipient must be vigilant for complications arising in any organ system.

Future Directions

Lung transplantation involves considerable risk and offers long-term survival and preservation of graft function for only a minority of patients.

Current immunosuppressive strategies expose patients to the risks of drug toxicity, infection, and malignancy while failing to prevent chronic rejection. Solutions to these shortcomings will likely emerge in the form of strategies to specifically manipulate the host immune system to be tolerant to the donor allograft without needing to induce a state of global immunosuppression. It is hoped that these strategies will ultimately transform lung transplantation into an enduring therapeutic option for patients with advanced pulmonary vascular disease.

References

1. Arcasoy SM, Kotloff RM: Lung transplantation. *N Engl J Med* 340:1081–1091, 1999.
2. Trulock EP, Edwards LB, Taylor DO, et al: The Registry of the International Society for Heart and Lung Transplantation: Twenty-first official adult lung and heart-lung transplant report—2004. *J Heart Lung Transplant* 23:804–815, 2004.
3. Reitz BA, Wallwork JL, Hunt SA, et al: Heart-lung transplantation: Successful therapy for patients with pulmonary vascular disease. *N Engl J Med* 306:557–564, 1982.
4. Boucek MM, Edwards LB, Keck BM, et al: Registry for the International Society for Heart and Lung Transplantation: Seventh official pediatric report—2004. *J Heart Lung Transplant* 23:933–947, 2004.
5. D'Alonzo GE, Barst RJ, Ayres SM, et al: Survival in patients with primary pulmonary hypertension. Results from a national prospective registry. *Ann Intern Med* 115:343–349, 1991.
6. Pierson RN, Milstone AP, Loyd JE, et al: Lung allocation in the United States, 1995-1997: An analysis of equity and utility. *J Heart Lung Transplant* 19:846–851, 2000.
7. McLaughlin VV, Genthner DE, Panella MM, et al: Reduction in pulmonary vascular resistance with long-term epoprostenol (prostacyclin) therapy in primary pulmonary hypertension. *N Engl J Med* 338:273–277, 1998.
8. Barst RJ, Rubin LJ, Long WA, et al: A comparison of continuous intravenous epoprostenol (prostacyclin) with conventional therapy for primary pulmonary hypertension. The Primary Pulmonary Hypertension Study Group. *N Engl J Med* 334:296–302, 1996.
9. Kuhn KP, Byrne DW, Arbogast PG, et al: Outcome in 91 consecutive patients with pulmonary arterial hypertension receiving epoprostenol. *Am J Respir Crit Care Med* 167:580–586, 2003.
10. Conte JV, Gaine SP, Orens JB, et al: The influence of continuous intravenous prostacyclin therapy for primary pulmonary hypertension on the timing and outcome of transplantation. *J Heart Lung Transplant* 17:679–685, 1998.
11. Sitbon O, Humbert M, Nunes H, et al: Long-term intravenous epoprostenol infusion in primary pulmonary hypertension: Prognostic factors and survival. *J Am Coll Cardiol* 40:780–788, 2002.
12. McLaughlin VV, Shillington A, Rich S: Survival in primary pulmonary hypertension: The impact of epoprostenol therapy. *Circulation* 106:1477–1482, 2002.
13. Wood P: The Eisenmenger syndrome or pulmonary hypertension with reversed central shunt. *Br Med J* 46:755–762, 1958.
14. Hopkins WE, Ochoa LL, Richardson GW, et al: Comparison of the hemodynamics and survival of adults with severe primary pulmonary hypertension or Eisenmenger syndrome. *J Heart Lung Transplant* 15:100–105, 1996.
15. Hopkins WE, Waggoner AD: Severe pulmonary hypertension without right ventricular failure: The unique hearts of patients with Eisenmenger syndrome. *Am J Cardiol* 89:34–38, 2002.
16. Oya H, Nagaya N, Uematsu M, et al: Poor prognosis and related factors in adults with Eisenmenger syndrome. *Am Heart J* 143:739–744, 2002.
17. Daliento L, Somerville J, Presbitero P, et al: Eisenmenger syndrome. Factors relating to deterioration and death. *Eur Heart J* 19:1845–1855, 1998.
18. Cantor WJ, Harrison DA, Moussadji JS, et al: Determinants of survival and length of survival in adults with Eisenmenger syndrome. *Am J Cardiol* 84:677–681, 1999.
19. Klepetko W, Mayer E, Sandoval J, et al: Interventional and surgical modalities of treatment for pulmonary arterial hypertension. *J Am Coll Cardiol* 43:73S–80S, 2004.
20. Cotler SJ, Jensen DM, Kesten S: Hepatitis C virus infection and lung transplantation: A survey of practices. *J Heart Lung Transplant* 18:456–459, 1999.
21. Hadjiliadis D, Duane Davis R, Steele MP, et al: Gastroesophageal reflux disease in lung transplant recipients. *Clin Transplant* 17:363–368, 2003.

22. Maurer JR, Frost AE, Estenne M, et al: International guidelines for the selection of lung transplant candidates. The International Society for Heart and Lung Transplantation, the American Thoracic Society, the American Society of Transplant Physicians, the European Respiratory Society. *J Heart Lung Trans- plant* 17:703–709, 1998.

23. Organ Procurement and Transplantation Network: Policy 3.7; Organ distribution: Allocation of thoracic organs: *http://www.unos.org/PoliciesandBylaws/policies/pdfs/policy_9.pdf,* 2004. Accessed December 23, 2005.

24. Dhillon GS, Doyle RL: The new UNOS lung transplantation allocation system. *Adv Pulm Hypertension* 4:12–13, 2005.

25. Pielsticker EJ, Martinez FJ, Rubenfire M: Lung and heart-lung transplant practice patterns in pulmonary hypertension centers. *J Heart Lung Transplant* 20:1297–1304, 2001.

26. Kramer MR, Valantine HA, Marshall SE, et al: Recovery of the right ventricle after single-lung transplantation in pulmonary hypertension. *Am J Cardiol* 73:494–500, 1994.

27. Bando K, Armitage JM, Paradis IL, et al: Indications for and results of single, bilateral, and heart-lung transplantation for pulmonary hypertension. *J Thorac Cardiovasc Surg* 108:1056–1065, 1994.

28. Moulton MJ, Creswell LL, Ungacta FF, et al: Magnetic resonance imaging provides evidence for remodeling of the right ventricle after single-lung transplantation for pulmonary hypertension. *Circulation* 94:II312–II319, 1996.

29. Levine SM: A survey of clinical practice of lung transplantation in North America. *Chest* 125:1224–1238, 2004.

30. Ueno T, Smith JA, Snell GI, et al: Bilateral sequential single lung transplantation for pulmonary hypertension and Eisenmenger's syndrome. *Ann Thorac Surg* 69:381–387, 2000.

31. Conte JV, Borja MJ, Patel CB, et al: Lung transplantation for primary and secondary pulmonary hypertension. *Ann Thorac Surg* 72:1673–1679; discussion 1679–1680, 2001.

32. Pasque MK, Trulock EP, Cooper JD, et al: Single lung transplantation for pulmonary hypertension. Single institution experience in 34 patients. *Circulation* 92:2252–2258, 1995.

33. Gammie JS, Keenan RJ, Pham SM, et al: Single- versus double-lung transplantation for pulmonary hypertension. *J Thorac Cardiovasc Surg* 115:397–402; discussion 402–403, 1998.

34. Mendeloff EN, Meyers BF, Sundt TM, et al: Lung transplantation for pulmonary vascular disease. *Ann Thorac Surg* 73:209–217; discussion 217–219, 2002.

35. Orens JB, Becker FS, Lynch JP, III, et al: Cardiopulmonary exercise testing following allogeneic lung transplantation for different underlying disease states. *Chest* 107:144–149, 1995.

36. Schwaiblmair M, Reichenspurner H, Muller C, et al: Cardiopulmonary exercise testing before and after lung and heart-lung transplantation. *Am J Respir Crit Care Med* 159:1277–1283, 1999.

37. Theodore J, Morris AJ, Burke CM, et al: Cardiopulmonary function at maximum tolerable constant work rate exercise following human heart-lung transplantation. *Chest* 92:433–439, 1987.

38. Oelberg DA, Systrom DM, Markowitz DH, et al: Exercise performance in cystic fibrosis before and after bilateral lung transplantation. *J Heart Lung Transplant* 17:1104–1112, 1998.

39. Levy RD, Ernst P, Levine SM, et al: Exercise performance after lung transplantation. *J Heart Lung Transplant* 12:27–33, 1993.

40. McKenna MJ, Fraser SF, Li JL, et al: Impaired muscle Ca^{2+} and K^+ regulation contribute to poor exercise performance post-lung transplantation. *J Appl Physiol* 95:1606–1616, 2003.

41. Tirdel GB, Girgis R, Fishman RS, et al: Metabolic myopathy as a cause of the exercise limitation in lung transplant recipients. *J Heart Lung Transplant* 17:1231–1237, 1998.

42. Mercier JG, Hokanson JF, Brooks GA: Effects of cyclosporine A on skeletal muscle mitochondrial respiration and endurance time in rats. *Am J Crit Care Med* 151:1532–1536, 1995.

43. Evans AB, Al-Himyary AJ, Hrovat MI, et al: Abnormal skeletal muscle oxidative capacity after lung transplantation by 31P-MRS. *Am J Respir Crit Care Med* 155:615–621, 1997.

44. TenVergert EM, Essink-Bot ML, Geertsma A, et al: The effect of lung transplantation on health-related quality of life: A longitudinal study. *Chest* 113:358–364, 1998.

45. MacNaughton KL, Rodrigue JR, Cicale M, et al: Health-related quality of life and symptom frequency before and after lung transplantation. *Clin Transplant* 12:320–323, 1998.

46. Vermeulen KM, Ouwens JP, van der Bij W, et al: Long-term quality of life in patients surviving at least 55 months after lung transplantation. *Gen Hosp Psychiatry* 25:95–102, 2003.

47. Lanuza DM, Lefaiver C, McCabe M, et al: Prospective study of functional status and quality of life before and after lung transplantation. *Chest* 118:115–122, 2000.

48. Kotloff RM, Ahya VN, Crawford SW: Pulmonary complications of solid organ and hematopoietic stem cell transplantation. *Am J Respir Crit Care Med* 170:22–48, 2004.

49. Christie JD, Kotloff RM, Pochettino A, et al: Clinical risk factors for primary graft failure fol-

lowing lung transplantation. *Chest* 124:1232–1241, 2003.

50. de Perrot M, Liu M, Waddell TK, et al: Ischemia-reperfusion-induced lung injury. *Am J Respir Crit Care Med* 167:490–511, 2003.

51. Thabut G, Vinatier I, Stern JB, et al: Primary graft failure following lung transplantation: Predictive factors of mortality. *Chest* 121:1876–1882, 2002.

52. Christie JD, Bavaria JE, Palevsky HI, et al: Primary graft failure following lung transplantation. *Chest* 114:51–60, 1998.

53. Meyers BF, Sundt TM, III, Henry S, et al: Selective use of extracorporeal membrane oxygenation is warranted after lung transplantation. *J Thorac Cardiovasc Surg* 120:20–26, 2000.

54. Gavazzeni V, Iapichino G, Mascheroni D, et al: Prolonged independent lung respiratory treatment after single lung transplantation in pulmonary emphysema. *Chest* 103:96–100, 1993.

55. Meade MO, Granton JT, Matte-Martyn A, et al: A randomized trial of inhaled nitric oxide to prevent ischemia-reperfusion injury after lung transplantation. *Am J Respir Crit Care Med* 167:1483–1489, 2003.

56. King RC, Binns OA, Rodriguez F, et al: Reperfusion injury significantly impacts clinical outcome after pulmonary transplantation. *Ann Thorac Surg* 69:1681–1685, 2000.

57. Novick RJ, Stitt LW, Al-Kattan K, et al: Pulmonary retransplantation: Predictors of graft function and survival in 230 patients. Pulmonary Retransplant Registry. *Ann Thorac Surg* 65:227–234, 1998.

58. Chhajed PN, Malouf MA, Tamm M, et al: Interventional bronchoscopy for the management of airway complications following lung transplantation. *Chest* 120:1894–1899, 2001.

59. Schmid RA, Boehler A, Speich R, et al: Bronchial anastomotic complications following lung transplantation: Still a major cause of morbidity? *Eur Respir J* 10:2872–2875, 1997.

60. Schroder C, Scholl F, Daon E, et al: A modified bronchial anastomosis technique for lung transplantation. *Ann Thorac Surg* 75:1697–1704, 2003.

61. Herrera JM, McNeil KD, Higgins RS, et al: Airway complications after lung transplantation: Treatment and long-term outcome. *Ann Thorac Surg* 71:989–993; discussion 993–994, 2001.

62. Hopkins PM, Aboyoun CL, Chhajed PN, et al: Prospective analysis of 1,235 transbronchial lung biopsies in lung transplant recipients. *J Heart Lung Transplant* 21:1062–1067, 2002.

63. Zuckermann A, Reichenspurner H, Birsan T: Cyclosporine A versus tacrolimus in combination with mycophenolate mofetil and steroids as primary immunosuppression after lung transplanta-tion: One-year results of a 2-center prospective ran-domized trial. *J Thorac Cardiovasc Surg* 125:891–900, 2003.

64. Schulman LL, Weinberg AD, McGregor C, et al: Mismatches at the HLA-DR and HLA-B loci are risk factors for acute rejection after lung transplantation. *Am J Respir Crit Care Med* 157:1833–1837, 1998.

65. Quantz MA, Bennett LE, Meyer DM, et al: Does human leukocyte antigen matching influence the outcome of lung transplantation? An analysis of 3,549 lung transplantations. *J Heart Lung Transplant* 19:473–479, 2000.

66. Yousem SA, Berry GJ, Cagle PT, et al: Revision of the 1990 working formulation for the classification of pulmonary allograft rejection: Lung Rejection Study Group. *J Heart Lung Transplant* 15:1–15, 1996.

67. Guilinger RA, Paradis IL, Dauber JH, et al: The importance of bronchoscopy with transbronchial biopsy and bronchoalveolar lavage in the manage-ment of lung transplant recipients. *Am J Respir Crit Care Med* 152:2037–2043, 1995.

68. Estenne M, Hertz MI: Bronchiolitis obliterans after human lung transplantation. *Am J Respir Crit Care Med* 166:440–444, 2002.

69. Reichenspurner H, Girgis RE, Robbins RC, et al: Stanford experience with obliterative bronchiolitis after lung and heart-lung transplantation. *Ann Thorac Surg* 62:1467–1473, 1996.

70. Girgis RE, Tu I, Berry GJ: Risk factors for the development of obliterative bronchiolitis after lung transplantation. *J Heart Lung Transplant* 15:1200–1208, 1996.

71. Estenne M, Maurer JR, Boehler A, et al: Bronchiolitis obliterans syndrome 2001: An update of the diag-nostic criteria. *J Heart Lung Transplant* 21:297–310, 2002.

72. Bando K, Paradis IL, Similo S, et al: Obliterative bronchiolitis after lung and heart-lung transplanta-tion: An analysis of risk factors and management. *J Thorac Cardiovasc Surg* 110:4–14, 1995.

73. Heng D, Sharples LD, McNeil K, et al: Bronchiolitis obliterans syndrome: Incidence, natural history, prognosis, and risk factors. *J Heart Lung Transplant* 17:1255–1263, 1998.

74. Sharples LD, McNeil K, Stewart S, et al: Risk factors for bronchiolitis obliterans: A systematic review of recent publications. *J Heart Lung Transplant* 21:271–281, 2002.

75. Bankier AA, Van Muylem A, Knoop C, et al: Bronchiolitis obliterans syndrome in heart-lung transplant recipients: Diagnosis with expiratory CT. *Radiology* 218:533–539, 2001.

76. Lee ES, Gotway MB, Reddy GP, et al: Early bronchi-olitis obliterans following lung transplantation:

Accuracy of expiratory thin-section CT for diagnosis. *Radiology* 216:472–477, 2000.

77. Leung AN, Fisher K, Valentine V, et al: Bronchiolitis obliterans after lung transplantation: Detection using expiratory HRCT. *Chest* 113:365–370, 1998.

78. Date H, Lynch JP, Sundaresan S, et al: The impact of cytolytic therapy on bronchiolitis obliterans syndrome. *J Heart Lung Transplant* 17:869–875, 1998.

79. Brugiere O, Pessione F, Thabut G, et al: Bronchiolitis obliterans syndrome after single-lung transplantation: Impact of time to onset on functional pattern and survival. *Chest* 121:1883–1889, 2002.

80. Iacono AT, Keenan RJ, Duncan SR, et al: Aerosolized cyclosporine in lung recipients with refractory chronic rejection. *Am J Respir Crit Care Med* 153:1451–1455, 1996.

81. Snell GI, Esmore DS, Williams TJ: Cytolytic therapy for the bronchiolitis obliterans syndrome complicating lung transplantation. *Chest* 109:874–878, 1996.

82. Kesten S, Chaparro C, Scavuzzo M, et al: Tacrolimus as rescue therapy for bronchiolitis obliterans syndrome. *J Heart Lung Transplant* 16:905–912, 1997.

83. Dusmet, M, Maurer, J, Winton, T, et al: Methotrexate can halt the progression of bronchiolitis obliterans syndrome in lung transplant recipients. *J Heart Lung Transplant* 15:948–954, 1996.

84. O'Hagan AR, Stillwell PC, Arroliga A, et al: Photopheresis in the treatment of refractory bronchiolitis obliterans complicating lung transplantation. *Chest* 115:1459–1462, 1999.

85. Kotloff RM: Lung retransplantation: All for one or one for all? *Chest* 123:1781–1782, 2003.

86. Kotloff RM, Ahya VN: Medical complications of lung transplantation. *Eur Respir J* 23:334–342, 2004.

87. Chan KM, Allen SA: Infectious pulmonary complications in lung transplant recipients. *Semin Respir Infect* 17:291–302, 2002.

88. Weill D, Dey GC, Hicks RA, et al: A positive donor gram stain does not predict outcome following lung transplantation. *J Heart Lung Transplant* 21:555–558, 2002.

89. Kramer MR, Marshall SE, Starnes VA, et al: Infectious complications in heart-lung transplanta-

tion. Analysis of 200 episodes. *Arch Intern Med* 153:2010–2016, 1993.

90. Maurer JR, Tullis DE, Grossman RF, et al: Infectious complications following isolated lung transplantation. *Chest* 101:1056–1059, 1992.

91. Boehler A, Estenne M: Post-transplant bronchiolitis obliterans. *Eur Respir J* 22:1007–1018, 2003.

92. Zamora MR: Cytomegalovirus and lung transplantation. *Am J Transplant* 4:1219–1226, 2004.

93. Khalifah AP, Hachem RR, Chakinala MM, et al: Respiratory viral infections are a distinct risk for bronchiolitis obliterans syndrome and death. *Am J Respir Crit Care Med* 170:181–187, 2004.

94. Mehrad B, Paciocco G, Martinez FJ, et al: Spectrum of *Aspergillus* infection in lung transplant recipients: Case series and review of the literature. *Chest* 119:169–175, 2001.

95. Birsan T, Taghavi S, Klepetko W: Treatment of aspergillus-related ulcerative tracheobronchitis in lung transplant recipients. *J Heart Lung Transplant* 17:437–438, 1998.

96. Cahill BC, Hibbs JR, Savik K, et al: *Aspergillus* airway colonization and invasive disease after lung transplantation. *Chest* 112:1160–1164, 1997.

97. Kessler R, Massard G, Warter A, et al: Bronchial-pulmonary artery fistula after unilateral lung transplantation: A case report. *J Heart Lung Transplant* 16:674–677, 1997.

98. Aris RM, Maia DM, Neuringer IP, et al: Post-transplantation lymphoproliferative disorder in the Epstein-Barr virus-naive lung transplant recipient. *Am J Respir Crit Care Med* 154:1712–1717, 1996.

99. Levine SM, Angel L, Anzueto A, et al: A low incidence of posttransplant lymphoproliferative disorder in 109 lung transplant recipients. *Chest* 116:1273–1277, 1999.

100. Paranjothi S, Yusen RD, Kraus MD, et al: Lymphoproliferative disease after lung transplantation: Comparison of presentation and outcome of early and late cases. *J Heart Lung Transplant* 20:1054–1063, 2001.

101. Loren AW, Porter DL, Stadtmauer EA, et al: Post-transplant lymphoproliferative disorder: A review. *Bone Marrow Transplant* 31:145–155, 2003.

Portopulmonary Hypertension

Karen L. Swanson, DO,

Michael J. Krowka, MD

Introduction

Patients with liver disease may develop pulmonary complications, including pleural effusions (hepatic hydrothorax), pulmonary vascular dilation with hypoxemia (hepatopulmonary syndrome), pulmonary hypertension from high cardiac output, and pulmonary hypertension from an increased pulmonary vascular resistance (portopulmonary hypertension [POPH]). POPH is defined hemodynamically as an elevated mean pulmonary artery pressure (mPAP > 25 mmHg at rest or > 30 mmHg with exercise), an increased pulmonary vascular resistance (PVR > 240 dynes·sec·cm^{-5}), and a normal pulmonary artery occlusion pressure (PAOP < 15 mm Hg) in a patient who has liver disease (TABLE 9-1).[1] No longer categorized as a "secondary" form of pulmonary hypertension, POPH is now classified by the World Health Organization under the category of pulmonary arterial hypertension (PAH), along with other forms of the disease such as idiopathic (formerly "primary") pulmonary arterial hypertension (IPAH) (TABLE 9-2).[2]

Previously, the pulmonary circulation was considered a passive conduit for blood as it acquired oxygen and disposed of carbon dioxide. The pulmonary vascular endothelium is, however, a complex, dynamic organ capable of producing a variety of vascular mediators and able to respond to significant changes in pulmonary blood flow. Aberrant vascular responses to flow conditions and abnormal levels of mediators may result in endothelial dysfunction. The pathogenesis of POPH is not entirely understood; however, it involves a vascular proliferative response in someone who has liver disease, most commonly portal hypertension. Because not all patients with portal hypertension, however, develop pulmonary hypertension, it is likely that POPH develops when elevated portal pressures occur in the setting of a genetic susceptibility, environmental exposure, or some other "second hit" that then triggers an abnormal pulmonary vascular proliferative response.

In order to interpret the hemodynamic abnormalities seen in POPH, it is important to recall the hemodynamic changes commonly observed in patients with liver disease but without pulmonary hypertension. Approximately 30-50 percent of patients with cirrhosis display a hyperdynamic circulation characterized by a high cardiac output, a low systemic vascular resistance, and a low PVR (FIGURE 9-1).[1-3] In these patients, pulmonary artery pressures may be elevated because of the increase in cardiac output and blood volume, but the PVR is normal or low. In POPH however, PVR is increased, as are pulmonary artery pressures. Cardiac output may be elevated initially due to the liver disease, but it often decreases as the severity of pulmonary hypertension progresses. Compared with patients with IPAH, those with POPH usually have a higher cardiac output. Both conditions, however, are characterized by an elevated PVR, differentiating them from patients with chronic liver disease alone.[4] These distinctions are important when orthotopic liver transplantation (OLT) is considered, because mild elevation of pulmonary artery pressures caused by increases in cardiac output in someone who has a normal or low PVR does not have the same deleterious effect on the outcome of transplantation.[5]

A 2004 consensus panel concluded that although the reported normal range of PVR has varied in the literature, a PVR greater than 240 dynes·sec·cm^{-5}

TABLE 9-1

Diagnostic Criteria for Portopulmonary Hypertension

Portal hypertension with or without cirrhosis
Pulmonary arterial hypertension defined at right heart catheterization
Increased mean pulmonary artery pressure (mPAP > 25 mmHg at rest, > 30 mmHg with exercise)
Increased pulmonary vascular resistance (PVR > 240 dynes·sec·cm^{-5})
Normal pulmonary artery occlusion pressure (PAOP < 15 mmHg)

The value used to define an abnormal elevation in PVR consistent with POPH has varied over time. Although some patients with POPH may have lower values, a PVR greater than 240 dynes·sec·cm^{-5} is definitively abnormal and usually clinically significant.

TABLE 9-2

Classification and Causes of Pulmonary Hypertension

1. Pulmonary Arterial Hypertension (PAH)
    1.1. Idiopathic (IPAH)
    1.2. Familial (FPAH)
    1.3. Associated with (APAH):
        1.3.1. Collagen vascular disease
        1.3.2. Congenital systemic-to-pulmonary shunts**
        1.3.3. Portal hypertension
        1.3.4. HIV infection
        1.3.5. Drugs and toxins
        1.3.6. Other (thyroid disorders, glycogen storage disease, Gaucher disease, hereditary hemorrhagic telangiectasia, hemoglobinopathies, myeloproliferative disorders, splenectomy)
    1.4. Associated with significant venous or capillary involvement
        1.4.1. Pulmonary veno-occlusive disease (PVOD)
        1.4.2. Pulmonary capillary hemangiomatosis (PCH)
    1.5. Persistent pulmonary hypertension of the newborn
2. Pulmonary hypertension with left-sided heart disease
    2.1. Left-sided atrial or ventricular heart disease
    2.2. Left-sided valvular heart disease
3. Pulmonary hypertension associated with lung diseases or hypoxemia
    3.1. Chronic obstructive pulmonary disease
    3.2. Interstitial lung disease
    3.3. Sleep-disordered breathing
    3.4. Alveolar hypoventilation disorders
    3.5. Long-term exposure to high altitude
    3.6. Developmental abnormalities
4. Pulmonary hypertension due to chronic thrombotic or embolic disease
    4.1. Thromboembolic obstruction of proximal pulmonary arteries
    4.2. Thromboembolic obstruction of distal pulmonary arteries
    4.3. Nonthrombotic pulmonary embolism (tumor, parasites, foreign material)
5. Miscellaneous (sarcoidosis, histiocytosis X, lymphangiomatosis, compression of pulmonary vessels [adenopathy, tumor, fibrosing mediastinitis])

HIV, *human immunodeficiency virus.*
Adapted from Ref. 2.

represents a definitive, clinically significant "cut-off."[1] Some patients with PVR values between 120 dynes·sec·cm^{-5} (a frequently used cut-off of normal) and 240 dynes·sec·cm^{-5} may have a constellation of findings consistent with POPH. The variation in definition requires attention in comparing the results of published studies with one another. The chosen cut-off is of particular importance as it is applied in determining patient candidacy for liver transplantation.

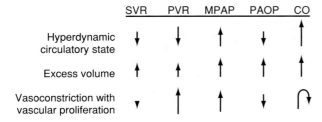

	SVR	PVR	MPAP	PAOP	CO
Hyperdynamic circulatory state	↓	↓	↑	↓	↑
Excess volume	↑	↑	↑	↑	↑
Vasoconstriction with vascular proliferation	▼	↑	↑	↓	↷

SVR - systemic vascular resistance;
PVR - pulmonary vascular resistance;
MPAP - mean pulmonary artery pressure;
PAOP - pulmonary artery occlusion pressure;
CO - cardiac output

Figure 9-1. Pulmonary Hemodynamic Patterns Associated With Advanced Liver Disease. *SVR,* systemic vascular resistance; *PVR,* pulmonary vascular resistance; *MPAP,* mean pulmonary artery pressure; *PAOP,* pulmonary artery occlusion pressure; *CO,* cardiac output.

Pathology

POPH is characterized by vasoconstrictive, proliferative, and obliterative changes in the pulmonary vascular bed. Pathologic vascular changes include plexiform lesions that consist of medial hypertrophy and endothelial and smooth muscle cell proliferation. The plexiform lesions seen in POPH are indistinguishable from those seen in IPAH (FIGURE 9-2).[6] In an autopsy study of 12 patients with POPH, four patterns of pulmonary artery disease were described: medial hypertrophy, thrombosis, plexiform lesions, and the coexistence of plexiform and thrombotic lesions.[7] Thrombotic lesions are believed to result from *in situ* clot formation caused by a combination of endothelial cell injury, platelet aggregation, and impaired blood flow, but in general are not caused directly by coagulation abnormalities.

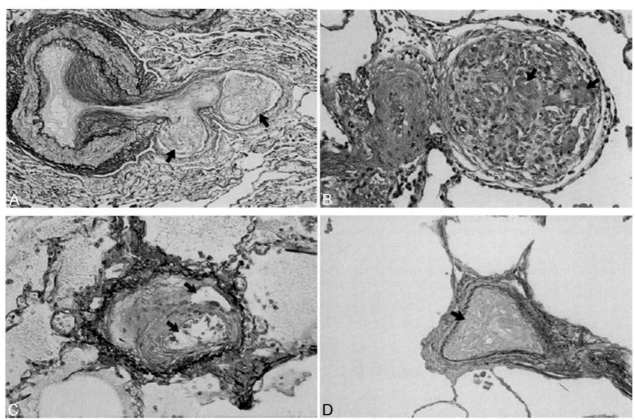

Figure 9-2. Pathologic findings in the pulmonary vasculature in portopulmonary hypertension: (**A**) plexogenic type (plexiform lesions: *arrows*); (**B**) obstructive plexiform lesion with occluding platelet-fibrin thrombi *(arrows)*; (**C**) thrombotic type: muscular pulmonary arteriole obstructed by recanalized thrombus *(arrows)*; (**D**) fibrotic type: pulmonary arteriole obstructed by dense fibrin plug. (From Krowka MJ, Edwards WD: A spectrum of pulmonary vascular pathology in portopulmonary hypertension. *Liver Transpl* 6:241-242, 2000.) (See Color Plate 10).

Although a thromboembolic source has been postulated, intrapulmonary thrombi typically are seen in the absence of evidence for systemic sources. The combination of vasoconstriction, obstruction to pulmonary vascular flow, and probable *in situ* microthrombosis results in the increase in PVR observed in patients with POPH.[8]

Pathogenesis

The pathogenesis of POPH is not completely understood. Possible mechanisms for the development of PAH in patients with liver disease include an imbalance of vascular mediators favoring vasoconstriction,[9-11] endothelial damage with vascular remodeling caused by excessive pulmonary blood flow,[12,13] and microvascular thrombosis.[8] The severity of liver disease or degree of portal hypertension does not appear to correlate with the severity of pulmonary hypertension.[3] Whether genetic mutations such as those identified in the bone morphogenetic protein receptor type 2 gene in familial PAH or in the activin receptor-like kinase gene in PAH and hereditary hemorrhagic telangiectasia also play a role in the development of POPH remains unknown.[14]

It is likely that a complex interaction of vascular mediators and endothelial and smooth muscle responses play a role in the development of POPH. Endothelin-1 (ET-1) is a potent vasoconstrictor in humans and has been implicated in the pathogenesis of IPAH. ET-1 levels are also increased in patients who have cirrhosis with refractory ascites.[15] Other mediators favoring vasoconstriction include serotonin, angiotensin II, and norepinephrine. Vascular mediators favoring vasodilation include nitric oxide and prostacyclin. Prostacyclin is a potent vasodilator normally found in high concentrations in the lungs. The expression of prostacyclin synthase, the enzyme responsible for production of prostacyclin, is decreased in the lungs of patients with POPH.[16] Decreased expression of such vasodilators may facilitate vascular remodeling and a proliferative vascular response, although the precise manner in which these and other mediators interact to produce POPH is not clear.

Portal hypertension induces changes that may influence the lung vasculature by altering the milieu of mediators to which it is exposed, or by affecting gene regulation in endothelial and smooth muscle cells. It is hypothesized that endotoxin or cytokines, or both, released from the splanchnic circulation bypass the liver and affect the pulmonary circulation.[17] In support of this hypothesis, patients with portosystemic shunting can develop pathologic changes of the pulmonary vascular bed similar to those seen in POPH. These changes normalize with reversal of shunting. To date however, no causative substance has been identified unequivocally.

Vascular remodeling provoked by shear stress from a hyperdynamic state (increased cardiac output) imposed upon the pulmonary endothelium also has been postulated to contribute to POPH. Studies are evaluating the role that bone marrow-derived progenitor cells might play in the pathogenesis of PAH. Because only a subset of patients with portal hypertension develops POPH, this suggests that genetic (and perhaps other) differences in susceptibility also play a role.

Epidemiology

The prevalence of POPH in patients with liver disease is not well defined. The reported prevalence of POPH in patients with cirrhosis generally ranges from 0.25–4.0 percent,[18-20] but one study of patients who had cirrhosis with refractory ascites estimated the prevalence of POPH to be 16.1 percent.[15] Many prevalence estimates have been made in patients evaluated for liver transplant and thus represent patients with more severe liver disease. A review of 1,205 consecutive patients who had received liver transplants estimated the prevalence of POPH to be 8.5 percent.[21] The incidence of POPH in patients with documented liver disease has not been well defined.

Clinical Features

In the early phases of POPH, patients may be asymptomatic or have symptoms caused by liver disease alone, which is why screening and a high clinical suspicion for pulmonary hypertension becomes critical in those being evaluated for liver transplantation. The most common initial symptom in patients with POPH is dyspnea on exertion. As the severity of pulmonary hypertension increases, symptoms can include peripheral edema, fatigue, dyspnea, abdominal bloating, and palpitations. As in other forms of PAH, chest discomfort and syncope are later, worrisome symptoms that indicate that disease probably is advanced.

Findings on physical examination depend upon the severity of pulmonary hypertension. In mild POPH, examination may be notable only for findings suggestive of liver disease and include spider telangiectases, jaundice, mild lower extremity edema, and ascites. As the severity of POPH increases, however, findings of right-sided heart pressure and volume overload may become more obvious. These include elevation of the jugular venous pressure, a right ventricular lift, a loud pulmonic valve closure, a tricuspid regurgitation or pulmonic insufficiency (Graham Steell) murmur, increased splitting of the second heart sound, a pulsatile liver, or a right-sided third or fourth heart sound.

Evaluation

Identification of POPH in patients with underlying liver disease is important not only to best direct medical therapy, but also to assess candidacy for liver transplantation. All patients undergoing evaluation for liver transplantation should be screened for POPH, because mortality in patients with moderate to severe POPH is increased during the intraoperative and immediate postoperative periods. Thus, the advisability and timing of transplantation may be influenced by POPH, and it is not acceptable to make the diagnosis after a pulmonary artery catheter is placed in the operating room during transplant.[5]

Patients with liver disease and complaints suggestive of pulmonary hypertension (most often dyspnea) should undergo a thorough history and physical examination. A transthoracic Doppler echocardiogram is the screening procedure of choice, although other focused testing should be considered. A chest radiograph may suggest POPH (enlarged central pulmonary arteries or cardiomegaly) and is useful in identifying other important causes of dyspnea, such as pleural effusions or interstitial lung disease. Pulmonary hypertension is suggested if evidence of right atrial or ventricular enlargement or a right bundle branch block pattern is seen on the electrocardiogram. Pulmonary function testing (PFT) results in patients with POPH are frequently normal and not diagnostic, although a reduced diffusing capacity may be present. PFT is important, however, to exclude significant airflow obstruction or restrictive lung disease.

Once the presence of pulmonary hypertension has been established, a ventilation-perfusion scan or, less optimally, a computed tomographic angiogram should be performed to exclude thromboembolic disease. A polysomnogram should be considered in patients with symptoms suggestive of obstructive sleep apnea and a screening overnight oximetry study performed in patients without a suggestive history. Blood testing is appropriate to screen for collagen vascular disease or human immunodeficiency virus infection. Human immunodeficiency virus testing may be of particular importance in patients with hepatitis acquired by intravenous drug use and those being considered for organ transplantation. Measurement of B-type natriuretic peptide (BNP) levels may be also be helpful. BNP is released from the ventricles under conditions of pressure or volume overload. Serial measurements of BNP may provide clinically useful information predictive of disease severity and response to management.[22] However, none of the abnormalities found on chest radiograph, electrocardiogram, PFT, or blood testing are diagnostic by themselves for PAH.

Transthoracic Doppler echocardiography is the screening procedure of choice and should be considered in all patients with liver disease and unexplained dyspnea, and performed in all patients undergoing evaluation for liver transplantation.[1] Findings on echocardiography suggestive of POPH include elevation of right ventricular systolic pressure (RVSP) calculated from the peak tricuspid regurgitant velocity (TRV) using the modified Bernoulli equation and an estimate of right atrial pressure:

$$RVSP = (4 \times TRV^2) + \text{right atrial pressure}$$

Right atrial pressure is estimated based on the filling characteristics of the inferior vena cava. Transthoracic Doppler echocardiography has a sensitivity of 97 percent and a specificity of 77 percent in the diagnosis of moderate to severe pulmonary hypertension in patients undergoing liver transplant evaluation.[24] When using an RVSP cutoff of 40 mmHg, Doppler echocardiography has a sensitivity of approximately 80 percent, specificity of 96 percent, positive predictive value of 60 percent, and negative predictive value of 98 percent.[24]

In an estimated 20 percent of cases, the TRV cannot be assessed adequately with Doppler echocardiography because of the lack of a tricuspid regurgitant jet. One study has proposed using pulmonary acceleration time, instead, of the estimated RVSP.[25] Pulmonary acceleration time is measured from the Doppler pulmonary artery flow velocity tracing as the time from the onset of ejection to peak flow velocity. Normal values are longer than 120 milliseconds. In POPH, pulmonary acceleration time was found to be shorter than 100 milliseconds, and the diagnostic accuracy 96 percent as compared with that of an estimated RVSP of 90 percent. This may be a useful measurement to determine which patients should undergo right heart catheterization for suspected POPH. A derived index of right ventricular myocardial performance (RIMP) using echocardiographic measurements is used in some centers, and it appears to be an independent predictor of cardiac death and need for transplantation in patients with PAH.[26] The RIMP is calculated by dividing the sum of the isovolumetric contraction and relaxation times by the ejection time. The RIMP is inversely related to right ventricular function. As pulmonary hypertension progresses, right ventricular dysfunction develops and the RIMP increases.

Regardless of the echocardiographic technique used to estimate the severity of pulmonary hypertension, however, echocardiography cannot differentiate between PAH (elevated PVR) and pulmonary hypertension caused by a hyperdynamic state (normal or low PVR). The diagnosis of POPH is confirmed with a right heart catheterization. This permits accurate measurement of pulmonary artery pressures, pulmonary artery occlusion (wedge) pressure (to exclude left heart dysfunction and volume overload), cardiac output (to exclude a high-output state as the cause of pulmonary hypertension), and documentation of an elevated PVR. PVR is calculated in dynes·sec·cm^{-5} as:

$$PVR = [(mPAP - PAOP) \div CO] \times 80$$

PVR normally is less than 240. One study of patients with decompensated cirrhosis and refractory ascites found that a right atrial pressure equal to 14 mmHg had a positive predictive value of 83 percent for pulmonary hypertension.[15] If indicated, a left heart catheterization can be performed at the same time to exclude significant coronary artery or left-sided valvular disease and directly measure left ventricular end-diastolic pressure; such information would also be of importance in the evaluation for transplantation.

A vasodilator trial should be performed in patients with moderate to severe pulmonary hypertension at the time of right heart catheterization. For vasodilator testing, a short-acting vasodilator such as nitric oxide, adenosine, or epoprostenol is administered to determine acute vasoreactivity. A positive vasodilator response generally is defined as a fall in mPAP by more than 10 mmHg and to a value of less than 40 mmHg, with no decrease in cardiac output, although an acute decrease in both mPAP and PVR of more than 20 percent from baseline without a fall in cardiac output has also been used.[1,27] Unlike in IPAH, a positive response to acute vasodilator testing in patients with POPH is not used to assess the potential utility of oral calcium channel antagonists, because such agents are not recommended in POPH. Acute vasodilator testing in POPH can help in assessing potential reversibility of hemodynamic abnormalities and therapeutic expectations. A positive vasodilator response cannot, however, predict survival either with or without liver transplantation.

Management

Mild POPH rarely requires management. Patients may have symptoms related to liver disease but are often without symptoms attributable to POPH. Patients with moderate to severe disease, however, may benefit symptomatically from treatment aimed at lowering pulmonary artery pressures and PVR. A management algorithm is shown in FIGURE 9-3.

Diuretics are employed almost universally in the management of POPH, both for associated cor pulmonale and to manage volume overload from liver disease. Diuretics are especially important if ascites or peripheral edema is present. Anticoagulation has been associated with improved survival in observational, nonrandomized trials involving patients with IPAH[28,29] but is often contraindicated in POPH because of gastroesophageal varices, thrombocytopenia, decreased coagulation factors, or other hemorrhagic diatheses related to liver disease. Patients with hypoxemia should be given supplemental oxygen to maintain oxygen saturation above 90 percent at all times.

Several classes of drugs with vasodilating and other vasomodulating effects can be employed to manage POPH, but randomized controlled trials specific to this population have not been performed. Most of the data regarding these medications come from clinical trials of patients with either IPAH or PAH associated with connective tissue disorders. Little information is available for their use in patients with POPH, and what data are available typically come from uncontrolled case reports or case series. Thus, the use of any of these pharmacologic agents in the management of POPH must be individualized according to the extent of liver disease and considerations for organ transplantation. In addition, psychosocial issues and the patient's ability to manage the challenges of

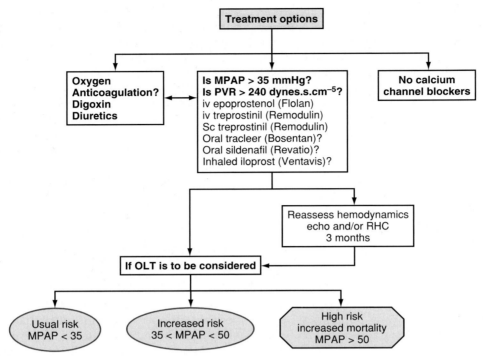

Figure 9-3. Management Algorithm for Portopulmonary Hypertension.

certain drug delivery systems (e.g., continuous intravenous or subcutaneous therapies) are also important considerations.

Even among acutely vasoreactive patients with POPH, many do not tolerate calcium channel antagonists due to worsening peripheral edema. Indeed, calcium channel antagonists generally are not recommended in patients with POPH, because they may increase the hepatic venous pressure gradient.[1,30,31]

Prostanoids such as epoprostenol (Flolan®) or treprostinil (Remodulin®) have been used successfully to lower pulmonary pressures in patients with POPH. Both require continuous 24-hour infusions via portable infusion pumps, and the intravenous forms require a permanent indwelling central venous catheter. Epoprostenol has a very short half-life, requires daily mixing, and must be kept cold with ice packs, making it a cumbersome therapy. Improvements in cardiopulmonary hemodynamics and exercise capacity in patients with POPH have been demonstrated following epoprostenol therapy, although a survival advantage has not been documented in this population.[32] Several case series have reported that some patients with POPH treated with intravenous epoprostenol to reduce pulmonary pressures have undergone successful OLT.[33-35] Complications of

intravenous epoprostenol therapy include central venous catheter thrombosis, infection, and infusion pump failure necessitating the availability of a back-up pump at all times. Epoprostenol is both a pulmonary and systemic vasodilator, as well as inhibitor of platelet aggregation. Patients with POPH treated with epoprostenol may develop progressive splenomegaly and thrombocytopenia, possibly caused by increased blood flow in the splanchnic circulation.[36]

Treprostinil has a longer half-life than epoprostenol and does not have to be kept chilled. The infusion pump used for subcutaneous and intravenous administration is smaller than that used with epoprostenol. The biggest disadvantage of subcutaneous treprostinil is local infusion site pain, which develops in up to 80 percent of patients and does not appear to be dosage related. Other prostacyclin-related side effects seen with both treprostinil and epoprostenol include flushing, diarrhea, jaw discomfort, and lower extremity pain. In 2004 the U.S. Food and Drug Administration (FDA) approved continuous intravenous administration of treprostinil, which might allow continuous infusion therapy that is less cumbersome than that of epoprostenol. An additional prostaglandin analogue, iloprost (Ventavis®) is administered as inhaled, nebulized therapy and received FDA approval in 2005 for the management of PAH. Inhaled iloprost has not been well studied in patients with POPH.

The dual endothelin receptor antagonist, bosentan (Tracleer®), is an oral agent approved by the FDA in 2002 for PAH management. Endothelin mediates vasoconstriction, cell proliferation, and inflammation; its binding to both endothelin A and B receptors is inhibited by bosentan. Because hepatotoxicity is an important adverse effect, bosentan has not been well studied in patients with liver disease. Several case reports have described its successful use, however, in patients with POPH.[37-40] In approximately 5-10 percent of patients, bosentan can cause elevations in transaminases, alkaline phosphatase, and bilirubin. The presumed mechanism is impairment of bile salt transport, leading to their accumulation within the liver.[41] Patients using bosentan must have monthly liver function testing performed.[43] The incidence of liver function abnormalities in patients with underlying liver disease using bosentan has not been well defined. Irreversible hepatic toxicity has not been documented; liver dysfunction in most patients returns to baseline levels upon discontinuing bosentan. Selective endothelin-A receptor antagonists (ambrisentan and sitaxsentan) are under study for the management of PAH and at the time of this writing are not FDA approved. These medications may cause less hepatotoxicity than bosentan.

Another oral agent with possible efficacy in POPH is the phosphodiesterase 5 inhibitor, sildenafil (Revatio®), which the FDA approved for PAH management in 2005. Sildenafil prolongs nitric oxide-mediated vasodilation by inhibiting the cyclic guanosine monophosphatase-specific phosphodiesterase type 5 enzyme that is found in large concentrations in pulmonary artery smooth muscle cells. In other forms of PAH, sildenafil increases cardiac output, and decreases pulmonary artery pressures and PVR without serious adverse events.[43-45] One case report showed that sildenafil decreased mPAP from 56 mmHg to 28-31 mmHg in a patient with POPH. The patient subsequently underwent successful liver transplantation.[46] Controlled studies regarding the use of sildenafil in POPH have not been performed.

Liver Transplantation

Liver transplantation may be beneficial in a highly selected subset of patients with POPH. However, POPH increases the risk for intraoperative and immediate postoperative complications of liver transplantation. As pulmonary artery pressure and PVR increase, so does mortality associated with transplantation. Potential candidates must be evaluated carefully at liver transplant centers experienced in the management of POPH, including medical management with well-defined protocols regarding the timing of OLT. In general, cadaveric liver transplantation is performed, although results of one successful living-related donor transplantation in a patient with POPH have been published.[47]

As mentioned above, all patients being considered for liver transplantation should have a screening transthoracic echocardiogram. Patients with an RVSP estimated as greater than 50 mmHg should be assessed further by right heart catheterization. Patients without evidence to suggest pulmonary hypertension on echocardiogram should be monitored with yearly repeat studies.[5] Patients with POPH on the OLT waiting list should have echocardiograms performed at 6-12 month intervals to ensure that pulmonary hypertension does not progress before proceeding with OLT.

Regardless of treatment, patients with POPH whose mPAP is between 35 and 50 mmHg have an increased mortality and may benefit from prolonged management of PAH.[5,48] Mortality is extremely high in patients with mPAP over 50 mm Hg, and such patients should not undergo OLT.

In the absence of pulmonary hypertension, right ventricular function is preserved through all phases of the liver transplant operation.[49] Patients with POPH, however, may develop hemodynamic instability during surgery. The most critical times during OLT include the induction of anesthesia, during and after graft reperfusion, and the immediate postoperative period.[50] Patients may need support intraoperatively with vasodilators if there is worsening pulmonary hypertension, or with inotropic medications to support right ventricular dysfunction and heart failure. In one study, eight patients with POPH diagnosed during anesthesia induction for OLT all required intraoperative vasodilator therapy because of marked increases in pulmonary artery pressures and PVR that occurred following graft reperfusion.[51] Both the increase in blood flow following reperfusion and the aggressive fluid administration often required during the perioperative period can worsen pulmonary hypertension. This may result in worsening right heart function and a backup of fluid into the transplanted liver. Infusion of 1 liter of crystalloid fluid over 10 minutes has been shown to increase mPAP and PAOP in OLT candidates without pulmonary hypertension,[52] and this response may be exaggerated in those with POPH. The usefulness of vasodilator therapy may be limited by either increased intrapulmonary shunting with consequent worsening in oxygenation, or by systemic hypotension.

A national database was initiated at 10 liver transplant centers to evaluate patients with POPH for OLT between 1996 and 2001.[53] The database showed that in-hospital liver transplant mortality was 36 percent (13/36) in patients with POPH, emphasizing the importance of accurately assessing the severity of PAH prior to attempting OLT.[48] Although transplant was denied to 45 percent (30/66) of referred patients because of the severity of POPH, transplant mortality during hospitalization occurred in 92 percent of those with a mPAP over 35 mmHg. Death in patients with severe POPH generally resulted from right ventricular failure. It is important to recognize, however, that although patients with severe POPH have a poor prognosis in general, some patients with moderate to severe POPH have been treated successfully with medications to lower pulmonary artery pressures and PVR such that OLT could be accomplished safely.

Some patients with POPH may exhibit resolution of pulmonary hypertension after OLT and may even been able to discontinue vasodilator medications.[35,45-47] Although OLT is the management of choice for hepatopulmonary syndrome, this is not true of POPH, and resolution of pulmonary hypertension after OLT is not universal. Many patients require continued therapy for POPH after OLT has been performed. PAH may resolve, persist, or even develop *de novo* following liver transplantation.[1] When PAH does resolve, it does so over months to years, suggesting that vascular remodeling, as opposed to simple reversal of vasoconstriction, is the probable explanation for the improvement.

Prognosis

Survival from the time POPH is diagnosed is difficult to predict. The natural history without management varies with the degree of liver disease and the severity of pulmonary hypertension. One retrospective study of 78 patients with POPH treated conservatively in the preprostanoid era found a median survival of 6 months, with a range from 0-84 months from the time of POPH diagnosis.[55] In the Mayo Clinic experience, survival after 1, 2, and 5 years in those with POPH is now approximately 71 percent, 58 percent, and 44 percent, respectively, regardless of whether liver transplantation has been performed (Swanson and Krowka, unpublished data). Causes of death include right-sided heart failure, sudden cardiac death, gastrointestinal bleeding, and small bowel perforation. In general, reports of outcomes with pharmacologic management of POPH with or without OLT consist of case series and retrospective reviews. Prospective studies of POPH management are lacking.

Cardiac index appears to be the most significant prognostic variable.[8] If right ventricular function is not impaired and the elevation in pulmonary arterial pressure is moderate (mPAP <35 mmHg), patients tend to do well with OLT.[20] Right ventricular impairment, however, is an ominous sign of advanced pulmonary hypertension and is associated with increased morbidity and mortality. Such patients may have elevated BNP levels from the increased pressure and volume overload of the right ventricle and a reduction in cardiac output. A persistently elevated BNP portends a poor prognosis in IPAH, especially among patients already receiving treatment for pulmonary hypertension.[22]

Summary

POPH is characterized by elevations in pulmonary artery pressure and PVR in patients with liver disease, most commonly with portal hypertension. Pathologic changes in the pulmonary vascular bed in patients with POPH are identical to those seen in IPAH. A high clinical suspicion for pulmonary hypertension is imperative, so that patients are diagnosed before the time of liver transplantation. All patients undergoing screening for OLT should have transthoracic Doppler echocardiography performed to exclude the possibility of POPH. Morbidity and mortality are increased in patients with moderate to severe POPH if OLT is performed. Pharmacologic treatment may be successful in lowering pulmonary artery pressures so that liver transplantation can be accomplished safely, if necessary. Studies specifically addressing the incidence, prevalence, and response to therapies in patients with POPH are lacking, but ultimately their results may be implemented to improve the pharmacologic strategies used with liver transplantation in these patients.

References

1. Rodriguez-Roisin R, Krowka MJ, Herve P, et al: Pulmonary-Hepatic Vascular Disorders Scientific Committee ERS Task Force. *Eur Respir J* 24:861-880, 2004.

2. Simonneau G, Galie N, Rubin LJ, et al: Clinical classification of pulmonary hypertension. *J Am Coll Cardiol* 43(12 Suppl S):5S-12S, 2004.

3. Hadengue A, Benhayoun MK, Lebrec D, et al: Pulmonary hypertension complicating portal hypertension: Prevalence and relation to splanchnic hemodynamics. *Gastroenterology* 100:520-528, 1991.

4. Kuo PC, Plotkin JS, Johnson LB, et al: Distinctive clinical features of portopulmonary hypertension. *Chest* 112:980-986, 1997.

5. Krowka MJ, Plevak DJ, Findlay JY, et al: Pulmonary hemodynamics and perioperative cardiopulmonary-related mortality in patients with portopulmonary hypertension undergoing liver transplantation. *Liver Transpl* 6:443-450, 2000.

6. Ramsay MA, Simpson BR, Nguyen AT, et al: Severe pulmonary hypertension in liver transplant candidates. *Liver Transpl Surg* 3:494-500, 1997.

7. Edwards BS, Weir EK, Edwards WD, et al: Coexistent pulmonary and portal hypertension: Morphologic and clinical features. *J Am Coll Cardiol* 10:1233-1238, 1987.

8. Herve P, Lebrec D, Brenot F, et al: Pulmonary vascular disorders in portal hypertension. *Eur Respir J* 11:1153-1166, 1998.

9. Kiely DG, Cargill RI, Struthers AD, et al: Cardiopulmonary effects of endothelin-1 in man. *Cardiovasc Res* 33:378-386, 1997.

10. Panos RJ, Baker SK: Mediators, cytokines, and growth factors in liver-lung interactions. *Clin Chest Med* 17:151-169, 1996.

11. Higgenbottam T: Pathophysiology of pulmonary hypertension. *Chest* 105(2 Suppl):7S-12S, 1994.

12. Krowka MJ: Hepatopulmonary syndrome and portopulmonary hypertension: Distinction and dilemmas. *Hepatology* 25:1282-1284, 1997.

13. Hongqun L, Lee SS: Cardiopulmonary dysfunction in cirrhosis. *Hepatology* 14:600-608, 2000.

14. Trembath RC, Thomson JR, Machado RD: Clinical and molecular genetic features of pulmonary hypertension in patients with hereditary hemorrhagic telangiectasia. *New Engl J Med* 345:325-34, 2001.

15. Benjaminov FS, Prentice M, Sniderman KW, et al: Portopulmonary hypertension in decompensated cirrhosis with refractory ascites. *Gut* 52:1355-1362, 2003.

16. Tuder RM, Cool CD, Geraci MW, et al: Prostacyclin synthase expression is decreased in lungs from patients with severe pulmonary hypertension. *Am J Respir Crit Care Med* 159:1925-1932, 1999.

17. Hoeper MM, Krowka MJ, Strassburg CP: Portopulmonary hypertension and hepatopulmonary syndrome. *Lancet* 363:1461-1468, 2004.

18. McDonnell PJ, Toye PJ, Hutchins GM: Primary pulmonary hypertension and cirrhosis: Are they related? *Am Rev Respir Dis* 127:437-441, 1983.

19. Cheng EY, Woehlck H: Pulmonary artery hypertension complicating anesthesia for liver transplantation. *Anesthesiology* 77:375-378, 1992.

20. Castro M, Krowka MJ, Schroeder DR, et al: Frequency and clinical implications of increased pulmonary artery pressures in liver transplantation. *Mayo Clin Proc* 71:543-551, 1996.

21. Ramsay MA, Simpson BR, Nguyen AT, et al: Severe pulmonary hypertension in liver transplant candidates. *Liver Transpl Surg* 3:494-500, 1997.

22. Leuchte HH, Holzapfel M, Baumgartner RA, et al: Characterization of brain natrivretic peptide in long-term follow-up of pulmonary arterial hypertension. *Chest* 128:2368–2374, 2005.

23. Kim WR, Krowka MJ, Plevak DJ, et al: Accuracy of Doppler echocardiography in the assessment of pulmonary hypertension in liver transplant candidates. *Liver Transpl* 6:453-458, 2000.

24. Colle IO, Moreau R, Godinho E, et al: Diagnosis of portopulmonary hypertension in candidates for liver transplantation: A prospective study. *Hepatology* 37:401-409, 2003.

25. Torregrosa M, Genesca J, Gonzalez A, et al: Role of Doppler echocardiography in the assessment of portopulmonary hypertension in liver transplantation candidates. *Transplantation* 71:572-574, 2001.

26. Yeo TC, Dujardin KS, Tei C, et al: Value of a Doppler-derived index combining systolic and diastolic time intervals in predicting outcome in primary pulmonary hypertension. *Am J Cardiol* 81:1157-1161, 1998.

27. Badesch DB, Abman SH, Ahearn GS, et al: Medical therapy for pulmonary arterial hypertension: ACCP evidence-based clinical practice guidelines. *Chest* 126(1 Suppl):35S-62S, 2004.

28. Fuster V, Steele PM, Edwards WD, et al: Primary pulmonary hypertension: Natural history and the importance of thrombosis. *Circulation* 70:580-587, 1984.

29. Rich S, Kaufmann E, Levy PS: The effect of high doses of calcium-channel blockers on survival in primary pulmonary hypertension. *N Engl J Med* 327:76-81, 1992.

30. Ota K, Shijo H, Kokawa H, et al: Effects of nifedipine on hepatic venous pressure gradient and portal vein blood flow in patients with cirrhosis. *J Gastroenterol Hepatol* 10:198-204, 1995.

31. Navasa M, Bosch J, Reichen J, et al: Effects of verapamil on hepatic and systemic hemodynamics and liver function in patients with cirrhosis and portal hypertension. *Hepatology* 8:850-854, 1988.

32. Swanson KL, McGoon MD, Krowka MJ: Survival in patients with portopulmonary hypertension. *Am J Respir Crit Care Med* 167:A693, 2003.

33. Kuo PC, Johnson LB, Plotkin JS, et al: Continuous intravenous infusion of epoprostenol for the treatment of portopulmonary hypertension. *Transplantation* 63:604-616, 1997.

34. Krowka MJ, Frantz RP, McGoon MD, et al: Improvement in pulmonary hemodynamics during intravenous epoprostenol (prostacyclin): A study of 15 patients with moderate to severe portopulmonary hypertension. *Hepatology* 30:641-648, 1999.

35. Kahler CM, Graziadei I, Wiedermann CJ, et al: Successful use of continuous intravenous prostacyclin in a patient with severe portopulmonary hypertension. *Wien Klin Wochenschr* 112:637-640, 2000.

36. Findlay JY, Plevak DJ, Krowka MJ, et al: Progressive splenomegaly after epoprostenol therapy in portopulmonary hypertension. *Liver Transpl Surg* 5:362-365, 1999.

37. Hinterhuber L, Graziadei IW, Kahler CM, et al: Endothelin-receptor antagonist treatment of portopulmonary hypertension. *Clin Gastroenterol Hepatol* 2:1039-1042, 2004.

38. Clift PF, Townend JN, Bramhall S, et al: Successful treatment of severe portopulmonary hypertension after liver transplantation by bosentan. *Transplantation* 77:1774-1775, 2004.

39. Halank M, Miehlke S, Hoeffken G, et al: Use of oral endothelin-receptor antagonist bosentan in the treatment of portopulmonary hypertension. *Transplantation* 77:1775-1776, 2004.

40. Kuntzen C, Gulberg V, Gerbes AL: Use of a mixed endothelin receptor antagonist in portopulmonary hypertension: A safe and effective therapy? *Gastroenterology* 128:164-168, 2005.

41. Fattinger K, Funk C, Pantze M, et al: The endothelin antagonist bosentan inhibits the canalicular bile salt export pump: A potential mechanism for hepatic adverse reactions. *Clin Pharmacol Ther* 69:223-231, 2001.

42. Rubin LJ, Roux S: Bosentan: A dual endothelin receptor antagonist. *Expert Opin Investig Drugs* 11:991-1002, 2002.

43. Watanabe H, Ohashi K, Takeuchi K, et al: Sildenafil for primary and secondary pulmonary hypertension. *Clin Pharmacol Ther* 71:398-402, 2002.

44. Michelakis E, Tymchak W, Lien D, et al: Oral sildenafil is an effective and specific pulmonary vasodilator in patients with pulmonary arterial hypertension: Comparison with inhaled nitric oxide. *Circulation* 105:2398-2403, 2002.

45. Ghofrani HA, Wiedemann R, Rose F, et al: Sildenafil for treatment of lung fibrosis and pulmonary hypertension: A randomised controlled trial. *Lancet* 360:895-900, 2002.

46. Makisalo H, Koivusalo A, Vakkuri A, et al: Sildenafil for portopulmonary hypertension in a patient undergoing liver transplantation. *Liver Transpl* 10:945-950, 2004.

47. Sulica R, Emre S, Poon M: Medical management of porto-pulmonary hypertension and right heart failure prior to living-related liver transplantation. *Congest Heart Fail* 10:192-194, 2004.

48. Krowka MJ, Mandell MS, Ramsay MA, et al: Hepatopulmonary syndrome and portopulmonary hypertension: A report of the multicenter liver transplant database. *Liver Transpl* 10:174-182, 2004.

49. De Wolf AM, Begliomini B, Gasior TA, et al: Right ventricular function during orthotopic liver transplantation. *Anesth Analg* 76:562-568, 1993.

50. Csete M: Intraoperative management of liver transplant patients with pulmonary hypertension. *Liver Transpl Surg* 3:454-455, 1997.

51. Taura P, Garcia-Valdecasas JC, Beltran J, et al: Moderate primary pulmonary hypertension in patients undergoing liver transplantation. *Anesth Analg* 83:675-680, 1996.

52. Kuo PC, Schroeder RA, Vagelos RH, et al: Volume-mediated pulmonary responses in liver transplant candidates. *Clin Transplant* 10:521-527, 1996.

53. Mandell MS, Krowka MJ: Formation of a national database on pulmonary hypertension and hepatopulmonary syndrome in chronic liver disease. *Anesthesiology* 87:450-451, 1997.

54. Robalino BD, Moodie DS: Association between primary pulmonary hypertension and portal hypertension: Analysis of its pathophysiology and clinical, laboratory and hemodynamic manifestations. *J Am Coll Cardiol* 17:492-498, 1991.

Pulmonary Hypertension Secondary to Chronic Respiratory Disease

Alicia Gerke, MD,

Jess Mandel, MD

Pulmonary hypertension associated with hypoxemia or parenchymal lung disease constitutes a large proportion of all patients with pulmonary hypertension. This population makes up one of the five categories in the 2003 Venice classification of pulmonary hypertension (TABLE 10-1). Diseases such as chronic obstructive pulmonary disease (COPD), interstitial lung disease, and sleep-disordered breathing have a relatively high prevalence in the general population, and associated pulmonary hypertension is a significant contributor to the morbidity and mortality of these conditions. Although development of pulmonary hypertension in each of these populations is multifactorial, they are linked by hypoxia-induced injury.

Hypoxia acts to constrict pulmonary arteries and, conversely, dilate the systemic circulation (see Chapter 1). Pulmonary vasoconstriction is a physiologic response to alveolar hypoxia that serves to minimize ventilation-perfusion ($\dot{V}/\dot{Q}$) mismatch, thereby increasing PaO_2 in arterial blood. However, during chronic hypoxia these physiologic mechanisms can become detrimental, leading to structural remodeling and sustained vasoconstriction by pulmonary arterial smooth muscle cells.[1] Both direct effects on the smooth muscle and indirect effects of endogenous vasoregulators appear to play a role in producing pulmonary hypertension. In most cases in which pulmonary hypertension results from alveolar hypoxia, management with oxygen can alleviate some of these deleterious effects and should be used as the primary therapy.

Chronic Obstructive Pulmonary Disease

Pulmonary hypertension is a well-established complication of COPD. Elevated pulmonary artery pressure correlates with worse outcomes, including shorter survival and increased use of hospital resources.[2,3] The presence of either pulmonary hypertension or documented right ventricular enlargement is a strong independent predictor of mortality in this population.[4-7]

The prevalence of pulmonary hypertension among patients with COPD has not been established definitively, but is thought to be quite high. Studies examining the hemodynamics of patients with COPD describe elevated pulmonary pressures in 20-35 percent of an unselected population, and report an even higher incidence in patients with hypoxemia.[2,8,9] A review of autopsies in a series of patients with COPD confirmed right ventricular hypertrophy in 40 percent of cases.

The severity of pulmonary hypertension progresses as airflow obstruction and hypoxemia worsen.[10] As with other causes of pulmonary hypertension, exercise-induced pulmonary hypertension often precedes the development of elevated pressures at rest, even in patients without resting hypoxemia.[11,12] Overall, the elevation in pulmonary pressures is mild to moderate in most patients, even when airflow obstruction is advanced. In most cases, there is an approximate elevation of 0.5 mmHg per year in mean pulmonary artery pressure from the onset of pulmonary hypertension in randomly selected patients followed over time.[8,12]

TABLE 10-1

Classification and Causes of Pulmonary Hypertension

1. Pulmonary Arterial Hypertension (PAH)
   1.1. Idiopathic (IPAH)
   1.2. Familial (FPAH)
   1.3. Associated with (APAH):
      1.3.1. Collagen vascular disease
      1.3.2. Congenital systemic-to-pulmonary shunts
      1.3.3. Portal hypertension
      1.3.4. Human Immunodeficiency Virus infection
      1.3.5. Drugs and toxins
      1.3.6. Other (thyroid disorders, glycogen storage disease, Gaucher disease, hereditary hemorrhagic telangiectasia, hemoglobinopathies, myeloproliferative disorders, splenectomy)
   1.4. Associated with significant venous or capillary involvement
      1.4.1. Pulmonary veno-occlusive disease (PVOD)
      1.4.2. Pulmonary capillary hemangiomatosis (PCH)
   1.5. Persistent pulmonary hypertension of the newborn
2. Pulmonary hypertension with left-sided heart disease
   2.1. Left-sided atrial or ventricular heart disease
   2.2. Left-sided valvular heart disease
3. Pulmonary hypertension associated with lung diseases or hypoxemia
   3.1. Chronic obstructive pulmonary disease
   3.2. Interstitial lung disease
   3.3. Sleep-disordered breathing
   3.4. Alveolar hypoventilation disorders
   3.5. Long-term exposure to high altitude
   3.6. Developmental abnormalities
4. Pulmonary hypertension due to chronic thrombotic or embolic disease
   4.1. Thromboembolic obstruction of proximal pulmonary arteries
   4.2. Thromboembolic obstruction of distal pulmonary arteries
   4.3. Nonthrombotic pulmonary embolism (tumor, parasites, foreign material)
5. Miscellaneous (sarcoidosis, histiocytosis X, lymphangiomatosis, compression of pulmonary vessels [adenopathy, tumor, fibrosing mediastinitis])

Adapted from Rubin LJ: Diagnosis and management of pulmonary arterial hypertension: ACCP evidence-based clinical practice guidelines. Chest 126:7S-10S, 2004.

The mean pulmonary artery pressure usually does not usually exceed 35-40 mmHg, and cardiac output, right atrial pressure, and pulmonary artery occlusion (wedge) pressure generally remain within normal limits.[2,9,13] The slow progression allows the right ventricle to adapt to the higher pressures and, therefore, right ventricular function often is well maintained. In stable patients, stroke volume and contractility remain normal, although the right ventricular ejection fraction may be reduced. In acute exacerbations, however, sudden rises of the pulmonary arterial pressure can decrease contractility and produce signs of right-sided heart failure, including elevated jugular venous pressures and peripheral edema, although measured cardiac output may be preserved.[14,15] Overall, severe pulmonary hypertension occurs infrequently, even in those with severe emphysema and poor lung function.[13,16] If severe pulmonary hypertension is encountered, it should not be attributed to COPD without careful exclusion of other possible contributors.[17] A number of patients are described as having "pulmonary hypertension out of proportion to the magnitude of COPD," but the degree to which they should be approached in an analogous manner as patients with idiopathic (formerly "primary") pulmonary arterial hypertension remains unclear (see Chapter 6).

Pathophysiology

The development of pulmonary hypertension in patients with COPD involves both parenchymal destruction and vascular remodeling. Hypoxic vasoconstriction is considered one of the primary causative factors. As a normal physiologic response, hypoxia induces transient pulmonary arteriolar constriction that limits blood flow to underventilated areas of the lung, resulting in improved $\dot{V}/\dot{Q}$ matching (see Chapter 1). This vasoconstriction promotes the release of vasoactive substances and increases cellular proliferation. Persistent vasoconstriction is hypothesized to lead to pulmonary hypertension. This process is believed to be propagated, in part, by alterations in endothelial cell function, including decreased production of nitric oxide and prostacyclin, and increased production and decreased clearance of endothelin-1.[1,18] Both the endothelial dysfunction and direct effects of hypoxic injury lead to vascular remodeling involving smooth muscle cell proliferation, intimal fibrosis, and the loss of collagen and elastic fibers. Together these changes result in a progressive loss of vascular compliance. Destruction of capillaries and precapillary arterioles also produces vascular stasis and congestion.

Histopathologic specimens show distal neomuscularization of the arterioles, intimal thickening, and medial hypertrophy. Abnormal collagen matrix deposition occurs within the adventitia.[19] Advanced grades of vascular pathology, such as thrombotic and plexogenic lesions that occur frequently with idiopathic pulmonary arterial hypertension (IPAH), are not usually observed in cases of COPD.

Although pathologic changes are strikingly evident in patients with severe pulmonary hypertension, they can also be present in COPD patients with only mildly altered hemodynamics. The degree of structural changes in the arterioles on pathologic viewing does not appear to correlate with the hemodynamic severity of pulmonary hypertension or responsiveness to oxygen.[19]

Furthermore, these changes have been noted in patients without hypoxemia and in smokers with normal lung function.[20] Hence, the central pathophysiologic mechanisms leading to pulmonary hypertension in this population are not entirely clear. Inflammation secondary to smoking may produce oxidative stress, direct vascular injury, and endothelial dysfunction, each of which may play a role.[21] Smoke injury increases the production of CD8+ lymphocytes, cytokines, and growth factors, and histopathologic specimens in patients with COPD can show an inflammatory infiltrate in the adventitia of pulmonary arteries.[20] Polycythemia may potentiate the process because of scavenging and inactivation of nitric oxide by excessive quantities of hemoglobin. In addition, an increased incidence of *in situ* thrombosis has been reported, likely due to thrombophilia associated with inflammation, although such lesions remain less common than those seen in IPAH.

Evaluation

Because the symptomatology of pulmonary hypertension is nonspecific, identification of COPD patients with elevated pulmonary artery pressures on clinical grounds is challenging. Patients initially seek treatment for fatigue or dyspnea that is difficult to discern from the primary disease process. Peripheral edema is a nonspecific sign that can be caused by a variety of mechanisms, including sympathetic activation of the renin-angiotensin system, increased vasopressin release, and increased venous congestion. Heart sounds may be difficult to hear because of hyperinflation, and the typical cardiac sounds associated with pulmonary hypertension (a tricuspid regurgitant murmur and a prominent pulmonic component of S_2) are appreciated inconsistently, especially in patients with mild disease.

Many common tests may suggest pulmonary hypertension, but they are neither sensitive nor specific. As examples, the chest radiograph may indicate hilar prominence or cardiomegaly, the electrocardiogram may show signs of right ventricular hypertrophy, right bundle branch block, or p-pulmonale, and arterial blood gas analysis may indicate hypoxemia and hypercapnia. Pulmonary function testing may identify patients with COPD, but is not of value in identifying the subgroup with pulmonary hypertension. The 6-minute walk test is performed routinely for functional assessment but cannot identify reliably those COPD patients with pulmonary hypertension. Cardiopulmonary exercise testing may be of use in precisely defining exercise capacity and may suggest pulmonary vascular abnormalities, but is not considered a method of choice for detecting pulmonary hypertension.

Echocardiography is a noninvasive and widely available tool to evaluate cardiac structure and estimate pulmonary artery pressures and can provide important prognostic information[4,22] (see Chapter 6). However, the technical quality of the study can be limited greatly by hyperinflation of the chest. More recent studies have employed transcutaneous measurement of jugular venous flow velocity by Doppler to estimate pulmonary artery pressures.[23] Magnetic resonance imaging is em- ployed in some centers and can provide detailed information on right ventricular dimensions, but its advantages over other modalities have not been established unequivocally.[24]

If there is clinical suspicion for pulmonary hypertension, several techniques can be employed to confirm the diagnosis. The gold standard is right heart catheterization, although is not routinely performed as an initial study in patients with COPD because of its invasive nature. By the 2003 Venice criteria, pulmonary hypertension is present if the mean pulmonary artery pressure exceeds 25 mmHg at rest or 30 mmHg with exertion, although a number of earlier studies have used a threshold value of 20 mmHg. Right heart catheterization is indicated when the diagnosis of pulmonary hypertension will influence management or significantly alter the potential risk-benefit ratio of therapies such as lung volume reduction surgery or lung transplantation.

Management

Oxygen

The mainstay of management for pulmonary hypertension associated with COPD is oxygen therapy. Hypoxemia worsens pulmonary vasoconstriction, increases pulmonary artery pressures, and can precipitate right-sided heart failure. Appropriate patients receiving long-term oxygen therapy have decreased mortality, improved quality of life, and a modest reduction in pulmonary vascular resistance. Oxygen therapy also can decrease exercise-induced pulmonary hypertension in patients with COPD.[25,26] Once hypoxemia develops, supplemental oxygen is recommended to keep arterial oxygenation 90 percent or greater (PaO_2 = 60 mmHg) in patients with COPD who have evidence of pulmonary hypertension. In the absence of pulmonary hypertension, cor pulmonale, or polycythemia, long-term oxygen therapy is not indicated for COPD management unless the oxygen saturation is 88 percent or lower or PaO_2 is 55 mmHg or lower.[27]

Oxygen therapy can halt and possibly reverse the progression of pulmonary hypertension, although it rarely returns the pulmonary artery pressure to the normal range.[26-29] The magnitude of reduction of pulmonary vascular resistance is usually small relative to the observed impact on mortality, suggesting that vascular remodeling and other qualitative changes in the vasculature may play a prominent role in the mechanism of action of oxygen therapy.[21] Therefore, patients treated late in the progression of the disease may not derive as much benefit as those with mild hypoxemia and early disease.[27] Despite overall improvements in survival on long-term oxygen therapy, patients with elevated pulmonary artery pressures remain at a higher risk of death.[7]

Management of airflow obstruction is also critical to improve gas exchange and to minimize hypoxia, as is smoking cessation to prevent ongoing damage to the lung parenchyma. Patients with COPD and persistent nocturnal desaturation caused by sleep apnea ("overlap syndrome") may benefit from the combination of noninvasive positive pressure ventilation and oxygen.[30,31]

Diuretics

Diuretic use in patients with COPD and right-sided heart failure is common because these medications can decrease ventricular preload and improve right ventricular function. However, diuretics should be used with caution, because they can induce a metabolic alkalosis, blunt the respiratory drive, and consequently worsen hypercapnia. In addition, an excessive decrease in intravascular volume may cause inadequate ventricular filling and ultimately decrease cardiac output. Finally, diuretics can aggravate polycythemia, which is associated with a higher pulmonary vascular resistance due to increased blood viscosity.[32-34]

Phlebotomy is another fluid removal technique that has been beneficial to patients with COPD, although no increase in length of survival has been demonstrated. Decreasing the viscosity and volume of blood can decrease pulmonary vascular resistance and pulmonary pressures, improving gas exchange and exercise capacity.[35] Furthermore, phlebotomy has symptomatic benefits, including fewer headaches and decreased fatigue, and may be used in a select group of patients. Phlebotomy should be considered in patients with a hematocrit greater than 55%, although when hypoxemia is alleviated, phlebotomy is usually not required.

Oral Vasodilators

No routine role for vasodilators such as calcium channel antagonists has been defined in patients with pulmonary hypertension associated with COPD. Administration of a calcium channel antagonist can decrease pulmonary artery pressure and increase cardiac output at rest and with exercise,[36-38] but it may also worsen $\dot{V}/\dot{Q}$ matching, presumably by interfering with hypoxic vasoconstriction.[39,40] In contrast, another study evaluating amlodipine and felodipine found that they decreased pulmonary pressures and increased oxygen delivery because cardiac output increased.[41] Despite this, the possible benefit of short-term increased cardiac output is overshadowed by the possibility of, worsened gas exchange,[42] and overall lack of proven long-term benefit.[43,44] Calcium channel antagonists should not be employed routinely in this patient population because of the absence of proven advantage and the risk of adverse effects such as systemic hypotension and cardiac conduction defects, in addition to those stated above.

Alternative vasodilators such as intravenous epoprostenol (prostacyclin) have not shown benefit in this subgroup, and they can lower PaO_2 in patients with COPD, probably due to worsened $\dot{V}/\dot{Q}$ matching.[45] Both prostanoids and endothelial receptor antagonists are believed to promote vascular remodeling in patients with IPAH, but it is unclear if similar beneficial effects can be produced in patients with COPD. Prostanoids, endothelin receptor antagonists, and phosphodiesterase 5 inhibitors such as sildenafil have not been approved for the management of pulmonary hypertension due to COPD.

Inhaled Vasodilators

Inhaled nitric oxide and inhaled prostanoids theoretically are attractive management options, because the drug is delivered directly to ventilated areas of the lung, thereby avoiding the undesirable systemic effects of oral vasodilators and serving to improve $\dot{V}/\dot{Q}$ matching, particularly during exercise.[18,46] This has led to the development of "spiked" or "pulsed" nitric oxide delivery that targets well-ventilated alveoli by fast delivery.[47] Some studies suggest that the combination of oxygen and nitric oxide can improve gas exchange and pulmonary arterial pressures in both acute and long-term situations. Pulmonary vascular resistance and pulmonary artery pressures can improve significantly without evidence of decreased arterial oxygenation.[48-50] Despite some encouraging preliminary data, large definitive trials have not been performed, and inhaled vasodilators cannot be recommended for the amelioration of pulmonary hypertension in patients with COPD.

Lung Volume Reduction Surgery and Transplantation

Lung volume reduction surgery (LVRS) has become an accepted treatment option for selected patients with severe COPD, although severe pulmonary hypertension is a contraindication to this procedure.[51,52] LVRS does not improve exercise-induced pulmonary hypertension in patients with severe COPD and may increase pulmonary arterial pressure at rest, although right ventricular systolic function sometimes is improved.[51,53] The lack of improvement in pulmonary pressures may be related to irreversible vascular remodeling, fibrosis of the small airways, destruction of the vasculature, or concurrent thromboembolism.[54,55] Because of the increased surgical risk associated with LVRS when pulmonary hypertension is present, lung transplantation frequently is a more appropriate management option.[52]

Additional Management

Digitalis is not prescribed routinely for pulmonary hypertension associated with COPD because of the potential for toxicity and the lack of established efficacy. Theophylline can decrease pulmonary vascular resistance and minimally reduce airflow obstruction, but its toxicities often outweigh the benefits of its use.[56]

INTERSTITIAL LUNG DISEASE

Interstitial lung disease (ILD) is a broad category of parenchymal disease of the lung that involves alveolar and interstitial inflammation, as well as fibrosis, and is associated with pulmonary hypertension. Examples include idiopathic pulmonary fibrosis, connective tissue diseases (e.g., scleroderma, systemic lupus erythematosus, rheumatoid arthritis, polymyositis-dermatomyositis, Sjögren syndrome, mixed connective tissue disease), and granulomatous disease, such as sarcoidosis[57] (TABLE 10-2).

TABLE 10-2

Clinical Classification of Interstitial Lung Disease

Connective Tissue Diseases

Scleroderma
Polymyositis-dermatomyositis
Systemic lupus erythematosus
Rheumatoid arthritis
Mixed connective tissue disease
Ankylosing spondylitis

(continued)

TABLE 10-2

Clinical Classification of Interstitial Lung Disease—cont'd

Treatment-related Disease

Antibiotics (e.g., nitrofurantoin, sulfasalazine)
Antiarrhythmic agents (e.g., amiodarone, tocainide, propranolol)
Antiinflammatory drugs (e.g., gold, penicillamine)
Anticonvulsant medications (e.g., phenytoin)
Antineoplastic agents (e.g., bleomycin, busulfan, cyclophosphamide, chlorambucil, methotrexate, azathioprine, carmustine)
Radiation therapy
Oxygen toxicity
Narcotics

Primary (Unclassified) Diseases

Sarcoidosis
Primary pulmonary Langerhans cell histiocytosis
Amyloidosis
Pulmonary vasculitis
Lipoid pneumonia
Lymphangitic carcinomatosis
Bronchoalveolar carcinoma
Pulmonary lymphoma
Gaucher disease
Niemann-Pick disease
Hermansky-Pudlak syndrome
Neurofibromatosis
Lymphangioleiomyomatosis
Tuberous sclerosis
Eosinophilic pneumonia
Alveolar proteinosis
Diffuse alveolar hemorrhage syndromes
Alveolar microlithiasis

Occupational and Environmental Diseases

Inorganic

Silicosis
Asbestosis
Hard metal pneumoconiosis
Coal worker's pneumoconiosis
Berylliosis
Aluminium oxide fibrosis
Talc pneumoconiosis
Siderosis
Stenosis

Organic

Bird fancier's lung
Farmer's lung
Other causes of hypersensitivity pneumonitis

Idiopathic Fibrotic Disorders

Acute interstitial pneumonitis (Hamman-Rich syndrome)
Idiopathic pulmonary fibrosis
Familial idiopathic pulmonary fibrosis
Desquamative interstitial pneumonitis
Respiratory bronchiolitis
Cryptogenic organizing pneumonitis
Nonspecific interstitial pneumonitis
Lymphocytic interstitial pneumonia (e.g., Sjögren syndrome, Hashimoto thyroiditis, connective tissue disease)
Autoimmune pulmonary fibrosis (e.g., inflammatory bowel disease, primary biliary cirrhosis, idiopathic thrombocytopenic purpura)

Adapted from King TE, Jr, Schwarz MI: Approach to the diagnosis and management of the idiopathic interstitial pneumonias. In: Mason RJ, Broaddus VC, Murray JF, et al, editors: Murray and Nadel's textbook of respiratory medicine. Philadelphia, 2005, Elsevier Saunders, p 1572.

It is predominantly the loss of functional surface area of the vascular bed that leads to pulmonary hypertension in ILD, although hypoxic vasoconstriction also may play a role. Both primary vascular disease and interstitial fibrotic disease lead to destruction of the capillaries and arterioles, increasing pulmonary vascular resistance. The pulmonary hypertension that evolves contributes to the high morbidity and mortality in many of these conditions and, unlike COPD, severe pulmonary hypertension is not unusual. Clinically, patients often note decreased exercise capacity as an early sign, which can progress to dyspnea on exertion and shortness of breath at rest. The symptoms are often confounded by anemia, musculoskeletal complaints, or restrictive ventilatory abnormalities.[58]

Given the prevalence of pulmonary hypertension in this population, there is increasing interest in early detection and management. Strong data in favor of such an approach, however, are thus far lacking except when pulmonary vascular disease, rather than ILD, is the primary process. Doppler echocardiography frequently is used as a noninvasive assessment tool, however, the accuracy of echocardiography is not universally accepted despite good correlation with catheterization pressures in some reports.[59] Brain natriuretic peptide levels may also be helpful in the diagnosis of pulmonary hypertension in patients with idiopathic pulmonary fibrosis.[60,61] Right heart catheterization usually is required to precisely measure pulmonary hemodynamics and exclude left-sided heart dysfunction.

ILD and pulmonary hypertension frequently coexist in both diffuse and limited cutaneous scleroderma (CREST syndrome [calcinosis, Raynaud phenomenon, oesophageal dysmotility, sclerodactyly, telangiectasia]).[57,62] Up to 30 percent of patients with scleroderma and one-half of patients with CREST syndrome develop pulmonary hypertension during the course of their disease.[63] Because of the high prevalence and considerable morbidity, it is standard that patients undergo annual monitoring with echocardiography to assess for pulmonary hypertension. Pulmonary hypertension in patients with systemic sclerosis can represent a complication of pulmonary fibrosis, or a more indolent process related to direct obliteration of the vasculature. Some patients exhibit combined features of these processes.[58,64] Patients with limited scleroderma are more likely to have isolated pulmonary arterial hypertension, while those with systemic sclerosis have pulmonary hypertension more often associated with fibrosis or restrictive lung disease.[65] Patients with rheumatoid arthritis and systemic lupus erythematosus also can have damage to the vascular bed caused by similar processes. Before the advent of effective therapies, patients with scleroderma-related pulmonary hypertension displayed a median survival as low as 50 percent at 1 year.[65,66] Survival has been significantly worse than that of patients with IPAH undergoing similar medical treatment.[67]

In patients with sarcoidosis, pulmonary hypertension also has been associated with poor outcomes.[68] As an example, pulmonary pressures in patients with sarcoidosis are an independent predictor of death in patients awaiting lung transplantation, with mean pressures of 41 mmHg versus 32 mmHg in nonsurvivors and survivors, respectively.[11] Of note, a significant proportion of patients without parenchymal disease or spirometric abnormalities have concurrent pulmonary hypertension; direct involvement of the pulmonary vasculature by a granulomatous vasculitis likely plays a role in these cases, although parenchymal fibrosis is a more important overall contributor among all patients with the disease. Extrinsic compression of the main pulmonary arteries or veins by lymph nodes is an additional cause of pulmonary hypertension in patients with sarcoidosis.[69]

Pulmonary vasoreactivity in response to vasodilator therapy has been reported, although vasodilator agents have not been evaluated in well-controlled trials of patients with sarcoidosis.[70-72] Nonetheless, pending additional negative trial results, it is reasonable to consider evaluation and treatment of these patients as outlined for those with IPAH (see Chapters 6 and 7). Given the poor prognosis of patients with sarcoidosis complicated by pulmonary hypertension, early referral for lung transplantation should be contemplated.[11]

Finally, idiopathic pulmonary fibrosis is a condition that is poorly understood, highly lethal, and in which pulmonary hypertension frequently occurs. To date, no management has proven effective for this disease. Because of laboratory data suggesting that therapy for pulmonary arterial hypertension, such as prostanoids, endothelin receptor antagonists, and phosphodiesterase 5 inhibitors, may reduce the progression of pulmonary fibrosis, there is intense interest in performing trials of these agents in human subjects.[73] Preliminary human trials have demonstrated some favorable results in hemodynamics and exercise tolerance, and more definitive trials with bosentan, inhaled iloprost, oral sildenafil, and other agents are underway[74-76] (FIGURE 10-1).

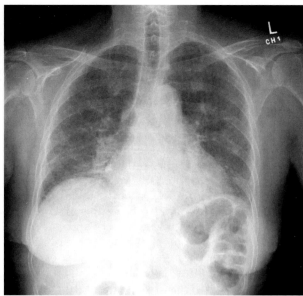

Figure 10-1. Coexistent Idiopathic Pulmonary Fibrosis and Pulmonary Hypertension. Posteoanterior chest radiograph from a 64-year-old man with biopsy-proven idiopathic pulmonary fibrosis, and a pulmonary artery pressure of 72/38 mmHg on cardiac catheterization, shows diffuse parenchymal lung disease and bilateral hilar prominence due to pulmonary hypertension and pulmonary artery enlargement.

Management

Oxygen therapy to minimize hypoxic vasoconstriction should be initiated if a patient is hypoxemic either at rest or with exertion. Identical criteria are used to determine eligibility for oxygen as are used with COPD patients, although data specifically from the ILD population validating these criteria are sparse. Diuretics may be required for those with severe right-sided heart failure, although they should be used with care in patients with scleroderma who may require high filling pressures for peripheral perfusion. Atrial septostomy has been performed in patients with systemic sclerosis, but is not advised because of the high morbidity and mortality associated with the procedure. It can be considered if all other medical management fails or as a bridge to transplantation.[77-79] Rheumatologic disease is no longer an absolute contraindication to lung transplantation, and this intervention should be considered (see Chapter 8).[80]

Preliminary data from several small trials have suggested that patients with ILD and pulmonary hypertension may benefit from management targeted at the latter process. Management is thought to improve the hypoxic vasoconstrictive component and to aid in vascular remodeling. As noted above, beneficial effects on the pathologic determinants that induce pulmonary fibrosis and inflammation have also been hypothesized.[73]

Systemic vasodilator therapy has been studied variably in this subgroup of patients. Treatment with calcium channel antagonists has been described in patients with scleroderma and idiopathic pulmonary fibrosis, and some small series have reported benefit.[81] Nonetheless, clinical experience with these agents has been largely unimpressive. More recently, management approaches similar to those employed for IPAH have been advocated, although a benefit of epoprostenol, bosentan, and other agents has been apparent mostly in ILD associated with the scleroderma spectrum of illness when ILD is mild (i.e., total lung capacity >70 percent of predicted values). Furthermore, no impact on mortality has been demonstrated directly.[82-84]

One concern with systemic therapy is that blood flow will be increased to poorly ventilated areas, thus worsening $\dot{V}/\dot{Q}$ mismatch and gas exchange. In addition, systemic therapy is associated with a variety of side effects, including hypotension and peripheral vasodilation. Inhaled agents such as prostacyclin, iloprost, and nitric oxide have been shown to decrease pulmonary arterial pressures in this population, and are thought to reduce the $\dot{V}/\dot{Q}$ mismatch induced by systemic therapy. As an example, one uncontrolled study of eight patients with pulmonary fibrosis from various causes and pulmonary hypertension found that inhaled iloprost significantly improved gas exchange and hemodynamics and was associated with sustained improvement in the one patient who received it on a long-term basis.[76,85]

Nonetheless, pending the completion of large high-quality clinical trials showing benefit to the aggressive treatment of pulmonary hypertension associated with ILD, this approach cannot be advocated.

Obstructive Sleep Apnea

Obstructive sleep apnea (OSA) may affect as much as 5-15 percent of the population and is being diagnosed with increasing frequency. It is associated with high morbidity from associated factors including hypertension, stroke, and cardiovascular disease.[86,87] Symptoms include prominent snoring and excessive daytime fatigue, and bed partners may witness nocturnal apneic episodes. Patients may report impaired work performance, poor concentration, depression, and memory impairment.[87]

OSA is a disorder of hypoventilation during sleep and can progress to chronic hypoxemia and hypercapnia. Decreased pharyngeal tone and reflexes combined with a large increase in airway resistance lead to recurrent episodes of hypopnea and apnea. Apnea occurs particularly during rapid eye movement sleep, when atonia of the respiratory muscles is maximal.[88] Apneic episodes induce a prominent sympathetic response, causing acute rises in systemic blood pressure, sometimes to values in excess of 200 mmHg.[89] Cardiac output decreases initially with apnea, then rises above baseline when the apnea ceases. Left ventricular afterload is further increased by the abnormal decrease in intrathoracic pressure.[90] Dysrhythmias are common during these periods, presumably as a consequence of the sympathetic response and hypoxia.[91] Periods of hypoxemia during the night cause vasoconstriction of the small pulmonary arteries and lead to repeated, transient elevations of pulmonary arterial pressures.[92] Pathologically, the mechanisms that cause pulmonary hypertension are thought to be similar to those of COPD and include hypoxic vasoconstriction, endothelial cell dysfunction and, over time, vascular remodeling. Chronic systemic hypertension has been associated with OSA, and consequent left ventricular dysfunction often complicates the diagnosis of pulmonary hypertension by producing an elevated pulmonary capillary wedge and left ventricular end-diastolic pressures.[93]

The prevalence of pulmonary hypertension in patients with OSA is estimated at 17-25 percent in the absence of concurrent lung disease.[94-99] In patients with concomitant pulmonary disease or marked obesity, the prevalence is greatly increased.[92,100-102] Exercise-induced pulmonary hypertension is seen in up to 80 percent of patients; this may be caused in part by an elevated pulmonary capillary occlusion pressure during exercise from coexistent left ventricular dysfunction.[89,97,101,103]

Frank cor pulmonale, defined by the presence of overt right ventricular dysfunction, develops in an estimated 12-18 percent of patients, although studies vary based on patient characteristics.[104,105] Hypoxemia appears to be a prominent feature of those with right ventricular dysfunction.[105] Right ventricular dysfunction occasionally appears to occur in the absence of pulmonary hypertension,[104]

possibly as a result of sympathetic activity-induced myocardial changes.[104,106,107]

Data suggest that the effect of OSA on pulmonary artery pressure is mild, with mean pulmonary artery pressures averaging 20-35 mmHg in most studies.[97,102] It is unclear if nighttime hypoxia alone is enough to cause severely elevated ventricular pressures and eventual cor pulmonale.[108] Most studies have failed to find a correlation between the severity of sleep apnea (as defined by the apnea-hypopnea index) and pulmonary hypertension.[104,109] Rather, chronic hypoxemia correlates more tightly with pulmonary hypertension.[97,100,102,105,109,110] Patients with severe right-sided heart failure and pulmonary hypertension with sleep apnea usually have coexisting daytime hypoxia from either chronic lung disease such as COPD, morbid obesity, or obesity hypoventilation syndrome. Unlike pulmonary hypertension, right ventricular dysfunction can be correlated with the severity of sleep apnea.[104]

OSA in combination with chronic lung disease is often called "overlap syndrome," and a much higher incidence of cor pulmonale is found in this subgroup.[100] Patients with daytime hypoventilation constitute 10-20 percent of the patients with OSA and also have a higher incidence of pulmonary hypertension and cor pulmonale.[111] Morbid obesity can cause restrictive lung disease, with decreased compliance and restriction of lung volumes that can account for daytime alveolar hypoventilation and chronic hypoxia. For both of these populations, although the daytime hypoxia may be mild (PaO_2 60-70 mmHg), the accompanying nocturnal hypoxia is generally much more severe.[97,99,102]

Management of sleep apnea is based on relieving the upper airway obstruction and decreasing the inspiratory resistance. Nasal continuous positive airway pressure (CPAP) has become the treatment of choice for these patients, because it improves oxygenation and decreases the frequency and severity of apneic and hypopneic episodes. Tracheostomy also reduces apnea, hypopnea, and hypoxemia in sleep apnea.[112] CPAP has been shown to decrease pulmonary arterial pressures and pulmonary vascular resistance in patients without coexistent lung disease after several months of use,[96,113] although the data are less clear in patients with concomitant lung disease.[114] It is recommended that patients with concomitant sleep apnea syndrome and chronic obstructive lung disease be treated with CPAP and supplemental oxygen to avoid worsening apnea with oxygen alone.[31]

Potential reasons for the decrease in pulmonary artery pressures seen in response to management include a decrease in pulmonary vascular constriction to hypoxia and a reversal of the structural changes of pulmonary vascular remodeling.[113] This concept is supported by an exaggerated pulmonary vascular responsiveness to hypoxia and hypercapnia seen in some patients with OSA that returns to normal after long-term treatment with CPAP.[102] In addition, management with nasal CPAP or tracheostomy decreases both daytime and nocturnal blood pressures, further suggesting a role of endothelial dysfunction in the pathogenesis of pulmonary and systemic hypertension. If poor oxygenation persists despite management with CPAP, oxygen therapy is indicated, especially in patients with overlap syndrome or daytime alveolar hypoventilation.[31] Weight loss also helps alleviate the disrupted hemodynamics and has been shown to decrease both systemic and pulmonary hypertension.[115] If OSA is managed successfully with CPAP, overall survival appears similar to that of the general population, although the prognosis of the subgroup of treated patients with pulmonary hypertension is less clearly defined.[116]

References

1. Shimoda LA, Sham JS, Sylvester JT: Altered pulmonary vasoreactivity in the chronically hypoxic lung. *Physiol Res* 49:549-560, 2000.
2. Weitzenblum E, Hirth C, Ducolone A, et al: Prognostic value of pulmonary artery pressure in chronic obstructive pulmonary disease. *Thorax* 36:752-758, 1981.
3. Kessler R, Faller M, Fourgaut G, et al: Predictive factors of hospitalization for acute exacerbation in a series of 64 patients with chronic obstructive pulmonary disease. *Am J Respir Crit Care Med* 159:158-164, 1999.
4. Burgess MI, Mogulkoc N, Bright-Thomas RJ, et al: Comparison of echocardiographic markers of right ventricular function in determining prognosis in chronic pulmonary disease. *J Am Soc Echocardiogr* 15:633-639, 2002.
5. Incalzi RA, Fuso L, De Rosa M, et al: Electro-cardiographic signs of chronic cor pulmonale: A negative prognostic finding in chronic obstructive pulmonary disease. *Circulation* 99:1600-1605, 1999.
6. Traver GA, Cline MG, Burrows B: Predictors of mortality in chronic obstructive pulmonary disease. A 15-year follow-up study. *Am Rev Respir Dis* 119:895-902, 1979.
7. Oswald-Mammosser M, Weitzenblum E, Quoix E, et al: Prognostic factors in COPD patients receiving long-term oxygen therapy. Importance of pulmonary artery pressure. *Chest* 107:1193-1198, 1995.
8. Weitzenblum E, Sautegeau A, Ehrhart M, et al: Long-term course of pulmonary arterial pressure in chronic obstructive pulmonary disease. *Am Rev Respir Dis* 130:993-998, 1984.
9. Burrows B, Kettel LJ, Niden AH, et al: Patterns of cardiovascular dysfunction in chronic obstructive lung disease. *N Engl J Med* 286:912-918, 1972.
10. Doi M, Nakano K, Hiramoto T, et al: Significance of pulmonary artery pressure in emphysema patients with mild-to-moderate hypoxemia. *Respir Med* 97:915-920, 2003.
11. Shorr AF, Davies DB, Nathan SD: Predicting mortality in patients with sarcoidosis awaiting lung transplantation. *Chest* 124:922-928, 2003.
12. Kessler R, Faller M, Weitzenblum E, et al: "Natural history" of pulmonary hypertension in a series of 131 patients with chronic obstructive lung disease. *Am J Respir Crit Care Med* 164:219-224, 2001.
13. Scharf SM, Iqbal M, Keller C, et al: Hemodynamic characterization of patients with severe emphysema. *Am J Respir Crit Care Med* 166:314-322, 2002.
14. Weitzenblum E, Apprill M, Oswald M, et al: Pulmonary hemodynamics in patients with chronic obstructive pulmonary disease before and during an episode of peripheral edema. *Chest* 105:1377-1382, 1994.
15. MacNee W, Wathen CG, Flenley DC, et al: The effects of controlled oxygen therapy on ventricular function in patients with stable and decompensated cor pulmonale. *Am Rev Respir Dis* 137:1289-1295, 1988.
16. Stevens D, Sharma K, Szidon P, et al: Severe pulmonary hypertension associated with COPD. *Ann Transplant* 5:8-12, 2000.
17. Chaouat A, Bugnet AS, Kadaoui N, et al: Severe pulmonary hypertension and chronic obstructive pulmonary disease. *Am J Respir Crit Care Med* 172:189-194, 2005.
18. Giaid A, Saleh D: Reduced expression of endothelial nitric oxide synthase in the lungs of patients with pulmonary hypertension. *N Engl J Med* 333:214-221, 1995.
19. Wright JL, Petty T, Thurlbeck WM: Analysis of the structure of the muscular pulmonary arteries in patients with pulmonary hypertension and COPD: National Institutes of Health nocturnal oxygen therapy trial. *Lung* 170:109-124, 1992.
20. Peinado VI, Barbera JA, Abate P, et al: Inflammatory reaction in pulmonary muscular arteries of patients with mild chronic obstructive pulmonary disease. *Am J Respir Crit Care Med* 159:1605-1611, 1999.

21. Hale KA, Niewoehner DE, Cosio MG: Morphologic changes in the muscular pulmonary arteries: Relationship to cigarette smoking, airway disease, and emphysema. *Am Rev Respir Dis* 122:273-278, 1980.

22. Burgess MI, Bright-Thomas R: Usefulness of transcutaneous Doppler jugular venous echo to predict pulmonary hypertension in COPD patients. *Eur Respir J* 19:382-383, 2002.

23. Matsuyama W, Ohkubo R, Michizono K, et al: Use fulness of transcutaneous Doppler jugular venous echo to predict pulmonary hypertension in COPD patients. *Eur Respir J* 17:1128-1131, 2001.

24. Kruger S, Haage P, Hoffmann R, et al: Diagnosis of pulmonary arterial hypertension and pulmonary embolism with magnetic resonance angiography. *Chest* 120:1556-1561, 2001.

25. Continuous or nocturnal oxygen therapy in hypoxemic chronic obstructive lung disease: A clinical trial. Nocturnal Oxygen Therapy Trial Group. *Ann Intern Med* 93:391-398, 1980.

26. Timms RM Khaja FU, Williams GW: Hemodynamic response to oxygen therapy in chronic obstructive pulmonary disease. *Ann Intern Med* 102:29-36, 1985.

27. Gorecka D, Gorzelak K, Sliwinski P, et al: Effect of long-term oxygen therapy on survival in patients with chronic obstructive pulmonary disease with moderate hypoxaemia. *Thorax* 52:674-679, 1997.

28. Zielinski J, Tobiasz M, Hawrylkiewicz I, et al: Effects of long-term oxygen therapy on pulmonary hemodynamics in COPD patients: A 6-year prospective study. *Chest* 113:65-70, 1998.

29. Weitzenblum E, Sautegeau A, Ehrhart M, et al: Long-term oxygen therapy can reverse the progression of pulmonary hypertension in patients with chronic obstructive pulmonary disease. *Am Rev Respir Dis* 131:493-498, 1985.

30. Diaz O, Iglesia R, Ferrer M, et al: Effects of noninvasive ventilation on pulmonary gas exchange and hemodynamics during acute hypercapnic exacerbations of chronic obstructive pulmonary disease. *Am J Respir Crit Care Med* 156:1840-1845, 1997.

31. Sampol G, Sagales MT, Roca A, et al: Nasal continuous positive airway pressure with supplemental oxygen in coexistent sleep apnoea-hypopnea syndrome and severe chronic obstructive pulmonary disease. *Eur Respir J* 9:111-116, 1996.

32. Defouilloy C, Teiger E, Sediame S, et al: Poly cythemia impairs vasodilator response to acetylcholine in patients with chronic hypoxemic lung disease. *Am J Respir Crit Care Med* 157:1452-1460, 1998.

33. Deem S, Swenson ER, Alberts MK, et al: Red-blood-cell augmentation of hypoxic pulmonary vasoconstriction: Hematocrit dependence and the importance of nitric oxide. *Am J Respir Crit Care Med* 157:1181-1186, 1998.

34. Vanier T, Dulfano J, Wu C, et al: Emphysema, hypoxia and the polycythemic response. *N Engl J Med* 269:169-178, 1963.

35. Borst MM, Leschke M, Konig U, et al: Repetitive hemodilution in chronic obstructive pulmonary disease and pulmonary hypertension: Effects on pulmonary hemodynamics, gas exchange, and exercise capacity. *Respiration* 66:225-232, 1999.

36. Gassner A, Sommer G, Fridrich L, et al: Differential therapy with calcium antagonists in pulmonary hypertension secondary to COPD. Hemodynamic effects of nifedipine, diltiazem, and verapamil. *Chest* 98:829-834, 1990.

37. Muramoto A, Caldwell J, Albert RK, et al: Nifedipine dilates the pulmonary vasculature without producing symptomatic systemic hypotension in upright resting and exercising patients with pulmonary hypertension secondary to chronic obstructive pulmonary disease. *Am Rev Respir Dis* 132:963-966, 1985.

38. Sajkov D, McEvoy RD, Cowie RJ, et al: Felodipine improves pulmonary hemodynamics in chronic obstructive pulmonary disease. *Chest* 103:1354-1361, 1993.

39. Bratel T, Hedenstierna G, Nyquist O, et al: The use of a vasodilator, felodipine, as an adjuvant to long-term oxygen treatment in COLD patients. *Eur Respir J* 3:46-54, 1990.

40. Simonneau G, Escourrou P, Duroux P, et al: Inhibition of hypoxic pulmonary vasoconstriction by nifedipine. *N Engl J Med* 304:1582-1585, 1981.

41. Sajkov D, Wang T, Frith PA, et al: A comparison of two long-acting vasoselective calcium antagonists in pulmonary hypertension secondary to COPD. *Chest* 111:1622-1630, 1997.

42. Barbera JA, Peinado VI, Santos S: Pulmonary hypertension in chronic obstructive pulmonary disease. *Eur Respir J* 21:892-905, 2003.

43. Saadjian AY, Philip-Joet FF, Vestri R, et al: Long-term treatment of chronic obstructive lung disease by nifedipine: An 18-month haemodynamic study. *Eur Respir J* 1:716-720, 1988.

44. Agostoni P, Doria E, Galli C, et al: Nifedipine reduces pulmonary pressure and vascular tone during short- but not long-term treatment of pulmonary hypertension in patients with chronic obstructive pulmonary disease. *Am Rev Respir Dis* 139:120-125, 1989.

45. Archer SL, Mike D, Crow J, et al: A placebo-controlled trial of prostacyclin in acute respiratory failure in COPD. *Chest* 109:750-755, 1996.

46. Jeremy JY, Rowe D, Emsley AM, et al: Nitric oxide and the proliferation of vascular smooth muscle cells. *Cardiovasc Res* 43:580-594, 1999.

47. Katayama Y, Higenbottam TW, Cremona G, et al: Minimizing the inhaled dose of NO with breath-by-breath delivery of spikes of concentrated gas. *Circulation* 98:2429-2432, 1998.

48. Yoshida M, Taguchi O, Gabazza EC, et al: Combined inhalation of nitric oxide and oxygen in chronic obstructive pulmonary disease. *Am J Respir Crit Care Med* 155:526-529, 1997.

49. Ashutosh K, Phadke K, Jackson JF, et al: Use of nitric oxide inhalation in chronic obstructive pulmonary disease. *Thorax* 55:109-113, 2000.

50. Vonbank K, Ziesche R, Higenbottam TW, et al: Controlled prospective randomised trial on the effects on pulmonary haemodynamics of the ambulatory long term use of nitric oxide and oxygen in patients with severe COPD. *Thorax* 58:289-293, 2003.

51. National Emphysema Treatment Research Group. Patients at high risk of death after lung-volume-reduction surgery. *N Engl J Med* 345:1075-1083, 2001.

52. Meyers BF, Patterson GA: Chronic obstructive pulmonary disease. 10: Bullectomy, lung volume reduction surgery, and transplantation for patients with chronic obstructive pulmonary disease. *Thorax* 58:634-638, 2003.

53. Weg IL, Rossoff L, McKeon K, et al: Development of pulmonary hypertension after lung volume reduction surgery. *Am J Respir Crit Care Med* 159:552-556, 1999.

54. Haniuda M, Kubo K, Fujimoto K, et al: Effects of pulmonary artery remodeling on pulmonary circulation after lung volume reduction surgery. *Thorac Cardiovasc Surg* 51:154-158, 2003.

55. Kubo K, Koizumi T, Fujimoto K, et al: Effects of lung volume reduction surgery on exercise pulmonary hemodynamics in severe emphysema. *Chest* 114:1575-1582, 1998.

56. Vaz Fragoso CA, Miller MA: Review of the clinical efficacy of theophylline in the treatment of chronic obstructive pulmonary disease. *Am Rev Respir Dis* 147:S40-S47, 1993.

57. Strange C, Highland KB: Interstitial lung disease in the patient who has connective tissue disease. *Clin Chest Med* 25:549-559, vii, 2004.

58. Denton CP, Black CM: Pulmonary hypertension in systemic sclerosis. *Rheum Dis Clin North Am* 29:335-349, vii, 2003.

59. Arcasoy SM, Christie JD, Ferrari VA, et al: Echocardiographic assessment of pulmonary hypertension in patients with advanced lung disease. *Am J Respir Crit Care Med* 167:735-740, 2003.

60. Hill NS: Brain natriuretic peptide: Is it helpful in detecting pulmonary hypertension in fibrotic lung disease? *Am J Respir Crit Care Med* 170:352-353, 2004.

61. Leuchte HH, Neurohr C, Baumgartner R, et al: Brain natriuretic peptide and exercise capacity in lung fibrosis and pulmonary hypertension. *Am J Respir Crit Care Med* 170:360-365, 2004.

62. Lee P, Langevitz P, Alderdice CA, et al: Mortality in systemic sclerosis (scleroderma). *Q J Med* 82:139-148, 1992.

63. Ungerer RG, Tashkin DP, Furst D, et al: Prevalence and clinical correlates of pulmonary arterial hypertension in progressive systemic sclerosis. *Am J Med* 75:65-74, 1983.

64. Chang B, Wigley FM, White B, et al: Scleroderma patients with combined pulmonary hypertension and interstitial lung disease. *J Rheumatol* 30:2398-2405, 2003.

65. Koh ET, Lee P, Gladman DD, et al: Pulmonary hypertension in systemic sclerosis: An analysis of 17 patients. *Br J Rheumatol* 35:989-993, 1996.

66. MacGregor AJ, Canavan R, Knight C, et al: Pulmonary hypertension in systemic sclerosis: Risk factors for progression and consequences for survival. *Rheumatology (Oxford)* 40:453-459, 2001.

67. Kawut SM, Taichman DB, Archer-Chicko CL, et al: Hemodynamics and survival in patients with pulmonary arterial hypertension related to systemic sclerosis. *Chest* 123:344-350, 2003.

68. Gluskowski J, Hawrylkiewicz I, Zych D, et al: Pulmonary haemodynamics at rest and during exercise in patients with sarcoidosis. *Respiration* 46:26-32, 1984.

69. Smith LJ, Lawrence JB, Katzenstein AA: Vascular sarcoidosis: A rare cause of pulmonary hypertension. *Am J Med Sci* 285:38-44, 1983.

70. Preston IR, Klinger JR, Landzberg MJ, et al: Vasoresponsiveness of sarcoidosis-associated pulmonary hypertension. *Chest* 120:866-872, 2001.

71. Barst RJ, Ratner SJ: Sarcoidosis and reactive pulmonary hypertension. *Arch Intern Med* 145:2112-2114, 1985.

72. Jones B, Fowler J: Membranous nephropathy associated with sarcoidosis. Response to prednisolone. *Nephron* 52:101-102, 1989.

73. Clozel M: Effects of bosentan on cellular processes involved in pulmonary arterial hypertension: Do they explain the long-term benefit? *Ann Med* 35:605-613, 2003.

74. Ghofrani HA, Wiedemann R, Rose F, et al: Combination therapy with oral sildenafil and inhaled iloprost for severe pulmonary hypertension. *Ann Intern Med* 136:515-522, 2002.

75. Ghofrani HA, Wiedemann R, Rose F, et al: Sildenafil for treatment of lung fibrosis and pulmonary hypertension: A randomised controlled trial. *Lancet* 360:895-900, 2002.

76. Olschewski H, Ghofrani HA, Walmrath D, et al: Inhaled prostacyclin and iloprost in severe pul-

monary hypertension secondary to lung fibrosis. *Am J Respir Crit Care Med* 160:600-607, 1999.

77. Klepetko W, Mayer E, Sandoval J, et al: Interventional and surgical modalities of treatment for pulmonary arterial hypertension. *J Am Coll Cardiol* 43(12 Suppl S):73S-80S, 2004.

78. Allcock RJ, O'Sullivan JJ, Corris PA: Palliation of systemic sclerosis-associated pulmonary hypertension by atrial septostomy. *Arthritis Rheum* 44:1660-1662, 2001.

79. Allcock RJ, O'Sullivan JJ, Corris PA: Atrial septostomy for pulmonary arterial hypertension. *Heart* 89:1344-1347, 2003.

80. Vassallo R, Thomas CF: Advances in the treatment of rheumatic interstitial lung disease. *Curr Opin Rheumatol* 16:186-191, 2004.

81. Sturani C, Papiris S, Galavotti V, et al: Pulmonary vascular responsiveness at rest and during exercise in idiopathic pulmonary fibrosis: Effects of oxygen and nifedipine. *Respiration* 50:117-129, 1986.

82. Badesch DB, Tapson VF, McGoon MD, et al: Continuous intravenous epoprostenol for pulmonary hypertension due to the scleroderma spectrum of disease. A randomized, controlled trial. *Ann Intern Med* 132:425-434, 2000.

83. Humbert M, Sanchez O, Fartoukh M, et al: Short-term and long-term epoprostenol (prostacyclin) therapy in pulmonary hypertension secondary to connective tissue diseases: Results of a pilot study. *Eur Respir J* 13:1351-1356, 1999.

84. Rubin LJ, Badesch DB, Barst RJ, et al: Bosentan therapy for pulmonary arterial hypertension. *N Engl J Med* 346:896-903, 2002.

85. de la Mata J, Gomez-Sanchez MA, Aranzana M, et al: Long-term iloprost infusion therapy for severe pulmonary hypertension in patients with connective tissue diseases. *Arthritis Rheum* 37:1528-1533, 1994.

86. Parish JM, Somers VK: Obstructive sleep apnea and cardiovascular disease. *Mayo Clin Proc* 79:1036-1046, 2004.

87. Roux F, D'Ambrosio C, Mohsenin V: Sleep-related breathing disorders and cardiovascular disease. *Am J Med* 108:396-402, 2000.

88. Gay PC: Chronic obstructive pulmonary disease and sleep. *Respir Care* 49:39-51; discussion 52, 2004.

89. Tilkian AG, Guilleminault C, Schroeder JS, et al: Hemodynamics in sleep-induced apnea. Studies during wakefulness and sleep. *Ann Intern Med* 85:714-719, 1976.

90. Bradley TD: Right and left ventricular functional impairment and sleep apnea. *Clin Chest Med* 13:459-479, 1992.

91. Guilleminault C, Connolly SJ, Winkle RA: Cardiac arrhythmia and conduction disturbances during sleep in 400 patients with sleep apnea syndrome. *Am J Cardiol* 52:490-494, 1983.

92. Kessler R, Chaouat A, Weitzenblum E, et al: Pulmonary hypertension in the obstructive sleep apnoea syndrome: Prevalence, causes and therapeutic consequences. *Eur Respir J* 9:787-794, 1996.

93. Hla KM, Young TB, Bidwell T, et al: Sleep apnea and hypertension. A population-based study. *Ann Intern Med* 120:382-388, 1994.

94. Sajkov D, Cowie RJ, Thornton AT, et al: Pulmonary hypertension and hypoxemia in obstructive sleep apnea syndrome. *Am J Respir Crit Care Med* 149:416-422, 1994.

95. Yamakawa H, Shiomi T, Sasanabe R, et al: Pulmonary hypertension in patients with severe obstructive sleep apnea. *Psychiatry Clin Neurosci* 56:311-312, 2002.

96. Alchanatis M, Tourkohoriti G, Kakouros S, et al: Daytime pulmonary hypertension in patients with obstructive sleep apnea: The effect of continuous positive airway pressure on pulmonary hemodynamics. *Respiration* 68:566-572, 2001.

97. Chaouat A, Weitzenblum E, Krieger J, et al: Pulmonary hemodynamics in the obstructive sleep apnea syndrome. Results in 220 consecutive patients. *Chest* 109:380-386, 1996.

98. Krieger J, Sforza E, Apprill M, et al: Pulmonary hypertension, hypoxemia, and hypercapnia in obstructive sleep apnea patients. *Chest* 96:729-737, 1989.

99. Weitzenblum E, Krieger J, Apprill M, et al: Daytime pulmonary hypertension in patients with obstructive sleep apnea syndrome. *Am Rev Respir Dis* 138:345-349, 1988.

100. Fletcher EC, Schaaf JW, Miller J, et al: Long-term cardiopulmonary sequelae in patients with sleep apnea and chronic lung disease. *Am Rev Respir Dis* 135:525-533, 1987.

101. Hawrylkiewicz I, Sliwinski P, Gorecka D, et al: Pulmonary haemodynamics in patients with OSAS or an overlap syndrome. *Monaldi Arch Chest Dis* 61:148-152, 2004.

102. Laks L, Lehrhaft B, Grunstein RR, et al: Pulmonary hypertension in obstructive sleep apnoea. *Eur Respir J* 8:537-541, 1995.

103. Hetzel M, Kochs M, Marx N, et al: Pulmonary hemodynamics in obstructive sleep apnea: Frequency and causes of pulmonary hypertension. *Lung* 181: 157-166, 2003.

104. Sanner BM, Konermann M, Sturm A, et al: Right ventricular dysfunction in patients with obstructive sleep apnoea syndrome. *Eur Respir J* 10:2079-2083, 1997.

105. Bradley TD, Rutherford R, Grossman RF, et al: Role of daytime hypoxemia in the pathogenesis of right heart failure in the obstructive sleep apnea syndrome. *Am Rev Respir Dis* 131:835-839, 1985.

106. Hedner J, Ejnell H, Sellgren J, et al: Is high and fluctuating muscle nerve sympathetic activity in the sleep apnoea syndrome of pathogenetic importance for the development of hypertension? *J Hypertens Suppl* 6:S529-S531, 1988.

107. Carlson JT, Hedner J, Elam M, et al: Augmented resting sympathetic activity in awake patients with obstructive sleep apnea. *Chest* 103:1763-1768, 1993.

108. Chaouat A, Weitzenblum E, Kessler R, et al: Sleep-related O_2 desaturation and daytime pulmonary haemodynamics in COPD patients with mild hypoxaemia. *Eur Respir J* 10:1730-1735, 1997.

109. Apprill M, Weitzenblum E, Krieger J, et al: Frequency and mechanism of daytime pulmonary hypertension in patients with obstructive sleep apnoea syndrome. *Cor Vasa* 33:42-49, 1991.

110. Weitzenblum E, Oswald M, Mirhom R, et al: Evolution of pulmonary haemodynamics in COLD patients under long-term oxygen therapy. *Eur Respir J* Suppl 7:669s-673s, 1989.

111. Weitzenblum E, Chaouat A, Kessler R, et al: Daytime hypoventilation in obstructive sleep apnoea syndrome. *Sleep Med Rev* 3:79-93, 1999.

112. Fletcher EC, Brown DL: Nocturnal oxyhemoglobin desaturation following tracheostomyp for obstructive sleep apnea. *Am J Med* 79:35-42, 1985.

113. Sajkov D, Wang T, Saunders NA, et al: Continuous positive airway pressure treatment improves pulmonary hemodynamics in patients with obstructive sleep apnea. *Am J Respir Crit Care Med* 165:152-158, 2002.

114. Chaouat A, Weitzenblum E, Kessler R, et al: Five-year effects of nasal continuous positive airway pressure in obstructive sleep apnoea syndrome. *Eur Respir J* 10:2578-2582, 1997.

115. Valencia-Flores M, Orea A, Herrera M, et al: Effect of bariatric surgery on obstructive sleep apnoea and hypopnea syndrome, electrocardiogram, and pulmonary arterial pressure. *Obes Surg* 14:755-762, 2004.

116. Chaouat A, Weitzenblum E, Krieger J, et al: Prognostic value of lung function and pulmonary haemodynamics in OSA patients treated with CPAP. *Eur Respir J* 13:1091-1096, 1999.

117. King TE, Jr, Schwarz MI: Approach to the diagnosis and management of the idiopathic interstitial pneumonias. In: Mason RJ, Broaddus VC, Murray JF, et al, editors: *Murray and Nadel's textbook of respiratory medicine*. Philadelphia, 2005, Elsevier Saunders, p 1572.

Chapter 11

Pulmonary Veno-occlusive Disease

Jess Mandel, MD

Pulmonary veno-occlusive disease (PVOD), also called "pulmonary occlusive venopathy," remains one of the most deadly and least understood pulmonary vascular disorders.[1,2] In contrast to the insights into pathophysiology and the advances in therapy that have characterized idiopathic pulmonary arterial hypertension (IPAH; formerly known as "primary" pulmonary hypertension) over the past decade, the understanding of PVOD remains primitive, diagnosis is problematic, and therapy is largely unsatisfactory.

Dr. Julius Höra at the University of Munich first described the clinicopathologic syndrome of PVOD in 1934.[3] The initial patient described was a 48-year-old previously healthy baker, who died a year after he had first sought treatment for progressive dyspnea, edema, and cyanosis. Before his death, the patient was assumed to be suffering from mitral stenosis, but at autopsy, diffuse obstruction of the pulmonary venules with loose fibrous tissue was noted, and there was no evidence of mitral valve disease or other causes of left atrial hypertension. Höra suspected that an infection, perhaps streptococcal, was responsible for the pathologic findings, but no organisms could be demonstrated on stains or cultures.

The condition was referred to as "isolated pulmonary venous sclerosis," "obstructive disease of the pulmonary veins," or "the venous form of primary pulmonary hypertension" for the next several decades, until the term "pulmonary veno-occlusive disease" was popularized in the mid-1960s by Heath, Brown, and others.[4-7] More recently, the term "pulmonary obstructive venopathy" has been suggested to describe the syndrome more accurately.[8]

PVOD does not include, and should be differentiated from, abnormalities that result from stenosis of one or more of the four main pulmonary veins. Stenosis of these large pulmonary veins may occur congenitally, or they may develop as a complication of cardiothoracic surgery or radiofrequency ablation for atrial fibrillation or other dysrhythmias.[9-13]

Epidemiology

The true incidence and prevalence of PVOD are challenging to measure precisely, because mild cases may not come to medical attention, and many cases probably are misclassified as IPAH because of the difficulty in distinguishing the two syndromes without tissue biopsy. However, an estimate of the annual incidence of PVOD can be extracted from analysis of several IPAH series in which the fractions of patients fulfilling criteria for PVOD were reported. Pooling of seven such series published between 1970 and 1991 and comprising a total of 465 patients suggests that the incidence of PVOD is approximately 10 percent of that of true IPAH.[14-21] If one accepts an annual incidence of IPAH of 1 to 2 cases per million persons in the general population, this suggests an annual incidence of PVOD of around 0.1 to 0.2 cases per million persons in the general population.[22,23] However, this may represent an underestimate, because a number of cases probably are misclassified as interstitial lung disease or heart failure because of similarities in radiographic findings. Unfortunately, no well-designed study has thoroughly examined the magnitude of this likely misclassification phenomenon.

Unlike IPAH, which appears to be far more common in women, there does not appear to be a clear gender imbalance among patients with PVOD.[2,24,25] The age at diagnosis has ranged from within 9 days of birth to the seventh decade of life.

Pathology

The proper pathologic characterization of pulmonary vasculopathy remains challenging, even for experienced pathologists. To minimize errors in interpretation, lung specimens should be fixed in a distended state, and at least five blocks from each lobe should be sampled and examined. In addition to hematoxylin and eosin staining, examination using Movat, Masson, Verhoeff-van Gieson, and Perls iron stains is recommended. Immunohistochemical markers for smooth muscle and endothelial antigens (e.g., factor VIII, CD31, CD34) may also be useful.[8]

The most prominent pathologic feature of PVOD is the extensive and diffuse obliteration of small pulmonary veins or venules by fibrous tissue, which may be either loose and edematous, or may be dense, sclerotic, and acellular.[2,8,14,26,27] Lesions within the venous system tend to be eccentric or trabeculated, similar to the changes that are observed in arterial structures that have undergone recanalization following thrombotic occlusion.[28] The media of the venules may undergo arterialization with an increase in elastic fibers, and these fibers become calcified in some cases (FIGURE 11-1). A foreign body giant cell response to these calcified fibers may be observed.[8]

Pulmonary arteriolar changes frequently accompany venous changes, although it is not clear if they develop concomitantly or develop later as a consequence of the venous abnormalities. In approximately 50 percent of patients with PVOD, pulmonary arterioles demonstrate marked medial hypertrophy, which may lead to an erroneous diagnosis of IPAH unless the venous structures are surveyed carefully. Capillaries become engorged and tortuous, occasionally leading to a misdiagnosis of pulmonary capillary hemangiomatosis (also called "pulmonary microvasculopathy").[10,29] Plexiform lesions are encountered less commonly than is the case in IPAH, and arteritis or venulitis are distinctly uncommon.[30,31] Pleural and parenchymal lymphatic channels can become markedly dilated, presumably because of increased volume of fluid moving from pulmonary capillaries to the interstitial space as a result of pulmonary venous hypertension.[32]

Areas of microscopic pulmonary hemorrhage and hemosiderosis are observed frequently and presumably develop as a consequence of capillary endothelial damage and extravasation of erythrocytes due to pulmonary capillary hypertension (FIGURE 11-2). Determining whether observed areas of pulmonary hemorrhage are caused by PVOD or reflect tissue disruption by biopsy procedures can be challenging. Patients with PVOD commonly demonstrate hemosiderin within alveolar macrophages or the interstitium, and in some cases this feature is sufficiently prominent that the diagnosis of idiopathic pulmonary hemosiderosis or a vasculitis (e.g., Wegener granulomatosis) is considered.[2,33]

In contrast to many other causes of pulmonary hypertension, pulmonary parenchymal abnormalities commonly are observed in PVOD. Interstitial edema is seen frequently and is particularly distinct within lobular septa. Collagen deposition in these areas, and occasionally also involving alveolar walls, can appear similar to changes observed in longstanding mitral stenosis.[34] Lymphocytes and monocytes are seen frequently within the

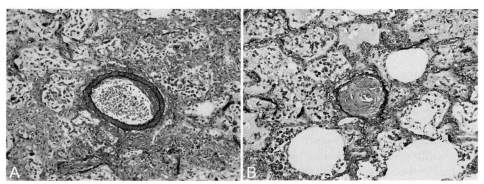

Figure 11-1. Pulmonary Veno-occlusive Disease. Elastic stain distinguishes a small artery (**A**) from an involved small vein (**B**) (20×). (Courtesy of Michelle Bianco, MD.) (See Color Plate 10).

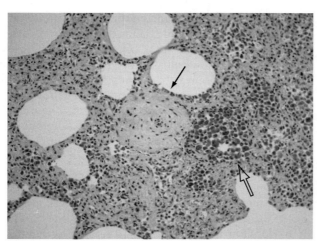

Figure 11-2. Pulmonary Veno-occlusive Disease. Hematoxylin and eosin staining shows obstructive intimal fibrosis of small vein (thin arrow) and extensive hemosiderin-laden intraalveolar macro-phages (thick arrow) (20×). (Courtesy of Michelle Bianco, MD.) (See Color Plate 10).

interstitium, and they may be sufficiently numerous to erroneously suggest usual interstitial pneumonitis as the primary diagnosis.[27]

Because of a number of shared features, it has been suggested that IPAH, PVOD, and pulmonary capillary hemangiomatosis may represent a continuous spectrum of manifestations of a single disease process termed "pulmonary vascular occlusive disease."[8] Advocates of this paradigm emphasize that obliterative pulmonary vascular lesions frequently are not limited to the arterial, capillary, or venous structures, but they can involve a number of different vascular areas within the same patient. In addition, bone morphogenic protein receptor type-2 (BMP-RII) abnormalities have been described in both IPAH and PVOD. Such a conceptualization has not yet found general acceptance, although at the Third World Health Organization Conference in Pulmonary Hypertension (Venice 2003) both PVOD and pulmonary capillary hemangiomatosis were classified together in the subcategory of "pulmonary arterial hypertension associated with significant venous or capillary involvement."[10]

ETIOLOGY

The etiology of PVOD remains unknown. No well-designed and adequately powered case control or cohort studies have been performed specifically to explore the causes of this condition. The situation is further complicated because PVOD may represent a final common clinicopathologic pathway triggered in a susceptible host by a number of discrete causes. Nonetheless, a variety of risk factors have been proposed, based upon case reports and small case series.

Genetic Susceptibility

Reports of PVOD developing in siblings have led to suspicion that a genetic predisposition may underlie development of the disease in some instances. Most cases involving siblings have developed before the third decade of life, and unaffected siblings have been detailed in a number of these families.[7,20,27,35,36] No definite genetic abnormality has been demonstrated in these sibling pairs, and the development of disease in these cases could reflect common environmental exposures to inciting agents, such as chemicals or infections.

Since the identification of mutations of the BMP-RII (*BMPR2*) gene as a major cause of familial PAH in 2000, there has been speculation that abnormalities at this site may also be involved in the pathogenesis of PVOD.[37–39] In 2003, a *BMPR2* mutation that resulted in a truncated and nonfunctional protein has been described in a patient who developed PVOD at age 36.[40] The patient's mother had died of pulmonary hypertension several decades earlier, but lung tissue had not been examined to determine if she suffered from PVOD. The authors reported that the index patient had been stable for 5 years while receiving continuous intravenous epoprostenol, a course that is somewhat atypical in those with PVOD.

The description of a *BMPR2* mutation in a patient with PVOD suggests the possibility that IPAH and PVOD may share a common genetic basis, and the pathologic phenotype that develops may be caused by modifier genes or differing environmental exposures. Loss of a functional *BMPR2* allele might contribute to the development of PVOD by diminishing the normal antiproliferative effects of bone morphogenic protein on pulmonary vascular endothelial and smooth muscle cells, resulting in unchecked proliferation in response to other ligands of the transforming growth factor-β family.[41]

A common *BMPR2* defect might also help explain the overlap in pathologic features found in IPAH and PVOD: development of scattered venous lesions found in some patients who have IPAH with predominantly precapillary disease, and the presence of precapillary lesions and abnormal precapillary resistance in many patients with

PVOD.[42,43] Expanded genotype profiling of patients with PVOD should help clarify these issues.

Infectious Agents

Since Höra's initial description of PVOD, some have postulated that infection plays an etiologic role in the disease.[3,44] Höra believed that streptococcal infection played a role in his patient's illness, but in the decades that followed, nonbacterial agents have been hypothesized more commonly as etiologic agents. An antecedent influenza-like illness or serologic evidence of recent infection with agents such as measles virus and *Toxoplasma gondii* have been documented at the time PVOD has been diagnosed, and some patients have had manifestations of Epstein-Barr or cytomegalovirus infection, such as lymphadenopathy, fever, and erythrophagocytosis.[4,5,45–47] Several cases have been reported among patients infected with the human immunodeficiency virus.[48–50]

It is difficult to reconcile the courses of acute infectious illnesses and PVOD, given that it requires months to years to develop right ventricular hypertrophy and the symptom complex for which patients with PVOD commonly seek treatment. More likely, the significance of an acute illness near the time of PVOD diagnosis is that it may bring an undiagnosed patient to medical attention and stimulate a diagnostic evaluation that ultimately demonstrates that PVOD is present. Human immunodeficiency virus and other lentiviruses could pursue a chronology of infection that is more congruent with the time required for the development of observed cardiovascular adaptations to PVOD, but viral inclusions or deoxyribonucleic acid have not been documented in the pulmonary vascular lesions of affected patients.

Toxic Exposures

An association between certain drugs or chemicals and the development of PVOD has been postulated. As an example, the disease developed in a 14-year-old boy with a 2-year history of ingesting and sniffing a powdered cleaning product containing silica, soda ash, dodecyl benzyl sulfonate, and trichloro-s-triazinetrione.[51]

As awareness developed that patients could manifest hepatic veno-occlusive disease following antineoplastic chemotherapy, reports began to emerge linking PVOD to these agents, as well. Many of the patients with PVOD diagnosed after the management of malignancy received radiation and a variety of antineoplastic drugs over several years, making identification of a specific culprit agent problematic; nonetheless, the most commonly implicated compounds have been bleomycin, mitomycin, carmustine (BCNU), and gemcitabine.[52–58] Anecdotal reports suggest that PVOD may be more common following either allogeneic or autologous bone marrow transplantation than following conventional cytoreductive chemotherapy; however, there are insufficient data to definitively test this assertion.[59]

The mechanism by which certain drugs might cause pulmonary venous remodeling is unknown. It is possible that these chemotherapeutic agents are metabolized to toxic intermediates in pulmonary capillaries and then cause damage to pulmonary venous structures.

Cocaine, amphetamines, and anorectic agents are associated with pulmonary arterial hypertension, but they have not been linked definitively to PVOD.[22,23] Similarly, "bush teas" containing pyrrolizidine alkaloids have been responsible for case clusters of hepatic veno-occlusive disease but have not been associated with PVOD.[60,61]

Thrombophilia

Because venules and small veins in PVOD have an appearance similar to recanalized, thrombotically occluded arteries, and because lung specimens occasionally have evidence of fresh thrombi in affected vessels, it has long been hypothesized that thrombophilia may play a role PVOD pathogenesis. Coagulation and rheologic parameters have not been assessed in patients with PVOD by state-of-the-art techniques, but several reports from the 1960s described increased platelet adhesiveness in patients with the disorder, in one case to a degree 4 standard deviations above the mean for normals.[4,62] A number of cases of PVOD have occurred in patients with risk factors for hypercoagulability, such as pregnancy or oral contraceptive use.[63,64]

However, although cases of PVOD have indeed occurred in patients with documented thrombophilia, such comorbidities are unusual.[65] The thrombophilia hypothesis also fails to explain why extrapulmonary venous or arterial thrombi, which would be expected to develop commonly in hypercoagulable states, occur infrequently in patients with PVOD. Finally, careful examination of lung specimens fails to demonstrate acute pulmonary venous thrombi in most patients with PVOD.[32]

Autoimmune Disorders

Venulitis, either primary or occurring secondary to an infectious vasculitis, followed by thrombosis, remodeling, or both, could presumably explain the pathologic changes seen in PVOD, but inflammation is not a typical feature of this disorder. Granulomatous venulitis rarely has been described to accompany sarcoidosis, and a similar vascular lesion has been described in a 21-year-old marijuana-smoking man with the clinical syndrome of PVOD.[31,66]

Although most patients with PVOD do not display manifestations of autoimmunity, a number of individuals who have developed PVOD have positive antinuclear antibodies, alopecia, myopathy, rheumatoid arthritis, Felty syndrome, systemic lupus erythematosus, or the scleroderma spectrum of conditions (including features such as calcinosis, Raynaud phenomenon, esophageal dysmotility, sclerodactyly, and telangiectasias).[67–77] However, only a minority of cases displays associated autoimmune findings, which argues against autoimmunity playing a fundamental role in the development of PVOD.

Clinical Manifestations

Most patients with PVOD come to medical attention with nonspecific symptoms of pulmonary hypertension, such as dyspnea on exertion and fatigue.[25] Patients may develop a chronic cough (either productive or nonproductive), and many patients are diagnosed initially with an acute respiratory infection; PVOD subsequently is found after they fail to improve significantly after treatment with antimicrobial agents.[5,47,78] As pulmonary hypertension worsens, patients may develop right upper quadrant pain (secondary to hepatic congestion), pedal edema, and exertional syncope. Orthopnea reportedly is more common and severe in patients with PVOD than in those with IPAH or other causes of pulmonary arterial hypertension.[33] Unusual clinical pictures of PVOD include symptomatic diffuse alveolar hemorrhage or sudden cardiac death.[79–81] Chronic subacute alveolar hemorrhage appears common on the basis of lung histopathologic findings, but massive and life-threatening hemoptysis rarely develops.[79]

Physical examination also tends to reveal nonspecific findings of pulmonary hypertension, with or without overt right ventricular failure, such as increased intensity of the pulmonic component of the second heart sound or a right ventricular heave or lift. Murmurs of tricuspid regurgitation and, less commonly, pulmonic insufficiency may be appreciated, and a right-sided fourth heart sound, elevated jugular venous pressure, hepatomegaly, and edema may also be apparent. Murmurs or gallops generally are augmented with inspiration, because increased venous return to the thorax increases turbulent flow through right-sided valvular defects.[82] Digital clubbing is sometimes present, and basilar rales are appreciated in some cases[47] (FIGURE 11-3).

Pleural effusions are relatively common in patients with PVOD, in contrast to their infrequent association with purely precapillary causes of pulmonary hypertension.[83,84] This is probably because PVOD and other postcapillary causes of pulmonary hypertension produce elevated pulmonary capillary and visceral pleural hydrostatic pressures, leading to transudation of fluid into the pleural space. In contrast, the predominant high-resistance areas of the pulmonary circulation are precapillary in IPAH, and thus pleural effusions generally do not accumulate until elevated hydrostatic pressure develops in the central systemic veins, leading to elevations in hydrostatic pressure within the parietal pleural capillaries.

Radiographic Findings

Chronic pulmonary capillary hypertension can produce transudation of fluid into the pulmonary interstitium, with consequent engorgement of pulmonary lymphatic vessels; this gives the

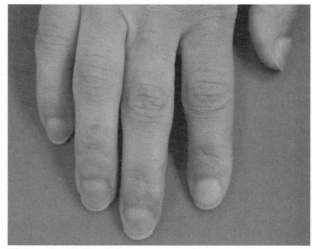

Figure 11-3. Prominent Clubbing of the Digits in a Patient With Pulmonary Veno-occlusive Disease. (Courtesy of Michelle Bianco, MD.)

radiographic appearance of Kerley B lines on plain chest radiographs (FIGURE 11-4). Central pulmonary arteries are visibly enlarged, peribronchial cuffing can be seen, and scattered parenchymal opacities may be present.[4,85] However, these findings are not pathognomonic of PVOD, and the absence of any or all of these findings does not eliminate the possibility that PVOD is present.[25,73,86,87]

Computed tomography images may display smooth thickening of the septae, diffuse or mosaic ground glass opacities, multiple well-defined or poorly defined small noncalcified nodules, pleural effusions, or areas of alveolar consolidation which may be gravity dependent[83,88–92] (FIGURE 11-5). The pathologic correlate of ground glass attenuation seen in these patients is not entirely clear, although alveolar hemorrhage, focal areas of hydrostatic edema, nonspecific interstitial inflammation, and alveolar septal thickening with associated epithelial hyperplasia have each been proposed to explain the finding. Importantly, the central pulmonary veins and the left atrium are not enlarged, in contrast to patients with mitral stenosis, cor triatriatum, left atrial myxoma, or large vein stenosis secondary to electrophysiologic ablation. Prominent mediastinal lymphadenopathy has been reported in several cases.[1,9,91–94]

Radionuclide ventilation-perfusion images display normal ventilation but commonly show multiple focal areas of hypoperfusion, sometimes

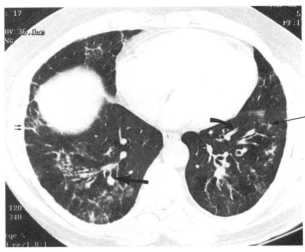

Figure 11-5. Computed tomographic image through the lung bases shows numerous thickened septal lines (*double arrow*) and patchy foci of ground-glass attenuation (*thin arrow*). The arteries are enlarged relative to bronchi (*thick arrow*), whereas pulmonary veins appear of normal caliber (*curved arrow*). (Used with permission from Mandel J, Mark E, Hales C: Pulmonary veno-occlusive disease. *Am J Respir Crit Care Med* 162:1964, 2000.)

approximating a segmental pattern.[95] This finding may be misinterpreted as supportive of the diagnosis of chronic thromboembolic pulmonary hypertension.[25,33,78,79,87,88,96–99]

Cardiac Catheterization

It is frequently difficult to obtain a satisfactory pulmonary artery occlusion (wedge) pressure in patients with PVOD. Flushing of the catheter when the distal port of the catheter is in the wedged position and the balloon is inflated results in a disproportionate rise in recorded pressure, which then falls extremely slowly to baseline. These phenomena reflect impaired run-off of infused saline due to diminished cross-sectional area of the pulmonary venules and small veins.[4,79,100] To document successful catheter wedging in this situation, it may be necessary to demonstrate that blood gas analysis of a sample drawn slowly from the distal catheter port while the balloon is inflated displays values similar to a specimen drawn simultaneously from an arterial source.

If a pulmonary artery occlusion pressure can be measured successfully, one should record values in several different locations to ensure that spurious

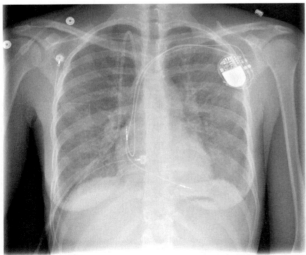

Figure 11-4. Pulmonary Veno-occlusive Disease. A posteroanterior chest radiograph from 28-year-old woman with pulmonary veno-occlusive disease demonstrated at autopsy shows increased interstitial markings diffusely and Kerley B lines that are most prominent in her lower lateral right chest.

values have not been obtained because of local phenomena. In patients with PVOD, the pulmonary artery occlusion pressure generally is normal or decreased, although postcapillary obstruction does produce pulmonary capillary hypertension.[47,101] The cause of this seeming paradox is that the pulmonary artery occlusion pressure is determined by left atrial pressures, not by hydrostatic pressures within the pulmonary capillaries, as the term "pulmonary capillary wedge pressure" is sometimes taken to imply. Rather, with the balloon inflated and the catheter in the wedged position, a static column of blood is created that extends from the catheter tip, through the pulmonary capillaries, venules, and veins to the left atrium, the latter of which determines the recorded pressure, and this pressure generally is normal in those with PVOD. Extensive stenosis of the small pulmonary veins in PVOD tends to dampen this pressure tracing to some degree, but does not alter the fact that left atrial pressures are the fundamental determinant of the pulmonary artery occlusion pressure.[102,103]

Short-acting pulmonary arterial vasodilators are administered routinely to patients with pulmonary hypertension at the time of cardiac catheterization to determine if pulmonary vasoreactivity is present.[23] However, in patients with PVOD, such medications may lead to acute life-threatening pulmonary edema.[47,94] Presumably pulmonary edema develops in this setting because of pulmonary arterial vasodilation without concomitant pulmonary venodilation, producing a rapid increase in transcapillary hydrostatic forces and transudation of fluid into the pulmonary interstitium and alveoli.

Other Studies

Patients with PVOD generally display normal spirometric values. The single-breath diffusing capacity for carbon monoxide (DL_{CO}) usually is reduced, and a mild to moderate restrictive ventilatory defect is observed in some cases.[47,87,88] Laboratory parameters usually are unremarkable, although isolated cases have displayed otherwise unexplained features such as microangiopathic hemolytic anemia,[56] heavy proteinuria,[5] or elevated immunoglobulin G (IgG) or IgM concentrations.[69]

Bronchoscopy may reveal intense hyperemia and longitudinal vascular engorgement of the lobar and segmental bronchi in patients with PVOD.[97] This finding is thought to result from engorgement of the bronchial arterial system, which in segmental and more distal bronchi normally drains into the pulmonary circulation, but which has poor distal run-off in PVOD. In this report, hyperemia was not seen in the trachea or main bronchi, where systemic bronchial veins are well developed.

Diagnosis

The triad of severe pulmonary hypertension, radiographic evidence of pulmonary edema, and a normal pulmonary artery occlusion pressure frequently is sufficient to warrant a clinical diagnosis of PVOD.[103] However, many patients with PVOD do not have all three components of this triad, and thus its absence cannot reliably exclude the diagnosis.

Delays in diagnosis are encountered almost universally by patients with PVOD, with many patients believed to suffer from heart failure because of radiographic evidence of pulmonary edema and pleural effusions, or chronic thromboembolic pulmonary hypertension because of nonresolving radionuclide perfusion defects. In cases of PVOD in which interstitial changes are radiographically or histologically prominent, alternative diagnoses of diffuse parenchymal lung diseases such as sarcoidosis, pneumoconioses, cystic fibrosis, or idiopathic pulmonary fibrosis may be considered.[104]

Definitive diagnosis is possible only by surgical lung biopsy, and this procedure should be contemplated to confirm the clinical suspicion of PVOD. Although the need for lung biopsy has been questioned because therapy for PVOD is so unsatisfactory, establishing the diagnosis has significant implications for prognosis, medical therapy, and timing of lung transplantation; therefore, biopsy should be considered in patients in whom the diagnosis is suspected and surgical risk is not prohibitive.

Demonstration of occult pulmonary hemorrhage by bronchoalveolar lavage in the proper clinical setting may support the diagnosis if lung tissue has not been obtained.[105] Transbronchial biopsy almost never yields enough tissue for a firm pathologic diagnosis and carries significant risks when performed in patients with pulmonary hypertension.

Prognosis and Management

The prognosis of PVOD is poor, with most patients dying within 2 years of diagnosis. However, cases have been reported in which individuals have survived for 5 years or more, generally when therapy with oral calcium channel antagonists or intravenous epoprostenol therapy have been well tolerated.[40,106,107]

Because PVOD is a rare disease, large treatment trials cannot be performed easily, and the degree to which any of the therapies influence survival and quality of life is speculative.[108] With the possible exceptions of lung transplantation and intravenous epoprostenol (if tolerated), the positive impact of therapies does not seem profound.

Calcium Channel Antagonists and Epoprostenol

A minority of patients with IPAH will display acute pulmonary vasoreactivity in response to vasodilator medications such as adenosine, epoprostenol, inhaled nitric oxide, or calcium channel antagonists.[109,110] (Pulmonary vasoreactivity was defined in older literature as a 20–25 percent decrease in mean pulmonary artery pressure and pulmonary vascular resistance, or more recently as a reduction in mean pulmonary artery pressure of >10 mmHg to a value of 40 mmHg or below, with a normal or high cardiac output.[111]) Vasoreactive patients tend to have an excellent prognosis when treated with calcium channel antagonists. In IPAH patients without an acute hemodynamic response and who thus cannot be treated with calcium channel antagonists, therapy with continuous intravenous epoprostenol has been associated with improved survival.[112] Therapy with treprostinil or endothelin-1 receptor antagonists such as bosentan likewise is associated with improved outcomes.[113,114]

The generalizability of such data to PVOD is unclear. Theoretically, a reduction in pulmonary arterial resistance without a concomitant reduction in pulmonary venous resistance could cause pulmonary edema, whereas a parallel decrease in both arterial and venous resistance should be well tolerated and advantageous.

The clinical experience with vasodilator/remodeling medications in patients with PVOD has been mixed. Modest improvements in hemodynamics and exercise tolerance have been reported in a small number of patients with nifedipine, hydralazine, and prazosin, but in general these benefits have not been well maintained.[107,115] Epoprostenol has had salutary effects on pulmonary hemodynamics and decreased vasomotor tone in pulmonary venules in some patients, but it has produced fulminant pulmonary edema and death in others.[40,47,94,106,116,117] There is limited experience with inhaled nitric oxide or iloprost in this condition, although initial descriptions of the use of these agents suggested that improvement in cardiac output resulted without pulmonary edema.[118]

Because the therapeutic options in PVOD are so limited, a cautious trial of epoprostenol generally is indicated. If tolerated, epoprostenol is initiated at a dosage of 2–4 ng/kg/min, then titrated upward by 1–2 ng/kg/min every 1–4 weeks as permitted by side effects. Whether endothelin-1 antagonists or phosphodiesterase 5 inhibitors exert a beneficial or detrimental effect has not been firmly established.

Lung Transplantation

Either single lung and double lung transplantation can be performed to manage PVOD.[119] Heart-lung transplantation rarely is required, because impaired right ventricular function usually improves following the transplantation of normal lungs.[119,120] Rare recurrence of PVOD after transplantation has been reported, although the risk of recurrence is difficult to estimate because the number of transplants performed for this diagnosis has been relatively small.[89,121,122]

Conventional Supportive Therapy

Patients with PVOD should receive conventional supportive therapy similar to that prescribed for patients with IPAH, unless contraindications are present (see Chapter 7).[110] Of note, none of these therapies has been documented in high-quality randomized trials to be efficacious in patients with pulmonary hypertension of any cause; they are employed because of theoretical consideration or case reports, case series, or retrospective analyses that have suggested possible benefit.

Warfarin generally is titrated to an International Normalized Ratio of approximately 2.0, based upon the suggestion of several nonrandomized studies in IPAH that length of survival may be improved modestly.[109,123] Episodic small-volume hemoptysis generally does not require discontinuation of anticoagulation, but the medication usually is stopped if more than 50 mL of blood is expectorated over a 24-hour period, if significant extrapulmonary hemorrhage occurs, or if syncope or other risk factors for head trauma develop.

Long-term oxygen therapy should be initiated if an oxygen saturation of 89 percent or less, or an arterial PO_2 of 59 mmHg or less, is documented. These recommendations are based on results of clinical trials of oxygen therapy in patients with chronic obstructive pulmonary disease rather than primary pulmonary vascular disease, and it should be appreciated that not all patients with pulmonary hypertension show improvement in pulmonary hemodynamics after oxygen therapy is begun.[124–126] Transtracheal oxygen therapy permits delivery of oxygen at higher flow rates than via nasal cannulae and may be considered when epistaxis is problematic, although local bleeding complications can occur.[127]

Diuretics should be used as necessary to maintain euvolemia. Both dehydration and hypervolemia should be avoided, and patients should monitor their weight daily. Based on the modest improvement in cardiac output described in patients with IPAH managed with digoxin, the drug is prescribed routinely to patients with PVOD unless contraindications are present.[128]

Immunosuppressive Agents

Immunosuppressive medications such as glucocorticoids and azathioprine have been employed occasionally in PVOD management, although protocols have been neither standardized nor randomized, making unequivocal conclusions about their effectiveness difficult. Nonetheless, only rare responses to therapy have been reported, and only a minority of these cases have shown sustained improvement.[69,77,129,130] Most patients do not have prominent autoimmune features or biochemical indices suggestive of an inflammatory process, and thus would not be expected to respond to such interventions.[2,104]

In general, immunosuppressive agents do not have a role in PVOD management, although a 4-week trial of 0.75–1.0 mg/kg of prednisone may be considered in patients with associated nonspecific interstitial pulmonary inflammation, or autoimmune features such as arthritis, alopecia, or an elevated erythrocyte sedimentation rate. If improvement is seen in symptoms, radiographs, diffusing capacity, or alveolar-arterial oxygen gradient, the dosage is then slowly tapered to 20–40 mg per day.

Experimental Therapies

Although endothelin-1 receptor antagonists, such as bosentan, and phosphodiesterase 5 inhibitors, such as sildenafil, are finding roles in management of pulmonary arterial hypertension, there is scant experience with these medications in PVOD management.[114,131–133] Both classes of medications could prove either beneficial or deleterious in PVOD for similar reasons as vasodilators, and no recommendation regarding their use can be made.

A number of experimental therapies have been investigated for hepatic veno-occlusive disease, such as defibrotide, recombinant tissue plasminogen activator, or antithrombin-III concentrate.[134,135] No data are available regarding the utility of these managements in PVOD, and given the likely differences in pathogenesis of the two conditions, none of these agents is recommended for patients with PVOD pending specific data supporting their efficacy.

Conclusion

PVOD remains a highly lethal and poorly understood syndrome, with basic and critical questions about its etiology and optimal management remaining unanswered, despite the seven decades since its initial description. Its diagnosis requires a high degree of clinical suspicion and frequently necessitates surgical lung biopsy, but the prognosis and management of PVOD is sufficiently different from other causes of pulmonary hypertension that such efforts generally are justified. In particular, the approaches to timing of lung transplantation and to optimal medical therapy are different than in IPAH, and significant harm or death may occur if PVOD goes unrecognized. Additional research is required to more precisely delineate risk factors for the syndrome and to define optimal therapy for it.

References

1. Veeraraghavan S, Koss M, Sharma O: Pulmonary veno-occlusive disease. *Curr Opin Pulm Med* 5:310, 1999.
2. Mandel J, Mark E, Hales C: Pulmonary veno-occlusive disease. *Am J Respir Crit Care Med* 162:1964, 2000.
3. Höra J: Zur histologie der klinischen "primaren Pulmonalsklerose." *Frankf Z Pathol* 47:100, 1934.
4. Brown C, Harrison C: Pulmonary veno-occlusive disease. *Lancet* 2:61, 1966.
5. Heath D, Segel N, Bishop J: Pulmonary veno-occlusive disease. *Circulation* 34:242, 1966.
6. Weisser K, Wyler F, Gloor F: Pulmonary veno-occlusive disease. *Arch Dis Child* 42:322, 1967.
7. Rosenthal A, Vawter G, Wagenvoort C: Intrapulmonary veno-occlusive disease. *Am J Cardiol* 31:78, 1973.
8. Pietra G, Capron F, Stewart S, et al: Pathologic assessment of vasculopathies in pulmonary hypertension. *J Am Coll Cardiol* 43:S25-S32, 2004.

9. Purerfellner H, Aichinger J, Martinek M, et al: Incidence, management, and outcome in significant pulmonary vein stenosis complicating ablation for atrial fibrillation. *Am J Cardiol* 93:1428–1431, 2004.

10. Simonneau G, Galie N, Rubin L, et al: Clinical classification of pulmonary hypertension. *J Am Coll Cardiol* 46:S5-S12, 2004.

11. Robbins I, Colvin E, Doyle T, et al: Pulmonary vein stenosis after catheter ablation of atrial fibrillation. *Circulation* 98:1769, 1998.

12. Arentz T, Jander N, von Rosenthal J, et al: Incidence of pulmonary vein stenosis 2 years after radiofrequency catheter ablation of refractory atrial fibrillation. *Eur Heart J* 24:963, 2003.

13. Spray T, Bridges N: Surgical management of congenital and acquired pulmonary vein stenosis. *Semin Thorac Cardiovasc Surg Pediatr Card Surg Annu* 2:177, 1999.

14. Pietra G, Edwards W, Kay J, et al: Histopathology of primary pulmonary hypertension: A qualitative and quantitative study of pulmonary blood vessels from 58 patients in the National Heart, Lung, and Blood Institute Primary Pulmonary Hypertension Registry. *Circulation* 80:1198, 1989.

15. Palevsky H, Schloo B, Pietra G, et al: Primary pulmonary hypertension. Vascular structure, morphometry, and responsiveness to vasodilator agents. *Circulation* 80:1207, 1989.

16. Wagenvoort C: Lung biopsy specimens in the evaluation of pulmonary vascular disease. *Chest* 77:614, 1980.

17. Kinare S, Deshpande J: Primary pulmonary hypertension in India (autopsy study of 26 cases). *Indian Heart J* 39:9, 1987.

18. Burke A, Farb A, Virmani R: The pathology of primary pulmonary hypertension. *Mod Pathol* 4:269, 1991.

19. Pietra G: The pathology of primary pulmonary hypertension. In: Rubin L, Rich S, editors: *Primary pulmonary hypertension,* New York, 1997, Marcel Dekker.

20. Bjornsson J, Edwards W: Primary pulmonary hypertension: A histopathologic study of 80 cases. *Mayo Clin Proc* 60:16, 1985.

21. Wagenvoort C, Wagenvoort N: Primary pulmonary hypertension: A pathologic study of the lung vessels in 156 clinically diagnosed cases. *Circulation* 42:1163, 1970.

22. Abenhaim L, Moride Y, Brenot F, et al: Appetite-suppressant drugs and the risk of primary pulmonary hypertension. *N Engl J Med* 335:609, 1996.

23. Rubin L: Primary pulmonary hypertension. *N Engl J Med* 336:111, 1997.

24. Wagenvoort C: Pulmonary veno-occlusive disease. Entity or syndrome? *Chest* 69:82, 1976.

25. Thadani U, Burrow C, Whitaker W, et al: Pulmonary veno-occlusive disease. *Q J Med* 64:133, 1975.

26. Rubin E, Farber J: The respiratory system. In: Rubin E, Farber J, editors: *Pathology,* Philadelphia, 1994, JB Lippincott, pp 557–617.

27. Wagenvoort C, Wagenvoort N: The pathology of pulmonary veno-occlusive disease. *Virchows Arch A Pathol Anat Histol* 364:69, 1974.

28. Chazova I, Robbins I, Loyd J, et al: Venous and arterial changes in pulmonary veno-occlusive disease, mitral stenosis and fibrosing mediastinitis. *Eur Respir J* 15:116, 2000.

29. Schraufnagel D, Sekosan M, McGee T, et al: Human alveolar capillaries undergo angiogenesis in pulmonary veno-occlusive disease. *Eur Respir J* 9:346, 1996.

30. Wagenvoort C, Wagenvoort N, Takahashi T: Pulmonary veno-occlusive disease: Involvement of pulmonary arteries and review of the literature. *Hum Pathol* 16:1033, 1985.

31. Crissman J, Koss M, Carson R: Pulmonary veno-occlusive disease secondary to granulomatous venulitis. *Am J Surg Pathol* 4:93, 1980.

32. Carrington C, Liebow A: Pulmonary veno-occlusive disease. *Hum Pathol* 1:322, 1970.

33. Glassroth J, Woodford D, Carrington C, et al: Pulmonary veno-occlusive disease in the middle-aged. *Respiration* 47:309, 1985.

34. Cortese D: Pulmonary function in mitral stenosis. *Mayo Clin Proc* 53:321, 1978.

35. Davies P, Reid L: Pulmonary veno-occlusive disease in siblings: Case reports and morphometric study. *Hum Pathol* 13:911, 1982.

36. Voordes C, Kuipers J, Elema J: Familial pulmonary veno-occlusive disease: A case report. *Thorax* 32:763, 1977.

37. Deng Z, Morse J, Slager S, et al: Familial primary pulmonary hypertension (gene *PPH1*) is caused by mutations in the bone morphogenetic protein receptor-II gene. *Am J Hum Genet* 67:737, 2000.

38. Thomas A, Carneal J, Markin C, et al: Specific bone morphogenic protein receptor II mutations found in primary pulmonary hypertension cause different biochemical phenotypes in vitro. *Chest* 121:83S, 2002.

39. Lane K, Machado R, Pauciulo M, et al: Heterozygous germline mutations in *BMPR2*, encoding a TGF-β receptor, cause familial primary pulmonary hypertension. The International PPH Consortium. *Nat Genet* 26:81, 2000.

40. Runo J, Vnencak-Jones C, Prince M, et al: Pulmonary veno-occlusive disease caused by an inherited mutation in bone morphogenetic protein receptor II. *Am J Respir Crit Care Med* 167:889, 2003.

41. Machado R, Pauciulo M, Thomson J, et al: *BMPR2* haploinsufficiency as the inherited molecular mech-

anism for primary pulmonary hypertension. *Am J Hum Genet* 68:92, 2001.

42. Chazova I, Loyd J, Zhdanov V, et al: Pulmonary artery adventitial changes and venous involvement in primary pulmonary hypertension. *Am J Pathol* 146:389, 1995.

43. Dorfmuller P, Humbert M, Sanchez O, et al: Significant occlusive lesions of pulmonary veins are common in patients with pulmonary hypertension associated to connective tissue diseases (abstract), American Thoracic Society 99th International Conference, Seattle, WA, May 16–21, 2003 (abstract).

44. Pulmonary veno-occlusive disease. *Br Med J* 3:369, 1972.

45. Stovin P, Mitchinson M: Pulmonary hypertension due to obstruction of the intrapulmonary veins. *Thorax* 20:106, 1965.

46. McDonnell P, Summer W, Hutchins G: Pulmonary veno-occlusive disease. Morphological changes suggesting a viral cause. *JAMA* 246:667, 1981.

47. Holcomb BJ, Loyd J, Ely E, et al: Pulmonary veno-occlusive disease. A case series and new observations. *Chest* 118:1671, 2000.

48. Ruchelli E, Nojadera G, Rutstein R, et al: Pulmonary veno-occlusive disease. Another vascular disorder associated with human immunodeficiency virus infection? *Arch Pathol Lab Med* 118:664, 1994.

49. Escamilla R, Hermant C, Berjaud J, et al: Pulmonary veno-occlusive disease in a HIV-infected intravenous drug abuser. *Eur Respir J* 8:1982, 1995.

50. Hourseau M, Capron F, Nunes H, et al: Pulmonary veno-occlusive disease in a patient with HIV infection. A case report with autopsy findings. *Ann Pathol* 22:472, 2002.

51. Liu L, Sackler J: A case of pulmonary veno-occlusive disease: Etiological and therapeutic appraisal. *Angiology* 23:299, 1973.

52. Doll D, Yarbro J: Vascular toxicity associated with chemotherapy and hormonotherapy. *Curr Opin Oncol* 6:345, 1994.

53. Joselson R, Warnock M: Pulmonary veno-occlusive disease after chemotherapy. *Hum Pathol* 14:88, 1983.

54. Knight B, Rose A: Pulmonary veno-occlusive disease after chemotherapy. *Thorax* 40:874, 1985.

55. Swift G, Gibbs A, Campbell I, et al: Pulmonary veno-occlusive disease and Hodgkin's lymphoma. *Eur Respir J* 6:596, 1993.

56. Waldhorn R, Tsou E, Smith F, et al: Pulmonary veno-occlusive disease associated with microangiopathic hemolytic anemia and chemotherapy of gastric adenocarcinoma. *Med Pediatr Oncol* 12:394, 1984.

57. Gagnadoux F, Capron F, Lebeau B: Pulmonary veno-occlusive disease after neoadjuvant mitomycin chemotherapy and surgery for lung carcinoma. *Lung Cancer* 36:213, 2002.

58. Vansteenkiste JF, Bomans P, Verbeken EK, et al: Fatal pulmonary veno-occlusive disease possibly related to gemcitabine. *Lung Cancer* 31:83, 2001.

59. Williams L, Fussell S, Veith R, et al: Pulmonary veno-occlusive disease in an adult following bone marrow transplantation. Case report and review of the literature. *Chest* 109:1388, 1996.

60. Kumana C, Ng M, Lin H, et al: Herbal tea induced hepatic veno-occlusive disease: Quantification of toxic alkaloid exposure in adults. *Gut* 26:101, 1985.

61. Tandon B, Tandon H, Tandon R, et al: An epidemic of veno-occlusive disease of the liver in central India. *Lancet* 2:271, 1976.

62. Clinicopathological conference: A case of veno-occlusive disease. Demonstrated at the Royal Postgraduate Medical School. *Br Med J* 1:818–822, 1968.

63. Tsou E, Waldhorn R, Kerwin D, et al: Pulmonary venoocclusive disease in pregnancy. *Obstet Gynecol* 64:281, 1984.

64. Townend J, Roberts D, Jones E, et al: Fatal pulmonary venoocclusive disease after use of oral contraceptives. *Am Heart J* 124:1643, 1992.

65. Hussein A, Trowitzsch E, Brockmann M: Pulmonary veno-occlusive disease, antiphospholipid antibody and pulmonary hypertension in an adolescent. *Klin Padiatr* 211:92, 1999.

66. Hoffstein V, Ranganathan N, Mullen J: Sarcoidosis simulating pulmonary veno-occlusive disease. *Am Rev Respir Dis* 134:809, 1986.

67. Scully R, Mark E, McNeely B: Case records of the Massachusetts General Hospital: Weekly clinicopathologic exercises. Case 14-1983: A 67-year-old woman with pulmonary hypertension. *N Engl J Med* 308:823, 1983.

68. Scully R, Mark E, McNeely W, et al: Case records of the Massachusetts General Hospital: Weekly clinicopathologic exercises. Case 37-1992: A 68-year-old woman with rheumatoid arthritis and pulmonary hypertension. *N Engl J Med* 327:873, 1992.

69. Sanderson J, Spiro S, Hendry A, et al: A case of pulmonary veno-occlusive disease responding to treatment with azathioprine. *Thorax* 32:140, 1977.

70. Morassut P, Walley V, Smith C: Pulmonary veno-occlusive disease and the CREST variant of scleroderma. *Can J Cardiol* 8:1055, 1992.

71. Kishida Y, Kanai Y, Kuramochi S, et al: Pulmonary venoocclusive disease in a patient with systemic lupus erythematosus. *J Rheumatol* 20:2161, 1993.

72. Katz D, Scalzetti E, Katzenstein A, et al: Pulmonary veno-occlusive disease presenting with thrombosis of pulmonary arteries. *Thorax* 50:699, 1995.

73. Leinonen H, Pohjola-Sintonen S, Krogerus L: Pulmonary veno-occlusive disease. *Acta Med Scand* 221:307, 1987.

74. Liang M, Stern S, Fortinn P, et al: Fatal pulmonary venoocclusive disease secondary to a generalized venopathy: A new syndrome presenting with facial swelling and pericardial tamponade. *Arthritis Rheum* 34:228, 1991.

75. Devereux G, Evans M, Kerr K, et al: Pulmonary veno-occlusive disease complicating Felty's syndrome. *Respir Med* 92:1089, 1998.

76. Andreassen A, Jahnsen F, Andersen R, et al: Pulmonal venookklusiv sykdom ved sklerodermi og CREST-syndrom. *Tidsskr Nor Laegeforen* 123:3391–3392, 2003.

77. Saito A, Takizawa H, Ito K, et al: A case of pulmonary veno-occlusive disease associated with systemic sclerosis. *Respirology* 8:383–385, 2003.

78. Calderon M, Burdine J: Pulmonary veno-occlusive disease. *J Nucl Med* 15:455, 1974.

79. Chawla S, Kittle C, Faber L, et al: Pulmonary venoocclusive disease. *Ann Thorac Surg* 22:249, 1976.

80. Bolster M, Hogan J, Bredin C: Pulmonary vascular occlusive disease presenting as sudden death. *Med Sci Law* 30:26, 1990.

81. Cagle P, Langston C: Pulmonary veno-occlusive disease as a cause of sudden infant death. *Arch Pathol Lab Med* 108:338, 1984.

82. Wiedemann H: Cor pulmonale. In: Rose B, editor: *UpToDate*, vol 13.3, Wellesley, MA, 2005, UpToDate.

83. Swensen S, Tashjian J, Myers J, et al: Pulmonary venoocclusive disease: CT findings in eight patients. *AJR Am J Roentgenol* 167:937, 1996.

84. Weiner-Kronish J, Goldstein R, Matthay R, et al: Lack of association of pleural effusion with chronic pulmonary arterial and right atrial hypertension. *Chest* 92:967, 1987.

85. Gluecker T, Capasso P, Schnyder P, et al: Clinical and radiographic features of pulmonary edema. *Radio-graphics* 19:1507, 1999.

86. Scheibel R, Dedeker K, Gleason D, et al: Radiographic and angiographic characteristics of pulmonary veno-occlusive disease. *Radiology* 103:47, 1972.

87. Elliott C, Colby T, Hill T, et al: Pulmonary venoocclusive disease associated with severe reduction of single-breath carbon monoxide diffusing capacity. *Respiration* 53:262, 1988.

88. Maltby J, Gouverne M: CT findings in pulmonary venoocclusive disease. *J Comput Assist Tomogr* 8:758, 1984.

89. Cassart M, Gevenois P, Kramer M, et al: Pulmonary venoocclusive disease: CT findings before and after single-lung transplantation. *AJR Am J Roentgenol* 160:759, 1993.

90. Worthy S, Müller N, Hartman T, et al: Mosaic attenuation pattern on thin section CT scans of the lung: Differentiation among infiltrative lung, airway, and vascular diseases as a cause. *Radiology* 205:465, 1997.

91. Resten A, Maitre S, Humbert M, et al: Pulmonary arterial hypertension: Thin section CT predictors of epoprostenol therapy failure. *Radiology* 222:782, 2002.

92. Resten A, Maitre S, Capron F, et al: Pulmonary hypertension: CT findings in pulmonary veno-occlusive disease. *J Radiol* 84:1739–1745, 2003.

93. Scully R, Mark E, McNeely W, et al: Case records of the Massachusetts General Hospital: Weekly clinicopathologic exercises. Case 48-1993: A 27-year-old woman with mediastinal lymphadenopathy and relentless cor pulmonale. *N Engl J Med* 329:1720, 1993.

94. Dufour B, Maitre S, Humbert M, et al: High-resolution CT of the chest in four patients with pulmonary capillary hemangiomatosis or pulmonary venoocclusive disease. *AJR Am J Roentgenol* 171:1321, 1998.

95. Bailey C, Channick R, Auger W, et al: "High probability" perfusion lung scans in pulmonary venoocclusive disease. *Chest* 162:1974, 2000.

96. Rich S, Pietra G, Kieras K, et al: Primary pulmonary hypertension: Radiographic and scintigraphic patterns of histologic subtypes. *Ann Intern Med* 105:499, 1986.

97. Matthews A, Buchanan R: A case of pulmonary veno-occlusive disease and a new bronchoscopic sign. *Respir Med* 84:503, 1990.

98. Nawaz S, Dobersen M, Blount SJ, et al: Florid pulmonary veno-occlusive disease. *Chest* 98:1037, 1990.

99. Shackelford G, Sacks E, Mullins J: Pulmonary venoocclusive disease: Case report and review of the literature. *AJR Am J Roentgenol* 128:643, 1977.

100. Rapidly progressive dyspnea in a teenage boy. Clinical pathological conference. *JAMA* 223:1243, 1973.

101. Schwarz M: Respiratory distress in woman who began complaining of dyspnea and cough 5 months ago. *Chest* 124:2388–2390, 2003.

102. Weed H: Pulmonary "capillary" wedge pressure not the pressure in the pulmonary capillaries. *Chest* 100:1138, 1991.

103. Rambihar V, Fallen E, Cairns J: Pulmonary venoocclusive disease: Antemortem diagnosis from roentgenographic and hemodynamic findings. *Can Med Assoc J* 120:1519, 1979.

104. De Vries T, Weening J, Roorda R: Pulmonary venoocclusive disease: A case report and a review of therapeutic possibilities. *Eur Respir J* 4:1029, 1991.

105. Rabiller A, Humbert M, Sitbon O, et al: Bronchoalveolar lavage (BAL) as a diagnostic tool in pulmonary hypertension: Occult alveolar haemorrhage is a common feature of pulmonary

veno-occlusive disease (PVOD), American Thoracic Society 99th International Conference, Seattle, WA, May 16–21, 2003 (abstract).

106. Okumura H, Nagaya N, Kyotani S, et al: Effects of continuous IV prostacyclin in a patient with pulmonary veno-occlusive disease. *Chest* 122:1096, 2002.

107. Salzman G, Rosa U: Prolonged survival in pulmonary veno-occlusive disease treated with nifedipine. *Chest* 95:1154, 1989.

108. Lagakos S: Clinical trials and rare diseases. *N Engl J Med* 348:2455, 2003.

109. Rich S, Kaufmann E, Levy P: The effect of high doses of calcium-channel blockers on survival in primary pulmonary hypertension. *N Engl J Med* 327:76, 1992.

110. Runo J, Loyd J: Primary pulmonary hypertension. *Lancet* 361:1533, 2003.

111. Barst R, McGoon M, Torbicki A, et al: Diagnosis and differential assessment of pulmonary arterial hypertension. *J Am Coll Cardiol* 16:40S-47S, 2004.

112. Barst R, Rubin L, Long W, et al: A comparison of continuous intravenous epoprostenol (prostacyclin) with conventional therapy for primary pulmonary hypertension: The Primary Pulmonary Hypertension Study Group. *N Engl J Med* 334:296, 1996.

113. Simonneau G, Barst R, Galie N, et al: Continuous subcutaneous infusion of treprostinil, a prostacyclin analogue, in patients with pulmonary arterial hypertension: A double-blind, randomized, placebo-controlled trial. *Am J Respir Crit Care Med* 165:800–804, 2002.

114. Rubin L, Badesch D, Barst R, et al: Bosentan therapy for pulmonary arterial hypertension. *N Engl J Med* 346:896, 2002.

115. Palevsky H, Pietra G, Fishman A: Pulmonary veno-occlusive disease and its response to vasodilator agents. *Am Rev Respir Dis* 142:426, 1990.

116. Davis L, deBoisblanc B, Glynn C, et al: Effect of prostacyclin on microvascular pressures in a patient with pulmonary veno-occlusive disease. *Chest* 108:1754, 1995.

117. Palmer S, Robinson L, Wang A, et al: Massive pulmonary edema and death after prostacyclin infusion in a patient with pulmonary veno-occlusive disease. *Chest* 113:237, 1998.

118. Hoeper M, Eschenbruch C, Zink-Wohlfart C, et al: Effects of inhaled nitric oxide and aerosolized iloprost in pulmonary veno-occlusive disease. *Respir Med* 93:62, 1999.

119. Gammie J, Keenan R, Pham S, et al: Single-versus double-lung transplantation for pulmonary hypertension. *J Thorac Cardiovasc Surg* 115:397, 1998.

120. Bando K, Armitage J, Paradis I, et al: Indications for and results of single, bilateral, and heart-lung transplantation for pulmonary hypertension. *J Thorac Cardiovasc Surg* 108:1056, 1994.

121. Kramer M, Estenne M, Berkman N, et al: Radiation-induced pulmonary veno-occlusive disease. *Chest* 104:1282, 1993.

122. Izbicki G, Shitrit D, Schechtman I, et al: Recurrence of pulmonary veno-occlusive disease after heart-lung transplantation. *J Heart Lung Transplant* 24:635–637, 2005.

123. Frank H, Mlczoch J, Huber K, et al: The effect of anticoagulant therapy in primary and anorectic drug-induced pulmonary hypertension. *Chest* 112:714, 1997.

124. Continuous or nocturnal oxygen therapy in hypoxemic chronic obstructive lung disease: A clinical trial. Nocturnal Oxygen Therapy Trial Group. *Ann Intern Med* 93:391, 1980.

125. Long term domiciliary oxygen therapy in chronic hypoxic cor pulmonale complicating chronic bronchitis and emphysema. Report of the Medical Research Council Working Party. *Lancet* 1:681, 1981.

126. Morgan J, Griffiths M, du Bois R, et al: Hypoxic pulmonary vasoconstriction in systemic sclerosis and primary pulmonary hypertension. *Chest* 99:551, 1991.

127. Eckmann D: Transtracheal oxygen delivery. *Crit Care Clin* 16:463, 2000.

128. Rich S, Seidlitz M, Dodin E, et al: The short-term effects of digoxin in patients with right ventricular dysfunction from pulmonary hypertension. *Chest* 114:787, 1998.

129. Hackman R, Madtes D, Petersen F, et al: Pulmonary venoocclusive disease following bone marrow transplantation. *Transplantation* 47:989, 1989.

130. Gilroy RJ, Teague M, Loyd J: Pulmonary veno-occlusive disease: Fatal progression of pulmonary hypertension despite steroid-induced remission of interstitial pneumonitis. *Am Rev Respir Dis* 143:1130, 1991.

131. Cheng J: Bosentan. *Heart Dis* 5:161, 2003.

132. Kothari S, Duggal B: Chronic oral sildenafil therapy in severe pulmonary artery hypertension. *Indian Heart J* 54:404, 2002.

133. Prasad S, Wilkinson J, Gatzoulis M: Sildenafil in primary pulmonary hypertension. *N Engl J Med* 343:1342, 2000 (letter).

134. Richardson P, Murakami C, Jin Z, et al: Multi-institutional use of defibrotide in 88 patients after stem cell transplantation with severe veno-occlusive disease and multisystem organ failure: Response without significant toxicity in a high-risk population and factors predictive of outcome. *Blood* 100:4337, 2002.

135. Willner I: Veno-occlusive disease. *Curr Treat Options Gastroenterol* 5:465, 2002.

Hemolytic Anemia Associated Pulmonary Hypertension

Roberto F. Machado, MD,

Mark T. Gladwin, MD

Advances in the care of patients with sickle cell disease, thalassemia, and other hemolytic anemias have led to a significant improvement in their life expectancy. Interventions that may have contributed to longevity include early detection, education, advances in red blood cell transfusion and iron chelation therapy, penicillin prophylaxis, vaccination, and hydroxyurea therapy. As this patient population ages, new chronic complications of these hemoglobinopathies develop. In this context, pulmonary arterial hypertension (PAH) is emerging as one of the leading causes of morbidity and mortality in adult patients with sickle cell disease and thalassemia, and likely in patients with other hemolytic disorders.

It is estimated that around 250,000 children worldwide are born with homozygous sickle cell anemia every year.[1] Approximately 0.15 percent of African Americans are homozygous for sickle cell disease, and 8 percent have sickle cell trait. Sickle cell disease occurs in individuals who are homozygous for a single nucleotide substitution in the β-globin gene that ultimately renders their hemoglobin (HbS) much less soluble than normal hemoglobin (HbA) when deoxygenated. This insolubility causes polymerization and aggregation of HbS inside sickled erythrocytes as they traverse the microcirculation. Rigid, dense, and sickled cells become entrapped in the microcirculation producing vascular obstruction, ischemia and reperfusion injury, and secondary vascular inflammation, thrombosis, and oxidant stress. Intracellular polymerization ultimately damages the membrane and depletes erythrocyte energy reserves, leading to chronic and episodic extravascular and intravascular hemolytic anemia.[2]

Thalassemia refers to a spectrum of diseases characterized by reduced or absent production of one or more α-globin or β-globin chains. β-Thalassemia is caused by impaired production of β-globin chains, which leads to a relative excess of α-globin chains. These excess α-globin chains are unstable, incapable of forming soluble tetramers on their own, and precipitate within the cell, leading to ineffective erythropoiesis and hemolytic anemia.[3] Thalassemia major, or homozygous β-thalassemia, is a severe disorder caused by inheritance of two β-thalassemia alleles. Starting during the first year of life, patients have severe and lifelong transfusion-dependent anemia, hepatosplenomegaly, and skeletal deformities from bone marrow expansion; they are prone to infection and skeletal fractures. β-Thalassemia minor, also called β-thalassemia trait, occurs in heterozygotes who have inherited a single gene leading to reduced β-globin production. Such patients are asymptomatic, may be only mildly anemic, and their disease usually is diagnosed when a blood cell count has been obtained for other reasons. β-Thalassemia intermedia occurs in patients with disease of intermediate severity, such as those who are compound heterozygotes of two thalassemic variants. Such patients may have the skeletal abnormalities and hepatosplenomegaly seen in thalassemia major. However, their hemoglobin concentrations usually range from 5 to 10 gm/dl and they usually require transfusions only when they have an intercurrent event that impairs erythropoiesis, such as an infection. Their clinical symptoms may not be apparent until well after the first year of life. People with hemoglobin E, which is the most common hemoglobin variant in the world, are mostly asymptomatic or have a mild microcytic anemia in its heterozygous or homozygous states. Because hemoglobin E is synthesized at a reduced rate, it can interact with β-thalassemia to produce a condition called hemoglobin E β-thalassemia. Around one-half of these patients are phenotypically similar to patients with thalassemia major and require regular transfusion therapy, with the other half having courses similar to thalassemia intermedia.

A common feature of these two diseases, intravascular hemolysis, produces a state of endothelial dysfunction, vascular proliferation, and pro-oxidant and proinflammatory stress.[4] These mechanisms ultimately can produce a systemic proliferative vasculopathy, a hallmark of which is pulmonary hypertension that develops during adulthood. In support of the role of hemolysis as an important contributing mechanism in this disorder, PAH is an increasingly recognized complication of chronic hereditary and acquired hemolytic anemias including sickle cell disease,[5-15] thalassemia,[16-25] paroxysmal nocturnal haemoglobinuria,[26,27] hereditary spherocytosis and stomatocytosis,[28-33] microangiopathic hemolytic anemias,[34-40] pyruvate kinase deficiency,[41] and possibly malaria.[42,43] Additionally, certain other conditions are associated with both intravascular hemolysis and risk of pulmonary hypertension, such as schistosomiasis,[44,45] and iatrogenic hemolysis from mechanical heart valves,[46,47] left ventricular assist devices, and cardiopulmonary bypass procedures.[48-52]

Epidemiology

Echocardiographic studies performed at tertiary care sickle cell disease centers have reported that 20-30 percent of screened adult patients with sickle cell anemia have pulmonary hypertension (mean pulmonary artery pressure [mPAP] = 25 mmHg).[7,8] More recent autopsy studies suggest that up to 75 percent of patients with sickle cell disease have histologic evidence of PAH at the time of death.[11] Similarly, retrospective studies have demonstrated that 40-50 percent of patients with thalassemia intermedia[23] and 10-75 percent of patients with thalassemia major have echocardiographic evidence of pulmonary hypertension.[18,20,22] Although there are no formal epidemiologic data on the prevalence of PAH in other hemolytic disorders, several case series of PAH have been reported in patients with other inherited or acquired hemolytic disorders.[26-41,44-52] Of note, a number of studies suggest that

PAH may be more common in patients with thalassemia intermedia and E thalassemia than in patients with thalassemia major. This observation emphasizes the importance of chronic hemolysis in PAH pathogenesis, because patients with thalassemia major are transfused repeatedly and have minimal intravascular hemolysis[125].

Patients with sickle cell disease and PAH exhibit a significantly increased mortality rate compared with patients without PAH. They survive only short periods after being diagnosed. Sutton and colleagues reported a 40 percent mortality rate after 22 months with an odds ratio for death of 7.86 when pulmonary hypertension was present.[7] Powars and colleagues reported a mean 2.5-year survival in sickle cell patients with chronic lung disease with pulmonary hypertension.[6] Castro and colleagues[12] similarly reported a 50 percent 2-year mortality rate in patients with sickle cell disease with pulmonary hypertension confirmed by right heart catheterization.

These data are consistent with the results of a National Institutes of Health (NIH) PAH screening study in patients with sickle cell disease.[14] This effort enrolled 195 adult patients with sickle cell disease who were screened with transthoracic Doppler echocardiography, and the tricuspid regurgitant jet velocity (TRV) was used to estimate the pulmonary artery systolic pressure. The Doppler echocardiogram can be used to measure the velocity of regurgitant blood across the tricuspid valve using the modified Bernoulli equation ($4 \times TRV^2$ plus central venous pressure estimate) in order to calculate the pulmonary artery systolic pressure (the method is described in detail elsewhere).[14] To avoid the more subjective estimation of central venous pressure in this study, pulmonary hypertension was defined prospectively by a specific Doppler TRV value of greater than or equal to 2.5 m/sec, and moderate to severe pulmonary hypertension defined by a TRV greater than or equal to 3.0 m/sec. Right heart catheterization was performed in consenting patients with TRV greater than or equal to 2.8 m/sec. Of patients with sickle cell disease, 32 percent had elevated pulmonary artery systolic pressures (defined TRV ≥ 2.5 m/sec), and 9 percent had moderate to severe pressure elevations (defined TRV ≥ 3.0 m/sec).

Univariate statistical analysis of the NIH cohort found that markers of hemolytic anemia, including reduced hemoglobin concentration and hematocrit, elevated aspartate aminotransferase but not alanine aminotransferase levels, and elevated lactate dehydrogenase (LDH) levels, were associated with elevated pulmonary artery pressures.

Increasing age was also a univariate predictor of a high TRV, and patients with PAH were significantly older than patients without PAH. Multiple logistic regression analysis identified a history of renal or cardiovascular complications, increased systemic systolic blood pressure, elevated plasma LDH alkaline phosphatase values, and reduced serum transferrin levels as independent predictors of PAH. In men, a history of priapism was also an independent associated factor.

These associations suggest that PAH represents a component of the systemic vasculopathy of sickle cell disease (systemic hypertension, renal failure, and priapism) and is mechanistically linked to hemolytic rate, iron overload, and cholestatic hepatic dysfunction. Interestingly, PAH was not associated with markers of inflammation, fetal hemoglobin level, or platelet count.

Consistent with retrospective studies suggesting that PAH is associated with a higher mortality, a measured TRV of at least 2.5 m/sec (as compared with a velocity of less than 2.5 m/sec) was associated with a marked increased risk of death (RR 10.1; 95 percent CI, 2.2-47; P < .001) and remained so after adjustment for other risk factors in proportional hazards regression analysis. The 18-month mortality was 16 percent for patients with a TRV of greater than or equal to 2.5 m/sec, but was less than 2 percent in patients without PAH. Follow-up data from this cohort continue to demonstrate that PAH is a strong independent risk factor for mortality, with a 40-month mortality rate of approximately 40 percent (FIGURE 12-1).

Similar results were reported in another prospective study of 60 patients systematically sampled at a comprehensive sickle cell treatment center, where the prevalence of PAH was 30 percent.[15] Other investigators have found a similar prevalence of PAH and a remarkably similar 17 percent 2-year mortality rate for such patients compared with approximately 2 percent for patients without PAH.[53] Taken together, the retrospective[6,7,12] and prospective studies[14,53,54] strongly support the hypothesis that PAH is the greatest risk factor facing the aging population of patients with sickle cell disease, as well as patients with other chronic hemolytic disorders.

Pathogenesis

Although the various hemolytic diseases have many unique clinical manifestations, the etiology of PAH in individuals with hemolytic disorders

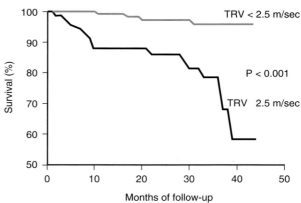

Figure 12-1. Kaplan-Meier Survival Curves According to the Tricuspid Regurgitant Jet Velocity. The survival rate is significantly higher among patients with a tricuspid regurgitant jet velocity of less than 2.5 meters per second than among those with a tricuspid regurgitant jet velocity of at least 2.5 meters per second (P < .001). (Updated from Gladwin MT, Sachdev V, Jison ML, et al: Pulmonary hypertension as a risk factor for death in patients with sickle cell disease. *N Engl J Med* 350(9):886-895, 2004, in April 2005.)

likely reflects mechanisms shared by all disorders. These are likely to include hemolysis, producing endothelial dysfunction and oxidant and inflammatory stress, chronic hypoxemia with activation of proliferative mediators, chronic thromboembolism and *in situ* thrombosis, chronic liver disease, iron overload, and asplenia (FIGURE 12-2).

Hemolysis

An apparent central process in PAH development is chronic intravascular hemolysis.[4,14,55,56] Cell-free plasma hemoglobin destroys nitric oxide at a rate 1,000-fold faster than does intraerythrocytic hemoglobin.[57-59] As a result of hemolysis, hemoglobin is released into plasma where it reacts with and destroys nitric oxide, resulting in abnormally high rates of nitric oxide consumption and a state of resistance to nitric oxide activity.[56,56b] Consequently, smooth muscle guanylyl cyclase is not activated and vasodilation is inhibited. In support of this mechanism, plasma from patients with sickle cell disease contains cell-free ferrous hemoglobin, which stoichiometrically consumes micromolar quantities of nitric oxide and abrogates forearm blood flow responses to nitric oxide donor infusions. Furthermore, oxidation of the plasma hemoglobin by therapeutic nitric oxide

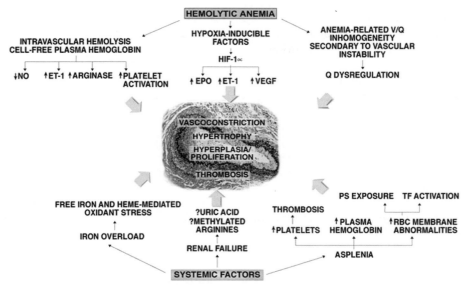

Figure 12-2. Pathogenesis of Pulmonary Arterial Hypertension in Patients With Hemolytic Disorders. The vessel shown in the figure is an autopsy specimen from a 55-year-old male with sickle cell disease and pulmonary arterial hypertension and demonstrates the intimal and medial pulmonary arterial proliferative vasculopathy characteristic of the disease. *EPO,* erythropoietin; *ET-1,* endothelin-1; *HIF,* hypoxia inducible factor; *NO,* nitric oxide; *PS,* phosphatidylserine; *TF,* tissue factor; *VEGF,* vascular endothelial growth factor. (Reproduced with permission from Machado RF, Gladwin MT: Chronic sickle cell lung disease: New insights into the diagnosis, pathogenesis and treatment of pulmonary hypertension. *Br J Haematol* 129(4):449-464, 2005.)

gas inhalation restores nitric oxide bioavailability.[56,56b,60] As such, plasma hemoglobin-free and oxygen-free radical–mediated consumption of nitric oxide produces a state of resistance to nitric oxide in patients with sickle cell disease.[56,58,61-65]

Downstream effects of hemolytic anemia include increased endothelin-1 expression, heme-mediated and free iron–mediated oxygen radical generation, platelet activation, and increased endothelial adhesion molecule expression.[4,56,66-68] In patients with sickle cell disease, plasma endothelin-1 levels are increased in steady state and during crisis.[69,70] *In vitro,* sickled erythrocytes increase endothelin-1 production by cultured human endothelial cells,[71,72] and endothelin receptor A antagonism abrogates the vasoconstrictive effects of conditioned media from pulmonary endothelial cells exposed to sickled erythrocytes on aortic rings.[69] In addition, endothelin-1 activates Gardos channels in human sickle erythrocytes, an effect that may promote sickle cell dehydration and facilitate red blood cell sickling and adhesion.[73]

Intravascular hemolysis also has the potential to promote a procoagulant state. Platelet activation is profoundly inhibited by nitric oxide and such

nitric oxide-dependent inhibition may in turn be blocked by plasma hemoglobin-mediated nitric oxide scavenging.[74-77] Additionally, hemolytic anemia is associated with hemoglobin desaturation and ventilation-perfusion inhomogeneity;[68,78] it is possible that such a hypoxic state can induce hypoxia-inducible factor-1-dependent factors such as erythropoietin, vascular endothelial growth factor, and endothelin. These mediators may produce a proliferative vasculopathy in the lung and other organs, such as the kidney.

In addition to hemoglobin decompartmentalization, hemolysis releases erythrocyte arginase, which converts L-arginine, the substrate for nitric oxide synthesis, to ornithine.[79–82,82b] Consistent with this observation, the arginine-to-ornithine ratio decreases significantly as pulmonary pressures increase in patients with sickle cell disease.[14,82b]

Asplenia

Functional or surgical asplenia may also contribute to PAH development in patients with hemolytic disorders. Splenectomy has been reported as a risk factor for pulmonary hypertension,[83] particularly among patients with hemolytic disorders.[25,30,41] It has been speculated that the loss of splenic function increases the circulation of platelet-derived mediators and that senescent and abnormal erythrocytes in the circulation trigger platelet activation, promoting pulmonary microthrombosis and red blood cell adhesion to the endothelium.[84] Intravenous injection of hemolysate promotes the formation of platelet-rich thrombi in the pulmonary vascular bed of rabbits after ligation of the splenic artery, whereas no thrombus formation was observed among animals without splenic artery ligation.[85]

A role for intensification of intravascular hemolysis by splenectomy has also been suggested by the demonstration of significantly higher plasma hemoglobin and erythrocyte-derived microvesicle levels in patients with thalassemia intermedia who have undergone splenectomy versus patients with the disease who have not had the procedure.[86] It is likely that the spleen subserves a critical function in the removal of senescent and damaged erythrocytes and that following splenectomy the rate of intravascular hemolysis increases, with secondary increases in plasma hemoglobin and red blood cell membranes with exposed phosphatidylserine.[87]

Hypoxia

In patients with sickle cell disease, chronic lung injury as a consequence of infection, bronchoconstriction, fat embolism, and undetected episodes of regional pulmonary hypoxia (resulting in sickling, increased vascular adhesion, and the production of vasoactive substances) may lead to chronic pulmonary fibrosis, disregulated vascular tone, vascular proliferation, regional hypoxia, and a consequent pulmonary vasculopathy. Interestingly, however, the number of episodes of acute chest syndrome (a potential cause of chronic lung disease and pulmonary fibrosis) was not associated with PAH in the NIH prospective prevalence study.[14] In addition, a similar prevalence of PAH in patients with thalassemia intermedia, who do not develop the acute chest syndrome, suggests that although acute lung injury may worsen pulmonary hypertension, it is not etiologic.

Interestingly, individuals with pulmonary hypertension have a higher incidence of restrictive lung disease and pulmonary fibrosis found with high-resolution chest computed tomography than age-matched and hemoglobin-matched patients with sickle cell disease but without PAH (Anthi

et al, manuscript in preparation). Restrictive ventilatory defects and pulmonary fibrosis have also been documented in patients with thalassemia.[88,89] Taken together, these data suggest that similar pathogenic proliferative mechanisms that lead to PAH may underlie the genesis of pulmonary fibrosis in these patients (see FIGURE 12-2).

Thrombosis

A hypercoagulable state, including relatively reduced levels of protein C and S, elevated levels of thrombin-antithrombin complexes and D-dimers, and increased activation of tissue factor, is observed in patients with sickle cell disease.[90-96] This hypercoagulable state may promote vascular obstruction. *In situ* thrombosis is observed in patients with idiopathic pulmonary arterial hypertension (IPAH) and in those with sickle cell disease.[97-99] Pulmonary thromboembolism is reported in patients with sickle cell disease,[98] thalassemia,[100] pyruvate kinase deficiency,[41] hereditary spherocytosis,[28,30] paroxysmal nocturnal hemoglobinuria,[27,101] and hereditary stomatocytosis.[29,31,32] However, differentiation between *in situ* and embolic thrombosis is not always explicit in these reports. Autopsy studies in patients with sickle cell disease suggest that much of the observed thrombosis is *in situ*, similar to what occurs in other forms PAH.[11] Whether thrombosis occurs secondary to preexisting PAH or serves as an initiating or propagating factor in its development is a subject of study (FIGURE 12-2).

Clinical Manifestations

Diagnosing PAH in patients with chronic hemolytic disorders can be challenging. Unlike those with IPAH, patients with sickle cell disease and other hemolytic disorders have multiorgan complications of their disease that limit exercise tolerance independent of elevations in pulmonary vascular resistance. As an example, exertional dyspnea, the most typical symptom of PAH, is also a cardinal symptom of chronic anemia. More specific symptoms such as angina, syncope, and lower extremity edema are uncommon and usually are associated with severe and advanced PAH, as are physical findings suggestive of right ventricular dysfunction such as jugular venous distention, right ventricular S_3 gallop, an accentuated pulmonary component of S_2, ascites, and peripheral edema. We have observed a high

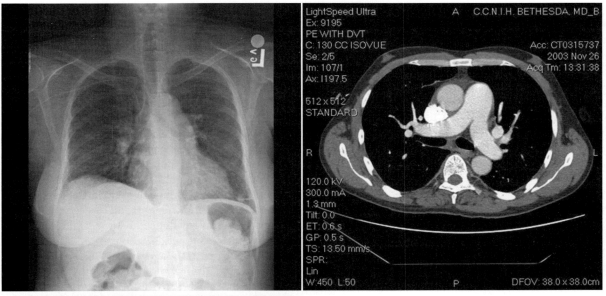

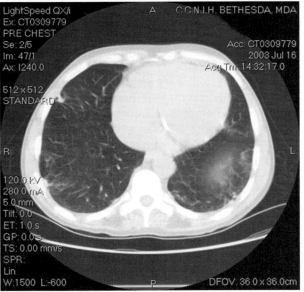

Figure 12-3. Radiographic Features of Sickle Cell Disease and Pulmonary Arterial Hypertension. **A,** Chest radiograph demonstrating enlargement of main pulmonary arteries and mild basilar pulmonary fibrosis. **B,** Enlargement of pulmonary arteries in severe PAH. **C,** Mild pulmonary fibrosis typical of patients with sickle cell disease and PAH.

prevalence of clubbing in sickle cell and thalassemia patients with PAH. Other conditions commonly present in these patients, such as left ventricular systolic or diastolic dysfunction, pulmonary fibrosis, and cirrhosis of the liver, can manifest in a similar fashion and but also contribute to pulmonary hypertension.

Patients with sickle cell disease and PAH tend to be older, have higher systolic arterial blood pressure, lower hemoglobin levels, higher indices of hemolysis, lower arterial oxyhemoglobin saturation, a greater degree of renal and liver dysfunction, and a higher number of lifetime red blood cell transfusions,[14] suggesting a greater burden of sickle cell disease and a generalized vasculopathy associated with chronic intravascular hemolysis.

In contrast to patients with traditional forms of PAH (e.g., IPAH or PAH associated with scleroderma), patients with chronic hemolytic disorders and PAH become symptomatic at a mild-to-moderate degree of elevation in pulmonary pressures (TABLE 12-1). Another peculiar finding seen in these patients is mild elevations in pulmonary capillary wedge pressure, a finding not seen in other forms of PAH, in which the pulmonary capillary wedge pressure is normal ($\leq$15 mmHg). This raises the question of a potential contribution of left-sided heart disease, in particular diastolic dysfunction and high-output biventricular failure, to the development of

TABLE 12-1

Hemodynamic Profiles in Patients With Sickle Cell Disease

	Without PAH	With PAH
PA systolic (mmHg)	31 ± 1	54 ± 2
PA diastolic (mmHg)	12 ± 1	26 ± 1
PA mean (mmHg)	19 ± 1	36 ± 1
RAP (mmHg)	8 ± 2	12 ± 1
PCWP (mmHg)	10 ± 1	17 ± 0.9
CO (L/min)	9 ± 0.8	9 ± 0.4
PVR (dynes/sec/cm⁻⁵)	93 ± 19	184 ± 26

CO, *cardiac output;* PA, *pulmonary artery;* PCWP, *pulmonary capillary wedge pressure;* PVR, *pulmonary vascular resistance;* RAP, *right atrial pressure.*
Reproduced with permission from Machado RF, Gladwin MT: *Chronic sickle cell lung disease: New insights into the diagnosis, pathogenesis and treatment of pulmonary hypertension.* Br J Haematol 129(4):449-464, 2005.

pulmonary hypertension. Although it has been observed that measures of left ventricular systolic and diastolic dysfunction were not associated with elevated pulmonary artery systolic pressures or mortality in patients with sickle cell disease and PAH,[14] it remains possible that there is a concomitant element of left-sided disease in a subgroup of affected patients.

It is important to emphasize that pulmonary hypertension in patients with sickle cell disease and other hemolytic diseases is clearly a different disorder than other forms of PAH because of the presence of chronic anemia, which requires a resting high cardiac output (usually around 10 L/min) to compensate for a decrease in blood oxygen carrying capacity. It is likely that in patients with critical anemia, any degree of PAH is poorly tolerated and results in significant morbidity and possibly mortality. Consistent with this hypothesis are the results of a study evaluating the cardiopulmonary function of patients with sickle cell disease.[102] When compared with age, gender, and hemoglobin-matched patients with sickle cell disease without PAH, individuals with PAH and mean pulmonary artery pressure of 36 mmHg had a significantly shorter mean 6-minute walk distance (427 meters versus 308 meters) and a very low peak oxygen consumption during cardiopulmonary exercise testing. In comparison, in a randomized trial evaluating the effects of the selective endothelin antagonist sitaxsentan in patients with idiopathic collagen vascular disease or intracardiac shunt-related PAH with mean pulmonary artery pressure of 54 mmHg, the mean baseline 6-minute walk distance was

398 meters.[103] Taken together these data suggest that in patients with chronic anemia, mild to moderate PAH has a severe adverse impact on functional and aerobic exercise capacity.

Diagnostic Evaluation

A unique feature of sickle cell disease, thalassemia, and possibly other hemolytic disorders that is also shared by patients with scleroderma, is the extremely high prevalence of PAH in the population (approximately one-third of all patients). Considering this high prevalence and the high associated mortality, universal echocardiographic screening of all adults with hemolytic disorders is generally recommended. In the case of sickle cell disease, it is important that such screening be performed in the absence of exacerbations or crises, because pressures rise during vaso-occlusive painful crises.[104]

Diagnostic evaluation of patients with hemolytic disorders suspected of having PAH should follow the same guidelines established for other causes of PAH.[105,106] We will review specific aspects of the diagnostic workup that are particularly relevant to patients with hemolytic disorders.

Symptom Evaluation and Functional Assessment

Quantification of the degree of symptomatic exercise limitation should be evaluated with the World Health Organization classification and could be used in evaluating response to therapy. The most commonly used exercise test in patients with PAH is the 6-minute walk test. Although this test has not been validated extensively in patients with hemolytic disorders, we have presented preliminary data in patients with sickle cell disease demonstrating that the 6-minute walk distance correlates directly with peak oxygen consumption and inversely with the degree of PAH, and that the 6-minute walk distance improves with therapy, suggesting that the test could be used in this patient population.[102] A recent study of sildenafil in patients with thalassemia also demonstrates improvement in 6-minute walk distance.[107]

Laboratory Tests

Minimally required tests to exclude other associated conditions include serologic testing to screen for collagen vascular disorders, human immunodeficiency virus, viral hepatitis, and liver function testing. In addition, the severity of iron-overload and hemolytic anemia should be assessed, because these are important comorbidities that require management.

Transthoracic Doppler Echocardiography

Doppler echocardiography provides essential information such as noninvasive estimation of pulmonary artery systolic pressure, valvular function, and right and left ventricular function (FIGURE 12-4). The use of echocardiography to estimate pulmonary artery systolic pressures has been validated in patients with sickle cell disease, and noninvasive assessment correlates reasonably well with the measurement of pulmonary arterial pressures by right heart catheterization.[14]

Because an elevated TRV also is seen with left-sided heart failure, the echocardiogram must be scrutinized for important information about left ventricular systolic dysfunction (observed in 2 percent of patients in the NIH cohort) and diastolic dysfunction (observed in 15 percent of patients in the NIH cohort). We have also observed increases in pulmonary artery pressures in these patients associated with mild exercise and vaso-occlusive painful crisis.[104]

It is important to recognize that patients with normal resting pulmonary pressures can have abnormal elevations in their pressures during exercise. For this reason, we recommend an exercise echocardiogram with assessment of pulmonary pressures to evaluate patients with significant exertional dyspnea and normal resting TRVs.

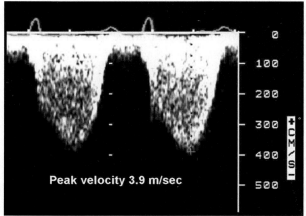

Figure 12-4. Tricuspid Regurgitant Jet Velocity and Pulmonary Artery Systolic Pressure Estimation by Doppler Echocardiogram.

Although the criteria for an abnormal response to exercise are not well established, in healthy untrained men TRV increases from an average baseline of 1.72 m/sec to an average of 2.46 m/sec at mid-level exercise and to 2.27 m/sec at peak exercise (240 W).[108]

Pulmonary Function Testing

Most adult patients with sickle cell disease develop abnormal pulmonary function characterized by restrictive lung disease, abnormal diffusing capacity, and hypoxemia.[6,109-113] In patients with thalassemia, restrictive ventilatory defects and pulmonary fibrosis have also been documented.[88,89] However, the degree of pulmonary function abnormalities in these patients is rarely severe enough to be a major contributor to their pulmonary hypertension.

Ventilation-perfusion Lung Scintigraphy

The lung ventilation-perfusion scan (FIGURE 12-5) is an indispensable component of the evaluation, because chronic thromboembolic pulmonary hypertension is a potential curable cause of pulmonary hypertension, and it can develop in patients with chronic hemolytic disorders. In our experience, however, scintigraphic evidence of thromboembolic disease has been unusual, and the most commonly observed abnormalities are patchy areas of abnormal perfusion, similar to nonspecific findings described in other forms of pulmonary hypertension.

Chronic thromboembolic pulmonary hypertension has been managed surgically with success in patients with sickle cell disease[114] and hereditary stomatocytosis.[32] As such, patients should undergo imaging studies and, if suggestive of chronic thromboembolic pulmonary hypertension, should undergo conventional angiography to determine is surgically manageable disease is present.

Screening Nocturnal and Exercise Oximetry

Severe sleep apnea syndrome that causes frequent episodes of nocturnal desaturation can lead to the development of pulmonary hypertension, and oximetry can provide clues to the diagnosis. More importantly, nighttime oxygen desaturation is a well-documented entity in children and adolescents with sickle cell disease.[115-117] Several lines of evidence suggest that nocturnal hypoxemia contributes to neurologic events and vaso-occlusive

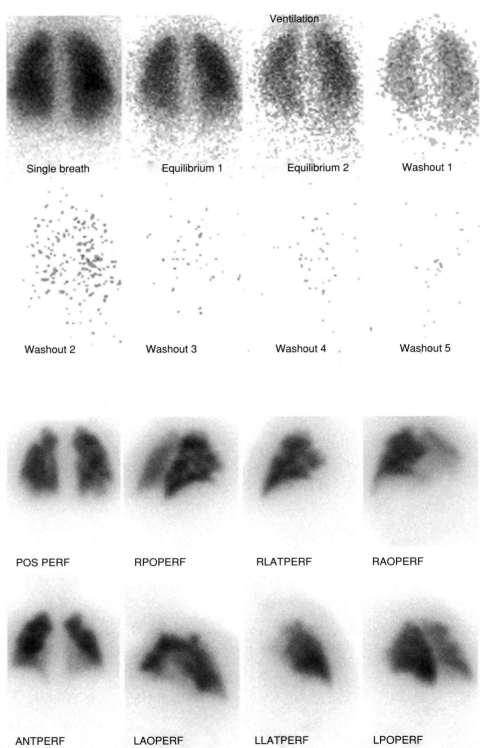

Ventilation

Single breath Equilibrium 1 Equilibrium 2 Washout 1

Washout 2 Washout 3 Washout 4 Washout 5

POS PERF RPOPERF RLATPERF RAOPERF

ANTPERF LAOPERF LLATPERF LPOPERF

Figure 12-5. Ventilation-perfusion Lung Scan in a Patient With Sickle Cell Disease and Pulmonary Arterial Hypertension. Although there are no discrete perfusion defects suggestive of thromboembolic disease, the perfusion scan demonstrates patchy areas of abnormal perfusion characteristically similar to those observed in patients with IPAH.

crisis via mechanisms that could involve upregulation of several cell-adhesion mediators.[68,116,118] These effects could also play a role in the vasculopathy associated with PAH. Several epidemiologic studies have linked hemolytic rate and low resting hemoglobin oxygen saturation, suggesting that hemolytic anemia may act to produce ventilation-perfusion heterogeneity.[68,119]

Right Heart Catheterization

Right heart catheterization is required to confirm the diagnosis and assess the severity of pulmonary hypertension, while excluding other contributors, such as left atrial hypertension. In our practice we routinely catheterize symptomatic patients with TRVs of 2.9 m/sec or greater. It is important to exclude by right heart catheterization diastolic or systolic left ventricular dysfunction as an independent cause of pulmonary hypertension or as a comorbidity. Although the pulmonary capillary wedge pressure has been reported to be high in patients with sickle cell disease and thalassemia, even in the absence of left ventricular dysfunction, an increased gradient between the pulmonary capillary wedge pressure and the pulmonary artery diastolic pressure (of 8 mmHg or greater) with an absolute pulmonary capillary wedge pressure of less than or equal to 18 mmHg supports the diagnosis of intrinsic pulmonary vascular disease. In our experience, approximately 50 percent of catheterized patients have PAH without diastolic dysfunction, 35 percent have a combination of diastolic dysfunction and PAH (evidenced by an elevated wedge pressure in association with an elevated pulmonary artery diastolic–to–wedge pressure gradient), and 15 percent have pure diastolic dysfunction.

Uncontrolled studies in patients with IPAH suggest that long-term treatment with calcium channel blockers prolongs survival in the small subgroup of patients who respond acutely to short-acting pulmonary vasodilators, such as inhaled nitric oxide, adenosine, or prostacyclin. The definition of a positive acute response includes a 10 mmHg decrease in mean pulmonary arterial pressure to reach a mean pulmonary artery pressure of less than or equal to 40 mmHg. The role of acute vasodilator challenge, however, is not established in patients with hemolytic diseases. Although acute vasodilator testing may be useful for prognostic information, we do not use calcium channel blockers in this population.

Management

There are limited data on the specific treatment of patients with hemolytic disorders and PAH. Most of the recommendations are based on expert opinion or extrapolated from data derived from other forms of PAH. Our general approach usually includes maximal treatment of the underlying hemoglobinopathy of sickle cell disease, management of associated cardiopulmonary conditions, and targeted therapy with pulmonary vasodilator-antiremodeling agents (FIGURE 12-6).

Maximal Management of Sickle Cell Disease

In sickle cell disease, a role for chronic intravascular hemolysis as a central mechanism in the development of PAH is supported by a correlation between markers of increased hemolytic rate and severity of PAH. Based on this observation, it is

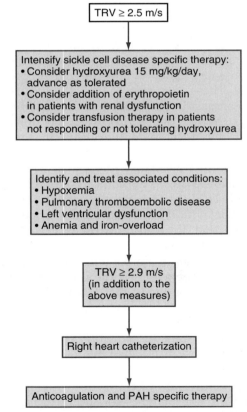

Figure 12-6. Treatment Algorithm in Patients With Sickle Cell Disease and Pulmonary Arterial Hypertension.

likely that maximization of standard managements targeted at decreasing hemolytic rate is beneficial.

As such, we recommend that all patients with sickle cell disease and PAH undergo maximization of therapy with hydroxyurea or simple exchange transfusions. Hydroxyurea decreases hemolytic rate, increases hemoglobin levels, decreased transfusion requirements, and decreases pain, incidence of acute chest syndrome, and overall mortality.[120,121] It is possible that some of the benefits seen in pulmonary and cardiovascular deaths could be related to an improvement in PAH. For patients with creatinine levels less than 1.0 g/dl, hydroxyurea usually is started at a dose of 15 mg/kg/day rounded to the nearest 500-mg tablet. Patients with renal dysfunction tend to tolerate poorly the myelosuppressant effects of hydroxyurea. In this situation, we recommend the addition of erythropoietin to the regimen.

Long-term transfusion therapy in patients with sickle cell disease reduces the synthesis of sickle cells and their pathologic effects. The risks of most complications of the disease are reduced, including the risks of pulmonary events and central nervous system vasculopathy.[122-124] It is also possible that exchange transfusion, targeted to a hemoglobin level of 10-12 g/dl and a hemoglobin S level of less than 30 percent, might improve cardiopulmonary function and prevent progression of PAH. These data have to be balanced with the lack of association between fetal hemoglobin levels and the use of hydroxyurea, and protection against the development of PAH in the NIH cohort study.[14]

Long-term transfusion therapy in severe thalassemia has changed the clinical course of the disease and is likely to have a favorable impact in individuals with PAH. This thesis is supported by a report that in well-transfused, iron-chelated patients with thalassemia major, PAH was prevented completely.[125] In patients with paroxysmal nocturnal hemoglobinuria, the use of eculizumab (a monoclonal antibody that blocks the cleavage of the complement component C5 and thus prevents complement-mediated red blood cell lysis) resulted in a dramatic reduction in intravascular hemolysis,[126] suggesting that this agent could be of benefit in patients with paroxysmal nocturnal hemoglobinuria and PAH.

Even if these therapies do not lower hemolytic rates sufficiently to prevent vasculopathy, a higher hemoglobin level and higher oxygen-carrying capacity are likely to reduce morbidity and possibly mortality by preventing comorbid events.

Management of Associated Conditions

An aggressive search for associated conditions such as iron overload, chronic liver disease (e.g., iron overload or viral hepatitis), human immunodeficiency virus infection, nocturnal hypoxemia, and thromboembolic disorders should always be undertaken because of the availability of specific therapies. Oxygen desaturation, especially unrecognized nocturnal hypoxemia, should be evaluated in patients with sickle cell disease.[68,116,118]

There is evidence of a beneficial mortality effect of warfarin anticoagulation in patients with IPAH, based on retrospective analyses.[127-129] The potential benefits of warfarin have to be weighed against the risk of hemorrhagic stroke in adults with sickle cell disease or hemorrhage in chronically anemic individuals. In the case of patients with sickle cell disease, we believe that the relatively low risk of hemorrhagic stroke (0.21 events per 100 patient years[130]) compared with the high risk of death in patients with TRVs greater than or equal to 3.0 m/sec (16-50 percent 2-year mortality[12,14,55]) supports the use of anticoagulation in such patients unless a specific contraindication is present.

Therapy Specific to PAH

There are limited data on the specific efficacy of selective pulmonary vasodilator-remodeling pharmacologic agents in patients with hemolytic disorders. Considering that there are likely 15,000-20,000 patients in the United States with sickle cell disease-associated PAH, compared with an estimated 15,000 patients with all other forms of PAH, a concerted effort to evaluate these drugs in this population is indicated. Similarly, thalassemic disorders are a major public health problem in the Middle East and Southeast Asia, as well as in the United States. As an example, the World Health Organization estimates that in Thailand more than 250,000 symptomatic patients will be diagnosed with thalassemia over the next few decades. At least 100,000 new cases of hemoglobin E β-thalassemia are expected.[131] There are an estimated 30 million people in Africa and 80 million people in Asia living with chronic hemolytic disorders. As such, hemolytic anemia may represent the most common cause of PAH in the world.

There is well-documented evidence for the beneficial effects of therapy with prostanoids,[132] endothelin antagonists,[133] and phosphodiesterase 5 inhibitors[134,134b] in patients with IPAH and related disorders. There are no long-term data on the specific management of PAH in patients with hemolytic disorders, and the choice of agents at this juncture is largely empiric and based on the safety profile of the drugs and physician preference.

Nonetheless, there are specific concerns regarding the use of these drugs in patients with hemolytic diseases:

- The systemic use of prostanoids produces significant systemic vasodilation and increases in cardiac output, raising the concern for potential high-output heart failure in anemic patients. In addition, the risk of chronic intravenous line-related complications such as thrombosis and sepsis is likely higher in patients with sickle cell disease.
- The main toxicity of endothelin-1 receptor antagonists is hepatocellular injury, which could limit their applicability in these patients who are at risk for liver dysfunction (e.g., iron overload, hepatitis C). Another class effect of these agents is a dosage-related decrease in hemoglobin levels usually in the range of 1.0 g/dl.[103]
- A concern related to the use of sildenafil and other phosphodiesterase 5 inhibitors by men with sickle cell disease is the potential for priapism.

Because alterations in nitric oxide bioavailability are likely to be involved in the pathogenesis of the PAH associated with chronic hemolytic disorders, therapeutic interventions that enhance nitric oxide effects, such as inhaled nitric oxide, L-arginine, and sildenafil, may be of benefit (FIGURE 12-7). Long-term inhaled nitric oxide could be beneficial because of its ability to selectively dilate the pulmonary vasculature and oxidatively inactivate

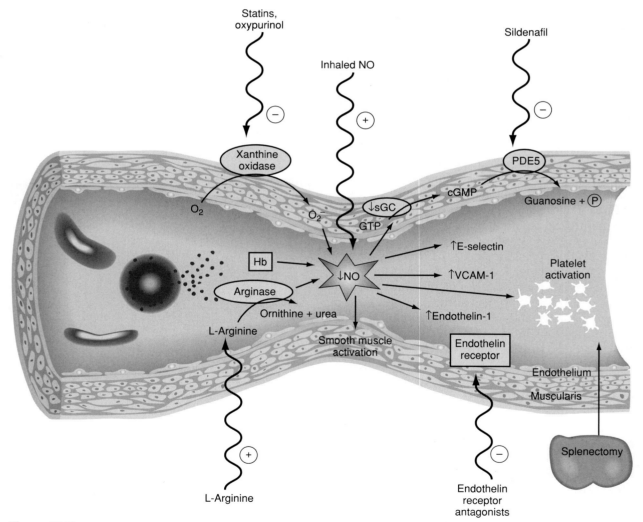

Figure 12-7. Therapeutic Targets in Hemolysis-associated Pulmonary Arterial Hypertension. (Reproduced with permission from Lin EE, Gladwin MT, Machado RF: Pulmonary hypertension in patients with hemoglobinopathies: Could a mechanism for dysfunction provide an avenue for novel therapeutics? *Haematologica* 90(4):441-444, 2005.)

circulating plasma hemoglobin.[56b] However, the long-term use of inhaled nitric oxide is investigational, potentially expensive, and requires relatively complicated delivery systems.[135]

L-arginine is a nitrogen donor for the production of nitric oxide by nitric oxide synthase. When given for 5 days to 10 patients with sickle cell disease and moderate to severe PAH, L-arginine (0.1 g/kg 3 times daily) decreased estimated pulmonary artery systolic pressure by a mean of 15 percent, suggesting that it may have a role in the long-term management of PAH in sickle cell disease.[81] In one case series,[107] seven patients with either thalassemia intermedia (n = 4), thalassemia major (n = 2), or sickle thalassemia (n = 1), and severe PAH with mean tricuspid regurgitant gradients of 45 mmHg at rest, were treated with sildenafil 50 mg twice daily for a period ranging from 4 weeks to 48 months. The tricuspid gradient decreased in all patients, and functional status as defined by World Health Organization class and 6-minute walk test improved. Sildenafil was well tolerated without any significant hemodynamic adverse effects, and there was no priapism observed in the one patient who had sickle cell disease. Sildenafil use also resulted in symptomatic improvement and near normalization of pulmonary pressures in one patient with thalassemia intermedia.[136]

The NIH experience with sildenafil in patients with sickle cell disease and PAH included the treatment of 12 patients (9 females and 3 males) with mean estimated pulmonary artery systolic pressure of 51 mmHg (mean TRV of 3.1 m/sec) for a mean of 6 months. Sildenafil therapy was associated with a 10-mmHg decrease in estimated pulmonary artery systolic pressure and a 78-meter improvement in 6-minute walk distance, an effect similar to that observed in a case series of sildenafil in other forms of PAH.[134b,137] Transient headaches occurred in two patients and transient periorbital edema occurred in four individuals. No episodes of priapism occurred in the three men enrolled in the study, but one male had prior erectile dysfunction and two males were on long-term exchange transfusion therapy.

We recommend specific pulmonary vasodilator-remodeling therapy for symptomatic patients with moderate to severe PAH (TRV of 2.9 m/sec or greater). Based on the lack of data from any long-term study we cannot recommend any specific agent, and the choice of regimen should be individualized to each patient. Careful monitoring for unanticipated adverse effects unique to this population is necessary. In patients with sickle cell disease, two multicenter clinical trials have begun or are planned: A trial of bosentan (Asset 1 and 2) and an NHLBI sponsored trial of sildenafil.

Conclusions and Future Directions

PAH is a common complication of adults with chronic hemolytic disorders that is associated with high morbidity and mortality. Based on this evidence, echocardiographic screening for PAH should be strongly considered in the adult patient population. Given the likely relationship between PAH and hemolysis, it is likely that intensification of hemoglobinopathy-specific therapy can limit the progression of the disease at its earliest stages and reduce the associated morbidity and mortality at later stages. In patients with more severe PAH, specific therapy with vasodilator-antiremodeling agents should be considered.

Further studies are necessary to understand fully the biology of PAH in patients with hemolytic disorders, such as the effects of mild elevations in pulmonary pressures on the cardiopulmonary function, mechanisms of increased mortality, and the contribution of the left ventricle to the elevations in pulmonary arterial pressures. Finally, large randomized trials evaluating the effects of specific therapy for PAH in these patients clearly are indicated.

References

1. Serjeant GR: Sickle-cell disease. *Lancet* 350:725-730, 1997.
2. Stuart MJ, Nagel RL: Sickle-cell disease. *Lancet* 364:1343-1360, 2004.
3. Weatherall DJ: The thalassaemias. *BMJ* 314:1675-1678, 1997.
4. Rother RP, Bell L, Hillmen P, et al: The clinical sequelae of intravascular hemolysis and extracellular plasma hemoglobin: A novel mechanism of human disease. *JAMA* 293:1653-1662, 2005.
5. Collins FS, Orringer EP: Pulmonary hypertension and cor pulmonale in the sickle hemoglobinopathies. *Am J Med* 73:814-821, 1982.
6. Powars D, Weidman JA, Odom-Maryon T, et al: Sickle cell chronic lung disease: Prior morbidity and the risk of pulmonary failure. *Medicine* 67:66-76, 1988.
7. Sutton LL, Castro O, Cross DJ, et al: Pulmonary hypertension in sickle cell disease. *Am J Cardiol* 74:626-628, 1994.
8. Castro O: Systemic fat embolism and pulmonary hypertension in sickle cell disease. *Hematol Oncol Clin North Am* 10:1289-1303, 1996.

9. Simmons BE, Santhanam V, Castaner A, et al: Sickle cell heart disease. Two-dimensional echo and Doppler ultrasonographic findings in the hearts of adult patients with sickle cell anemia. *Arch Intern Med* 148:1526-1528, 1988.

10. Aboubakr SE, Girgis R, Swerldow P: Pulmonary hypertension in sickle cell disease. *Am J Respir Crit Care Med* 160:A144, 1999 (abstract).

11. Haque AK, Gokhale S, Rampy BA, et al: Pulmonary hypertension in sickle cell hemoglobinopathy: A clinicopathologic study of 20 cases. *Hum Pathol* 33:1037-1043, 2002.

12. Castro O, Hoque M, Brown BD: Pulmonary hypertension in sickle cell disease: Cardiac catheterization results and survival. *Blood* 101:1257-1261, 2003.

13. Boussaada R, Boubaker K, Mourali S, et al: [Pulmonary hypertension in sickle cell anemia. A case report.] *Tunis Med* 82 Suppl 1:180-184, 2004.

14. Gladwin MT, Sachdev V, Jison ML, et al: Pulmonary hypertension as a risk factor for death in patients with sickle cell disease. *N Engl J Med* 350:886-895, 2004.

15. Ataga KI, Sood N, De Gent G, et al: Pulmonary hypertension in sickle cell disease. *Am J Med* 117:665-669, 2004.

16. Wu TJ, Tseng CD, Tseng YZ, et al: [A case of β-thalassemia major with mediastinal hematopoietic tumor and pulmonary hypertension.] *Taiwan Yi Xue Hui Za Zhi* 85:315-320, 1986.

17. Aessopos A, Stamatelos G, Skoumas V, et al: Pulmonary hypertension and right heart failure in patients with β-thalassemia intermedia. *Chest* 107:50-53, 1995.

18. Du ZD, Roguin N, Milgram E, et al: Pulmonary hypertension in patients with thalassemia major. *Am Heart J* 134:532-537, 1997.

19. Jootar P, Fucharoen S: Cardiac involvement in β-thalassemia/hemoglobin E disease: Clinical and hemodynamic findings. *Southeast Asian J Trop Med Public Health* 21:269-273, 1990.

20. Grisaru D, Rachmilewitz EA, Mosseri M, et al: Cardiopulmonary assessment in β-thalassemia major. *Chest* 98:1138-1142, 1990.

21. Finazzo M, Midiri M, D'Angelo P, et al: [The heart of the patient with β thalassemia major. Study with magnetic resonance.] *Radiol Med (Torino)* 96:462-465, 1998.

22. Derchi G, Fonti A, Forni GL, et al: Pulmonary hypertension in patients with thalassemia major. *Am Heart J* 138:384, 1999.

23. Aessopos A, Farmakis D, Karagiorga M, et al: Cardiac involvement in thalassemia intermedia: A multicenter study. *Blood* 97:3411-3416, 2001.

24. Zakynthinos E, Vassilakopoulos T, Kaltsas P, et al: Pulmonary hypertension, interstitial lung fibrosis, and lung iron deposition in thalassaemia major. *Thorax* 56:737-739, 2001.

25. Atichartakarn V, Likittanasombat K, Chuncharunee S, et al: Pulmonary arterial hypertension in previously splenectomized patients with β-thalassemic disorders. *Int J Hematol* 78:139-145, 2003.

26. Uchida T, Miyake T, Matsuno M, et al: Fatal pulmonary thromboembolism in a patient with paroxysmal nocturnal hemoglobinuria. *Rinsho Ketsueki* 39:150-152, 1998.

27. Heller PG, Grinberg AR, Lencioni M, et al: Pulmonary hypertension in paroxysmal nocturnal hemoglobinuria. *Chest* 102:642-643, 1992.

28. Verresen D, De Backer W, Van Meerbeeck J, et al: Spherocytosis and pulmonary hypertension coincidental occurrence or causal relationship? *Eur Respir J* 4:629-631, 1991.

29. Stewart GW, Amess JA, Eber SW, et al: Thromboembolic disease after splenectomy for hereditary stomatocytosis. *Br J Haematol* 93:303-310, 1996.

30. Hayag-Barin JE, Smith RE, Tucker FC, Jr: Hereditary spherocytosis, thrombocytosis, and chronic pulmonary emboli: A case report and review of the literature. *Am J Hematol* 57:82-84, 1998.

31. Jais X, Till SJ, Cynober T, et al: An extreme consequence of splenectomy in dehydrated hereditary stomatocytosis: Gradual thrombo-embolic pulmonary hypertension and lung-heart transplantation. *Hemoglobin* 27:139-147, 2003.

32. Murali B, Drain A, Seller D, et al: Pulmonary thromboendarterectomy in a case of hereditary stomatocytosis. *Br J Anaesth* 91:739-741, 2003.

33. Jardine DL, Laing AD: Delayed pulmonary hypertension following splenectomy for congenital spherocytosis. *Intern Med J* 34:214-216, 2004.

34. Stuard ID, Heusinkveld RS, Moss AJ: Microangiopathic hemolytic anemia and thrombocytopenia in primary pulmonary hypertension. *N Engl J Med* 287:869-870, 1972.

35. McCarthy JT, Staats BA: Pulmonary hypertension, hemolytic anemia, and renal failure. A mitomycin-associated syndrome. *Chest* 89:608-611, 1986.

36. Jubelirer SJ: Primary pulmonary hypertension. Its association with microangiopathic hemolytic anemia and thrombocytopenia. *Arch Intern Med* 151:1221-1223, 1991.

37. Suzuki H, Nakasato M, Sato S, et al: Microangiopathic hemolytic anemia and thrombocytopenia in a child with atrial septal defect and pulmonary hypertension. *Tohoku J Exp Med* 181:379-384, 1997.

38. Labrune P, Zittoun J, Duvaltier I, et al: Haemolytic uraemic syndrome and pulmonary hypertension in a patient with methionine synthase deficiency. *Eur J Pediatr* 158:734-739, 1999.

39. Fischer EG, Marek JM, Morris A, et al: Cholesterol granulomas of the lungs associated with micro-angiopathic hemolytic anemia and thrombocytopenia in pulmonary hypertension. *Arch Pathol Lab Med* 124:1813-1815, 2000.

40. Alvarez Navascues R, Marin R: [Severe maternal complications associated with pre-eclampsia: An almost forgotten pathology?] *Nefrologia* 21:565-573, 2001.

41. Chou R, DeLoughery TG: Recurrent thromboembolic disease following splenectomy for pyruvate kinase deficiency. *Am J Hematol* 67:197-199, 2001.

42. Huchzermeyer FW: Avian pulmonary hypertension syndrome. IV. Increased right ventricular mass in turkeys experimentally infected with *Plasmodium durae. Onderstepoort J Vet Res* 55:107-108, 1988.

43. Saissy JM, Rouvin B, Koulmann P: [Severe malaria in intensive care units in 2003.] *Med Trop (Mars)* 63:258-266, 2003.

44. Strauss E, Da Costa Gayotto LC, Antonelli R, et al: Systemic surgical shunts and splenomegaly as causes of haemolysis in portal hypertension in mansonic schistosomiasis. Evaluation through serum levels of haptoglobin, hemopexin and bilirubins. *J Hepatol* 2:340-350, 1986.

45. de Cleva R, Herman P, Pugliese V, et al: Prevalence of pulmonary hypertension in patients with hepatosplenic Mansonic schistosomiasis—prospective study. *Hepatogastroenterology* 50:2028-2030, 2003.

46. Kyllonen K, Mattila T, Hartikainen M, et al: Mitral valve replacement with ball and tilting disc valve prosthesis. A clinical and haemodynamic study. *Scand J Thorac Cardiovasc Surg* 10:15-20, 1976.

47. Iwaki H, Kuraoka S, Tatebe S: [Hemolytic anemia due to aortic valve regurgitation after mitral valve replacement.] *Kyobu Geka* 56:124-128, 2003.

48. Chukwuemeka AO, Turtle MR, Trivedi UH, et al: A clinical evaluation of platelet function, haemolysis and oxygen transfer during cardiopulmonary bypass comparing the Quantum HF-6700 to the HF-5700 hollow fibre membrane oxygenator. *Perfusion* 15:479-484, 2000.

49. Pierangeli A, Masieri V, Bruzzi F, et al: Haemolysis during cardiopulmonary bypass: How to reduce the free haemoglobin by managing the suctioned blood separately. *Perfusion* 16:519-524, 2001.

50. Gerrah R, Shargal Y, Elami A: Impaired oxygenation and increased hemolysis after cardiopulmonary bypass in patients with glucose-6-phosphate dehydrogenase deficiency. *Ann Thorac Surg* 76:523-527, 2003.

51. Philippidis P, Mason JC, Evans BJ, et al: Hemoglobin scavenger receptor CD163 mediates interleukin-10 release and heme oxygenase-1 synthesis: Antiinflammatory monocyte-macrophage responses *in vitro*, in resolving skin blisters *in vivo*, and after cardiopulmonary bypass surgery. *Circ Res* 94:119-126, 2004.

52. Takami Y, Makinouchi K, Nakazawa T, et al: Hemolytic characteristics of a pivot bearing supported Gyro centrifugal pump (C1E3) simulating various clinical applications. *Artif Organs* 20:1042-1049, 1996.

53. De Castro LM, Jonassiant JC, Graham FL, et al: Pulmonary hypertension in SS, SC and Sβ thalassemia: Prevalence, associated clinical syndromes, and mortality. *Blood* 104:462a, 2004.

54. Ataga K, Jones S, Olajide O, et al: The relationship of pulmonary hypertension and survival in sickle cell disease. *Blood* 104:463a, 2004.

55. Jison ML, Gladwin MT: Hemolytic anemia-associated pulmonary hypertension of sickle cell disease and the nitric oxide/arginine pathway. *Am J Respir Crit Care Med* 168:3-4, 2003.

56. Reiter CD, Wang X, Tanus-Santos JE, et al: Cell-free hemoglobin limits nitric oxide bioavailability in sickle-cell disease. *Nat Med* 8:1383-1389, 2002.

56b. Minneci PC, Deans KJ, Zhi H, et al. Hemolysis-associated endothelial dysfunction mediated by accelerated NO inactivation by decompartmentalized oxyhemoglobin. *J Clin Invest* 2005; 115:3409–17.

57. Gladwin MT, Crawford JH, Patel RP: The biochemistry of nitric oxide, nitrite, and hemoglobin: Role in blood flow regulation. *Free Radic Biol Med* 36:707-717, 2004.

58. Gladwin MT, Lancaster JR, Jr, Freeman BA, et al: Nitric oxide's reactions with hemoglobin: A view through the SNO-storm. *Nat Med* 9:496-500, 2003.

59. Schechter AN, Gladwin MT: Hemoglobin and the paracrine and endocrine functions of nitric oxide. *N Engl J Med* 348:1483-1485, 2003.

60. Gladwin MT, Schechter AN, Shelhamer JH, et al: Inhaled nitric oxide augments nitric oxide transport on sickle cell hemoglobin without affecting oxygen affinity. *J Clin Invest* 104:937-945, 1999.

61. Aslan M, Ryan TM, Adler B, et al: Oxygen radical inhibition of nitric oxide-dependent vascular function in sickle cell disease. *Proc Natl Acad Sci U S A* 98:15215-15220, 2001.

62. Aslan M, Ryan TM, Townes TM, et al: Nitric oxide-dependent generation of reactive species in sickle cell disease. Actin tyrosine induces defective cytoskeletal polymerization. *J Biol Chem* 278:4194-4204, 2003.

63. Eberhardt RT, McMahon L, Duffy SJ, et al: Sickle cell anemia is associated with reduced nitric oxide bioactivity in peripheral conduit and resistance vessels. *Am J Hematol* 74:104-111, 2003.

64. Nath KA, Katusic ZS, Gladwin MT: The perfusion paradox and vascular instability in sickle cell disease. *Microcirculation* 11:179-193, 2004.

65. Reiter CD, Gladwin MT: An emerging role for nitric oxide in sickle cell disease vascular homeostasis and therapy. *Curr Opin Hematol* 10:99-107, 2003.

66. Gladwin MT, Schechter AN, Ognibene FP, et al: Divergent nitric oxide bioavailability in men and women with sickle cell disease. *Circulation* 107:271-278, 2003.

67. Hebbel RP: Auto-oxidation and a membrane-associated "Fenton reagent": A possible explanation for development of membrane lesions in sickle erythrocytes. *Clin Haematol* 14:129-140, 1985.

68. Setty BN, Stuart MJ, Dampier C, et al: Hypoxaemia in sickle cell disease: Biomarker modulation and relevance to pathophysiology. *Lancet* 362:1450-1455, 2003.

69. Ergul S, Brunson CY, Hutchinson J, et al: Vasoactive factors in sickle cell disease: *In vitro* evidence for endothelin-1-mediated vasoconstriction. *Am J Hematol* 76:245-251, 2004.

70. Graido-Gonzalez E, Doherty JC, Bergreen EW, et al: Plasma endothelin-1, cytokine, and prostaglandin E2 levels in sickle cell disease and acute vaso-occlusive sickle crisis. *Blood* 92:2551-2555, 1998.

71. Phelan M, Perrine SP, Brauer M, et al: Sickle erythrocytes, after sickling, regulate the expression of the endothelin-1 gene and protein in human endothelial cells in culture. *J Clin Invest* 96:1145-1151, 1995.

72. Shiu YT, McIntire LV, Udden MM: Sickle erythrocytes increase prostacyclin and endothelin-1 production by cultured human endothelial cells under flow conditions. *Eur J Haematol* 68:163-169, 2002.

73. Rivera A, Jarolim P, Brugnara C: Modulation of Gardos channel activity by cytokines in sickle erythrocytes. *Blood* 99:357-603, 2002.

74. Keh D, Gerlach M, Kurer I, et al: Reduction of platelet trapping in membrane oxygenators by transmembraneous application of gaseous nitric oxide. *Int J Artif Organs* 19:291-293, 1996.

75. Michelson AD, Benoit SE, Furman MI, et al: Effects of nitric oxide/EDRF on platelet surface glycoproteins. *Am J Physiol* 270:H1640-1648, 1996.

76. Radomski MW, Palmer RM, Moncada S: Endogenous nitric oxide inhibits human platelet adhesion to vascular endothelium. *Lancet* 2:1057-1058, 1987.

77. Radomski MW, Vallance P, Whitley G, et al: Platelet adhesion to human vascular endothelium is modulated by constitutive and cytokine induced nitric oxide. *Cardiovasc Res* 27:1380-1382, 1993.

78. Gladwin MT, Rodgers GP: Pathogenesis and treatment of acute chest syndrome of sickle-cell anaemia. *Lancet* 355:1476-1478, 2000.

79. Azizi E, Dror Y, Wallis K: Arginase activity in erythrocytes of healthy and ill children. *Clin Chim Acta* 28:391-396, 1970.

80. Belfiore F: [Enzymatic activities of the blood serum in thalassemia and in thalassodrepanocytosis.] *Riforma Med* 78:1052-1055, 1964.

81. Morris CR, Morris SM, Jr, Hagar W, et al: Arginine therapy: A new treatment for pulmonary hypertension in sickle cell disease? *Am J Respir Crit Care Med* 168:63-69, 2003.

82. Schnog JJ, Jager EH, van der Dijs FP, et al: Evidence for a metabolic shift of arginine metabolism in sickle cell disease. *Ann Hematol* 83:371-375, 2004.

82b. Morris CR, Kato GJ, Poljakovic M, et al. Dysregulated arginine metabolism, hemolysis-associated pulmonary hypertension, and mortality in sickle cell disease. *Jama* 2005; 294:81–90.

83. Hoeper MM, Niedermeyer J, Hoffmeyer F, et al: Pulmonary hypertension after splenectomy? *Ann Intern Med* 130:506-509, 1999.

84. Atichartakarn V, Angchaisuksiri P, Aryurachai K, et al: *In vivo* platelet activation and hyperaggregation in hemoglobin E/β-thalassemia: A consequence of splenectomy. *Int J Hematol* 77:299-303, 2003.

85. Kisanuki A, Kietthubthew S, Asada Y, et al: Intravenous injection of sonicated blood induces pulmonary microthromboembolism in rabbits with ligation of the splenic artery. *Thromb Res* 85:95-103, 1997.

86. Westerman M, Pizzey A, Hirschman J, et al: Plasma "free" Hb is related to red cell derived vesicle numbers in sickle cell anemia and thalassemia intermedia: Implications for nitric oxide (NO) scavenging and pulmonary hypertension. *Blood* 104:465a, 2004.

87. Atichartakarn V, Angchaisuksiri P, Aryurachai K, et al: Relationship between hypercoagulable state and erythrocyte phosphatidylserine exposure in splenectomized haemoglobin E/β-thalassaemic patients. *Br J Haematol* 118:893-898, 2002.

88. Carnelli V, D'Angelo E, Pecchiari M, et al: Pulmonary dysfunction in transfusion-dependent patients with thalassemia major. *Am J Respir Crit Care Med* 168:180-184, 2003.

89. Tai DY, Wang YT, Lou J, et al: Lungs in thalassaemia major patients receiving regular transfusion. *Eur Respir J* 9:1389-1394, 1996.

90. Berney SI, Ridler CD, Stephens AD, et al: Enhanced platelet reactivity and hypercoagulability in the steady state of sickle cell anaemia. *Am J Hematol* 40:290-294, 1992.

91. el-Hazmi MA, Warsy AS, Bahakim H: Blood proteins C and S in sickle cell disease. *Acta Haematol* 90:114-119, 1993.

92. Hagger D, Wolff S, Owen J, et al: Changes in coagulation and fibrinolysis in patients with sickle cell disease compared with healthy black controls. *Blood Coagul Fibrinolysis* 6:93-99, 1995.

93. Kurantsin-Mills J, Ofosu FA, Safa TK, et al: Plasma factor VII and thrombin-antithrombin III levels

indicate increased tissue factor activity in sickle cell patients. *Br J Haematol* 81:539-544, 1992.

94. Marfaing-Koka A, Boyer-Neumann C, Wolf M, et al: Decreased protein S activity in sickle cell disease. *Nouv Rev Fr Hematol* 35:425-430, 1993.

95. Peters M, Plaat BE, ten Cate H, et al: Enhanced thrombin generation in children with sickle cell disease. *Thromb Haemost* 71:169-172, 1994.

96. Shet AS, Aras O, Gupta K, et al: Sickle blood contains tissue factor-positive microparticles derived from endothelial cells and monocytes. *Blood* 102: 2678-2683, 2003.

97. Adedeji MO, Cespedes J, Allen K, et al: Pulmonary thrombotic arteriopathy in patients with sickle cell disease. *Arch Pathol Lab Med* 125:1436-1441, 2001.

98. Manci EA, Culberson DE, Yang YM, et al: Causes of death in sickle cell disease: An autopsy study. *Br J Haematol* 123:359-365, 2003.

99. Vichinsky EP: Pulmonary hypertension in sickle cell disease. *N Engl J Med* 350:857-859, 2004.

100. Taher A, Abou-Mourad Y, Abchee A, et al: Pulmonary thromboembolism in β-thalassemia intermedia: Are we aware of this complication? *Hemoglobin* 26:107-112, 2002.

101. Uchida T, Miyake T, Matsuno M, et al: [Fatal pulmonary thromboembolism in a patient with paroxysmal nocturnal hemoglobinuria.] *Rinsho Ketsueki* 39:150-152, 1998.

102. Machado RF, Martyr SE, Anthi A, et al: Pulmonary hypertension in sickle cell disease: Cardiopulmonary evaluation and response to chronic phosphodiesterase 5 inhibitor therapy. *Blood* 104:71a, 2004.

103. Barst RJ, Langleben D, Frost A, et al: Sitaxsentan therapy for pulmonary arterial hypertension. *Am J Respir Crit Care Med* 169:441-447, 2004.

104. Kato GJ, Martyr S, Machado RF, et al: Acute and chronic pulmonary hypertension in patients with sickle cell disease. *Blood* 104:464a, 2004.

105. Barst RJ, McGoon M, Torbicki A, et al: Diagnosis and differential assessment of pulmonary arterial hypertension. *J Am Coll Cardiol* 43(12 Suppl S): 40S-47S, 2004.

106. McGoon M, Gutterman D, Steen V, et al: Screening, early detection, and diagnosis of pulmonary arterial hypertension: ACCP evidence-based clinical practice guidelines. *Chest* 126(1 Suppl):14S-34S, 2004.

107. Derchi G, Forni GL, Formisano F, et al: Efficacy and safety of sildenafil in the treatment of severe pulmonary hypertension in patients with hemoglobinopathies. *Haematologica* 90:452-458, 2005.

108. Bossone E, Rubenfire M, Bach DS, et al: Range of tricuspid regurgitation velocity at rest and during exercise in normal adult men: Implications for the diagnosis of pulmonary hypertension. *J Am Coll Cardiol* 33:1662-1666, 1999.

109. Koumbourlis AC, Hurlet-Jensen A, Bye MR: Lung function in infants with sickle cell disease. *Pediatr Pulmonol* 24:277-281, 1997.

110. Koumbourlis AC, Zar HJ, Hurlet-Jensen A, et al: Prevalence and reversibility of lower airway obstruction in children with sickle cell disease. *J Pediatr* 138:188-192, 2001.

111. Lonsdorfer J, Bogui P, Otayeck A, et al: Cardiorespiratory adjustments in chronic sickle cell anemia. *Bull Eur Physiopathol Respir* 19:339-344, 1983.

112. Santoli F, Zerah F, Vasile N, et al: Pulmonary function in sickle cell disease with or without acute chest syndrome. *Eur Respir J* 12:1124-1129, 1998.

113. Young RC, Jr, Rachal RE, Reindorf CA, et al: Lung function in sickle cell hemoglobinopathy patients compared with healthy subjects. *J Nat Med Assoc* 80:509-514, 1988.

114. Yung GL, Channick RN, Fedullo PF, et al: Successful pulmonary thromboendarterectomy in two patients with sickle cell disease. *Am J Respir Crit Care Med* 157:1690-1693, 1998.

115. Castele RJ, Strohl KP, Chester CS, et al: Oxygen saturation with sleep in patients with sickle cell disease. *Arch Intern Med* 146:722-725, 1986.

116. Hargrave DR, Wade A, Evans JP, et al: Nocturnal oxygen saturation and painful sickle cell crises in children. *Blood* 101:846-884, 2003.

117. Needleman JP, Franco ME, Varlotta L, et al: Mechanisms of nocturnal oxyhemoglobin desaturation in children and adolescents with sickle cell disease. *Pediatr Pulmonol* 28:418-422, 1999.

118. Kirkham FJ, Hewes DK, Prengler M, et al: Nocturnal hypoxaemia and central-nervous-system events in sickle-cell disease. *Lancet* 357:1656-1659, 2001.

119. Quinn CT, Ahmad N: Prevalence and predictors of steady state hypoxemia in sickle cell disease. *Br J Haematol* 131:129-134, 2005.

120. Steinberg MH, Barton F, Castro O, et al: Effect of hydroxyurea on mortality and morbidity in adult sickle cell anemia: Risks and benefits up to 9 years of treatment. *JAMA* 289:1645-1651, 2003.

121. Charache S, Terrin ML, Moore RD, et al: Effect of hydroxyurea on the frequency of painful crises in sickle cell anemia. Investigators of the Multicenter Study of Hydroxyurea in Sickle Cell Anemia. *N Engl J Med* 332:1317-1322, 1995.

122. Adams RJ, McKie VC, Hsu L, et al: Prevention of a first stroke by transfusions in children with sickle cell anemia and abnormal results on transcranial Doppler ultrasonography. *N Engl J Med* 339:5-11, 1998.

123. Koshy M, Burd L, Wallace D, et al: Prophylactic red-cell transfusions in pregnant patients with sickle

cell disease. A randomized cooperative study. *N Engl J Med* 319:1447-1452, 1988.

124. Pegelow CH, Adams RJ, McKie V, et al: Risk of recurrent stroke in patients with sickle cell disease treated with erythrocyte transfusions. *J Pediatr* 126:896-899, 1995.

125. Aessopos A, Farmakis D, Hatziliami A, et al: Cardiac status in well-treated patients with thalassemia major. *Eur J Haematol* 73:359-366, 2004.

126. Hillmen P, Hall C, Marsh JC, et al: Effect of eculizumab on hemolysis and transfusion requirements in patients with paroxysmal nocturnal hemoglobinuria. *N Engl J Med* 350:552-559, 2004.

127. Frank H, Mlczoch J, Huber K, et al: The effect of anticoagulant therapy in primary and anorectic drug-induced pulmonary hypertension. *Chest* 112:714-721, 1997.

128. Fuster V, Steele PM, Edwards WD, et al: Primary pulmonary hypertension: Natural history and the importance of thrombosis. *Circulation* 70:580-587, 1984.

129. Rich S, Kaufmann E, Levy PS: The effect of high doses of calcium-channel blockers on survival in primary pulmonary hypertension. *N Engl J Med* 327:76-81, 1992.

130. Ohene-Frempong K, Weiner SJ, Sleeper LA, et al: Cerebrovascular accidents in sickle cell disease: Rates and risk factors. *Blood* 91:288-294, 1998.

131. Cohen AR, Galanello R, Pennell DJ, et al: Thalassemia. *Hematology (Am Soc Hematol Educ Program)* 14-34, 2004.

132. Badesch DB, McLaughlin VV, Delcroix M, et al: Prostanoid therapy for pulmonary arterial hypertension. *J Am Coll Cardiol* 43(12 Suppl S):56S-61S, 2004.

133. Channick RN, Sitbon O, Barst RJ, et al: Endothelin receptor antagonists in pulmonary arterial hypertension. *J Am Coll Cardiol* 43(12 Suppl S):62S-67S, 2004.

134. Ghofrani HA, Pepke-Zaba J, Barbera JA, et al: Nitric oxide pathway and phosphodiesterase inhibitors in pulmonary arterial hypertension. *J Am Coll Cardiol* 43(12 Suppl S):68S-72S, 2004.

134b. Galie N, Ghofrani HA, Torbicki A, et al. Sildenafil citrate therapy for pulmonary arterial hypertension. *N Engl J Med* 2005; 353:2148-57.

135. Channick RN, Newhart JW, Johnson FW, et al: Pulsed delivery of inhaled nitric oxide to patients with primary pulmonary hypertension: An ambulatory delivery system and initial clinical tests. *Chest* 109:1545-1549, 1996.

136. Littera R, La Nasa G, Derchi G, et al: Long-term treatment with sildenafil in a thalassemic patient with pulmonary hypertension. *Blood* 100:1516-1517, 2002.

137. Machado RF, Martyr S, Kato GJ, et al: Sildenafil therapy in patients with sickle disease and pulmonary hypertension. *Br J Haematol* 130:445-453, 2005.

138. Machado RF, Gladwin MT: Chronic sickle cell lung disease: New insights into the diagnosis, pathogenesis and treatment of pulmonary hypertension. *Br J Haematol* 129:449-464, 2005.

139. Lin EE, Gladwin MT, Machado RF: Pulmonary hypertension in patients with hemoglobinopathies: Could a mechanism for dysfunction provide an avenue for novel therapeutics? *Haematologica* 90:441-444, 2005.

Chronic Thromboembolic Pulmonary Hypertension

Kelly M. Chin, MD,

Peter F. Fedullo, MD

Substantial advances have occurred over the past two decades in the evaluative, surgical, and postoperative care of patients afflicted with chronic thromboembolic pulmonary hypertension.[1-7] Thromboendarterectomy for chronic thromboembolic pulmonary hypertension was first proposed in 1958, and the first successful bilateral procedure via sternotomy was performed in 1961.[8-9] By 1984, the aggregate world experience encompassed only 85 operated patients with a perioperative mortality rate of 22 percent.[10] Although exact figures are not available, approximately 3,000 thromboendarterectomy procedures have now been performed worldwide, most at the University of California, San Diego (UCSD) Medical Center. Accompanying this increased experience, mortality rates reported by established programs with the requisite clinical experience in the evaluation and treatment of patients with this disease process have fallen to the 4 to 8 percent range.[11-13] In the absence of such experience, mortality rates may be several-fold higher[11,14-16] (TABLE 13-1).

Lagging behind these clinical advances, however, has been a comprehensive understanding of the epidemiology of the disease and the pathophysiologic mechanisms involved in its initiation and progression. Recent data would suggest that the disease process is more common than previously thought, affecting as many as 3 percent of those following an initial episode of pulmonary embolism and up to 13 percent following recurrent venous thromboembolism.[17] Assuming 400,000 embolic survivors annually in the United States, these figures would suggest that the diagnosis is being overlooked in a substantial number of patients or these patients are not receiving appropriate medical care.[18] Additionally, the most feared complications of thromboendarterectomy, residual pulmonary hypertension and reperfusion pulmonary edema, remain enigmatic in terms of their pathogenesis, prevention, and therapy. Ongoing investigative efforts into these areas of uncertainty are essential, both to decrease the prevalence of the disease and, when surgical intervention is necessary, to decrease the morbidity and mortality from the procedure.

Pathogenesis and Risk Factors

Although the thromboembolic basis of chronic thromboembolic pulmonary hypertension has been questioned, clinical experience and studies of the natural history of acute pulmonary embolic events suggest that incomplete resolution, with or without recurrent thromboembolic episodes, is the primary inciting event.[19,20]

On an acute basis, approximately 30-percent obstruction of the pulmonary vascular bed is necessary to cause pulmonary hypertension.[21] It is not uncommon for patients with an acute pulmonary embolism to display elevated pulmonary arterial pressures at the time of diagnosis.[21,22] Over the next 4-6 weeks, abnormalities on echocardiogram and lung perfusion scan improve and often fully resolve. Improvement may be incomplete, however, and echocardiographic abnormalities that remain at 4-6 weeks predict continued echocardiographic abnormalities after 1 year; perfusion scan

TABLE 13-1

Published Results for Pulmonary Thromboendarterectomy Since 1996

Year	Author	Location	Patients (N)	Preoperative PVR	Postoperative PVR	Mortality (%)
1997	Nakajima[69]	Japan	30	937 ± 45	299 ± 16	13.3
1997	Mayer[70]	Germany	32	967 ± 238	301 ± 151	9.3
1998	Gilbert[71]	Baltimore	17	≈700 ± 200*	≈170 ± 180*	23.5
1998	Miller[72]	Philadelphia	25	Not known	Not known	24.0
1999	Dartevelle[73]	France	68	1,174 ± 416	519 ± 250	13.2
1999	Ando[15]	Japan	24	1,066 ± 250	268 ± 141	20.8
2000	Jamieson[6]	San Diego	457	877 ± 452	267 ± 192	7.0
2000	Mares[74]	Austria	33	1,478 ± 107**	975 ± 93**	9.1
2000	Mares[74]	Austria	14	1,334 ±135**	759 ± 99**	21.4
2000	Rubens[12]	Canada	21	765 ± 372	208 ± 92	4.8
2000	D'Armini[13]	Italy	33	1,056 ± 344	196 ± 39†	9.1
2001	Tscholl[75]	Germany	69	988 ± 554	324 ± 188	10.1
2001	Masuda[16]	Japan	50	869 ± 299‡	344 ± 174‡	18.0
2003	Hagl[76]	Germany	30	873 ± 248	290 ± 117	10.0
2003	Jamieson[11]	San Diego	500	893 ± 444	285 ± 214	4.4

*Estimate derived from graph.
**Results expressed as pulmonary vascular resistance index.
†Data in 23 patients at 3-month follow-up.
‡34 patients by sternotomy, 16 patients by thoracotomy.
PVR, pulmonary vascular resistance in dynes·sec·cm^{-5}.

results may continue to improve for 3 to 6 months.[23,24]

The frequency and significance of this incomplete resolution has been debated. Based on the relatively small number of patients referred annually for pulmonary thromboendarterectomy, experts previously suggested that as few as 0.01-0.1 percent of pulmonary embolism survivors develop chronic thromboembolic pulmonary hypertension.[25] More rigorous follow-up studies of patients with acute pulmonary embolism are challenging this view, and it now appears that chronic thromboembolic pulmonary hypertension develops more frequently. A 1999 study that followed survivors of an acute pulmonary embolism found that echocardiogram findings remained abnormal in 44 percent of patients after 1 year. Although "normal" was defined rather conservatively, and confirmatory cardiac catheterization data were not reported, 3 of 78 patients underwent pulmonary thromboendarterectomy over the next 5 years, suggesting that progression to chronic thromboembolic pulmonary hypertension is not uncommon.[26]

Another study of patients with acute pulmonary embolism reported more comprehensive follow-up data and obtained similar results. All patients were asked routinely about dyspnea, and any patient with unexplained dyspnea underwent right heart catheterization. Seven of 223 (3.1 percent) patients

with a first pulmonary embolism and 11 of 82 (13.4 percent) patients with a recurrent pulmonary embolism (or prior deep venous thrombosis) developed symptomatic chronic thromboembolic pulmonary hypertension, confirmed by catheterization. Median follow-up was 38 months, and all occurrences of chronic thromboembolic pulmonary hypertension were detected during the first 2 years of follow-up. Risk factors for chronic thromboembolic pulmonary hypertension in this study included younger age, larger perfusion defect, idiopathic pulmonary embolism, and multiple pulmonary embolic episodes.[17]

Patients with anatomically massive pulmonary embolism, defined as greater than 50 percent obstruction of the pulmonary vascular bed, may be at even higher risk. In one 2003 study of patients meeting criteria for anatomically massive pulmonary embolism and undergoing treatment with thrombolytic agents, 46 of 227 patients (20.2 percent) developed chronic thromboembolic pulmonary hypertension.[27] Factors associated with an adverse long-term outcome in this study related to anatomic and hemodynamic abnormalities following the administration of thrombolytic agents, including a pulmonary artery systolic pressure greater than 50 mmHg, greater than 30 percent pulmonary vascular obstruction, and evidence of right ventricular dysfunction.

The cause for the variable natural history after an acute pulmonary embolic event is not well understood. It is possible, albeit somewhat simplistic, that chronic thromboembolic pulmonary hypertension represents part of the normal spectrum of disease associated with pulmonary embolism: complete anatomic and hemodynamic resolution in a minority of patients, partial resolution associated with normal exercise capacity in most, and progression to pulmonary hypertension in the remaining few.

Although antiphospholipid antibodies occur in 10-20 percent of patients with chronic thromboembolic pulmonary hypertension, most patients have not had identifiable coagulopathic tendencies. Rates of antithrombin III deficiency, protein C or S deficiency, and factor V Leiden have not been higher than in the general population, and major deficiencies in the fibrinolytic system have not been identified.[28-31] One study reported elevated plasma concentrations of factor VIII in 122 patients with chronic thromboembolic pulmonary hypertension (41 percent, versus 5 percent of controls), while another small study found increased rates of hyperhomocysteinemia.[32,33] If confirmed, these findings suggest that a greater percentage of patients may have an impairment of thrombotic or fibrinolytic mechanisms than previously appreciated.

Clinical Picture

The clinical picture of patients with chronic thromboembolic pulmonary hypertension is similar to that of patients with other forms of pulmonary hypertension. Symptoms typically begin with dyspnea on exertion that progresses over months or years. Patients accustomed to higher levels of activity on a daily basis recognize the decline in exercise capacity at an earlier point than those who lead a sedentary lifestyle. Later in the course of the disease, presyncopal symptoms and a chronic nonproductive cough may develop. Patients often complain of lightheadedness and increased dyspnea when bending from the waist, perhaps related to a transient decrease in venous return and cardiac output. Syncopal events, often precipitated by a bout of coughing, and exertional chest pain develop late in the course of the disease, as right coronary artery perfusion and right ventricular function become incapable of responding to increased metabolic demands.

Most patients provide a history of a documented venous thromboembolic event or an incident consistent with that diagnosis, such as a remote episode of pleurisy, lower extremity edema, or hemoptysis. In the absence of a history consistent with embolism, patients may describe a prolonged atypical pneumonia, a complicated hospitalization, or a surgical procedure following which they did not return to their baseline cardiopulmonary status. Given data that document the frequency with which venous thromboembolism is overlooked in the population at large, it is not surprising that an episode of venous thromboembolism may have been undiagnosed or misdiagnosed.[34,35]

It is also important to recognize that a considerable delay, extending from several months to as long as a decade, may exist between the documented or suspected embolic event and the onset of clinical symptoms. The degree to which this symptomatic and hemodynamic decline is related to recurrent embolic events, *in situ* thrombosis, changes in the pulmonary microvasculature, or loss of right ventricular adaptive mechanisms is one of the most compelling enigmas surrounding this disease process.[20] There is evidence, based on lung biopsy obtained at the time of thromboendarterectomy, that changes in the microvasculature, similar to those encountered in other variants of pulmonary hypertension, may account for the progressive decline in many patients.[36] Supporting this hypothesis has been the finding of progressive symptomatic and hemodynamic decline in the presence of an abnormal but unchanged perfusion scan, suggesting that the distal pulmonary vascular bed rather than major vessel *in situ* thrombosis or recurrent embolism is responsible for the progression of pulmonary hypertension.

Diagnostic delay following symptom onset, often of a prolonged duration, is common. This is in part attributable to the often nonspecific symptoms of the disease process and, early in its natural history, the subtlety of its physical examination findings. However, it is also attributable in some cases to limitations on patient referral to subspecialty care, specifically pulmonary and cardiac specialists who are most familiar with the clinical picture and its appropriate diagnostic evaluation. Diagnostic delays are most common when there is no history of acute thromboembolism. The progressive dyspnea and exercise intolerance are often erroneously attributed to asthma, physical deconditioning, advancing age, interstitial lung disease, coronary artery disease, or psychogenic factors.

Physical Examination

Physical examination findings are dependent on the level of pulmonary hypertension when the patient is evaluated. Early in the course of the disease, the physical examination findings may be surprisingly normal, thereby contributing to diagnostic delay. Before significant right ventricular hypertrophy or overt right ventricular failure develops, abnormalities can be limited to a widening of the second heart sound or a subtle accentuation of its pulmonic component. As the disease progresses, classic findings of pulmonary hypertension develop and include a right ventricular lift, fixed splitting of the second heart sound with an accentuated pulmonic component, a right-sided ventricular S_4 gallop, and varying degrees of tricuspid regurgitation. Even at this stage of the disease, however, physical findings can be deceptive, particularly for physicians unfamiliar with the physical diagnostic manifestations of pulmonary hypertension and in patients who are obese or who have coexisting cardiopulmonary disease. Eventually, as right ventricular failure ensues, jugular venous distention, a right-sided S_3, lower extremity edema, hepatomegaly, ascites, and cyanosis may develop. The intensity of the tricuspid regurgitant murmur may diminish as the tricuspid annulus dilates and the transvalvular pressure gradient decreases. Lower extremity edema may be the result of right-sided heart failure or venous outflow obstruction related to residual venous thrombosis. Findings consistent with the postphlebitic syndrome may be present. Finally, an important physical diagnostic finding in approximately 30 percent of patients with chronic thromboembolic disease is pulmonary flow murmurs.[37] These bruits, which appear to result from turbulent flow across partially obstructed pulmonary vascular segments, are high pitched and blowing in quality, audible over the anterior and posterior lung fields rather than the precordium, and are most apparent during an inspiratory breath-holding maneuver. These flow murmurs are not unique to chronic thromboembolic disease and have been described in other disease states associated with focal narrowing of large pulmonary arteries, such as congenital branch stenosis and pulmonary arteritis. However, they have not been described in idiopathic pulmonary arterial hypertension (IPAH), the most common competing diagnosis.

Laboratory Studies

Routine laboratory studies, including hematology, blood chemistry, and liver function study results, are usually unremarkable. Mild elevations of transaminases, alkaline phosphatase, or bilirubin levels may suggest passive hepatic congestion. A prolonged activated partial thromboplastin time in the absence of heparin therapy or a decreased platelet count may suggest a lupus anticoagulant or anticardiolipin antibody.[30] As in other variants of pulmonary hypertension, elevated uric acid levels and brain natriuretic peptide levels are also encountered commonly and appear to correlate positively with the level of mean right atrial pressure and inversely with the level of the cardiac output.[38-40]

Although the arterial PO_2 may be within normal limits, the alveolar-arterial oxygen gradient typically is widened, and most patients experience a decrease in the arterial PO_2 with exercise. Dead space ventilation (V_D/V_T) often is increased at rest and worsens with exercise. Hypoxemia appears to be the consequence of moderate ventilation-perfusion inequality and a limited cardiac output which depresses mixed venous PO_2.[41] Oxygen desaturation during exercise appears to be related to the inability of the right ventricle to augment cardiac output when there is increased systemic oxygen demand, resulting in further depression of the mixed venous PO_2. In patients with a patent foramen ovale, exercise-related hypoxemia may result from an increase in the right-to-left shunt fraction.

Diagnostic Evaluation

Patients with suspected chronic thromboembolic pulmonary hypertension undergo evaluation with the goals of establishing the severity of pulmonary hypertension, determining whether surgically accessible chronic thromboemboli are present, and evaluating comorbidities that may affect surgical risk. Routine testing includes pulmonary function testing, chest radiograph, echocardiogram, ventilation-perfusion scan (or occasionally computed tomography [CT] angiography) and pulmonary angiography. In select cases, pulmonary angioscopy and a technique to "partition" the pulmonary vascular resistance are used, as well.

Chest Radiography

Chest radiography, although results are often normal, may demonstrate one or more findings that suggest the diagnosis of pulmonary hypertension. Asymmetry in the size of the central pulmonary arteries or enlargement of both pulmonary arteries may be present (FIGURE 13-1). Areas of hypoperfusion and hyperperfusion may also be appreciated. The areas of hyperperfusion may be so dramatic as to suggest a focal infiltrate or interstitial disease, and pleural-based scars, consistent with prior infarcts, may be visualized.[42,43] The cardiac silhouette may reflect obvious right atrial or right ventricular enlargement; more commonly, right ventricular enlargement is suggested only on the lateral film by encroachment on the retrosternal space. Lower extremity duplex ultrasonography demonstrates findings consistent with prior venous thrombosis in approximately 45 percent of patients.

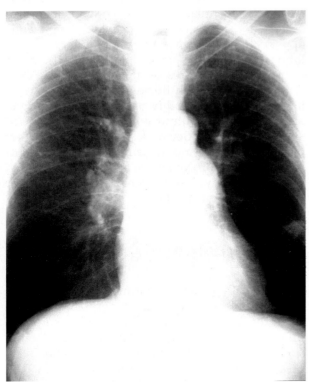

Figure 13-1. Chest Radiograph in a Patient With Chronic Thromboembolic Pulmonary Hypertension. Asymmetry of the central pulmonary arteries, enlargement of the right pulmonary artery, and absence of the left descending pulmonary artery are seen along with a left-sided opacity most likely from a prior pulmonary infarct.

Echocardiography

When pulmonary hypertension is suspected, echocardiography is a very useful test early in the diagnostic workup. In centers with experienced practitioners where simultaneous or sequential cardiac catheterization has been performed, directly measured pulmonary artery systolic pressure and estimated pulmonary artery systolic pressures using the tricuspid regurgitant jet velocity have correlated closely.[44,45] Additional findings, albeit nonspecific ones, include enlargement of the right cardiac chambers, flattening or paradoxical motion of the interventricular septum, and abnormally low mitral early to late atrial diastolic filling velocity (E/A) ratios (<1.25).[46] Contrast echocardiography is useful in detecting interatrial or interventricular shunts, such as a patent foramen ovale or septal defect, and should be performed routinely when echocardiographic evidence of pulmonary hypertension is present.

One limitation of echocardiography is that not all patients have a measurable tricuspid regurgitant jet, particularly patients with mild pulmonary hypertension. Also, modest overestimation and underestimation of pulmonary pressures can occur. Thus although a normal echocardiogram generally excludes moderate or severe pulmonary hypertension, abnormally elevated pressures must be confirmed by right heart catheterization. Furthermore, echocardiography can not exclude mild or exercise-associated pulmonary hypertension, and is not capable of differentiating among the various causes of pulmonary hypertension.[47]

Pulmonary Function Testing

Pulmonary function testing is useful mainly to exclude coexisting obstructive or restrictive lung disease. Mild to moderate restriction is seen in approximately 20 percent of patients with chronic thromboembolic pulmonary hypertension and has been strongly associated with the degree of parenchymal scarring, possibly related to infarction accompanying acute pulmonary embolism.[42] As is the case in IPAH, the most common pulmonary function test abnormality is a reduction in the diffusing capacity of carbon monoxide (DL_{CO}).[48] A normal DL_{CO} does not exclude chronic thromboembolic pulmonary hypertension; severe reductions are uncommon and should lead to the consideration of possible alternative diagnoses. Interestingly, the reduction in DL_{CO} does not appear to resolve following surgery despite improvements in pulmonary artery pressure, cardiac output, and pulmonary perfusion.[49]

Ventilation-Perfusion Radionuclide Scan

Once a diagnosis of pulmonary hypertension is established or strongly suspected, determining whether surgically accessible chronic thromboembolic disease is present should be the next step in the diagnostic sequence. Ventilation-perfusion scanning is the test most commonly used for this purpose. Patients with chronic thromboembolic pulmonary hypertension typically demonstrate multiple segmental or larger perfusion defects[43,50,51] (FIGURE 13-2). In contrast, perfusion scan findings in patients with IPAH are either normal or exhibit a "mottled" appearance characterized by subsegmental defects. Occasionally, the perfusion scan pattern in small vessel pulmonary hypertension demonstrates a basilar redistribution of flow, suggesting obstruction of the upper and middle lobe arteries. This pattern of flow, however, is nonsegmental and inconsistent with the usual lower lobar distribution of pulmonary emboli, and angiography demonstrates that patent proximal vessels are present.

Although clinical studies are limited, ventilation-perfusion scanning is believed to be very sensitive but less specific for chronic thromboembolic pulmonary hypertension. In one study of 75 patients undergoing evaluation for pulmonary hypertension, 24 of 25 patients with chronic thromboembolic pulmonary hypertension had high-probability scan results while 1 patient had an intermediate-probability scan findings. The specificity of an intermediate-probability or high-probability scan result was 86 percent, requiring that patients with a suggestive ventilation-perfusion scan undergo pulmonary angiography to confirm surgically accessible thromboembolic disease.[52]

Causes of mismatched segmental defects in a patient with pulmonary hypertension other than thromboembolic obstruction include pulmonary artery sarcoma, large vessel pulmonary vasculitides, extrinsic vascular compression by mediastinal adenopathy or fibrosis and, on occasion, pulmonary veno-occlusive disease. Unlike scan findings in patients with acute pulmonary embolism, the size and number of defects do not accurately predict hemodynamics in chronic thromboembolic pulmonary hypertension, and perfusion scans often underestimate the degree of obstruction.[53,54] This is thought to be due to partial recanalization of obstructed vessels, allowing the radioisotopic agent to reach the periphery of the lung. Therefore, in a patient with pulmonary hypertension, even a single, mismatched, segmental ventilation-perfusion scan defect should raise concerns of a potential thromboembolic basis, regardless of whether this defect appears disproportionate to the extent of the pulmonary hypertension.

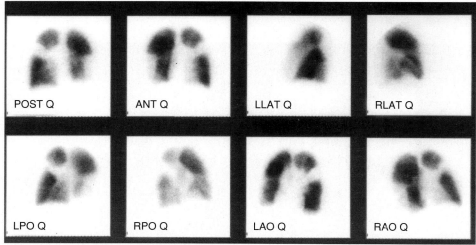

Figure 13-2. Representative Perfusion Scan in a Patient With Chronic Thromboembolic Pulmonary Hypertension. Perfusion scan demonstrates multiple mismatched segmental and larger defects. The ventilation scan results in this patient were normal.

Computerized Tomography

CT and magnetic resonance imaging have been advocated as screening techniques for the diagnosis of chronic thromboembolic disease.[55-57] Thrombus within the central pulmonary arteries can be demonstrated by helical tomography, although the absence of thrombus proximal to the segmental arteries does not preclude the possibility of surgical intervention. Helical tomography is less sensitive in detecting chronic thrombus that is mural rather than intraluminal. A variety of computed tomographic abnormalities have been described in patients with chronic thromboembolic pulmonary hypertension: right ventricular enlargement, dilated central pulmonary arteries, chronic thromboembolic material within the central pulmonary arteries, bronchial artery collateral flow, parenchymal abnormalities consistent with prior infarcts, and mosaic attenuation of the pulmonary parenchyma. CT appears most useful in the small subset of patients with unilateral or predominantly unilateral vascular occlusion in whom the probability of other diagnostic possibilities (sarcoma, vasculitis, malignancy, and mediastinal fibrosis) is increased[58] (FIGURE 13-3).

Contrast-enhanced magnetic resonance angiography has also proven useful in defining the extent of pulmonary vascular obstruction to the level of the subsegmental arteries. However, it is not capable of providing accurate hemodynamic data that are essential to timing appropriate surgical referral, and the overall performance of magnetic resonance angiography compared with CT angiography was reported as only "equally effective" at identifying the direct and indirect signs of chronic thromboembolic disease.[59,60]

Right Heart Catheterization, Pulmonary Angiography, and Pulmonary Angioscopy

Right heart catheterization and pulmonary angiography are essential to define the degree of pulmonary hypertension, to establish the presence of chronic thromboembolic obstruction, and to define its surgical accessibility, as well as to help exclude competing diagnostic possibilities. If hemodynamic measurements at rest demonstrate only modest degrees of pulmonary hypertension, measurements should be obtained following a short period of symptom-limited exercise.[61] In patients with chronic thromboembolic obstruction of a magnitude sufficient to abolish normal compensatory mechanisms, exercise results in a submaximal increase in cardiac output with an almost linear elevation of the pulmonary artery pressure.

The angiographic appearance of chronic thromboembolic disease bears little resemblance to that of acute pulmonary embolism.[62] Five distinct angiographic patterns have been described that correlate with the finding of chronic thromboembolic material at the time of surgery: (1) pouch defects, (2) pulmonary artery webs or bands, (3) intimal irregularities, (4) abrupt, often angular narrowing of the major pulmonary arteries, and (5) complete obstruction of main, lobar or segmental vessels at their point of origin (FIGURE 13-4). In most patients with extensive chronic thromboembolic disease, two or more of these angiographic findings are present. Competing diagnoses exist with angiographic findings similar to those encountered in chronic thromboembolic disease. Bandlike narrowing can be a feature of medium or large vessel pulmonary arteritis or can be seen with

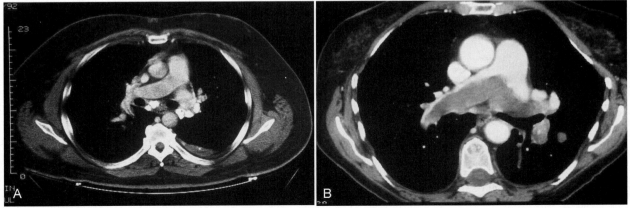

Figure 13-3. Computed Tomography (CT) Scans in Patients With Nonthromboembolic Causes of Pulmonary Artery Obstruction. **A**, CT scan demonstrating multiple calcified, enlarged mediastinal lymph nodes due to fibrosing mediastinitis. Several lymph nodes surround and narrow the left main pulmonary artery. **B**, CT scan demonstrating a large pulmonary artery sarcoma within the pulmonary trunk.

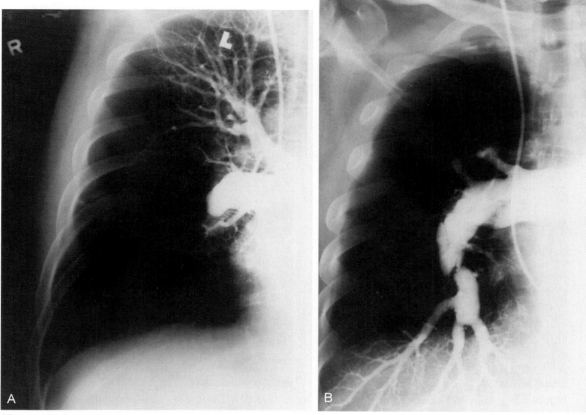

Figure 13-4. Representative Angiograms in Patients With Chronic Thromboembolic Pulmonary Hypertension. **A**, Right-sided pulmonary angiogram (anterior view) demonstrating a prominent "pouch" defect in the right interlobar artery. **B**, Right-sided pulmonary angiogram (anterior view) demonstrating a pulmonary artery "web" in the right lower lobe pulmonary artery, a right upper lobe artery that is cut off abruptly, and irregularity of the lateral wall of the interlobar and lower lobe arteries.

congenital pulmonary artery stenosis. Total or partial obstruction of central pulmonary arteries can be the consequence of an intravascular process such as a primary pulmonary artery tumor, or an extravascular process such as mediastinal or hilar lymphadenopathy, lung carcinoma, or fibrosing mediastinitis.

Pulmonary angiography can be performed safely even when pulmonary hypertension is severe.[63,64] The widespread perception of risk of pulmonary angiography in these patients cannot be supported by studies. Precautions taken to minimize the risk of the procedure include: (1) use of a single injection of nonionic contrast material into the right and left pulmonary arteries, (2) modification of the contrast volume and infusion rate based on the cardiac output, (3) careful patient monitoring and supplemental oxygen administration during the procedure, and (4) avoidance of repeated, selective injections.

In terms of angiographic technique, cut-film biplane acquisition appears to be optimal. On occasion, areas of central recanalization have been obscured on digital subtraction studies. Routine use of the lateral projection has proven invaluable in providing a much more detailed view of the lobar and segmental branches and minimizing artifacts resulting from dilated, overlapping vessels (FIGURE 13-5).

Pulmonary angioscopy is performed in selected cases to confirm the presence of thromboembolic disease and to determine whether it is amenable to surgical intervention.[65,67] The angioscope, a fiberoptic device 120 centimeters in length and 3.0 millimeters in external diameter, is introduced through a vascular sheath, preferably via a right internal jugular approach, and passed into the pulmonary arteries under fluoroscopic guidance. Inflation of the distal balloon with carbon dioxide obstructs pulmonary artery blood flow and allows visualization of the arterial walls. The features of organized chronic emboli consist of roughening or pitting of the intimal surface, bands and webs traversing the vascular lumen, pitted masses of

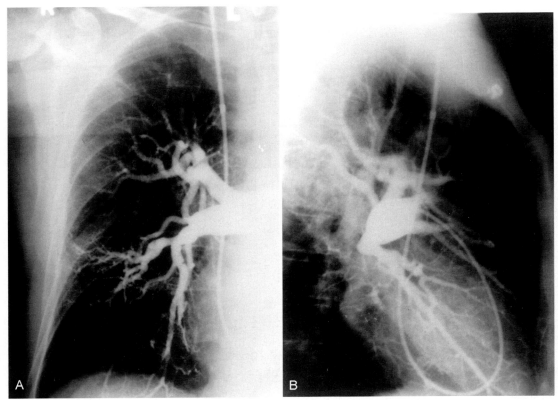

Figure 13-5. Pulmonary Angiogram, Anterior and Lateral Views. **A,** Right-sided pulmonary angiogram (anterior view) demonstrating abrupt narrowing and intimal irregularities in the right upper and lower lobe vessels. **B,** Same patient as in *A*, lateral view. The lateral projection is very useful in this case, demonstrating the nearly complete lack of patent vessels to the lower lobe and to the apical and anterior upper lobe segments.

chronic embolic material within the lumen, and partial recanalization (FIGURE 13-6). During the early experience with evaluation of the disease, angioscopy was performed in approximately 25 percent of patients undergoing evaluation at UCSD Medical Center.[66] Improvements in imaging techniques and interpretation have reduced the need for the procedure to approximately 10 percent of those undergoing evaluation. The procedure remains useful in predicting a beneficial hemodynamic outcome in selected patients with relatively modest levels of pulmonary hypertension and angiographic findings that do not precisely define the proximal extent of the thromboembolic disease. It also is useful for confirming operability in patients with severe pulmonary hypertension who would not have been referred to surgery based on angiographic findings alone.

A primary focus in the evaluation of patients with chronic thromboembolic pulmonary hypertension is differentiating the resistance conferred by the central, accessible component of the thromboembolic disease and that arising from the distal pulmonary vascular bed.[68] Persistent pulmonary hypertension after pulmonary thromboendarterectomy surgery remains a common cause of subsequent morbidity and mortality. Most patients experiencing this complication appear to have undergone successful removal of the central thromboembolic obstruction, with the residual vascular resistance arising from an arteriopathy affecting the distal pulmonary vascular bed. Preoperative identification of these patients can be difficult. An elevated pulmonary vascular resistance that appears out of proportion to the angiographic findings may lead to a clinical suspicion of significant small vessel disease, but diagnostic uncertainty often remains.

Surgical Management

Surgical Selection

The decision to proceed to pulmonary thromboendarterectomy can be a complex one. The central

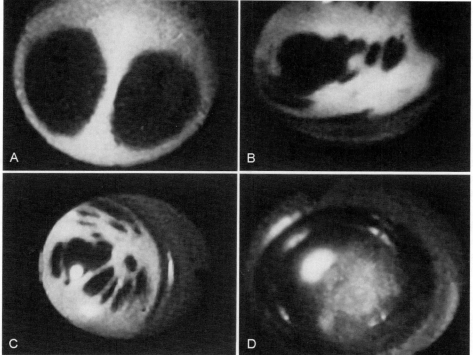

Figure 13-6. Pulmonary Angioscopy. **A,** Normal angioscopic view of a segmental pulmonary artery. Note the symmetric bifurcation and smooth vascular wall. **B** and **C,** Angioscopic views of chronic thromboembolism. Note the complex patters of organization and recanalization resulting in vessel narrowing. **D,** Angioscopic view of a subacute thrombus. Note the pitted, mass-like lesion partially obstructing the vessel lumen.

goals of the evaluative process are to establish the need for surgical intervention, to determine the surgical accessibility of the chronic thromboemboli, and to estimate the risk of the procedure as well as the anticipated hemodynamic outcome in the individual patient.

Most patients who undergo thromboendarterectomy exhibit a pulmonary vascular resistance greater than 300 dynes·sec·cm^{-5}. Preoperative pulmonary vascular resistance is typically in the range of 700 to 1100 dynes·sec·cm^{-5}.[11-13,69-76] At this level of pulmonary hypertension, patient impairment at rest and with exercise can be considerable. The need to intervene at this advanced stage of pulmonary hypertension is in part a consequence of the delay in diagnosis and referral which, in many patients, can be months to years after symptom onset.

Occasional patients without substantially altered pulmonary hemodynamics, such as those with involvement of one main pulmonary artery, those with unusually vigorous lifestyle expectations, and those who live at altitude, may also be considered for surgery to alleviate the exercise impairment associated with their high dead space and minute ventilatory demands. Surgery is also offered to patients with normal pulmonary hemodynamics or only mild levels of pulmonary hypertension at rest who develop significant levels of pulmonary hypertension with exercise.

An absolute criterion for surgery is accessible chronic thrombi as assessed by pulmonary angiography or angioscopy. Surgical techniques allow removal of organized thrombi whose proximal extent is in the main and lobar arteries and, depending on surgical skill and experience, those involving the proximal segmental arteries. Not only is the proximal location of the occluding thromboemboli of importance, also is the extent of accessible thromboembolic disease in relation to the degree of hemodynamic impairment. As experience with this disease process has grown, it has become apparent that the increased pulmonary vascular resistance associated with chronic thromboembolic disease arises not only from the central, surgically accessible chronic thromboembolic obstruction but also from the distal, surgically inaccessible obstruction and the resistance arising from a secondary, small vessel arteriopathy. Thromboendarterectomy will relieve only that portion of the pulmonary hypertension that arises from the accessible component. A primary focus of the preoperative evaluation, therefore, is attempting to partition the proximal component of the elevated vascular resistance from the distal, inaccessible component and, by extension, estimating the anticipated hemodynamic outcome. With experience in hemodynamic-anatomic correlation, this determination can be made with reasonable accuracy and is an important one. Failure to lower pulmonary vascular resistance, particularly in patients with severe pulmonary hypertension and right ventricular dysfunction, may be associated with severe hemodynamic instability and death during the early postoperative period.

A technique to partition the pulmonary vascular resistance into "proximal" (surgically accessible) and "distal" (surgically inaccessible) pulmonary vascular abnormalities using a modified Swan-Ganz pulmonary artery catheter has been developed and may be a useful adjunctive test in the evaluation of surgical candidacy. This technique was developed with the intention of measuring pulmonary capillary pressures, but experimental evidence suggested that pressures in the small pulmonary arterioles contributed.[77] This technique involves a computer generated "upstream resistance percentage" calculated from the decay curve between the pulmonary artery and pulmonary capillary wedge pressures. Using this approach, investigators have shown that the average upstream resistance percentage is higher in chronic thromboembolic pulmonary hypertension than in pulmonary arterial hypertension, while patients with pulmonary veno-occlusive disease have the lowest upstream resistance percentages. However, significant overlap exists among these three forms of pulmonary hypertension, and as a single test it can not differentiate between chronic thromboembolic pulmonary hypertension and pulmonary arterial hypertension.[78] However, one study of 26 patients undergoing pulmonary thromboendarterectomy suggests that the technique may be useful in identifying patients who are unlikely to improve with surgery. Postoperative hemodynamics correlated closely with preoperative upstream resistance measurements, and all four deaths occurred in patients who had very low upstream resistance percentages and significant postoperative residual pulmonary hypertension.[79]

Comorbid conditions that may adversely affect perioperative mortality or morbidity as well as long-term survival must also be considered before surgical referral. Determining surgical risk requires a careful assessment of hemodynamics, age, and medical comorbidities. This assessment is separate from the determination of operability. Coexisting coronary artery disease, parenchymal lung disease, renal insufficiency, or hepatic dysfunction may substantially complicate management during the postoperative period. However, advanced age or the presence of collateral disease does not represent an absolute contraindication to pulmonary thromboendarterectomy, although these factors do influence risk assessment. The prognosis from advanced chronic thromboembolic pulmonary hypertension is generally so poor that surgery may be considered even in high-risk patients. The one exception to this guideline is severe underlying obstructive or restrictive parenchymal lung disease. The postoperative course in these patients frequently is complicated by the need for prolonged ventilatory support. Furthermore, the hemodynamic benefits of thromboendarterectomy often result in minimal symptomatic improvement.

Surgical Approach

Details of the surgical approach to chronic thromboembolic pulmonary hypertension have been described extensively elsewhere.[6,80] However, several features of the procedure should be emphasized. Although a thoracotomy incision has been used in the past, the standard approach now involves median sternotomy and cardiopulmonary bypass. Given that the disease is rarely unilateral, a sternotomy approach provides access to the central pulmonary vessels of both lungs. A sternotomy approach also avoids the potential for disruption of the extensive bronchial collateral circulation and pulmonary adhesions that may develop following pulmonary artery obstruction and provides adequate exposure for any additional procedures that need to be performed. In a review of 1,190 patients undergoing thromboendarterectomy at UCSD Medical Center, 90 patients (7.6 percent) required a combined procedure other than of solitary closure of a patent foramen ovale (which is performed in approximately 30 percent of thromboendarterectomy procedures). Of these 90 patients, 83 underwent coronary bypass graft surgery, 3 underwent tricuspid valve repair, 2 underwent mitral valve repair, and 2 underwent aortic valve replacement.[81]

The thromboendarterectomy procedure involves periods of complete hypothermic circulatory arrest to assure a bloodless operative field and optimal exposure of the pulmonary vascular intima. Circulatory arrest periods are limited to 20 minutes, with resumption of blood flow and restoration of mixed venous O_2 saturation during each interruption.

The procedure is a true thromboendarterectomy, not an embolectomy. The chronic thromboembolic material is fibrotic and incorporated into the native vascular lumen (FIGURE 13-7). The

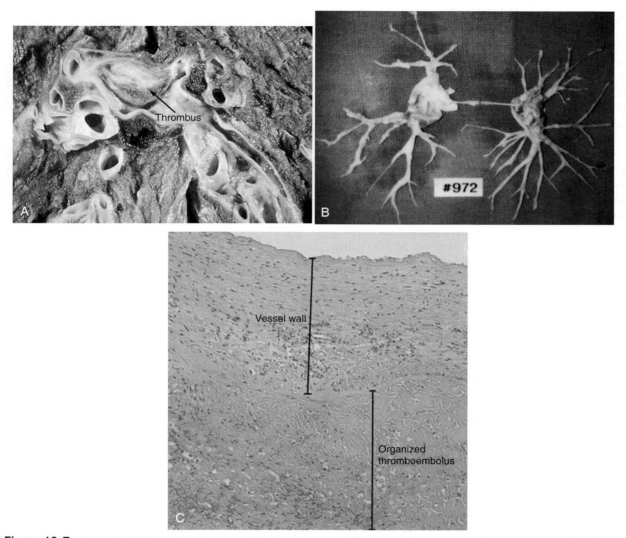

Figure 13-7. Organized Clot and Its Removal at Pulmonary Artery Thromboendarterectomy. **A,** An organized thrombus as seen within the lung at autopsy occluding a lobar pulmonary artery in a patient with chronic thromboembolic pulmonary hypertension. (Courtesy of Dr. Giuseppe G. Pietra.) **B,** Right and left pulmonary artery specimens removed at thromboendarterectomy. Note fibrotic nature of dissected tissue. **C,** Low-power photomicrograph of a specimen removed at the time of pulmonary thromboendarterectomy showing that the vascular intima, as well as organized thrombus, has been removed. (Hematoxylin and eosin stain.) (Courtesy of Dr. Giuseppe G. Pietra.)

neointima must be dissected meticulously away from the native intima, and considerable surgical experience with this procedure is required to identify the correct operative plane. Removal of non-adherent, partially organized thrombus within the lumen of the central pulmonary arteries is ineffective in reducing right ventricular afterload; creation of too deep a plane poses the risk of pulmonary artery perforation and massive pulmonary hemorrhage when cardiopulmonary bypass is discontinued.

Modifications of the surgical approach, intended to decrease risk or improve hemodynamic outcome, continue to be explored. These include intraoperative video-assisted angioscopy to increase visibility in the distal pulmonary arteries, thereby permitting surgical intervention in patients with previously inaccessible disease, division rather than retraction of the superior vena cava, selective antegrade cerebral perfusion to decrease the risk of neurologic sequelae, and bronchial artery occlusion to minimize retrograde bronchial artery flow.[73,80,82-84]

Postoperative Care

The approach to the postoperative care of patients undergoing pulmonary thromboendarterectomy must take into consideration the acute physiologic changes that occur as a result of the procedure.[6,85,86] The contractile state, preload, and afterload of the right ventricle (rather than the left ventricle) tend to determine cardiovascular function during the immediate postoperative period.

Careful postoperative management is essential for a successful outcome following thromboendarterectomy. Although most patients show an immediate improvement in pulmonary hemodynamics, the postoperative course can be complex. In addition to complications common to other forms of cardiac surgery (bleeding, dysrhythmias, atelectasis, wound infection, pericardial effusions, delirium, nosocomial pneumonia), patients undergoing pulmonary thromboendarterectomy often experience two unique complications that may adversely affect gas exchange in the postoperative period: pulmonary artery "steal" and reperfusion pulmonary edema.

Pulmonary artery "steal" represents a postoperative redistribution of pulmonary arterial blood flow away from previously well-perfused segments and into the newly endarterectomized segments. Although the basis for this phenomenon is uncertain, clinically relevant observations regarding "steal" are that it occurs commonly following pulmonary thromboendarterectomy, that it does not involve thrombosis of the nonoperated pulmonary segments, and that the distribution of pulmonary blood flow improves over time in most patients.[87,88]

The acute injury that may occur following thromboendarterectomy appears to represent a localized form of high-permeability lung injury.[89] Although often referred to as "reperfusion pulmonary edema," it has not yet been defined whether the phenomenon is related to ischemia-reperfusion, the effects of cardiopulmonary bypass, effects of the surgical procedure itself, or to some other combination of causes. Whatever the basis, acute lung injury following thromboendarterectomy can appear immediately after termination of cardiopulmonary bypass or as long as 72 hours after surgery. It is highly variable in severity, ranging from a mild form resulting in postoperative hypoxemia to an acute, hemorrhagic, and fatal form (FIGURE 13-8). One unique aspect of this form of lung injury is that it is limited to those areas from which proximal thromboembolic obstructions have been removed.

Reperfusion injury can represent a significant postoperative challenge in terms of ventilator

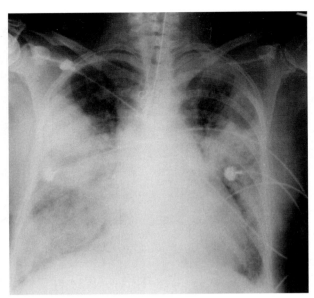

Figure 13-8. Reperfusion Pulmonary Edema. Chest radiograph demonstrates severe opacities due to reperfusion pulmonary edema in a patient who had undergone pulmonary thromboendarterectomy.

management. This is especially true in those with coincident pulmonary artery "steal." Under this circumstance, most pulmonary blood flow is shunted into areas of lung that have low compliance and are poorly ventilated, thereby resulting in transpulmonary shunting and hypoxemia. Management of reperfusion edema, as with other forms of acute lung injury, is supportive until resolution occurs. High-dose glucocorticoid therapy has been used to modulate the inflammatory component of the process, although its effectiveness is unpredictable and, frequently, minimal. In one randomized trial of 51 patients, the intraoperative and early postoperative administration of a selectin-mediated neutrophil adhesion blocking agent reduced the relative risk of reperfusion injury by 50 percent but had no impact on mortality, number of ventilator days, or number of days in the intensive care unit.[90]

It is unclear whether postoperative ventilator and inotropic strategies can reduce occurrence of this complication. An uncontrolled study found that low tidal volume ventilation (<8 ml/kg) and avoidance of inotropic support resulted in lower mortality than higher tidal volume ventilation (10-15 ml/kg) and routine inotropic support, but the two strategies were used at separate institutions, making it difficult to control for confounders.[75] In adult respiratory distress syndrome, low tidal volume ventilation often worsens oxygenation slightly, and it is possible that this effect may be magnified in patients with concomitant pulmonary artery "steal."[91] Thus, extrapolation of data from medical patients with acute lung injury to those who have this unique postsurgical condition should be done cautiously, and clinical studies in this specific patient population are needed.

Inhaled nitric oxide has been reported to improve gas exchange, although in our experience this effect is transient and does not affect disease progression.[92-95] In extreme situations, extracorporeal support has been used successfully in patients when aggressive conventional measures have failed to maintain adequate gas exchange.

Patients posing the most difficult management problem following thromboendarterectomy are those with persistent pulmonary hypertension. Even patients with well-compensated right ventricular function before the procedure may experience postoperative hemodynamic instability as a result of the depressant effects of cardiopulmonary bypass, deep hypothermia, acidosis, and hypoxemia. Management goals include minimizing systemic oxygen consumption, optimizing right ventricular preload, and providing aggressive inotropic support. Afterload reduction in this patient population may have adverse consequences. Cardiac output and pulmonary vascular resistance are commonly fixed, and attempts at pharmacologic manipulation of right ventricular afterload (sodium nitroprusside, calcium channel blockers) may simply decrease systemic vascular resistance, systemic blood pressure, and right coronary artery perfusion pressure. Inhaled nitric oxide is theoretically ideal for this circumstance because it has negligible systemic effects. However, experience with this intervention in those with persistent postoperative pulmonary hypertension has been disappointing.

Persistent pulmonary hypertension during the postoperative period remains a major cause of mortality in patients undergoing thromboendarterectomy, notwithstanding attempts at aggressive management. Mortality from this cause will not be diminished by advances in the operating suite or intensive care unit but by improved methods of preoperative evaluation and surgical referral.

Outcome

In reported series of patients undergoing thromboendarterectomy since 1996, in-hospital mortality rates have ranged between 4.4 and 23.5 percent (see TABLE 13-1). Factors affecting perioperative mortality have not been completely defined.

Several studies have suggested that World Health Organization (WHO) functional class IV status, age greater than 70 years, the presence of comorbid conditions, the severity of preoperative pulmonary vascular resistance, the presence of right ventricular failure as manifested by high right atrial pressures, and perhaps the duration of pulmonary hypertension may adversely influence outcome.[11,75,96]

Of these factors, the severity of the preoperative and postoperative pulmonary vascular resistance appears to have the greatest prognostic power. In a series of 500 patients undergoing pulmonary thromboendarterectomy at the UCSD Medical Center between 1998 and 2002, hospital mortality was 4.4 percent. In individuals in whom the preoperative pulmonary vascular resistance was less than 1,000 dynes·sec·cm^{-5}, the mortality rate was 1.3 percent, while those with a preoperative pulmonary vascular resistance greater than 1,000 dynes·sec·cm^{-5} had a mortality rate of 10.1 percent.[11] This effect of preoperative pulmonary vascular resistance on outcome has been confirmed by others.[84] In terms of postoperative pulmonary vascular resistance, patients with a resistance higher than 500 dynes·sec·cm^{-5}, a group encompassing approximately 10 percent of those undergoing the procedure, had a mortality rate of 30.6 percent, whereas individuals with a postoperative pulmonary vascular resistance less than 500 dynes·sec·cm^{-5} had a mortality rate of 0.9 percent.[11] Given what is known about the natural history of the disease and the progressive nature of the pulmonary hypertension associated with it, these findings suggest that early referral is preferable unless the possibility of a recent embolic event exists. Under this circumstance, a period of 3 months of conventional therapy is recommended to allow optimal thrombus resolution. Beyond this period, further improvement in the level of pulmonary hypertension cannot be achieved with anticoagulation alone.[26]

Experience with the evaluation and treatment of this patient population would also appear to affect outcome. The operative mortality rate was 17 percent for the first 200 patients operated on at UCSD between 1970 and 1990. The perioperative mortality rate has since declined steadily to 8.8 percent for the 500 individuals who had the operation between 1994 and 1998, and to 4.4 percent for the 500 patients operated on between 1998 and 2002. It is possible that increased physician recognition of the disease resulting in referral before secondary arteriopathy develops or right ventricular failure begins has contributed to this decline in mortality. However, it is also reasonable to suggest that a strong relationship between number of procedures performed and outcome may exist, as has been demonstrated with other high-risk surgical procedures.[97,98] In the case of thromboendarterectomy, this may be related to consistency of patient evaluation, surgical experience, uniform delivery of postoperative care, and dedicated resources for dealing with postoperative complications.

In most patients undergoing thromboendarterectomy, both the short-term and long-term hemodynamic outcomes are favorable. Dramatic reduction, and at times normalization, of the pulmonary artery pressure and pulmonary vascular resistance can be achieved. In published series, the mean reduction in pulmonary vascular resistance has approximated 70 percent and a final pulmonary vascular resistance in the range of 200 to 350 dynes·sec·cm^{-5} can be achieved (see TABLE 13-1). A corresponding improvement in right ventricular function determined by echocardiography, gas exchange, exercise capacity, and quality of life also has been reported.[99-105] Most patients initially in WHO functional class III or IV preoperatively return postoperatively to WHO class I or II and are able to resume normal activities.

Lifelong anticoagulation is strongly recommended following thromboendarterectomy. A second thromboendarterectomy has been necessary in several patients in whom anticoagulation was discontinued or maintained at a subtherapeutic level. Repeat thromboendarterectomy has also been performed successfully in a number of patients who initially underwent an inadequate procedure, either by way of thoracotomy or sternotomy approach. A second procedure can be performed with morbidity and mortality comparable to those of the primary procedure, but the consequent improvements in hemodynamics have been less impressive.[106]

Medical Management

Survival of patients with chronic thromboembolic disease managed with anticoagulation alone has been very poor. In one study, the 5-year survival rate was 30 percent when the mean pulmonary artery pressure exceeded 40 mmHg and 10 percent when it exceeded 50 mmHg.[107] In another study, patients with a mean pulmonary artery pressure above 30 mmHg had a survival of less than 20 percent after 3 years.[108]

More recently, medications investigated for use in IPAH have been used in a number of clinical settings. Potential indications for long-term use of these drugs include inoperable or distal chronic thromboembolic pulmonary hypertension and postoperative use for patients with residual pulmonary hypertension after pulmonary thromboendarterectomy. Perioperative medical therapy can be considered for patients with a pulmonary vascular resistance greater than 1,000 dynes·sec·cm^{-5}.

Significant numbers of patients with chronic thromboembolic pulmonary hypertension have been included in only one randomized clinical trial of medical therapy; inhaled iloprost was the agent used. This study included patients with IPAH (n = 102), pulmonary arterial hypertension associated with other conditions (n = 44), and patients with inoperable chronic thromboembolic pulmonary hypertension (n = 57), randomized to inhaled iloprost or placebo for a 12-week period.[109] Treated patients showed improvement in hemodynamics, WHO class, and quality of life compared with placebo patients, and were less likely to drop out of the study early. Subgroup data is reported for the patients non-IPAH only as a group (101 patients), with overall less improvement in this group than in those with IPAH.

Patients with chronic thromboembolic pulmonary hypertension have also been included in a number of nonrandomized studies, including studies of intravenous epoprostenol (prostacyclin),[110-112] oral beraprost,[113,114] and oral sildenafil.[115] These studies reported statistically significant improvement in clinical status, hemodynamics, and exercise capacity compared with baseline. Two studies reported a possible survival benefit, but the lack of a randomized control group makes interpretation of this type of information difficult.

The limited amount of information from clinical trials is reflected in a 2004 American College of Chest Physicians practice guideline on chronic thromboembolic pulmonary hypertension. The guideline states that medical therapy for inoperable chronic thromboembolic pulmonary hypertension "may be considered," with the level of evidence reported as low, the benefit small and weak, and the grade of recommendation a "C."[116]

Additional evidence from studies of mediators, pathologic specimens, and animal studies is suggestive of a role for progressive small vessel arteriopathy in patients with chronic thromboembolic pulmonary hypertension. Hemodynamics in patients who do not undergo pulmonary thromboendarterectomy worsen over time despite stability or even improvement in ventilation-perfusion scan results.[117] Lung biopsy specimens from patients with chronic thromboembolic pulmonary hypertension show the full range of pulmonary hypertensive lesions. Intimal thickening of even the small pulmonary arteries occurs, and well-formed plexogenic lesions that are indistinguishable from those of patients with IPAH occur in some patients.[36,118] Finally, patients with chronic thromboembolic pulmonary hypertension, like those with pulmonary arterial hypertension, have abnormally increased levels of both endothelin-1 and angiopoietin-1, two mediators of smooth muscle cell growth.[119-121] Although no large clinical trial with endothelin receptor antagonists has been performed in patients with chronic thromboembolic pulmonary hypertension, bosentan prevents increases in pulmonary artery wall thickness in an animal model of embolic pulmonary hypertension.[122]

Most patients with inoperable chronic thromboembolic pulmonary hypertension or with residual pulmonary hypertension after surgery should be offered a trial of medical therapy given the lack of alternatives and the clinical trial evidence suggestive of a possible beneficial effect. Medical therapy usually is considered when the postoperative pulmonary vascular resistance is greater than 500 dynes·sec·cm^{-5}. Patients with modest elevations in their pulmonary vascular resistance (between 300 and 500 dynes·sec·cm^{-5}) should be followed with annual echocardiography and clinical evaluation, and may be considered for treatment if progressive symptoms and hemodynamic decline are seen.

Another area in which medical therapy has been considered is the preoperative treatment of patients with surgically accessible thromboembolic disease but very high pulmonary vascular resistance. It is possible, although not proven, that lowering the pulmonary vascular resistance through pharmacologic intervention before thromboendarterectomy could reduce surgical mortality, either by reducing the severity of concomitant small vessel disease or through improved right heart function.

In one study of 12 patients with severe chronic thromboembolic pulmonary hypertension (pulmonary vascular resistance >1,200 dynes·sec·cm^{-5}), all patients showed improvement in hemodynamics and clinical status after treatment with intravenous epoprostenol, and 11 of 12 patients showed further improvement after pulmonary thromboendarterectomy. The remaining patient died from persistent pulmonary hypertension.[123] In another study involving nine patients with a median pulmonary vascular resistance of 1,031 dynes·sec·cm^{-5}, treatment with intravenous epoprostenol yielded more variable results.[124] Six patients demonstrated clinical and hemodynamic stability or improvement, including three patients with stable hemodynamics over

22-26 months of treatment. The remaining three patients worsened clinically and hemodynamically, with two showing increases in pulmonary arterial pressure and pulmonary vascular resistance, and a third patient showing evidence of right heart failure despite a modest decline in pulmonary vascular resistance. Surgical results were more consistently favorable, with hemodynamic improvement seen in all patients after pulmonary thromboendarterectomy. Seven of nine patients were able to be weaned off epoprostenol shortly after surgery, while the remaining two patients tolerated decreases in dosage. Finally, in a hemodynamic study of the acute effects of inhaled iloprost given to 10 patients during the immediate preoperative and postoperative periods, no improvement was seen in preoperative pulmonary hemodynamics (cardiac index, mean pulmonary artery pressure, pulmonary vascular resistance), and systemic arterial pressure fell significantly, requiring two patients to be placed on vasopressors.[125]

Overall, it remains uncertain whether the high-risk patients in the two studies above showed good outcomes because of preoperative medical therapy, or whether surgery alone would have led to similar results. If medical therapy is chosen, dosage increases should be implemented cautiously, because the systemic vascular bed may be more vasoreactive than the pulmonary vascular bed, as shown in the inhaled iloprost study above. Interestingly, patients in this same study were also given inhaled iloprost during the immediate postoperative period, and the hemodynamic results were much better than the preoperative results, with an improvement in the cardiac index, mean pulmonary artery pressure, and right atrial pressure, while systemic blood pressure remained stable.

In summary, medical therapy is most appropriately considered in patients with inoperable or distal chronic thromboembolic pulmonary hypertension, and in the long-term treatment of patients with residual pulmonary hypertension following pulmonary thromboendarterectomy. Use of intravenous epoprostenol during the preoperative period is sometimes considered, but it remains unclear whether the potential benefits outweigh the risk of disease progression during the delay to surgical intervention.

Conclusion

Substantial progress has occurred in the diagnostic and therapeutic approaches to patients with chronic thromboembolic pulmonary hypertension.

However, a great deal remains to be accomplished. The development of chronic thromboembolic pulmonary hypertension represents a failure, at least in certain patients, in the prevention or initial diagnosis of venous thromboembolism and in the treatment and follow-up surveillance of those with documented disease. It is unlikely that the increase in surgical experience reflects an increased prevalence of disease but instead represents a heightened awareness of the disease as a correctable form of pulmonary hypertension. Given estimates of the incidence of the disease following acute embolism, it is probable that the disease continues to escape diagnosis in a substantial number of patients and contributes to their premature deaths.

A great deal also remains unknown about the early natural history of the disease. The level of pulmonary hypertension encountered in these patients at the time of initial clinical recognition cannot occur on an acute basis, and clinical experience would suggest that hemodynamic progression occurs in the absence of recurrent embolic events. The progressive nature of the disease may involve interplay among the extent of obstruction of the pulmonary vascular bed, the effects of circulating vasoconstrictors, the development of a hypertensive pulmonary arteriopathy, an individual genetic predisposition to pulmonary hypertension, the compensatory adaptations of the right ventricle, or to other, as-yet-unidentified factors. Early detection of persistent pulmonary hypertension following an acute thromboembolic event could serve to identify patients at risk of further hemodynamic impairment and shed light on the pathophysiologic mechanisms involved in the progression of their disease. Improved diagnostic and hemodynamic partitioning techniques are necessary to identify patients at risk for persistent postoperative pulmonary hypertension. Despite a broad experiential base, prognostic uncertainty exists in approximately 10 percent of patients before operative intervention. Because many of these patients will benefit from the procedure, and because many are ineligible for reason of age or other restriction for transplantation, it has been our belief that surgery should be offered to these patients, although at an assumed higher risk. To not do so would mean denying a potentially lifesaving procedure from many who would benefit and who might be left without an effective therapeutic alternative. However, the introduction of potentially effective, pharmacologic interventions might mandate a change in that approach. Investigation into the efficacy of pulmonary vascular dilating or antiproliferative agents, alone or combined with surgical intervention, needs to be conducted.

Finally, a principal challenge in this patient population lies in the prevention and management of reperfusion lung injury. This patient population offers a unique opportunity to enhance our understanding of the pathophysiologic mechanisms involved in acute lung injury and to evaluate the effects of prophylactic and therapeutic interventions.

References

1. Carroll D: Chronic obstruction of major pulmonary arteries. *Am J Med* 9:175-185, 1950.
2. Jamieson SW, Auger WR, Fedullo PF, et al: Experience and results with 150 pulmonary thromboendarterectomy operations over a 29-month period. *J Thorac Cardiovasc Surg* 106:116-127, 1993.
3. Fedullo PF, Auger WR, Channick RN, et al: Chronic thromboembolic pulmonary hypertension. *Clin Chest Med* 16:353-374, 1995.
4. Daily PO, Auger WR: Historical perspective: Surgery for chronic thromboembolic disease. *Semin Thorac Cardiovasc Surg* 11:143-151, 1999.
5. Daily PO, Dembitsky WP, Jamieson SW: The evolution and the current state of the art of pulmonary thromboendarterectomy. *Semin Thorac Cardiovasc Surg* 11:152-163, 1999.
6. Jamieson SW, Kapelanski DP: Pulmonary endarterectomy. *Curr Probl Surg* 37:165-252, 2000.
7. Kapelanski DP, Macoviak JA, Jamieson SW: Surgical intervention in the treatment of pulmonary embolism and chronic thromboembolic pulmonary hypertension. In: Oudkerk M, van Beek EJR, ten Cate JW, editors: *Pulmonary embolism,* Berlin, 1999, Blackwell Science, pp 382-397.
8. Hollister LE, Cull VL: The syndrome of chronic thrombosis of major pulmonary arteries. *Am J Med* 21:312-320, 1956.
9. Houk VN, Hufnagel CA, McClenathan JE, et al: Chronic thrombotic obstruction of major pulmonary arteries: Report of a case successfully treated by thromboendarterectomy, and a review of the literature. *Am J Med* 35:269-282, 1963.
10. Chitwood WR, Lyerly HK, Sabiston DC: Surgical management of chronic pulmonary embolism. *Ann Surg* 201:11-26, 1985.
11. Jamieson SW, Kapelanski DP, Sakakibara N, et al: Pulmonary endarterectomy: Experience and lessons learned in 1,500 cases. *Ann Thorac Surg* 76:1457-1462, 2003.

12. Rubens F, Wells P, Bencze S, et al: Surgical treatment of chronic thromboembolic pulmonary hypertension. *Can Respir J* 7:49-57, 2000.

13. D'Armini AM, Cattadori B, Monterosso C, et al: Pulmonary thromboendarterectomy in patients with chronic thromboembolic pulmonary hypertension: Hemodynamic characteristics and changes. *Eur J Cardiothorac Surg* 18:696-702, 2000.

14. Fedullo PF, Auger WR, Kerr KM, et al: Chronic thromboembolic pulmonary hypertension. *New Engl J Med* 345:1465-1472, 2001.

15. Ando M, Okita Y, Tagusari O, et al: Surgical treatment for chronic thromboembolic pulmonary hypertension under profound hypothermia and circulatory arrest in 24 patients. *J Card Surg* 14:377-385, 1999.

16. Masuda M, Nakajima N: Our experience of surgical treatment for chronic pulmonary thromboembolism. *Ann Thorac Cardiovasc Surg* 7:261-265, 2001.

17. Pengo V, Lensing AW, Prins MH, et al: Incidence of chronic thromboembolic pulmonary hypertension after pulmonary embolism. *N Engl J Med* 350:2257-2264, 2004.

18. Dalen JE, Alpert JS: Natural history of pulmonary embolism. *Prog Cardiovasc Dis* 17:259-270, 1975.

19. Egermayer P, Peacock AJ: Is pulmonary embolism a common cause of pulmonary hypertension? Limitations of the embolic hypothesis. *Eur Respir J* 15:440-448, 2000.

20. Fedullo PF, Rubin LJ, Kerr KM, et al: The natural history of acute and chronic thromboembolic disease: The search for the missing link. *Eur Respir J* 15:435-437, 2000 (editorial).

21. McIntyre KM, Sasahara AA: The hemodynamic response to pulmonary embolism in patients without prior cardiopulmonary disease. *Am J Cardiol* 28:288-294, 1971.

22. Wolfe MW, Lee RT, Feldstein ML, et al: Prognostic significance of right ventricular hypokinesis and perfusion lung scan defects in pulmonary embolism. *Am Heart J* 127:1371-1375, 1994.

23. Wartski M, Collignon MA: Incomplete recovery of lung perfusion after 3 months in patients with acute pulmonary embolism treated with antithrombotic agents. *J Nucl Med* 41:1043-1048, 2000.

24. Ribeiro A, Lindmarker P, Johnsson H, et al: Pulmonary embolism: A follow-up study of the relation between the degree of right ventricular overload and the extent of perfusion defects. *J Int Med* 245:601-610, 1999.

25. Moser KM, Auger WR, Fedullo PF: Chronic major-vessel thromboembolic pulmonary hypertension. *Circulation* 81:1735-1743, 1990.

26. Ribeiro A, Lindmarker P, Johnsson H, et al: Pulmonary embolism: One-year follow-up with echocardiography Doppler and 5-year survival analysis. *Circulation* 99:1325-1330, 1999.

27. Liu P, Meneveau N, Schiele F, et al: Predictors of long-term clinical outcome of patients with acute massive pulmonary embolism after thrombolytic therapy. *Chin Med J (Engl)* 116:503-509, 2003.

28. Naudziunas A, Miliauskas S: Factor V Leiden and post thromboembolic pulmonary hypertension. *Medicina (Kaunas)* 39:1171-1174, 2003.

29. Wolf M, Boyer-Neumann C, Parent F, et al: Thrombotic risk factors in pulmonary hypertension. *Eur Respir J* 15:395-399, 2000.

30. Auger WR, Permpikul P, Moser KM: Lupus anticoagulant, heparin use, and thrombocytopenia in patients with chronic thromboembolic pulmonary hypertension: A preliminary report. *Am J Med* 99:392-396, 1995.

31. Olman MA, Marsh JJ, Lang IM, et al: Endogenous fibrinolytic system in chronic large-vessel thromboembolic pulmonary hypertension. *Circulation* 86:1241-1248, 1992.

32. Bonderman D, Turecek PL, Jakowitsch J, et al: High prevalence of elevated clotting factor VIII in chronic thromboembolic pulmonary hypertension. *Thromb Haemost* 90:372-376, 2003.

33. Colorio CC, Martinuzzo ME, Forastiero RR, et al: Thrombophilic tendencies in chronic thromboembolic pulmonary hypertension. *Blood Coagul Fibrinolysis* 12:427-432, 2001.

34. Meignan M, Rosso J, Gauthier H, et al: Systematic lung scans reveal a high frequency of silent pulmonary embolism in patients with proximal deep venous thrombosis. *Arch Intern Med* 160:159-164, 2000.

35. Karwinski B, Svendsen E: Comparison of clinical and postmortem diagnosis of pulmonary embolism. *J Clin Pathol* 42:135-139, 1989.

36. Moser KM, Bloor CM: Pulmonary vascular lesions occurring in patients with chronic major-vessel thromboembolic pulmonary hypertension. *Chest* 103:684-692, 1993.

37. Auger WR, Moser KM: Pulmonary flow murmurs: A distinctive physical sign found in chronic pulmonary thromboembolic disease. *Clin Res* 37:145A, 1989.

38. Nagaya N, Uematsu M, Satoh T, et al: Serum uric acid levels correlate with the severity and the mortality of primary pulmonary hypertension. *Am J Respir Crit Care Med* 160:487-492, 1999.

39. Voelkel MA, Wynne KM, Badesch DB, et al: Hyperuricemia in severe pulmonary hypertension. *Chest* 117:19-24, 2000.

40. Nagaya N, Ando M, Oya H, et al: Plasma brain natriuretic peptide as a noninvasive marker for efficacy of pulmonary thromboendarterectomy. *Ann Thorac Surg* 74:180-184, 2002.

41. Kapitan KS, Buchbinder M, Wagner PD, et al: Mechanisms of hypoxemia in chronic thromboembolic pulmonary hypertension. *Am Rev Respir Dis* 139:1149-1154, 1989.

42. Morris TA, Auger WR, Ysrael MZ, et al: Parenchymal scarring is associated with restrictive spirometric defects in patients with chronic thromboembolic pulmonary hypertension. *Chest* 110:399-403, 1996.

43. D'Alonzo GE, Bower JS, Dantzker DR: Differentiation of patients with primary and thromboembolic pulmonary hypertension. *Chest* 85:457-461, 1984.

44. Currie PJ, Seward JB, Chan KL, et al: Continuous wave Doppler determination of right ventricular pressure: A simultaneous Doppler-catheterization study in 127 patients. *J Am Coll Cardiol* 6:750-756, 1985.

45. Berger M, Haimowitz A, Van Tosh A, et al: Quantitative assessment of pulmonary hypertension in patients with tricuspid regurgitation using continuous wave Doppler ultrasound. *J Am Coll Cardiol* 6:359-365, 1985.

46. Mahmud E, Raisinghani A, Hassankhani A, et al: Correlation of left ventricular diastolic filling characteristics with right ventricular overload and pulmonary artery pressure in chronic thromboembolic pulmonary hypertension. *J Am Coll Cardiol* 40:318-324, 2002.

47. Ghio S, Raineri C, Scelsi L, et al: Usefulness and limits of transthoracic echocardiography in the evaluation of patients with primary and chronic thromboembolic pulmonary hypertension. *J Am Soc Echocardiogr* 15:1374-1380, 2002.

48. Sun XG, Hansen JE, Oudiz RJ, et al: Pulmonary function in primary pulmonary hypertension. *J Am Coll Cardiol* 41:1028-1035, 2003.

49. Bernstein RJ, Ford RL, Clausen JL, et al: Membrane diffusion and capillary blood volume in chronic thromboembolic pulmonary hypertension. *Chest* 110:1430-1436, 1996.

50. Fishman AJ, Moser KM, Fedullo PF: Perfusion lung scans vs. pulmonary angiography in evaluation of suspected primary pulmonary hypertension. *Chest* 84:679-683, 1983.

51. Lisbona R, Kreisman H, Novales-Diaz J, et al: Perfusion lung scanning: Differentiation of primary from thromboembolic pulmonary hypertension. *Am J Roentgenol* 144:27-30, 1985.

52. Worsley DF, Palevsky HI, Alavi A: Ventilation-perfusion lung scanning in the evaluation of pulmonary hypertension. *J Nucl Med* 35:793-796, 1994.

53. Azarian R, Wartski M, Collignon MA, et al: Lung perfusion scans and hemodynamics in acute and chronic pulmonary embolism. *J Nucl Med* 38:980-983, 1997.

54. Ryan KL, Fedullo PF, Davis GB, et al: Perfusion scan findings understate the severity of angiographic and hemodynamic compromise in chronic thromboembolic pulmonary hypertension. *Chest* 93:1180-1185, 1988.

55. Bergin CJ, Sirlin CB, Hauschildt JP, et al: Chronic thromboembolism: Diagnosis with helical CT and MR imaging with angiographic and surgical correlation. *Radiology* 204:695-702, 1997.

56. King MA, Ysrael M, Bergin CJ: Chronic thromboembolic pulmonary hypertension: CT findings. *Am J Roentgenol* 170:955-960, 1998.

57. Bergin CJ, Rios G, King MA, et al: Accuracy of high-resolution CT in identifying chronic pulmonary thromboembolic disease. *Am J Roentgenol* 166:1371-1377, 1996.

58. Bergin CJ, Hauschildt JP, Brown MA, et al: Identifying the cause of unilateral hypoperfusion in patients suspected to have chronic pulmonary thromboembolism: Diagnostic accuracy of helical CT and conventional angiography. *Radiology* 213:743-749, 1999.

59. Kreitner KF, Ley S, Kauczor HU, et al: Chronic thromboembolic pulmonary hypertension: Pre- and postoperative assessment with breath-hold MR imaging techniques. *Radiology* 232:535-543, 2004.

60. Ley S, Kauczor HU, Heussel CP, et al: Value of contrast-enhanced MR angiography and helical CT angiography in chronic thromboembolic pulmonary hypertension. *Eur Radiol* 13:2365-2371, 2003.

61. Fedullo PF, Auger WR, Moser KM, et al: Hemodynamic response to exercise in patients with chronic, major vessel thromboembolic pulmonary hypertension. *Am Rev Respir Dis* 141:A-890, 1990 (abstract).

62. Auger WR, Fedullo PF, Moser KM, et al: Chronic major-vessel chronic thromboembolic pulmonary artery obstruction: Appearance of angiography. *Radiology* 182:393-398, 1992.

63. Pitton MB, Duber C, Mayer E, et al: Hemodynamic effects of nonionic contrast bolus injection and oxygen inhalation during pulmonary angiography in patients with chronic major-vessel thromboembolic pulmonary hypertension. *Circulation* 94:2485-2491, 1996.

64. Nicod P, Peterson K, Levine M, et al: Pulmonary angiography in severe chronic pulmonary hypertension. *Ann Intern Med* 107:565-568, 1987.

65. Shure D, Gregoratos G, Moser KM: Fiberoptic angioscopy: Role in the diagnosis of chronic pulmonary artery obstruction. *Ann Intern Med* 103:844-850, 1985.

66. Sompradeekul S, Fedullo PF, Kerr KM, et al: The role of pulmonary angioscopy in the preoperative assessment of patients with thromboembolic pulmonary hypertension (CTEPH). *Am J Respir Crit Care Med* 159:A-456, 1999 (abstract).

67. Channick RN, Auger WR, Fedullo PF, et al: Angioscopy. In: Feinsilver SH, Fein AM, editors: *Textbook of bronchoscopy*, 1995, Baltimore, MD: Williams and Wilkins, pp 477-485.

68. Fedullo PF, Auger WR, Channick RN, et al: Chronic thromboembolic pulmonary hypertension. *Clin Chest Med* 22:561-583, 2001.

69. Nakajima N, Masuda M, Mogi K: The surgical treatment for chronic pulmonary thromboembolism. Our experience and current review of the literature. *Ann Thorac Cardiovasc Surg* 3:15-21, 1997.

70. Mayer E, Kramm T, Dahm M, et al: Early results of pulmonary thromboendarterectomy in chronic thromboembolic pulmonary hypertension. *Z Kardiol* 86:920-927, 1997.

71. Gilbert TB, Gaine SP, Rubin LJ, et al: Short-term outcome and predictors of adverse events following pulmonary thromboendarterectomy. *World J Surg* 22:1029-1032, 1998.

72. Miller WT, Osiason AW, Langlotz CP, et al: Reperfusion edema after thromboendarterectomy: Radiographic patterns of disease. *J Thorac Imaging* 13:178-183, 1998.

73. Dartevelle P, Fadel E, Chapelier A, et al: Angioscopic video-assisted pulmonary endarterectomy for post-embolic pulmonary hypertension. *Eur J Cardiothorac Surg* 16:38-43, 1999.

74. Mares P, Gilbert TB, Tschernko EM, et al: Pulmonary artery thromboendarterectomy: A comparison of two different postoperative treatment strategies. *Anesth Analg* 90:267-273, 2000.

75. Tscholl D, Langer F, Wendler O, et al: Pulmonary thromboendarterectomy—risk factors for early survival and hemodynamic improvement. *Eur J Cardiothorac Surg* 19:771-776, 2001.

76. Hagl C, Khaladj N, Peters T, et al: Technical advances in pulmonary thromboendarterectomy for chronic thromboembolic pulmonary hypertension. *Eur J Cardiothorac Surg* 23:776-781, 2003.

77. Kafi SA, Mélot C, Vachiéry JL, et al: Partitioning of the pulmonary vascular resistance in primary pulmonary hypertension. *J Am Coll Cardiol* 31:1372-1376, 1998.

78. Fesler P, Pagnamenta A, Vachiery JL, et al: Single arterial occlusion to locate resistance in patients with pulmonary hypertension. *Eur Respir J* 21:31-36, 2003.

79. Kim NH, Fesler P, Channick RN, et al: Preoperative partitioning of pulmonary vascular resistance corre-

lates with early outcome after thromboendarterectomy for chronic thromboembolic pulmonary hypertension. *Circulation* 109:18-22, 2004.

80. Hartz RS: Surgery for chronic thromboembolic pulmonary hypertension. *World J Surg* 23:1137-1147, 1999.

81. Thistlethwaite PA, Auger WR, Madani MM, et al: Pulmonary thromboendarterectomy combined with other cardiac operations: Indications, surgical approach, and outcome. *Ann Thorac Surg* 72:13-19, 2001.

82. Zeebregts CJ, Dossche KM, Morshuis WJ, et al: Surgical thromboendarterectomy for chronic thromboembolic pulmonary hypertension using circulatory arrest with selective antegrade cerebral perfusion. *Acta Chir Belg* 98:95-97, 1998.

83. Zund G, Pretre R, Niederhauser U, et al: Improved exposure of the pulmonary arteries for thromboendarterectomy. *Ann Thorac Surg* 66:1821-1823, 1998.

84. Dartevelle P, Fadel E, Mussot S, et al: Chronic thromboembolic pulmonary hypertension. *Eur Respir J* 23:637-648, 2004.

85. Kapelanski DP, Macoviak JA, Jamieson SW: Surgical interventions in the treatment of pulmonary embolism and chronic thromboembolic pulmonary hypertension. In: Oudkerk M, van Beels EJR, ten Cate JW, editors: *Pulmonary embolism,* Berlin, 1999, Blackwell Science, pp 382-397.

86. Fedullo PF, Auger WR, Dembitsky WP: Postoperative management of the patient undergoing pulmonary thromboendarterectomy. *Semin Thorac Cardiovasc Surg* 11:172-178, 1999.

87. Olman MA, Auger WR, Fedullo PF, et al: Pulmonary vascular steal in chronic thromboembolic pulmonary hypertension. *Chest* 98:1430-1434, 1990.

88. Moser KM, Metersky ML, Auger WR, et al: Resolution of vascular steal after pulmonary thromboendarterectomy. *Chest* 104:1441-1444, 1993.

89. Levinson RM, Shure D, Moser KM: Reperfusion pulmonary edema after pulmonary artery thromboendarterectomy. *Am Rev Respir Dis* 134:1241-1245, 1986.

90. Kerr KM, Auger WR, Marsh J, et al: The use of Cylexin (CY-1503) in prevention of reperfusion lung injury in patients undergoing pulmonary thromboendarterectomy. *Am J Respir Crit Care Med* 162:14-20, 2000.

91. The acute respiratory distress syndrome network. Ventilation with lower tidal volumes as compared with traditional tidal volumes for acute lung injury and the acute respiratory distress syndrome. *N Engl J Med* 342:1301-1308, 2000.

92. Dupont H, Le Corre F, Fierobe L, et al: Efficiency of inhaled nitric oxide as rescue therapy during severe

ARDS: Survival and factors associated with the first response. *J Crit Care* 14:107-113, 1999.

93. Pinelli G, Mertes PM, Carteaux JP, et al: Inhaled nitric oxide as an adjunct to pulmonary thromboendarterectomy. *Ann Thorac Surg* 61:227-229, 1996.

94. Gardeback M, Larsen FF, Radegran K: Nitric oxide improves hypoxaemia following reperfusion oedema after pulmonary thromboendarterectomy. *Br J Anaesth* 75:798-800, 1995.

95. Troncy E, Collet JP, Shapiro S, et al: Inhaled nitric oxide in acute respiratory distress syndrome: A pilot randomized controlled study. *Am J Respir Crit Care Med* 157:1483-1488, 1998.

96. Hartz RS, Byrne JG, Levitsky S, et al: Predictors of mortality in pulmonary thromboendarterectomy. *Ann Thorac Surg* 62:1255-1259, 1996.

97. Birkmeyer JD, Siewers AE, Finlayson EV, et al: Hospital volume and surgical mortality in the United States. *N Engl J Med* 346:1128-1137, 2002.

98. Birkmeyer JD, Stukel TA, Siewers AE, et al: Surgeon volume and operative mortality in the United States. *N Engl J Med* 349:2117-2127, 2003.

99. Moser KM, Auger WR, Fedullo PF, et al: Chronic thromboembolic pulmonary hypertension: Clinical picture and surgical treatment. *Eur Respir J* 5:334-342, 1992.

100. Kramm T, Mayer E, Dahm M, et al: Long-term results after thromboendarterectomy for chronic pulmonary embolism. *Eur J Cardiothorac Surg* 15:579-584, 1999.

101. Kapitan KS, Clausen JL, Moser KM: Gas exchange in chronic thromboembolism after pulmonary thromboendarterectomy. *Chest* 98:14-19, 1990.

102. Tanabe N, Okada O, Nakagawa Y, et al: The efficacy of pulmonary thromboendarterectomy on long-term gas exchange. *Eur Respir J* 10:2066-2072, 1997.

103. Menzel T, Kramm T, Bruckner A, et al: Quantitative assessment of right ventricular volumes in severe chronic thromboembolic pulmonary hypertension using transthoracic three-dimensional echocardiography: Changes due to pulmonary thromboendarterectomy. *Eur J Echocardiogr* 3:67-72, 2002.

104. Archibald CJ, Auger WR, Fedullo PF, et al: Long-term outcome after pulmonary thromboendarterectomy. *Am J Respir Crit Care Med* 160:523-528, 1999.

105. Zoia MC, D'Armini AM, Beccaria M, et al: Pavia Thromboendarterectomy Group. Mid term effects of pulmonary thromboendarterectomy on clinical and cardiopulmonary function status. *Thorax* 57:608-612, 2002.

106. Mo M, Kapelanski DP, Mitruka SN, et al: Reoperative pulmonary thromboendarterectomy. *Ann Thorac Surg* 68:1770-1776, 1999.

107. Riedel M, Stanek V, Widimsky J, et al: Long-term follow-up of patients with pulmonary thromboembolism: Late prognosis and evolution of hemodynamic and respiratory data. *Chest* 81:151-158, 1982.

108. Lewczuk J, Piszko P, Jagas J, et al: Prognostic factors in medically treated patients with chronic pulmonary embolism. *Chest* 119:818-823, 2001.

109. Olschewski H, Simonneau G, Galie N, et al: Inhaled iloprost for severe pulmonary hypertension. *N Engl J Med* 347:322-329, 2002.

110. Higenbottam T, Butt AY, McMahon A, et al: Long-term intravenous prostaglandin (epoprostenol or iloprost) for treatment of severe pulmonary hypertension. *Heart* 80:151-155, 1998.

111. McLaughlin VV, Genthner DE, Panella MM, et al: Compassionate use of continuous prostacyclin in the management of secondary pulmonary hypertension: A case series. *Ann Intern Med* 130:740-743, 1999.

112. Scelsi L, Ghio S, Campana C, et al: Epoprostenol in chronic thromboembolic pulmonary hypertension with distal lesions. *Ital Heart J* 8:618-623, 2004.

113. Ono F, Nagaya N, Okumura H, et al: Effect of orally active prostacyclin analogue on survival in patients with chronic thromboembolic pulmonary hypertension without major vessel obstruction. *Chest* 123:1583-1588, 2003.

114. Nagaya N, Shimizu Y, Satoh T, et al: Oral beraprost sodium improves exercise capacity and ventilatory efficacy in patients with primary or thromboembolic pulmonary hypertension. *Heart* 87:340-345, 2002.

115. Ghofrani HA, Schermuly RT, Rose F, et al: Sildenafil for long-term treatment of nonoperable chronic thromboembolic pulmonary hypertension. *Am J Respir Crit Care Med* 167:1139-1141, 2003.

116. Doyle RL, McCrory D, Channick RN, et al: Surgical treatments/interventions for pulmonary artery hypertension. ACCP evidence-based clinical practice guidelines. *Chest* 126:63S-71S, 2004.

117. Skoro-Sajer N, Becherer A, Klepetko W, et al: Longitudinal analysis of perfusion lung scintigrams of patients with unoperated chronic thromboembolic pulmonary hypertension. *Thromb Haemost* 92:201-207, 2004.

118. Yi ES, Kim H, Ahn H, et al: Distribution of obstructive intimal lesions and their cellular phenotypes in chronic pulmonary hypertension. *Am J Respir Crit Care Med* 162:1577-1586, 2000.

119. Bauer M, Wilkens H, Langer F, et al: Selective upregulation of endothelin B receptor gene expression in severe pulmonary hypertension. *Circulation* 105:1034-1036, 2002.

120. Giaid A, Yanagisawa M, Langleben D, et al: Expression of endothelin-1 in the lungs of patients

with pulmonary hypertension. *N Engl J Med* 328: 1732-1739, 1993.

121. Du L, Sullivan C, Chu D, et al: Signaling molecules in nonfamilial pulmonary hypertension. *N Engl J Med* 348:500-509, 2003.

122. Kim H, Yung GL, Marsh JJ, et al: Endothelin mediates pulmonary vascular remodelling in a canine model of chronic embolic pulmonary hypertension. *Eur Respir J* 15:640-648, 2000.

123. Nagaya N, Sasaki N, Ando M, et al: Prostacyclin therapy before pulmonary thromboendarterectomy in patients with chronic thromboembolic pulmonary hypertension. *Chest* 123:338-343, 2003.

124. Bresser P, Fedullo PF, Auger WR, et al: Continuous intravenous epoprostenol for chronic thromboembolic pulmonary hypertension. *Eur Respir J* 23: 595-600, 2004.

125. Kramm T, Eberle B, Krummenauer F, et al: Inhaled iloprost in patients with chronic thromboembolic pulmonary hypertension: Effects before and after pulmonary thromboendarterectomy. *Ann Thorac Surg* 76:711-718, 2003.

14 Chapter

Pulmonary Vascular Tumors and Malformations

Karl W. Thomas, MD

Tumors and malformations of the pulmonary vasculature and lymphatic channels are among the most challenging diseases to diagnose and manage. The symptoms and radiographic findings are often indistinguishable from more common diseases such as pulmonary embolism, pulmonary hypertension, and cardiomyopathy. Management often is delayed by diagnostic uncertainty, and even if the correct diagnosis has been established long-term outcomes are frequently poor. The low prevalence and incidence of these diseases has limited research to individual case reports and small case series. Nevertheless, pulmonary vascular tumors and malformations have subtle and unique features that, if recognized, permit early, appropriate, and more effective management.

Pulmonary vascular tumors and malformations may arise from the pulmonary arteries, capillaries, veins, or lymphatic channels. Metastatic growth from distant primary tumors may also involve the vascular wall and lumen of the pulmonary vessels. The anatomic location, cellular characteristics, and physiologic effects of pulmonary vascular tumors or malformations will affect their clinical pictures, diagnostic procedure results and, ultimately, outcomes from management. This review will cover primary tumors of both the pulmonary arteries and veins, as well as secondary metastatic tumors that involve the pulmonary vasculature. Malformations including hereditary hemorrhagic telangiectasia, pulmonary capillary hemangiomatosis (PCH), and pulmonary artery aneurysms will be discussed. Finally, lymphatic disorders of the thoracic and pulmonary lymphatic channels will be reviewed.

Primary Tumors of the Pulmonary Vasculature

The most common vascular tumors are sarcomas and leiomyosarcomas. These may arise from the inferior vena cava, aorta, pulmonary arteries and veins, as well as smaller peripheral vessels. Only approximately 300 to 400 cases of these tumors arising in any vascular location have been reported.[1-3] Primary tumors of the pulmonary vasculature are an even more infrequent subset, with fewer than 200 reported cases worldwide. As with other vascular tumors, most tumors arising directly from the pulmonary vasculature are sarcomas or leiomyosarcomas. In general, these tumors are usually undifferentiated or poorly differentiated with leiomyosarcomatous, rhabdomyosarcomatous, or angiosarcomatous features. Other rare tumors, including pulmonary epithelioid hemangioendothelioma (EHE) and choriocarcinoma, have also been described with similar clinical and radiographic features. As the result of nonspecific symptoms and an insidious growth pattern, these tumors may be large at the time of examination and most will have metastasized before diagnosis.

In many cases, the final diagnosis in any of these disorders often is not suspected before failed management for other diseases, particularly pulmonary thromboembolism. Primary management involves surgical resection when possible for cure and occasionally for palliation. Although long-term survival has been reported, most patients with primary vascular neoplasms of the pulmonary arteries, veins, or capillaries die as the result of local disease effects or distant metastatic disease. The clinical approach to patients with suspected pulmonary vascular tumors should include specific attention to the clinical and radiographic features which favor these diagnoses over other conditions such as pulmonary thromboembolism.

Pulmonary Artery Sarcomas

Anatomic and Pathologic Features

Primary tumors of the pulmonary arteries are thought to arise from fibroblasts or myofibroblasts in the vascular media and intima. More specifically, several investigators have postulated that most of these tumors of the pulmonary arteries arise from mesenchymal cells of the muscle anlage of the bulbus cordis in the pulmonary trunk.[4-6] These tumors have been classified most commonly as undifferentiated sarcomas, followed by leiomyosarcoma, spindle cell sarcoma, fibrosarcoma, malignant fibrous histiocytoma, and rhabdomyosarcoma (TABLE 14-1). A wide range of other histologic subtypes including chondrosarcoma, mesenchymoma, myxosarcoma, and myosarcoma may occur rarely.[7,8] In general, these tumors may display a wide range of mitotic rates, cellular atypia, and myxoid tumor matrix characteristics. Although the tumors found in adult populations have malignant histologic and clinical characteristics, single case reports in children have also described tumors with benign histologic features such as pulmonary artery fibromas or myxomas.[9]

Pulmonary artery sarcomas usually display positive immunohistochemical staining for vimentin but show variable reactivity to desmin and smooth muscle actin. All primary pulmonary vascular tumors may fail to react to endothelial and epithelial cell markers.[5,10] Because so few patients have been compared prospectively and only a fraction of the patients with these tumors have been diagnosed antemortem, it is not apparent that the histologic type, grade, or location has a significant impact on clinical features or prognosis.[11,12]

Most pulmonary artery tumors are found in the pulmonary trunk in close proximity to the pulmonic valve. The next most frequent locations include the main pulmonary arteries. Although significantly less common, the tumors have also been described in association with lobar, segmental, or subsegmental vessels. These tumors may propagate in a retrograde manner and extend into the right ventricular

TABLE 14-1

Histologic Classification of Primary Pulmonary Arterial Tumors

Histologic Classification	Reported Frequency Range (Percent)
Undifferentiated sarcoma	20-31
Leiomyosarcoma	16-20
Spindle cell sarcoma	14-16
Fibrosarcoma	5-6
Fibromyxosarcoma	4-6
Rhabdomyosarcoma	4-6
Chondrosarcoma	4
Malignant fibrous histiocytoma	2-7
Mesenchymoma	3-4
Osteosarcoma	2-3
Myxosarcoma	2
Hemangiopericytoma	1-2
Angiosarcoma	1
Osteoid chondrosarcoma	1
Myosarcoma	1
Fibroleiomyosarcoma	1
Angiofibromyosarcoma	1
Hemangioendothelioma	1

From Cox JE, Chiles C, Aquino SL, et al: Pulmonary artery sarcomas: A review of clinical and radiologic features. J Comput Assist Tomogr 21(5):750-755, 1997; Kruger I, Borowski A, Horst M, et al: Symptoms, diagnosis, and therapy of primary sarcomas of the pulmonary artery. Thorac Cardiovasc Surg 38(2):91-95, 1990; and Parish JM, Rosenow EC, III, Swensen SJ, et al: Pulmonary artery sarcoma. Clinical features. Chest 110(6):1480-1488, 1996.

outflow tract or right ventricle. Morphologically these tumors appear as large smooth, multinodular or polypoid masses that encroach and spread over the pulmonary arteries. Commonly there is associated thrombosis, and on cut section many tumors display necrosis or hemorrhage.

Metastatic disease occurs in more than one-half of patients with pulmonary artery sarcomas. The most common sites of metastasis include the lung, regional lymph nodes, liver, brain, adrenal glands, kidneys, and skin. Rare metastatic locations include pancreas, mesentery, thyroid gland, and tongue.[8,13]

Clinical Features

The clinical characteristics of patients who develop pulmonary artery sarcomas are nonspecific and share many common features of patients with thromboembolic, cardiac valvular, or pulmonary parenchymal disease. The mean age of patients with pulmonary arterial sarcomas is 50-55 years, with a range from 13 to 86.[7,11,14,15] Although early case series and reviews described a female predominance, this has not been confirmed in more recent observations.

The most frequent symptoms at initial evaluation include chest pain, hemoptysis, dyspnea and palpitations. Less common symptoms include cough, syncope, voice changes, as well as constitutional symptoms such as fatigue, weight loss, and fever. Although the duration of reported symptoms has ranged from days to approximately 1 year, the average duration before diagnosis is 4-5 months. Physical findings may be absent, or they may relate to right ventricular failure. Peripheral edema, prominent jugular venous distention, and hepatomegaly may develop with advanced disease that produces significant obstruction of the right ventricular outflow tract or pulmonary trunk. Although not consistently reported, pulmonary vascular bruits, pulmonary friction rubs, a diminished or absent pulmonic component of the second heart sound (P_2), or systolic murmurs may be found on auscultation of the chest. Although many of these findings can occur in thromboembolic disease, subacute and chronic pulmonary symptoms accompanied by systemic symptoms such as weight loss or fatigue increase the probability of pulmonary artery tumor. Because of nonspecific symptoms and physical findings, the differential diagnosis for pulmonary arterial tumors includes acute thromboembolic disease, chronic thromboembolic disease, pulmonary hypertension from a variety of causes, congenital pulmonic stenosis, fibrosing mediastinitis, vasculitis, tuberculosis, and parenchymal lung carcinomas.[13,14,16,17]

Radiographic Characteristics

Although radiographic findings in patients with pulmonary vascular tumors usually are nonspecific, a number of characteristics suggest the diagnosis of tumor rather than thromboembolism or other vascular diseases. Posteroanterior and lateral chest radiographs may demonstrate normal findings or a wide range of abnormalities including central mass lesions, peripheral nodules or masses, atelectasis, postobstructive pneumonitis, or pleural effusions. Computed tomography (CT) with intravenous contrast enhancement may demonstrate intravascular filling defects or mass-like lesions associated with pulmonary vessels. Nonspecific findings may include a mosaic pattern of hypoperfusion, peripheral metastatic nodules, or focal peripheral consolidation. The masses have intermediate density comparable to skeletal muscle and typically contain areas of hypodensity consistent with necrosis. These neoplasms may produce mass effect, with displacement of surrounding structures or effacement of tissue planes from local invasion. Mass effects and effacement of tissue planes by pulmonary artery sarcomas are specific findings and, if present, permit differentiation from thromboembolic disease.

As CT scanning is used more frequently in the evaluation of patients with suspected pulmonary embolism and as the resolution of CT images improves, additional unique features of pulmonary artery tumors have been recognized. An analysis of a small cohort of 7 patients with pulmonary artery tumors and 40 patients with thromboembolic disease suggests that pulmonary artery tumors can be identified by low-attenuation filling defects that occupy the entire diameter of the pulmonary artery. In this cohort of patients, thromboembolism did not produce occlusion of the entire vascular lumen. Additional characteristics from this study that favored the diagnosis of pulmonary vascular tumor included expansion of the diameter of the involved arteries, evidence for extravascular invasion, stippled or focal nodular calcification, and presence only in the pulmonary trunk or main pulmonary arteries with sparing of the segmental and subsegmental branches.[18] Other published findings of clinically useful CT features for the diagnosis of pulmonary artery tumors include persistence or growth of the lesion despite anticoagulation or thrombolytic therapy and unilateral defects without evidence for contralateral disease.[17,19]

Lung scintigraphy (ventilation-perfusion scanning) is obtained frequently in patients with pulmonary vascular tumors before diagnosis to evaluate for suspected thromboembolic disease.

Although segmental perfusion abnormalities may be found, typical patterns include unilateral absence of perfusion or severe lobar perfusion defects.[20] Similarly, pulmonary angiography may demonstrate unilateral findings, but these cannot differentiate between thromboembolic and neoplastic disease. In some cases, magnetic resonance imaging (MRI) may demonstrate heterogenous soft tissue density that enhances following the administration of gadolinium-labeled contrast material (FIGURE 14-1).

Because thrombus does not enhance on MRI, this is considered a reliable method to distinguish tumor from thromboembolism; however, not all tumors have demonstrated uptake of paramagnetic contrast agents. Three-dimensional reconstruction imaging with either CT or MRI has been particularly useful in the preoperative and staging evaluations of patients with these tumors.[19,21,22] A single report of positron-emission tomographic imaging with fluorine 18-2-deoxy-D-glucose has demonstrated increased uptake in a pulmonary artery sarcoma.[23]

Clinical Diagnosis

Diagnosis of a pulmonary artery tumor is particularly challenging and often is delayed for months or not established until postmortem examination.[8,14] With advancements in imaging quality, particularly high-resolution CT and echocardiography, there has been a trend toward more frequent antemortem recognition and diagnosis. Because many tumors have pedunculated or polypoid features that may project in a retrograde manner, the presence of a mobile mass lesion extending through the pulmonic valve from the right ventricular outflow tract on echocardiography is highly suggestive of the diagnosis.[11] Histologic confirmation of the diagnosis may be obtained by bronchoscopy in a small number of cases with large central lesions or with visible endobronchial extension of the tumor.[20] Embolectomy suction catheters have also been employed to diagnose these tumors.[24] Unfortunately, the definitive antemortem diagnosis for most patients has required thoracotomy and surgical excision through arteriotomy, embolectomy, endarterectomy, pneumonectomy, or combinations of these procedures. Not all patients can withstand these operations. Metastatic disease or unresectable disease often is identified only at the time of surgery. Frequently both surgical and embolectomy catheter biopsy procedures are initiated for the management of other diseases such as thromboembolic disease. Thus, the diagnosis for pulmonary artery sarcomas often occurs only after failed diagnosis or management for thromboembolism.

Management and Outcome

At the time of diagnosis, many patients have unresectable disease, decompensated heart failure from right ventricular dysfunction, secondary hypoxemia, or evidence of metastasis. As the result of delayed diagnosis, metastatic disease, and the technical challenges of surgical resection, most patients die as the result of uncontrolled primary tumor. Unlike many other tumors, histologic subtype, grade, and differentiation characteristics have not been associated consistently with disease outcome. The natural history and survival rates for patients who do not have surgical resection are particularly poor, with a median survival time of 1.5 months and a 1-year survival rate of only 5 percent. For younger patients without comorbid conditions who undergo complete surgical resection, long-term survival and cure have been reported.[25]

Surgical resection is the management of choice and on average this may increase the 1-year survival rate to approximately 30 percent. However, the reported 5-year survival rates for patients who have surgical resection drops off significantly and varies between 6 percent and 20-30 percent.[7,12,20] The role of chemotherapy and radiotherapy alone or in conjunction with surgical resection has not been established. Although specific regimens used for pulmonary artery sarcomas vary significantly, most authors suggest that these managements may be beneficial in achieving short-term control of primary and metastatic disease.[12]

Primary Tumors of the Pulmonary Veins

Sarcomas of the pulmonary veins are among the rarest tumors affecting humans. Fewer than 20 cases have been reported worldwide, and very few clinical centers have significant experience in the diagnosis and management of these tumors.[1,26] Most of these cases have been described as leiomyosarcomas, although single cases of pulmonary vein angiosarcoma, lipomyosarcoma, alveolar soft part sarcoma, and leiomyoma have been described.[1] These tumors may affect any portion of the pulmonary veins and frequently extend into the left atrium or, less frequently, into the pulmonary parenchyma. The histologic features include moderate to poor differentiation with variable degrees of mitotic activity. These tumors typically have significant necrosis and usually stain positive for vimentin, desmin, and actin on immunohistochemical analysis.[3,26]

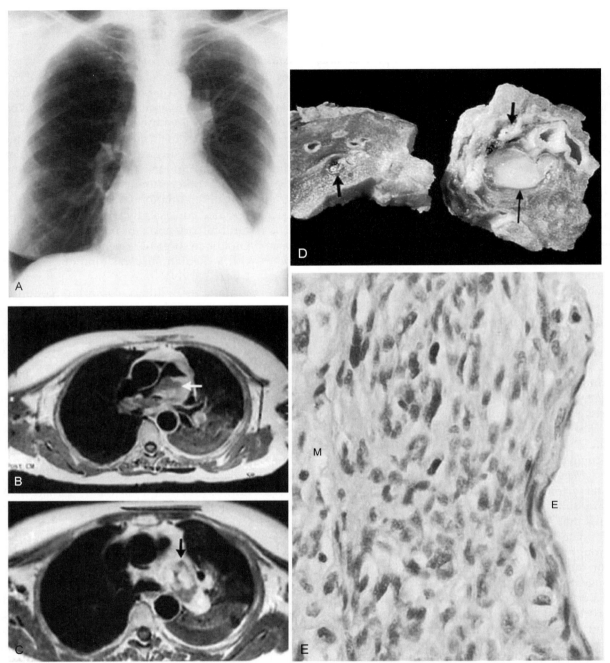

Figure 14-1. Pulmonary Artery Sarcoma. Chest radiograph (**A**) from a 69-year-old woman with a subacute history of cough, dyspnea, and left pleuritic chest pain shows left hilar prominence and a left pleural effusion. Magnetic resonance imaging of the chest (**B** and **C**) shows a mass in the left pulmonary artery, with extension into the main and right pulmonary arteries, that displays enhancement after the administration of gadolinium contrast material. Specimens obtained at thoracotomy (**D**) showed segmental *(long arrow)* and subsegmental arteries *(short arrows)* to be distended by white tumor. Histopathologic examination (**E**) revealed a pulmonary artery sarcoma composed of spindle cells with hyperchromatic nuclei in the intima. (Hematoxylin and eosin stain; original magnification, × 400). E, endothelial surface; M, media. (From Case records of the Massachusetts General Hospital. Weekly clinicopathological exercises. Case 25-2000: A 69-year-old woman with pleuritic pain and a pulmonary arterial obstruction. *N Engl J Med* 343(7):493-500, 2000, with permission.)

Patients with pulmonary vein leiomyosarcomas most commonly seek treatment for dyspnea, hemoptysis, and cough. Other symptoms and findings include chest pain, weight loss, palpitations, left-sided congestive heart failure, altered mental status, dizziness, weight loss, pleural effusion, and tachyarrhythmias. The average age of patients with this disease is 50 years, although a broad range from 27 to 74 years has been described. Most patients have had nondiagnostic imaging studies as the result of limited resolution for the pulmonary veins in most imaging modalities. Lung scintigraphy may demonstrate severe hypoperfusion of the affected lung. Echocardiography may disclose a pedunculated mass extending into the left atrium, and cardiac catheterization may demonstrate pulmonary hypertension. In most reported cases, the diagnosis has been established at the time of surgery or autopsy.[27] Surgical resection may be carried out for palliation or cure. Reported survival times for patients who have had resection range from 2 months to 21 years, with a 75 percent survival after 6 months and 20 percent after 5 years. The role for external beam radiotherapy and chemotherapy has not been studied systematically, but approximately 50 percent of reported patients developed local recurrence or distant metastasis following resection, suggesting a potential role for adjuvant therapy.[1,3]

Pulmonary Epithelioid Hemangioendothelioma

In 1975, Dail and Liebow described a series of 20 patients who developed atypical, aggressive tumors that invaded pulmonary blood vessels and produced pulmonary parenchymal nodules. Based on cellular characteristics that were similar to bronchoalveolar tumor cells and the multifocal nature of disease in most patients, the term "intravascular bronchoalveolar tumor"[1,3] was proposed to describe the condition.[28,29]

Since that time, at least 30 additional cases that primarily involve the pulmonary vasculature have been described. As the number of carefully investigated cases has increased, immunohistochemical and electron microscopic analysis has demonstrated that the tumor has vascular endothelial cell characteristics and does not originate from the alveolar epithelium.[30,31] Furthermore, intravascular bronchioloalveolar tumor (IVBAT) shares immunohistochemical, morphologic and anatomic features with other intravascular tumors that occur in a variety of organs. As the result of these findings, IVBAT has been renamed "epithelioid hemangioendothelioma" to reflect the origin of the malignant cells and its consistent appearance regardless of the organ involved.[32]

When present in the lung, EHE typically produces macroscopic pulmonary nodules from growth patterns that involve both intravascular proliferation and invasion of the surrounding alveolar structures. The tumor cells typically aggregate in the alveolar spaces, and larger nodules may develop central necrosis. EHEs may have varying grades of histologic atypia and mitotic indices but do not produce significant inflammation or effacement of the alveolar septa.

EHE may originate in the pulmonary vasculature, bone, liver, or other soft tissues. Both primary EHE and metastatic EHE to the lung have been recognized. Unlike most other tumors that involve the pulmonary vasculature, patients are often asymptomatic at the time of diagnosis or have minor dyspnea or cough. The tumor is more common in women and occurs at an earlier age than primary lung carcinoma, with almost one-half of patients less than 40 years of age at the time of diagnosis. Typical radiographic findings include peripheral, multiple, noncalcified, and bilateral lung nodules that typically range from 0.5 to 2.0 centimeters in diameter. High-resolution CT scanning features may also include ground glass opacities and interlobular septal thickening. In the first 20 cases of reported pulmonary EHE, Dail reported that 25 percent of patients had more than 20 nodules.[29] Given this appearance, most patients should receive extensive evaluation to rule out more common metastatic tumors, vasculitis, or granulomatous diseases. The tumor may metastasize to the mediastinal lymph nodes or result in malignant pleural effusion. Although transbronchial biopsy and fine-needle aspiration biopsy were diagnostic in a single reported case, the diagnosis most often is obtained by thoracoscopic or open lung biopsy.[31,33]

Although spontaneous regression of the tumor has been described, most patients have received treatment with chemotherapeutic regimens including interferon, carboplatin plus etoposide, or gemcitabine and docetaxel.[31,34] The prognosis for patients with this tumor remains highly variable, with reported survival rates of only 1-2 years for patients with pleural, mediastinal, or hepatic metastasis, whereas survival has been reported up to 15 years in other patients with asymptomatic nodules.

Primary Choriocarcinoma of the Pulmonary Artery

In 1959, Bagshawe and Brooks described a patient with choriocarcinoma involving the pulmonary arteries who did not have evidence for a primary abdominal or pelvic primary tumor.[35] Since that time, at least four additional cases have been described with similar clinical and histopathologic findings.

The clinical features of patients with these gestational trophoblastic tumors are remarkably similar and included female gender, premenopausal age, and markedly elevated serum β-human chorionic gonadotropin levels. The initial symptoms included subacute dyspnea, chest pain, and cough. Imaging findings included wedge-shaped peripheral densities consistent with infarction, as well as nodules and intravascular filling defects. A single patient underwent both pulmonary angiography and fluoro-2-deoxy-D-glucose positron-emission tomography that demonstrated occlusion of peripheral branches of the pulmonary artery and significant increased metabolic activity, respectively. Pressure recordings in the pulmonary artery of a single patient also suggested mild pulmonary hypertension.

Although one patient died from the disease, four patients have been treated successfully with systemic chemotherapy and achieved complete responses.[36-38] Although this tumor is rare, it should be considered in premenopausal women who have signs and symptoms of pulmonary thromboembolic disease or pulmonary arterial hypertension.

Secondary Tumors of the Pulmonary Vasculature

Pulmonary Tumor Embolism

Metastatic spread of tumor from distant sites is far more common than are primary tumors of the vessels. Terms that have been used to describe the clinical and pathologic findings of metastasis to the pulmonary vasculature include carcinomatous arteriopathy, pulmonary tumor thrombotic microangiopathy, carcinomatous endarteritis, embolic carcinomatosis, vascular intimal carcinomatosis, and vasculitis carcinomatosa. This wide range of nomenclature reflects the spectrum of clinical and histologic appearances of metastatic pulmonary vascular disease. For general purposes, pulmonary vascular tumor embolism is defined as the presence of isolated cells or clusters of tumor cells within the pulmonary vascular system, including pulmonary arteries and septal capillaries, that do not extend directly from other extravascular, metastatic, or parenchymal foci.[39,40]

The symptoms and distinguishing clinical findings in these secondary tumors of the pulmonary vessels are nonspecific and, as with primary tumors, the diagnosis frequently is not known before death. In many instances, patients with pulmonary tumor embolism have pathophysiologic features that cannot be distinguished from any other disease that causes cor pulmonale. In 1937, Brill and Robertson described a patient with subacute dyspnea, tachypnea, and cardiac collapse who on autopsy was found to have diffuse occlusion of the pulmonary arteries by metastatic carcinoma. This led to the conclusion that tumor embolism to the pulmonary vasculature should be considered when "rapid development of signs and symptoms of strain of the right side of the heart [develop] in a patient who gives no history of antecedent cardiopulmonary disease or other condition known to be capable of producing strain of the right side of the heart."[41] Since this early pathophysiologic description of disease, pulmonary tumor embolism has been well recognized as an infrequently occurring condition that produces subacute cor pulmonale. Explicit and careful attention to the duration of symptoms, clinical features, and the results of imaging or invasive testing may provide clues and permit the diagnosis to be established when management options still exist.

Incidence and Frequency

A large variety of primary tumors have been described in association with embolic and metastatic involvement of the pulmonary vasculature. The most common tumor origins include breast, lung, prostate, pancreas, and stomach malignancies (TABLE 14-2). Adenocarcinoma metastatic from abdominal and pelvic organs, particularly the stomach, is the single most common histologic subtype of disease.[42] Autopsy studies have shown a broad range of incidence rates of tumor embolism to the pulmonary vasculature in patients with known carcinoma, ranging between 2 percent and 26 percent.[39,40,42,43] A single prospective study of 222 consecutive autopsies of patients with cancer determined an incidence rate of 8.5 percent for arterial tumor embolism. Most patients in this autopsy series had had known metastatic disease elsewhere or were classified with advanced clinical

TABLE 14-2

Histologic Classification of Pulmonary Vascular Tumor Embolism and Approximate Frequency of Primary Tumors

Primary Malignancy	Reported Range (Percent)
Breast	27-30
Lung	10-16
Stomach	9-11
Prostate	7-13
Liver	7-8
Pancreas	2-6
Cervix	3-4
Kidney	2-4
Bladder	3
Ovary	2-3
Melanoma	2
Mesothelioma	2
Bone	2
Undifferentiated or unknown	4
Other	7

From Soares FA, Pinto AP, Landell GA, et al: Pulmonary tumor embolism to arterial vessels and carcinomatous lymphangitis. A comparative clinicopathological study. Arch Pathol Lab Med 117(8):827-831, 1993; Bassiri AG, Haghighi B, Doyle RL, et al: Pulmonary tumor embolism. Am J Respir Crit Care Med 155(6):2089-2095, 1997; and Roberts KE, Hamele-Bena D, Saqi A, et al: Pulmonary tumor embolism: A review of the literature. Am J Med 115(3):228-232, 2003.

disease but did not have recognized pulmonary vascular tumor embolism antemortem.[39]

Anatomic and Pathologic Features

As the large number of terms used to describe metastatic pulmonary vascular disease suggests, a broad spectrum of pathologic features has been observed. From a clinical standpoint, there are four general patterns in which metastatic disease may involve the pulmonary vasculature[44,45]:

- Large proximal embolization
- Generalized lymphatic invasion
- Small arterial and microvascular disease
- A combination of these types

The histologic appearance may be subclassified further on the basis of changes within the mural structure of the vessels and the characteristics of the cellular accumulations in the lumen of the vessels.[40] The content of the occlusive material in the vascular lumen represents a spectrum from aggregates of pure tumor cells to accumulation of secondary reactive thrombus composed of acellular fibrin and platelets. The vascular walls may be essentially unaffected by the tumor cells or may develop fibrointimal proliferation and medial hypertrophy, as well as other pulmonary vascular remodeling changes associated with pulmonary arterial hyper-

tension. There is considerable overlap of the histologic appearance of the mural changes associated with tumor embolism and other diseases that produce pulmonary hypertension, with the exception that plexiform lesions are not commonly observed in metastatic disease.[44] Autopsy findings of right ventricular hypertrophy, right ventricular dilation, or pulmonary infarction frequently coexist in patients with pulmonary vascular tumor embolism and may result from tumor cell occlusion or coexisting thromboembolic disease.[39]

Although the molecular and cellular processes by which metastatic cells induce these vascular mural changes has not been characterized fully, tumor cells are thought to produce local and direct damage to the vascular endothelium, interstitium, and elastic lamina. This damage occurs in areas of replacement of the endothelium by tumor cells, areas of adhesion of tumor cells to the endothelium, and induction of a fibroproliferative response within the vascular media. The tumor cells also alter the local microenvironment of the coagulation cascade to favor initiation of coagulation, thrombus formation, and associated inflammatory cytokine release and immune activation (FIGURE 14-2).

There is significant overlap between tumors which involve the pulmonary arteries or capillaries and those which produce lymphatic invasion. In one series, 18 of 21 cases with pulmonary vascular metastasis also had histologic evidence of lymphangiosis carcinomatosa, suggesting a common biologic propensity for both lymphangitic and vascular metastasis.[42]

Clinical Features

The clinical signs and symptoms of metastatic tumor embolism to the pulmonary vasculature are nonspecific and share considerable overlap with many diseases of the cardiovascular and pulmonary systems. No clinical features are specific to the disease. The most common initial symptom is subacute dyspnea developing over days to months, which develops in 50 to 100 percent of patients. Additional initial symptoms include chest pain, cough, hemoptysis, and cardiopulmonary arrest. Constitutional symptoms and other evidence of focal metastatic disease are frequent. Symptoms related to pulmonary tumor embolism often are attributed initially to adverse effects of systemic chemotherapy, such as opportunistic or infectious lung disease or pulmonary edema.

Finally, the clinical picture of pulmonary thromboembolism and paraneoplastic thrombophilia cannot be distinguished easily from tumor embolization. One feature of tumor embolism that may help differentiate it from acute pulmonary thromboembolism is subacute but relentlessly progressive dyspnea. Other characteristics that favor a diagnosis of pulmonary tumor embolism over other causes of pulmonary vascular disease include systemic symptoms related to malignancy and the failure of symptoms to improve with thrombolysis or anticoagulation.

The physical examination and results of laboratory and imaging studies of patients with pulmonary vascular tumor embolism also overlap considerably with other diseases of the cardiopulmonary system. If present for sufficient time, metastatic pulmonary tumor embolism may produce sustained right heart strain and secondary changes of pulmonary hypertension and cor pulmonale. Tachypnea, cyanosis, jugular venous engorgement, peripheral edema, tachycardia, and an accentuated pulmonic component of the second heart sound have all been described.

Arterial blood gas analysis typically shows hypoxemia and respiratory alkalosis, although normal values do not exclude the diagnosis. In accordance with the intravascular rather than intraparenchymal location of tumor metastasis, an unremarkable chest radiograph is the most common finding.[40,45] Other radiographic features may be attributed to either the effects on the pulmonary vasculature or other complications of metastatic disease, and include prominent pulmonary arteries, cardiomegaly, atelectasis, alveolar infiltrates, and pleural effusions. High-resolution CT may demonstrate a beaded and dilated appearance of the peripheral vasculature in multiple lobes.[46] In one study, 63 percent of patients with arterial tumor embolism also had evidence of nodular pulmonary parenchymal metastasis, suggesting that more typical patterns of pulmonary nodules may exist concurrently.[39]

Ventilation-perfusion scanning may demonstrate multiple segmental or subsegmental perfusion defects with normal ventilation. Compared with thromboembolic disease, the defects have been described as more commonly bilateral, numerous, and symmetric. Normal perfusion scans, focal segmental defects, and unilateral complete absence of perfusion can also be observed.

In distinction to acute thromboembolic disease, tumor embolism may cause significant and physiologically compensated pulmonary hypertension. Echocardiographic estimates or catheter-based measurements generally demonstrate markedly elevated systolic pulmonary artery pressures ranging between 40 mmHg and 100 mmHg.[42,43] The finding of severe pulmonary hypertension in a patient with a clinical picture of acute thromboembolic disease should raise the possibility of pulmonary vascular tumor embolism.

Diagnosis

The diagnosis of pulmonary vascular tumor embolism requires a high clinical suspicion and histologic or cytologic confirmation of tumor cells in the pulmonary vasculature. Although a significant number of diagnoses become apparent only after autopsy, antemortem diagnosis may be established through open or thoracoscopic lung biopsy. Transbronchial biopsies occasionally produce diagnostic specimens, but they are relatively contraindicated because of respiratory distress or significant pulmonary hypertension. Pulmonary artery catheterization with angiography has both a poor sensitivity and specificity for tumor embolism and in many cases does not demonstrate abnormal filling of the pulmonary arteries. As an example, in 13 of 15 reported cases with confirmed tumor embolism, pulmonary arteriography demonstrated no evidence of it.[43]

Pulmonary arterial catheterization with a balloon-tipped catheter may provide a less invasive means for cytologic sampling of the pulmonary capillary blood, as was first described in 1989 in a small series of eight patients who had lymphangitic carcinomatosis.[47] Through the cytologic examination of 5-10 ml of blood aspirated while the catheter was wedged in the pulmonary artery, a diagnosis of lymphangitic carcinomatosis was established in seven of the eight patients. Additional findings suggestive of metastatic disease using this balloon-tipped catheter technique in patients with tumor embolism include an elevated number of megakaryocytes and vascular epithelial cells.[48] Unfortunately, wedge aspiration of pulmonary artery blood has yielded false-positive results in patients with diffuse hepatic metastatic disease, pulmonary infarction, and in cases in which endothelial cell aggregates or abnormally appearing megakaryocytes are interpreted incorrectly as evidence for tumor embolism.[49]

Management and Outcome

Data regarding the effectiveness of early diagnosis and management of pulmonary tumor embolism derives only from case reports. Most information regarding the natural history and outcome of this disease has been obtained retrospectively from patients found to have pulmonary vascular tumor embolism at the time of autopsy. In general, pulmonary vascular tumor embolism signifies metastatic and incurable disease. Given the coexistence of significant pulmonary and cardiac disease with metastatic malignancy, few patients would be expected to tolerate aggressive therapy. However, some patients with lymphangitic carcinomatosis involving the lung may respond to systemic chemotherapy and achieve significant short-term survival, suggesting that even in advanced metastatic disease not all efforts are futile.[50,51] Several reports have described long-term survival following surgical embolectomy and resection for metastatic renal cell carcinoma.[52] For many patients in whom the diagnosis is established antemortem, a significant benefit may include avoiding unnecessary anticoagulation therapy for suspected pulmonary thromboembolism.[43]

Intravascular Lymphomatosis

Intravascular lymphomatosis is a non-Hodgkin lymphoma characterized by the endoluminal accumulation of mononuclear lymphoid cells within arteries, veins, and capillaries. Pfleger and Tappeiner first described this disease as "systemic proliferative angioendotheliomatosis" in 1959.[53] Since that time, this condition has been recognized as a rare malignant neoplasm with approximately 200 cases reported. Also referred to as malignant angioendotheliomatosis or angiotropic large cell lymphoma, the disease often manifests with nonspecific systemic symptoms, and the vasculature of multiple organs may be involved. Typically, patients have evidence of cutaneous or neurologic involvement; however, 14 cases have been described in which the initial clinical findings were related primarily to pulmonary vascular involvement.[54-56] On histologic examination, intravascular lymphomatosis is characterized by the accumulation of lymphoid cells within the lumen of small arteries, veins, or capillaries. The cells have scant cytoplasm, high nuclear-to-cytoplasmic ratio, prominent nucleoli, and typically have positive immunohistochemical stains for lymphocyte common antigen, CD20, and CD45.[57] Approximately 85 percent of the cases are typically of B-cell origin.[55,58] Autopsy evaluations suggest that the most common organs involved include lymph nodes, bone marrow, skin, brain, kidneys, and lungs.

There are no established risk factors for the disease, which typically affects patients aged 40 to 70 years. The most common initial symptoms of intravascular lymphomatosis include fever, night sweats, weight loss, rash, nodular cutaneous lesions, and neurologic deficits. Patients who develop pulmonary vascular disease may have a dry, nonproductive cough and slowly progressive dyspnea. The symptoms typically have a duration of 3-4 months before diagnosis; approximately one-half of cases are not diagnosed antemortem. With the exception of neurologic deficits and cutaneous findings, there are relatively few physical signs of the disease. Pulmonary examination findings are typically normal, although tachypnea and basilar crackles have been described.

Radiographically, multiple nonspecific patterns have been described, including normal lung fields, alveolar infiltrates, ground glass opacities, reticulonodular infiltrates, and pleural effusions. A single case of mosaic pattern alveolar infiltrate has been described in a patient who also had spirometric evidence of airflow obstruction.[56] A single case report has also described multiple, peripheral, mismatched segmental perfusion defects on ventilation-perfusion scanning.[54] Nonspecific laboratory findings of inflammation such as the elevations in erythrocyte sedimentation or lactic dehydrogenase may be noted. Spirometry may show a normal, restrictive, or obstructive pattern. Pulmonary hypertension and cor pulmonale resulting from pulmonary vascular involvement has been described and may improve with prostanoid management.[59,60]

Although open or thoracoscopic biopsy provides optimal specimens for histologic examination of lung tissue, the diagnosis also has been established from transbronchial forceps biopsy specimens.[56] From both clinical and pathologic standpoints, the major differential diagnosis for intravascular lymphomatosis includes systemic vasculitis syndromes, carcinomatous emboli, and angiocentric lymphoma. The distinguishing features of intravascular lymphomatosis include absence of thrombus, inflammation, or extravascular accumulation of malignant cells, as well as its unique immunohistochemical findings. Intravascular lymphomatosis is unique in that neither lymphadenopathy nor primary mass lesions are present in most cases.

Management regimens for intravascular lymphomatosis should include systemic chemotherapy with or without radiotherapy. Commonly described regimens include cyclophosphamide, doxorubicin, vincristine, and prednisone (CHOP); and bleomycin, doxorubicin, cyclophosphamide, vincristine, and prednisone (BACOP). Approximately one-half of patients will have no response or only a partial response to chemotherapy, although cases of complete remission and favorable long-term survival also have been observed.[61]

Direct Growth and Extension of Tumor Into Pulmonary Vasculature

Tumor invasion of the pulmonary artery may occur not only by distant metastasis, but also by direct intravascular extension of a distant primary tumor from its original location. Two cases of intravenous uterine leiomyomatosis, one case of renal cell carcinoma, and two cases of lung carcinoma have been reported to cause direct extension into the vasculature leading to occlusion of the pulmonary arteries.[62-64] Uterine leiomyomatosis is a common uterine tumor that has benign histopathologic features but may cause extensive intravascular proliferation and secondary vascular occlusion; several patients have been reported in whom a primary uterine leiomyoma proliferated through the inferior vena cava, to the right atrium and ventricle, and into the pulmonary artery.[62,64] One patient came to medical attention with circulatory collapse, the other with subacute dyspnea. Echocardiography revealed a mobile intracardiac mass extending to the pulmonary artery, while CT scans revealed the intravascular growth and extension from the pelvic origin of the tumor to the pulmonary artery. In these cases, the initial clinical appearance and evaluation began with a focus directed toward thromboembolic and myocardial disease. The diagnosis in these cases was strongly

suggested when intracardiac mass was detected by echocardiography. Surgical resection was the preferred management.

In a related manner, non–small cell lung carcinoma may also invade and proliferate within the pulmonary arteries. Significant intravenous growth of tumor can result in dyspnea and cardiac compromise.[65] As with intravenous leiomyomata, the primary tumor location generally is not immediately known or suspected. The preferred management is surgical resection.

Pulmonary Vascular Malformations and Aneurysms

As with tumors of the pulmonary vasculature, pulmonary vascular malformations and aneurysms occur infrequently, have nonspecific manifestations, but may become life threatening. These pulmonary vascular abnormalities may be classified as diseases of capillary proliferation, arteriovenous malformations, or aneurysmal vascular dilations, such as pulmonary artery aneurysms. All of these lesions may be congenital or acquired, and patients may be symptomatic or entirely asymptomatic.

Pulmonary Capillary Hemangiomatosis

Wagenvoort described the first case of PCH in 1978.[66] Most subsequent cases have been characterized by severe idiopathic proliferation of pulmonary capillaries associated with pulmonary arterial hypertension.[67-69] The histopathologic changes in patients with PCH typically include pulmonary microvasculopathy, including bilateral and multifocal proliferation of capillaries within the alveolar septa, perivascular sheaths, pleura, peribronchial connective tissue, and lymph nodes.[144] The disease is entirely confined to the lungs; no cases of extrathoracic disease have been reported.

There is no general agreement on the cause of this disease, although most authors have concluded that it represents a low-grade neoplasm. Case reports of PCH in association with other affected family members, vasculitis, and collagen vascular diseases have suggested that genetic predisposition, autoimmune disease, and inflammation may play a role in development or propagation of the disease.[70-73] Histologic evaluation of the pulmonary veins and venules in patients with PCH may reveal narrowing and obliteration similar to that seen in pulmonary occlusive venopathy, the pathologic findings most often associated with pulmonary veno-occlusive disease.[144] Similarly, muscular pulmonary arteries may show medial hypertrophy but rarely contain plexiform lesions.[16]

Most patients with PCH develop pulmonary hypertension, which is attributed to obstruction of pulmonary arterioles and capillaries by the growth of pathologic proliferating capillaries.[74] A wide and clinically unrecognized spectrum of disease in PCH likely exists. Although most cases reported have been symptomatic and progressed to death, one autopsy series demonstrated eight cases of well-localized PCH-like capillary proliferation without clinical evidence for pulmonary dysfunction, pulmonary hypertension, or contribution to the death of the patient.[75]

Patients with progressive and symptomatic PCH have an age distribution from 6 to 71 years, with the highest incidence in the fourth decade. The most common initial symptoms are nonspecific and include dyspnea, massive hemoptysis, weight gain, leg swelling, and abdominal bloating. Physical examination may reveal clubbing, cyanosis, pulmonary crackles, elevated jugular venous pressure, ascites, and peripheral edema.[67] Arterial blood gas analysis may reveal profound hypoxemia. Radiograph findings in patients with PCH may be normal but typically show a diffuse reticulonodular pattern with enlarged central arteries. Multiple peripheral nodules and pleural effusions may also be present.[76]

Patients with PCH frequently undergo diagnostic evaluations directed toward pulmonary thromboembolism, cor pulmonale, and more common forms of pulmonary arterial hypertension. Pulmonary arterial catheterization usually confirms moderate to severe pulmonary hypertension. Lung perfusion scintigraphy may show a heterogeneous pattern with focal areas of increased uptake in close proximity to areas of low uptake; this is attributed to the abnormal capillaries and compression of vascular structures, respectively.

Given these nonspecific symptoms and findings, the diagnosis of PCH requires histopathologic demonstration of pulmonary microvasculopathy. Because the proliferating capillaries may have a patchy distribution, multiple biopsy locations or large resection specimens may be required to accurately establish the diagnosis. Less than one-half of patients have been diagnosed antemortem. Most commonly, patients with PCH have been misdiagnosed with pulmonary veno-occlusive disease, pulmonary embolism, arteriovenous fistula,

lymphangiectasia, or hemangioendotheliomatosis.[68] Other than lung transplantation, there is no effective management for PCH. Epoprostenol does not produce consistent benefit and has been associated with clinical deterioration in some cases.[77] Although interferon-α has resulted in clinical improvement and stabilization, these results have not been widely confirmed.[78] Most patients with PCH have died as the result of progressive cor pulmonale, general multisystem decline, or massive hemoptysis. There is a wide range of survival times from 2 to 12 years, with a median survival of 3 years.[68]

Arteriovenous Malformations and Hereditary Hemorrhagic Telangiectasia

Pulmonary arteriovenous malformations (PAVMs) result from abnormal connections between pulmonary arteries and veins that permit blood flow to the systemic arterial circulation without passage through pulmonary capillary networks. These malformations are characterized as either simple or complex on the basis of the number of feeding arteries. Most PAVMs are characterized as simple and have a single feeding artery, usually derived from the pulmonary artery, and drain into the left atrium.[79] Less commonly, PAVMs are complex and have more than one feeding artery or are supplied directly from a systemic arterial source. The lesions may occasionally be solitary but more commonly are multiple. PAVMs typically occur in the lower lobes and are bilateral.[80,81]

Morbidity and mortality from these communications result from physiologic shunting of deoxygenated blood directly to the systemic arterial system. Additionally, PAVMs may cause systemic embolization of venous blood contaminants such as thrombosis and bacteria, resulting in tissue infarction and abscess formation. Finally, arteriovenous malformations lack normal structural integrity and may rupture spontaneously, causing hemorrhagic complications. Evaluation of patients with PAVMs involves screening for those at highest risk for developing these lesions, evaluating the physiologic consequences of the shunt, and preventing known complications to the degree possible.

A wide range of acquired diseases may result in PAVMs, but most arise from congenital disease. The most common congenital cause is hereditary hemorrhagic telangiectasia (HHT), also known as the Rendu-Osler-Weber syndrome, which accounts for 50-70 percent of all PAVMs.[81,82] Other causes include trauma, mitral stenosis, actinomycosis,

Fanconi syndrome, hepatic cirrhosis, systemic amyloidosis, and schistosomiasis.[83] Rarely, PAVMs may arise in patients with congenital heart disease who have undergone surgical aortopulmonary or cavopulmonary shunt procedures.[84] Although the etiology for these secondary PAVMs has not been established, it likely involves distinctly different pathways than those implicated in HHT. Analysis of lung biopsy specimens obtained from a small number of children who underwent cavopulmonary bypass procedures for complex congenital cyanotic heart disease has demonstrated an increased density of thin-walled vessels that have increased expression of vascular endothelial growth factor.[85,86] These findings, however, may apply only to patients in whom there is a disruption of the normal flow of venous blood from the liver through the lungs and may not adequately account for the other causes of secondary PAVMs.[84]

Hereditary Hemorrhagic Telangiectasia

HHT is an autosomal dominant disorder characterized by the clinical syndrome of mucocutaneous telangiectasias, PAVMs, cerebral arteriovenous malformations, and hemorrhage. The disease results from mutations in genes encoding vascular endothelial cell surface receptor and signal transduction proteins. These abnormal receptor proteins belong to the transforming growth factor-β (TGF-β) superfamily and mediate cell growth and proliferation. Mutations in the genes that encode endoglin (ENG), a TGF-β binding protein, and activin receptor-like kinase-1 (ALK-1), a serine-threonine kinase that binds TGF-β, are implicated in linkage and association studies as the causes of HHT. Mutations in the related intracellular mediator SMAD4 have also been associated in an overlap syndrome of HHT and juvenile polyposis.[87] An additional as-yet-unidentified mutation that does not map to either the ENG or ALK-1 locus has also been suggested in some linkage analysis studies.[88] Systematic sequencing studies to characterize the specific mutations in the abnormal HHT genes has confirmed the existence of at least 74 distinct mutations in ENG and 50 distinct mutations in ALK-1 in patients and families with HHT.[89,90] The presence of the multiple genotypes in HHT patients has been associated with some variability of disease phenotypes. Trembath and colleagues have demonstrated linkage in patients with combined HHT and pathophysiologic features indistinguishable from idiopathic pulmonary arterial hypertension to the ALK-1 gene on chromosome 12q13.[91] ENG mutations are more commonly associated with PAVMs than are ALK-1 mutations.[92]

HHT is a clinical diagnosis that depends on the presence of multiple features. The diagnostic certainty or probability increases as the number of suggestive clinical features increases for any single patient (TABLE 14-3). Because many mutations in multiple genes have been described, genetic screening or testing has a limited role outside the context of research. The primary features of HHT include mucocutaneous telangiectasias, arteriovenous malformations, bleeding from mucosal surfaces, and family history suggestive of HHT. Telangiectasias may develop on the fingers, lips, oral mucosa, nasal mucosa, alimentary tract, lungs,

---

TABLE 14-3

Clinical Diagnostic Criteria for Hereditary Hemorrhagic Telangiectasia

Probability of Hereditary Hemorrhagic Telangiectasia

Definite	If 3 criteria are present
Possible or suspected	If 2 criteria are present
Unlikely	If fewer than 2 criteria present

Criteria

Epistaxis	Spontaneous and recurrent at least twice
Telangiectases	Characteristic sites include lips, oral cavity, fingers, or nose
Visceral lesions	Evidence for arteriovenous malformations occurring in the lungs, liver, brain, or spine
Family history	First-degree relative with definite HHT by these criteria

HHT, hereditary hemorrhagic telangiectasia.
Adapted from Shovlin CL, Guttmacher AE, Buscarini E, et al: Diagnostic criteria for hereditary hemorrhagic telangiectasia (Rendu-Osler-Weber syndrome). Am J Med Genet 91(1):66-67, 2000

and virtually any visceral organ. Arteriovenous malformations may be present in the lungs, liver, spine, and brain. The most common bleeding manifestations include epistaxis and gastrointestinal hemorrhage, which increase in frequency with age.

Many patients with HHT report a family history of severe epistaxis, gastrointestinal hemorrhage, or arteriovenous malformations. There is considerable variability in the severity and penetrance of these disease manifestations. Although arteriovenous malformations may be present at birth, the telangiectasias may accumulate and grow with age. Bleeding or iron deficiency anemia often does not become apparent until adulthood. Given the large number of and variation in genetic and clinical disease manifestations, an attempt has been made to standardize the diagnostic approach to HHT based upon clinical probability of disease. A 2000 consensus statement by researchers in the field proposed that uniform criteria be used to determine the clinical probability of disease, ranging from definite to possible to unlikely (see TABLE 14-3).[93]

Clinical Features of PAVMs

As the result of nonspecific symptoms and multiple causes, it has been difficult to establish the incidence and prevalence of PAVMs. One study conducted during the 1950s of 15,000 consecutive autopsies described only three patients with PAVMs.[94] Long-term follow-up in a series of 91 patients who had undergone Glenn procedures (anastomosis of the superior vena cava to the pulmonary artery) for management of congenital defects such as tricuspid atresia found 18 patients (20 percent) who had developed pulmonary arteriovenous fistulas.[95] The estimated population prevalence of HHT in a Japanese community was 1:8,000 to 1:5,000. Of the patients found to have HHT, 16 of 32 (50 percent) were also found to have PAVMs.[96] The prevalence of HHT in a single county in Denmark was 15.6:100,000, with an overall prevalence rate of PAVMs of 24 percent in patients with HHT.[97,98] These observations are generally supported by investigations that have consistently demonstrated PAVMs in between 15 and 33 percent of patients with HHT.[99-101]

Among patients with PAVMs both with and without HHT, a greater female-to-male ratio has been reported in some, but not all, series.[81,83] Although patients may develop symptoms at any age, the most common age at diagnosis is between 40 and 50 years. For both primary and secondary

PAVMs, a large number of patients are entirely asymptomatic and come to medical attention during the evaluation for other unrelated disease, or as the result of screening in patients with HHT.[80,82,83,101] Symptoms of PAVMs may include dyspnea, hemoptysis, fatigue, cough, palpitations, and chest pain. Most patients have moderate to severe dyspnea (World Health Organization functional classes II to IV). Although patients who have a single PAVM may have significant dyspnea, patients with multiple and bilateral PAVMs more frequently develop this symptom.[82,102,103] Manifestations of PAVMs may also include headache, syncope, paresis, vertigo, and other symptoms of focal neurologic disease,[80,98] and 10-40 percent of patients with PAVMs experience systemic embolism or rupture of the lesions. Cerebral infarction, cerebral abscess, seizures, high-output cardiac failure, and hemoptysis may ensue. Any patient who has findings consistent with an unexplained cerebral abscess should undergo screening for PAVM. Both platypnea (dyspnea with erect posture relieved by lying flat) and orthodeoxia (decrease in oxygen saturation after shifting from horizontal to upright body position) have been well-documented findings in patients with PAVMs and are thought to result from an increase in blood flow to the lung bases where PAVMs frequently are located. Cohort and population findings are inconsistent for the rates of platypnea and orthopnea.[102,104]

As with symptoms, physical findings of PAVMs have a wide spectrum, from none to cyanosis, clubbing, and extracardiac murmurs. Murmurs or bruits typically are heard over the site of the PAVM and may be detected in up to 46 percent of patients.[82] Additional features of chronic hypoxemia, including polycythemia and congestive heart failure, may also develop late in the disease.

PAVMs have characteristic radiographic and physiologic features that distinguish them from other pulmonary vascular disorders. Shunt physiology and hypoxemia refractory to supplemental oxygen correlates with right heart failure and paradoxical embolus. In one series of 93 patients with a mean age of 40 years, the average PaO_2 before management was 56 mmHg. In another cohort of patients identified through the screening of family members of patients with HHT, all patients with PAVMs had significant hypoxemia based on an age-based correction for normal levels.[100] However, in one study of 25 patients with HHT who underwent confirmatory testing with pulmonary angiography, only 9 had abnormal SaO_2 values.[102]

Similarly, the arterial-alveolar (a-A) oxygen gradient may be elevated in patients with PAVM. In one cohort of 51 patients with PAVMs detected by screening among 105 patients with HHT, the sensitivity, specificity, and positive predictive value of an abnormal a-A gradient for the presence of PAVM were 68 percent, 98 percent, and 97 percent, respectively, suggesting that arterial hypoxemia is a common but not constant finding.[103] Both symptomatic and asymptomatic patients may have significant arterial hypoxemia and calculated shunt; however, the degree and reliability of these clinical studies depends on the posture of the patient (supine versus upright), age, and the presence or absence of other comorbid conditions. By using direct measurements of the arterial and mixed venous PO_2 in patients with PAVMs, the shunt fraction may be calculated. In most patients with clinically significant PAVMs, the shunt fraction is elevated and typically ranges between 5 to 40 percent of the cardiac output (as compared with the normal of 3 to 8 percent).

Considerable variability exists in the methodology and mathematical assumptions used to determine shunt fraction; however, the most widely accepted technique includes obtaining measurements in the upright position after 15-20 minutes of breathing 100 percent oxygen. If the venous blood oxygen content is not measured directly, it is assumed to be 5 ml O_2 per 100 ml blood lower than the arterial oxygen content, and the shunt fraction is estimated with the following formula[82,105,106]:

$$\text{Shunt fraction} = (Cc'O_2 - CaO_2) \div (Cc'O_2 - CaO_2 + 5)$$

in which $Cc'O_2$ and CaO_2 represent the capillary and systemic arterial blood oxygen content, respectively. Alternative methods to measure the shunt fraction include infusion of radiolabeled microaggregated albumin with subsequent measurement of regional lung and kidney uptake. Shunt fraction may then be calculated based on the differential radiotracer activity in the pulmonary and renal vascular beds. Although the 100 percent oxygen breathing calculation and the radiolabeled microalbumin methods may produce different results, serial measurements with a single test in individual patients are helpful in determining the physiologic effect of the PAVM and response to therapy.[106]

The radiographic appearance and echocardiographic features of PAVMs have considerable overlap with those of other pulmonary vascular diseases; however, some characteristic features allow the diagnosis to be established reliably.

Posteroanterior chest radiographs may demonstrate nodular densities consistent with PAVM in 60-98 percent of patients.[81,82] Typical findings include well-circumscribed, lobulated, homogenous densities that are lower lobe predominant and usually 1-2 centimeters in diameter but may range up to 6 centimeters. The finding on chest radiograph of a feeding artery arising from the hilum and efferent vessel draining to the left atrium is highly suggestive of a PAVM and is a feature that is useful for distinguishing these from other parenchymal nodules. Typical CT, MRI, and magnetic resonance angiography findings that are virtually diagnostic of PAVMs include a homogenous nodular density that enhances uniformly with intravenous contrast and demonstrates both afferent arterial supply and efferent venous drainage. Rarely, a PAVM may cause pleural effusion secondary to rupture and atraumatic hemothorax.

Contrast echocardiography provides complementary and confirmatory evidence of PAVMs in most patients. Contrast echocardiography usually is performed by venous injection of agitated saline solution with microscopic bubbles. In the presence of PAVMs, contrast appears in the left atrium and ventricle after a delay of 3-10 cardiac cycles. In distinction, contrast appears after 1-3 cardiac cycles when there is an atrial or ventricular septal defect with right-to-left shunting.

Neither radiography nor echocardiography performs well as a single diagnostic test for PAVMs. Although radiographic imaging, particularly advanced three-dimensional CT or MRI reconstruction images, may be highly suggestive of disease, it cannot confirm the presence of a physiologic shunt. Similarly, although echocardiography may demonstrate right-to-left shunting, it cannot by itself demonstrate the location of the shunt and lacks complete specificity.[82,99]

Diagnosis

The diagnosis of PAVMs depends upon the presence of both clinical and physiologic features. An elevated index of suspicion for the presence of PAVMs should be maintained in any patient with pulmonary nodules, telangiectasias, and dyspnea or hypoxemia that is out of proportion to the radiographic features. Similarly, pulmonary nodules and hypoxemia, hemoptysis, clubbing, and neurologic disease should raise the clinical suspicion for disease.

The initial diagnostic approach to patients with suspected PAVM should include both radiographic and physiologic characterization (FIGURE 14-3). In addition to chest radiographs, CT with

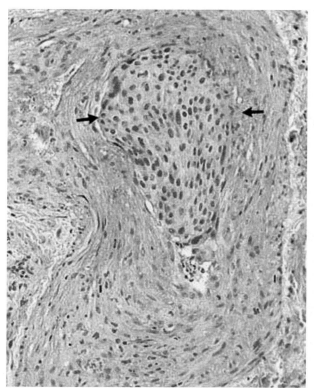

Figure 14-2. Embolus of Transitional-cell Carcinoma *(between arrows)* in the Lumen of an Artery. The embolus has elicited marked intimal proliferation. (Hematoxylin and eosin stain; original magnification, × 250.) (From Markowitz DH, Mark EJ: Case records of the Massachusetts General Hospital. Weekly clinicopathological exercises. Case 13-2002: A 43-year-old man with renal carcinoma and worsening dyspnea. *N Engl J Med* 46(17):1309-1317, 2002, with permission.)

three-dimensional reconstruction imaging and selective pulmonary angiography should be pursued to anatomically define the lesion (FIGURE 14-4). Shunt fraction calculation or measurement with radionuclide scanning provides complementary data and establishes a baseline to assess response to management. Echocardiography with intravenous contrast may also be useful in confirming the presence of an extracardiac shunt and ruling out primary or secondary cardiac disease. Finally, given the numerous and potentially devastating consequences of cerebral disease from thromboembolism, abscess, or arteriovenous malformations, patients with HHT generally should undergo neuroimaging with CT or MRI.

The results of routine screening of patients with HHT for PAVMs support the use of multiple and complementary clinical testing modalities. In population-based screening studies, chest radiography, peripheral oximetry, contrast echocardiography, shunt fraction calculations, and PaO_2 measurements on room air and while breathing 100 percent oxygen were compared systematically with the gold standard testing of pulmonary angiography. Chest radiography, oximetry, room air PaO_2 measurement, and shunt fraction calculations all demonstrated limited sensitivity as single tests. Although contrast echocardiography and PaO_2 less than 500 mmHg on 100 percent oxygen demonstrated very high sensitivities, these tests were limited significantly by low specificity and positive predictive values.[102,103] The use of both radiographic and echocardiographic testing together or radiographic and pulse oximetry testing together in a stepped approach appears to produce the highest sensitivity and specificity for detection of PAVMs in patients with HHT (FIGURE 14-3). In families with an established diagnosis of HHT or known genetic defect, all members should be offered clinical examination and screening for PAVMs if any disease manifestations are present. Although commercial genetic testing for known HHT mutations is not available or routinely performed, any patient with multiple affected family members should be considered for genetic screening and characterization in an HHT Center of Excellence (*http://www.hht.org/web/treatment_centers/*).

Management

The natural history of PAVMs may include rupture and pulmonary hemorrhage, cerebral abscess, stroke, and increased morbidity and mortality directly related to the underlying etiology. Overall, approximately 1-14 percent of patients will experience morbidity or mortality related to PAVMs. When only complications immediately related to the PAVM, such as stroke, brain abscess, hemithorax, and hemoptysis are considered, the attributed morbidity and mortality in unmanaged disease ranges from 0 to 12 percent.[82]

As the result of these elevated risks, all patients with clinically significant PAVM should be considered for management to occlude or remove the lesions. The management of choice is endovascular, catheter-based placement of occlusive metal coils or balloons to induce thrombosis in the supply artery and minimize shunting. These procedures are associated with few major procedure-related complications (1-3 percent) and have high initial success rates (98-100 percent). For technical reasons, embolization generally is limited to vessels 3 millimeters or greater in diameter. The frequency of minor complications, including pleuritic chest

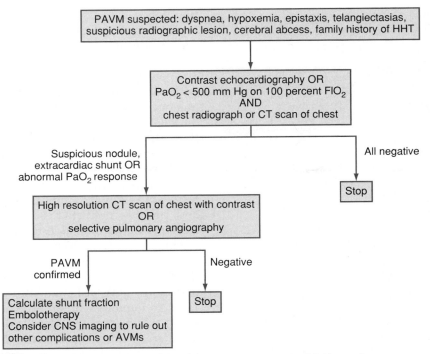

Figure 14-3. Clinical Evaluation for Suspected Pulmonary Arteriovenous Malformation.

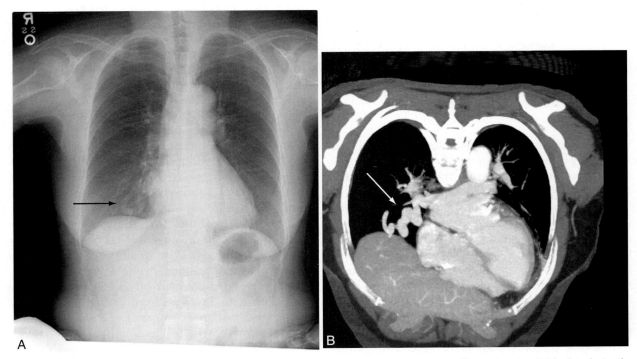

Figure 14-4. Pulmonary Arteriovenous Malformation. A pulmonary arteriovenous malformation is visible faintly in the right diaphragmatic area on posteroanterior chest radiograph (arrow) (A). A CT scan with contrast displays the dilated tortuous feeding vessel of the lesion (arrows) (B-F). (Courtesy of Dr. Steven Weinberger.)

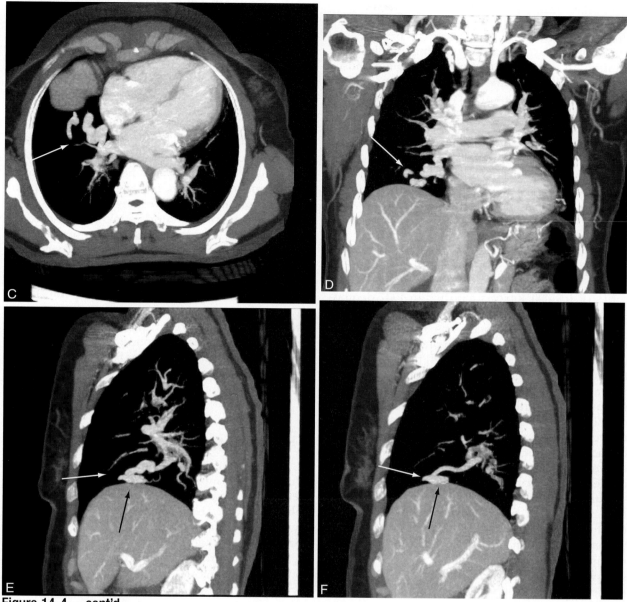

Figure 14-4.—cont'd

pain, angina, and paradoxical embolism of the coils or balloons, ranges from approximately 10 to 35 percent. Following embolization, physiologic parameters including SaO_2, shunt fraction, and exercise capacity improve in almost all patients and may return to normal in up to 33 percent.[80,82] Despite the improvement in physiologic parameters, however, many patients including those with excellent technical results will continue to have evidence of shunting with abnormal shunt fraction calculations or positive contrast echocardiography.[107] These findings suggest that microscopic and small vessel disease not immediately apparent on radiographic studies or pulmonary angiography is frequently present in patients with larger PAVMs who have undergone embolization. Patients with clinical evidence of persistent shunt should continue to receive periodic radiographic reevaluations for progression of their lesions. In some cases, such as patients with large central feeding arteries, multiple feeding arteries, uncontrolled massive hemoptysis, or multiple or diffuse small vessel disease, embolization therapy may be technically difficult or impossible. In these situations, surgical resection with lobectomy or pneumonectomy can be considered.

Pulmonary Artery Aneurysms

Pulmonary artery aneurysms may be present congenitally or may be acquired during childhood or adulthood. Although infrequent, the main causes of acquired pulmonary artery aneurysm include atherosclerosis, inflammatory vasculitis such as Behçet syndrome, pulmonary hypertension, pulmonary artery catheterization, cystic medial necrosis, Marfan syndrome, trauma, tuberculosis, syphilis, and septic emboli.[108] Poststenotic dilation of the pulmonary artery may also be seen in congenital pulmonic valve stenosis or in association with structurally abnormal pulmonary valves.[109-111] Mycotic aneurysms may occur with bacterial endocarditis or pneumonia.

Pulmonary artery aneurysms occur infrequently, and no firm population-based information exists regarding frequency. Review of an autopsy series of 109,000 subjects reported in 1947 demonstrated only 8 cases.[112]

Pulmonary artery aneurysms may be divided into two categories based on the presence or absence of an anatomic connection through the aneurysm to the draining capillaries and veins. Some aneurysms may appear as diverticulum-like, saccular dilations of the pulmonary artery without direct connection to draining vessels, as in mycotic aneurysms. Alternatively, circumferential aneurysms may appear as a dilation of the entire vessel with preserved direct communication to the draining capillary bed, as in congenital or vasculitis-related disease.[108]

Pulmonary artery aneurysms are rarely symptomatic and often are discovered incidentally on chest radiographic imaging. When symptoms are present, they often are attributed to compression of surrounding vessels or airways. When present, symptoms of pulmonary artery aneurysm are nonspecific and include dyspnea, cough, and chest pain. Cardiac murmurs, both diastolic and systolic, may be appreciated, as well as findings of right ventricular failure or right-to-left shunting, such as edema, ascites, cyanosis, clubbing, or paradoxical embolism.[108] Other findings include a prominent right ventricular impulse and pulsations palpated lateral to the left upper sternal border. Posteroanterior and lateral chest radiographs may demonstrate an apparent hilar mass lesion indistinguishable from neoplastic disease.

Aneurysms range in size from several millimeters to more than 10 centimeters in diameter and most commonly involve the main pulmonary arteries.[109] CT and MRI with intravenous contrast may establish the diagnosis and demonstrate the contrast-filled aneurysm in direct connection with the main, right, left, or segmental pulmonary artery. Without intravenous contrast, pulmonary artery aneurysms may be indistinguishable from soft tissue lesions or lymph nodes. Although conventional angiography remains the gold standard for diagnosis, this technique is used primarily in conjunction with catheter-directed management interventions.

The natural history of pulmonary artery aneurysms and patient prognosis depend on factors including growth rate, pulmonary hypertension, cardiovascular complications, and underlying etiology. Many patients do not require treatment or specific intervention. In patients with no apparent complications and without evidence of an infectious or inflammatory etiology, conservative management with serial observation may be pursued.[110,111,113] Indications for surgical correction with synthetic graft interposition or aneurysmorrhaphy include hemoptysis, evidence of continuing growth or expansion, and refractory hypoxemia as the result of right-to-left shunting through the aneurysm. Alternative strategies including embolization, lobectomy, banding, and endovascular grafting have been reported, but there is less experience with their use than with surgical resection.

Pulmonary Lymphatic Channel Diseases

Pulmonary lymphatic channel lesions are characterized by the proliferation or dilation of the lymphatic spaces. They are presumed to result from lymphatic ducts that are congenitally absent, or become inadequate or obstructed.[114,115] Thoracic lymphatic disorders may be grouped clinically into one of four categories that include lymphangioma, lymphangiomatosis, lymphangiectasis, and lymphatic dysplasia syndromes.[116] Lymphangioma are single and localized lesions that result in morbidity and mortality through direct local tissue effects. Lymphangiomatosis, lymphangiectasis, and the lymphatic dysplasia syndromes all represent multifocal or multisystem diseases characterized by progressive and often fatal natural histories related to chronic, multiple organ dysfunction (TABLE 14-4).

Lymphangioma

Lymphangiomas are solitary lesions that consist of dilated lymphatic or capillary tissue spaces that have either direct or interrupted connections with lymphatic channels. Although lymphangiomas may be diagnosed during adulthood, most are apparent in childhood and are believed to arise from congenital abnormalities of lymphatic duct development. These lesions have histologically benign features and are characterized by bizarre, irregular, and ectatic lymphatic channels lined by endothelial cells that range in size form less than 1 centimeter to 15 centimeters in their greatest dimension. Based upon histologic and structural appearances, lymphangiomas may be characterized further as capillary, cavernous, or cystic types. Lymphangiomas may be filled with lymphatic fluid, but following trauma or surgical disruption they may contain serum or blood.

Radiographically, these lesions appear as mediastinal masses, parenchymal nodules, or chest wall masses, may have a lobulated, thin-walled or thick-walled appearance, and may have a multiseptate appearance with central water density. In the mediastinum, the appearance may be indistinguishable from thymomas, lymphomas, or granulomatous lymphadenopathy.[117-119] Lymphangiomas may occur along the pleural surface or chest wall as isolated lesions or as one manifestation of Klippel-Trenaunay syndrome, a systemic disease characterized by soft tissue and bony hypertrophy of the extremities, skin changes, hemangiomas, and lymphangiomas.[120,121] Other rare cases of idiopathic isolated or solitary lymphangiomas occurring in the pulmonary parenchyma and airways have been described in both children and adults.[122-126]

In one series of 14 cases of lymphangioma, one-half of the subjects were children while the other half were adults; ages ranged from 3 to 76 years.[119] Although patients may be asymptomatic, the clinical picture and findings of patients with lymphangioma may include respiratory distress in newborns, subacute or chronic dyspnea, chest pain, mass effects including tracheal deviation, superior vena cava syndrome, postobstructive pneumonitis, or recurrent chylous pleural effusion.

Curative management for lymphangiomas is complete surgical excision. As a result of the often extensive nature of lymphangiomas that envelop the great vessels, trachea, heart and other vital structures, surgical excision is technically challenging and frequently incomplete.[119,123,127,128] Patients in whom complete surgical excision cannot be achieved may experience a progressive course, with complications and death from invasion or impairment of vital organs. Alternative therapies for local control such as interferon-α, external beam radiotherapy, cytotoxic chemotherapy, direct sclerosant injection, and radiofrequency ablation have been attempted with limited success when surgical resection cannot be accomplished.[129,130]

Lymphangiomatosis

Lymphangiomatosis is a congenital disorder that usually becomes apparent during adolescence or early adulthood. It is distinguished from lymphangioma by the development of multifocal or multisystem lymphangiomas. Pathologically, lymphangiomatosis has an appearance similar to that of solitary lymphangioma but is characterized by the proliferation of multiple, complex lymphatic channels and may involve both lungs. In approximately 75 percent of cases, the disease also involves multiple organs, particularly bone. The remainder of cases are characterized by complex, multifocal disease within a single organ or body region.[116]

Pulmonary lymphangiomatosis typically is accompanied by other clinical findings including recurrent chylothorax, chylous ascites, pericardial effusion, and lymphangiomas of the skin, bone, kidney, pancreas, retroperitoneum, mesentery, liver, spleen, and extremities.[119,131,132] Symptoms may include wheezing, chest pain, and dyspnea. Chyloptysis, hemoptysis, and peripheral lymphedema may also be present. Other symptoms are attributed to the various sites of organ involvement, including skeletal and abdominal disease.

The clinical evaluation of patients with suspected lymphangiomatosis should include a careful review for multiorgan disease and complete thoracic and abdominal high-resolution imaging with CT or MRI to determine the extent and distribution of lesions. The clinical course of the disease varies widely. In adults the prognosis is favorable with low mortality, whereas children frequently have progressive and relentless disease.[133] When present in early childhood, lymphangiomatosis often is associated with severe pulmonary impairment and respiratory failure. When technically possible, management is directed toward surgical debulking of large or symptomatic lesions that compress surrounding structures. Otherwise a program of drainage for symptomatic fluid collections and low-fat, high-protein diets with supplemental medium-chain triglycerides is advocated.

Lymphangiectasis

Unlike lymphangiomas or lymphangiomatosis, lymphangiectasis is characterized by diffuse, pathologic dilations of the lymphatic channels

TABLE 14-4

Distinguishing Features of Pulmonary Lymphatic Disorders

	Lymphangioma	Lymphangiomatosis	Lymphangiectasis	Lymphatic Dysplasia
Pathologic Features	Single, continuous lesion. Dilated lymphatic channels lined by epithelium without cellular atypia. Less common features include indiscrete margins or multiloculated cysts. May arise in mediastinum, pulmonary parenchyma or chest wall.	Proliferation of multiple, dilated lymphatic channels that may involve both lungs and commonly is present in multiple organs. Lung and bone common sites of organ involvement.	Dilated and cystic lymphatic channels without proliferation. May be present diffusely throughout lungs. Commonly present in mediastinum, liver, spleen, and retroperitoneum.	Heterogeneous group of disorders characterized by obstruction of proximal lymphatic vessels, hyperplastic or hypoplastic lymphatic channels, or incompetent lymphatic valves.
Etiology	Most are congenital developmental abnormality. May occur following chronic lymphatic obstruction.	Congenital developmental abnormality.	Primary congenital forms exist. May occur in association with complex congenital disease syndromes. May occur secondary to trauma, surgery, infection, or radiation.	Idiopathic, congenital, or developmental disorders.
Clinical Features	Affects adults, infants, and older children. May be asymptomatic. Swelling of head, neck, or face; tracheal deviation. Cough, dyspnea. May be discovered as incidental radiographic finding.	Affects both adults and children. Symptoms include wheezing, chest pain, dyspnea, cutaneous lesions, bone pain, ascites. Hemoptysis, chyloptysis, peripheral lymphedema.	May manifest as fetal demise or immediately after birth with respiratory distress. Chylothorax may be present.	Chylous pleural effusion in infancy or childhood, dyspnea.
Radiographic Features	Parenchymal or mediastinal mass with fluid density, pericardial or pleural effusions.	Pleural or pericardial effusions, ascites. Lymphangiomas present in mediastinum, chest wall, pleura.	Localized or multifocal pulmonary infiltrates, hyperinflation, pleural effusion.	Pleural effusion.
Management	Surgical excision. Injection of sclerosant.	Surgical debulking when necessary, drainage of symptomatic fluid collections. High-protein, low-fat diet, medium-chain triglyceride supplementation.	High-protein, low-fat diet, medium-chain triglyceride supplementation. Drainage of symptomatic fluid collections.	Drainage of symptomatic pleural effusion. Frequent antibiotics may be necessary. High-protein, low-fat diet, medium-chain triglyceride supplementation.

Adapted in part from Faul JL, Berry GJ, Colby TV, et al: Thoracic lymphangiomas, lymphangiectasis, lymphangiomatosis, and lymphatic dysplasia syndrome. Am J Respir Crit Care Med 161(3 Pt 1):1037-1046, 2000.

without proliferation of lymphatic tissue, large fluid collections, septations, or significant stromal tissue components. Both primary (or congenital) and secondary (or acquired) forms of this disease have been described. Primary lymphangiectasis may occur as an isolated finding or within the context of complex congenital disorders including Noonan, Ullrich-Turner, Ehlers-Danlos, and Down syndromes.[116] Primary thoracic lymphangiectasis may result in stillbirth or is frequently fatal during the neonatal period from severe hypoxemia and pulmonary congestion.[134] Lymphangiography and autopsy study have shown that primary lymphangiectasis may be present in many organs including lung, liver, spleen, retroperitoneal structures, and the alimentary canal.[135] Secondary thoracic lymphangiectasis may occur with any disease that obstructs pulmonary venous return, with congenital heart defects, and occasionally following a surgical manipulation of the lung and mediastinal structures. The common cause is presumed to arise from obstruction of thoracic lymphatic drainage.

Clinical features of lymphangiectasis include respiratory distress, dyspnea, failure to thrive, and chylothorax. Radiographic features include alveolar or interstitial infiltrates, hyperinflation, pleural effusion, and increased interstitial lung markings.[136] In patients who survive infancy, the symptoms and clinical course often improve, and long-term survival has been described.[134,137] There is no definitive management for lymphangiectasis, but patients may benefit from dietary modifications including high-protein, low-fat, enhanced medium-chain triglyceride diets.[138] Octreotide may be of some use in controlling abdominal organ disease manifestations such as protein-losing enteropathy, but its role in management of thoracic disease has not been established.[139]

Lymphatic Dysplasia

Lymphatic dysplasia syndromes of the thorax and lungs are a heterogenous group of disorders that include idiopathic lymphedema syndromes, idiopathic recurring chylous effusions, and the yellow nail syndrome. Pathologically and radiographically, these disorders may be characterized by obstruction of proximal lymphatic vessels, hyperplastic or hypoplastic lymphatic channels, or incompetent lymphatic valves. The common features of these syndromes are persistent and refractory accumulation of chyle and edema within the soft tissues and in the chest by chylous pleural or, rarely, pericardial effusions. Immunodeficiency

from immunoglobulin loss may be present if pleural effusions are recurrent.

In neonates and children, lymphatic dysplasia frequently results in "idiopathic" chylous effusions. Dyspnea, cough, respiratory distress, and peripheral lymphedema may be present. The most well-recognized disease manifestation in adults is the yellow nail syndrome, which is characterized by lymphedema, yellowed and dystrophic nails, and idiopathic pleural effusions.[140] In addition to hemodynamic aspects of persistent pleural fluid loss, these patients may develop protein deficiency and immunosuppression, as well as recurrent pulmonary infections from immunoglobulin and protein losses.[141,142] Pleural effusions must be managed with thoracentesis as necessary, frequent antibiotics given for pulmonary infection, and the same dietary modifications prescribed for patients with lymphangiomatosis and lymphangiectasis.[116] Patients with massive or frequently recurring pleural effusions may require pleurovenous or pleuroperitoneal shunts.[143]

References

1. Okuno T, Matsuda K, Ueyama K, et al: Leiomyosarcoma of the pulmonary vein. *Pathol Int* 50: 839-846, 2000.

2. Szekely E, Kulka J, Miklos I, et al: Leiomyosarcomas of great vessels. *Pathol Oncol Res* 6(3):233-236, 2000.

3. Oliai BR, Tazelaar HD, Lloyd RV, et al: Leiomyosarcoma of the pulmonary veins. *Am J Surg Pathol* 23:1082-1088, 1999.

4. Bleisch VR, Kraus FT: Polypoid sarcoma of the pulmonary trunk: Analysis of the literature and report of a case with leptomeric organelles and ultrastructural features of rhabdomyosarcoma. *Cancer* 46:314-324, 1980.

5. Gaumann A, Petrow P, Mentzel T, et al: Osteopontin expression in primary sarcomas of the pulmonary artery. *Virchows Arch* 439:668-674, 2001.

6. Burke AP, Virmani R: Sarcomas of the great vessels. A clinicopathologic study. *Cancer* 71:1761-1773, 1993.

7. Cox JE, Chiles C, Aquino SL, et al: Pulmonary artery sarcomas: A review of clinical and radiologic features. *J Comput Assist Tomogr* 21:750-755, 1997.

8. Kruger I, Borowski A, Horst M, et al: Symptoms, diagnosis, and therapy of primary sarcomas of the pulmonary artery. *Thorac Cardiovasc Surg* 38:91-95, 1990.

9. Schroeder JK, Srinivasan V: Intraluminal pulmonary artery fibroma in a 7-year-old boy. *Pediatr Cardiol* 21:480-482, 2000.

10. Mayer E, Kriegsmann J, Gaumann A, et al: Surgical treatment of pulmonary artery sarcoma. *J Thorac Cardiovasc Surg* 121:77-82, 2001.

11. Parish JM, Rosenow EC, III, Swensen SJ, et al: Pulmonary artery sarcoma. Clinical features. *Chest* 110:1480-1488, 1996.

12. Genoni M, Biraima AM, Bode B, et al: Combined resection and adjuvant therapy improves prognosis of sarcomas of the pulmonary trunk. *J Cardiovasc Surg (Torino)* 42:829-833, 2001.

13. Govender D, Pillay SV: Right pulmonary artery sarcoma. *Pathology* 33:243-245, 2001.

14. Nonomura A, Kurumaya H, Kono N, et al: Primary pulmonary artery sarcoma. Report of two autopsy cases studied by immunohistochemistry and electron microscopy, and review of 110 cases reported in the literature. *Acta Pathol Jpn* 38:883-896, 1988.

15. Choi EY, Yoon YW, Kwon HM, et al: A case of pulmonary artery intimal sarcoma diagnosed with multislice CT scan with 3D reconstruction. *Yonsei Med J* 45:547-551, 2004.

16. Yi ES: Tumors of the pulmonary vasculature. *Cardiol Clin* 22:431-440, vi-vii, 2004.

17. Simpson WL, Jr, Mendelson DS: Pulmonary artery and aortic sarcomas: Cross-sectional imaging. *J Thorac Imaging* 15:290-294, 2000.

18. Yi CA, Lee KS, Choe YH, et al: Computed tomography in pulmonary artery sarcoma: Distinguishing features from pulmonary embolic disease. *J Comput Assist Tomogr* 28:34-39, 2004.

19. Shimono T, Yuasa H, Yuasa U, et al: Pulmonary leiomyosarcoma extending into left atrium or pulmonary trunk: Complete resection with cardiopulmonary bypass. *J Thorac Cardiovasc Surg* 115:460-461, 1998.

20. Pui MH, Yu SP, Chen JD: Primary intrathoracic malignant fibrous histiocytoma and angiosarcoma. *Australas Radiol* 43:3-6, 1999.

21. Mader MT, Poulton TB, White RD: Malignant tumors of the heart and great vessels: MR imaging appearance. *Radiographics* 17:145-153, 1997.

22. Kacl GM, Bruder E, Pfammatter T, et al: Primary angiosarcoma of the pulmonary arteries: Dynamic contrast-enhanced MRI. *J Comput Assist Tomogr* 22:687-691, 1998.

23. Thurer RL, Thorsen A, Parker JA, et al: FDG imaging of a pulmonary artery sarcoma. *Ann Thorac Surg* 70:1414-1415, 2000.

24. Yamada N, Kamei S, Yasuda F, et al: Primary leiomyosarcoma of the pulmonary artery confirmed by catheter suction biopsy. *Chest* 113:555-556, 1998.

25. Mattoo A, Fedullo PF, Kapelanski D, et al: Pulmonary artery sarcoma: A case report of surgical cure and 5-year follow-up. *Chest* 122:745-747, 2002.

26. Laroia ST, Potti A, Rabbani M, et al: Unusual pulmonary lesions. Case 3: Pulmonary vein leiomyosarcoma presenting as a left atrial mass. *J Clin Oncol* 20:2749-2751, 2002.

27. Gyhra AS, Santander CK, Alarcon EC, et al: Leiomyosarcoma of the pulmonary veins with extension to the left atrium. *Ann Thorac Surg* 61:1840-1841, 1996.

28. Dail DH, Liebow AA: Intravascular bronchoalveolar tumor. *Am J Pathol* 78:6a, 1975 (abstract).

29. Dail DH, Liebow AA, Gmelich JT, et al: Intravascular, bronchiolar, and alveolar tumor of the lung (IVBAT). An analysis of twenty cases of a peculiar sclerosing endothelial tumor. *Cancer* 51:452-464, 1983.

30. Weldon-Linne CM, Victor TA, Christ ML, et al: Angiogenic nature of the "intravascular bronchioloalveolar tumor" of the lung: An electron microscopic study. *Arch Pathol Lab Med* 105:174-179, 1981.

31. Cronin P, Arenberg D: Pulmonary epithelioid hemangioendothelioma: An unusual case and a review of the literature. *Chest* 125:789-793, 2004.

32. Weiss SW, Enzinger FM: Epithelioid hemangioendothelioma: A vascular tumor often mistaken for a carcinoma. *Cancer* 50:970-981, 1982.

33. Mhoyan A, Weidner N, Shabaik A: Epithelioid hemangioendothelioma of the lung diagnosed by transesophageal endoscopic ultrasound-guided fine needle aspiration: A case report. *Acta Cytol* 48:555-559, 2004.

34. Pinet C, Magnan A, Garbe L, et al: Aggressive form of pleural epithelioid haemangioendothelioma: Complete response after chemotherapy. *Eur Respir J* 14:237-238, 1999.

35. Bagshawe KD, Brooks WD: Subacute pulmonary hypertension due to chorionepithelioma. *Lancet* 1:653-658, 1959.

36. Seckl MJ, Rustin GJ, Newlands ES, et al: Pulmonary embolism, pulmonary hypertension, and choriocarcinoma. *Lancet* 338:1313-1315, 1991.

37. Watanabe S, Shimokawa S, Sakasegawa K, et al: Choriocarcinoma in the pulmonary artery treated with emergency pulmonary embolectomy. *Chest* 121:654-656, 2002.

38. Trubenbach J, Pereira PL, Huppert PE, et al: Primary choriocarcinoma of the pulmonary artery mimicking pulmonary embolism. *Br J Radiol* 70:843-845, 1997.

39. Soares FA, Pinto AP, Landell GA, et al: Pulmonary tumor embolism to arterial vessels and carcinomatous lymphangitis. A comparative clinicopathological study. *Arch Pathol Lab Med* 117:827-831, 1993.

40. Bassiri AG, Haghighi B, Doyle RL, et al: Pulmonary tumor embolism. *Am J Respir Crit Care Med* 155:2089-2095, 1997.

41. Brill IC, Robertson TD: Subacute cor pulmonale. *Arch Int Med* 60:1043-1057, 1937.

42. von Herbay A, Illes A, Waldherr R, et al: Pulmonary tumor thrombotic microangiopathy with pulmonary hypertension. *Cancer* 66:587-592, 1990.

43. Schriner RW, Ryu JH, Edwards WD: Microscopic pulmonary tumor embolism causing subacute cor pulmonale: A difficult antemortem diagnosis. *Mayo Clin Proc* 66:143-148, 1991.

44. Roberts KE, Hamele-Bena D, Saqi A, et al: Pulmonary tumor embolism: A review of the literature. *Am J Med* 115:228-232, 2003.

45. Kane RD, Hawkins HK, Miller JA, et al: Microscopic pulmonary tumor emboli associated with dyspnea. *Cancer* 36:1473-1482, 1975.

46. Shepard JA, Moore EH, Templeton PA, et al: Pulmonary intravascular tumor emboli: Dilated and beaded peripheral pulmonary arteries at CT. *Radiology* 187:797-801, 1993.

47. Masson RG, Krikorian J, Lukl P, et al: Pulmonary microvascular cytology in the diagnosis of lymphangitic carcinomatosis. *N Engl J Med* 321:71-76, 1989.

48. Soares FA: Increased numbers of pulmonary megakaryocytes in patients with arterial pulmonary tumour embolism and with lung metastases seen at necropsy. *J Clin Pathol* 45:140-142, 1992.

49. Lukl P: Pulmonary microvascular cytology in the dyspneic cancer patient. Merits and caution. *Arch Pathol Lab Med* 116:129-130, 1992.

50. Sadoff L, Grossman J, Weiner H: Lymphangitic pulmonary metastases secondary to breast cancer with normal chest x-rays and abnormal perfusion lung scans. *Oncology* 31:164-171, 1975.

51. Ikezoe J, Godwin JD, Hunt KJ, et al: Pulmonary lymphangitic carcinomatosis: Chronicity of radiographic findings in long-term survivors. *AJR Am J Roentgenol* 165:49-52, 1995.

52. Isringhaus H, Naber M, Kopper B: Successful treatment of tumor embolism of a hypernephroma with complete occlusion of the left pulmonary artery. *Thorac Cardiovasc Surg* 35:65-66, 1987.

53. Pfleger L, Tappeiner J: [On the recognition of systematized endotheliomatosis of the cutaneous blood vessels (reticuloendotheliosis)] *Hautarzt* 10:359-363, 1959.

54. Chim CS, Choy C, Ooi GC, et al: Two unusual lymphomas. Case 2: Pulmonary intravascular lymphomatosis. *J Clin Oncol* 18:3733-3735, 2000.

55. Ko YH, Han JH, Go JH, et al: Intravascular lymphomatosis: A clinicopathological study of two cases presenting as an interstitial lung disease. *Histopathology* 31:555-562, 1997.

56. Walls JG, Hong YG, Cox JE, et al: Pulmonary intravascular lymphomatosis: Presentation with dyspnea and air trapping. *Chest* 115:1207-1210, 1999.

57. Yamagata T, Okamoto Y, Ota K, et al: A case of pulmonary intravascular lymphomatosis diagnosed by thoracoscopic lung biopsy. *Respiration* 70:414-418, 2003.

58. Sepp N, Schuler G, Romani N, et al: "Intravascular lymphomatosis" (angioendotheliomatosis): Evidence for a T-cell origin in two cases. *Hum Pathol* 21:1051-1058, 1990.

59. Owa M, Koyama J, Asakawa K, et al: Intravascular lymphomatosis presenting as reversible severe pulmonary hypertension. *Int J Cardiol* 75:283-284, 2000.

60. Snyder LS, Harmon KR, Estensen RD: Intravascular lymphomatosis (malignant angioendotheliomatosis) presenting as pulmonary hypertension. *Chest* 96:1199-1200, 1989.

61. DiGiuseppe JA, Nelson WG, Seifter EJ, et al: Intravascular lymphomatosis: A clinicopathologic study of 10 cases and assessment of response to chemotherapy. *J Clin Oncol* 12:2573-2579, 1994.

62. Burke M, Opeskin K: Death due to intravenous leiomyomatosis extending to the right pulmonary artery. *Pathology* 36:202-203, 2004.

63. Wieder JA, Laks H, Freitas D, et al: Renal cell carcinoma with tumor thrombus extension into the proximal pulmonary artery. *J Urol* 169:2296-2297, 2003.

64. Nishizawa J, Matsumoto M, Sugita T, et al: Intravenous leiomyomatosis extending into the right ventricle associated with pulmonary metastasis and extensive arteriovenous fistula. *J Am Coll Surg* 198:842-843, 2004.

65. Yamaguchi T, Suzuki K, Asamura H, et al: Lung carcinoma with polypoid growth in the main pulmonary artery: Report of two cases. *Jpn J Clin Oncol* 30:358-361, 2000.

66. Wagenvoort CA, Beetstra A, Spijker J: Capillary haemangiomatosis of the lungs. *Histopathology* 2:401-406, 1978.

67. Eltorky MA, Headley AS, Winer-Muram H, et al: Pulmonary capillary hemangiomatosis: A clinicopathologic review. *Ann Thorac Surg* 57:772-776, 1994.

68. Almagro P, Julia J, Sanjaume M, et al: Pulmonary capillary hemangiomatosis associated with primary pulmonary hypertension: Report of 2 new cases and review of 35 cases from the literature. *Medicine (Baltimore)* 81:417-424, 2002.

69. de Perrot M, Waddell TK, Chamberlain D, et al: De novo pulmonary capillary hemangiomatosis occurring rapidly after bilateral lung transplantation. *J Heart Lung Transplant* 22:698-700, 2003.

70. Langleben D, Heneghan JM, Batten AP, et al: Familial pulmonary capillary hemangiomatosis

resulting in primary pulmonary hypertension. *Ann Intern Med* 109:106-109, 1988.

71. Kakkar N, Vasishta RK, Banerjee AK, et al: Pulmonary capillary haemangiomatosis as a cause of pulmonary hypertension in Takayasu's aortoarteritis. *Respiration* 64:381-383, 1997.

72. Gugnani MK, Pierson C, Vanderheide R, et al: Pulmonary edema complicating prostacyclin therapy in pulmonary hypertension associated with scleroderma: A case of pulmonary capillary hemangiomatosis. *Arthritis Rheum* 43:699-703, 2000.

73. Fernandez-Alonso J, Zulueta T, Reyes-Ramirez JR, et al: Pulmonary capillary hemangiomatosis as cause of pulmonary hypertension in a young woman with systemic lupus erythematosus. *J Rheumatol* 26:231-233, 1999.

74. Umezu H, Naito M, Yagisawa K, et al: An autopsy case of pulmonary capillary hemangiomatosis without evidence of pulmonary hypertension. *Virchows Arch* 439:586-592, 2001.

75. Havlik DM, Massie LW, Williams WL, et al: Pulmonary capillary hemangiomatosis-like foci. An autopsy study of 8 cases. *Am J Clin Pathol* 113:655-662, 2000.

76. Lippert JL, White CS, Cameron EW, et al: Pulmonary capillary hemangiomatosis: Radiographic appearance. *J Thorac Imaging* 13:49-51, 1998.

77. Ito K, Ichiki T, Ohi K, et al: Pulmonary capillary hemangiomatosis with severe pulmonary hypertension. *Circ J* 67:793-795, 2003.

78. White CW, Wolf SJ, Korones DN, et al: Treatment of childhood angiomatous diseases with recombinant interferon alfa-2a. *J Pediatr* 118:59-66, 1991.

79. Remy J, Remy-Jardin M, Giraud F, et al: Angioarchitecture of pulmonary arteriovenous malformations: Clinical utility of three-dimensional helical CT. *Radiology* 191:657-664, 1994.

80. Gupta P, Mordin C, Curtis J, et al: Pulmonary arteriovenous malformations: Effect of embolization on right-to-left shunt, hypoxemia, and exercise tolerance in 66 patients. *AJR Am J Roentgenol* 179:347-355, 2002.

81. Swanson KL, Prakash UB, Stanson AW: Pulmonary arteriovenous fistulas: Mayo Clinic experience, 1982-1997. *Mayo Clin Proc* 74:671-680, 1999.

82. Gossage JR, Kanj G: Pulmonary arteriovenous malformations. A state of the art review. *Am J Respir Crit Care Med* 158:643-661, 1998.

83. Pick A, Deschamps C, Stanson AW: Pulmonary arteriovenous fistula: Presentation, diagnosis, and treatment. *World J Surg* 23:1118-1122, 1999.

84. Srivastava D, Preminger T, Lock JE, et al: Hepatic venous blood and the development of pulmonary arteriovenous malformations in congenital heart disease. *Circulation* 92:1217-1222, 1995.

85. Starnes SL, Duncan BW, Kneebone JM, et al: Angiogenic proteins in the lungs of children after cavopulmonary anastomosis. *J Thorac Cardiovasc Surg* 122:518-523, 2001.

86. Duncan BW, Kneebone JM, Chi EY, et al: A detailed histologic analysis of pulmonary arteriovenous malformations in children with cyanotic congenital heart disease. *J Thorac Cardiovasc Surg* 117:931-938, 1999.

87. Gallione CJ, Repetto GM, Legius E, et al: A combined syndrome of juvenile polyposis and hereditary haemorrhagic telangiectasia associated with mutations in MADH4 (SMAD4). *Lancet* 363:852-859, 2004.

88. Wallace GM, Shovlin CL: A hereditary haemorrhagic telangiectasia family with pulmonary involvement is unlinked to the known HHT genes, endoglin and ALK-1. *Thorax* 55:685-690, 2000.

89. Cymerman U, Vera S, Karabegovic A, et al: Characterization of 17 novel endoglin mutations associated with hereditary hemorrhagic telangiectasia. *Hum Mutat* 21:482-492, 2003.

90. Abdalla SA, Pece-Barbara N, Vera S, et al: Analysis of ALK-1 and endoglin in newborns from families with hereditary hemorrhagic telangiectasia type 2. *Hum Mol Genet* 9:1227-1237, 2000.

91. Trembath RC, Thomson JR, Machado RD, et al: Clinical and molecular genetic features of pulmonary hypertension in patients with hereditary hemorrhagic telangiectasia. *N Engl J Med* 345:325-334, 2001.

92. Berg JN, Guttmacher AE, Marchuk DA, et al: Clinical heterogeneity in hereditary haemorrhagic telangiectasia: Are pulmonary arteriovenous malformations more common in families linked to endoglin? *J Med Genet* 33:256-257, 1996.

93. Shovlin CL, Guttmacher AE, Buscarini E, et al: Diagnostic criteria for hereditary hemorrhagic telangiectasia (Rendu-Osler-Weber syndrome). *Am J Med Genet* 91:66-67, 2000.

94. Sloan RD, Cooley RN: Congenital pulmonary arteriovenous aneurysm. *Am J Radiol* 70:183-210, 1953.

95. Kopf GS, Laks H, Stansel HC, et al: Thirty-year follow-up of superior vena cava-pulmonary artery (Glenn) shunts. *J Thorac Cardiovasc Surg* 100:662-670, discussion 70-71, 1990.

96. Dakeishi M, Shioya T, Wada Y, et al: Genetic epidemiology of hereditary hemorrhagic telangiectasia in a local community in the northern part of Japan. *Hum Mutat* 19:140-148, 2002.

97. Kjeldsen AD, Vase P, Green A: Hereditary haemorrhagic telangiectasia: A population-based study of prevalence and mortality in Danish patients. *J Intern Med* 245:31-39, 1999.

98. Kjeldsen AD, Oxhoj H, Andersen PE, et al: Prevalence of pulmonary arteriovenous malformations (PAVMs) and occurrence of neurological symptoms in patients with hereditary haemorrhagic telangiectasia (HHT). *J Intern Med* 248:255-262, 2000.

99. Nanthakumar K, Graham AT, Robinson TI, et al: Contrast echocardiography for detection of pulmonary arteriovenous malformations. *Am Heart J* 141:243-246, 2001.

100. Haitjema T, Disch F, Overtoom TT, et al: Screening family members of patients with hereditary hemorrhagic telangiectasia. *Am J Med* 99:519-524, 1995.

101. Shovlin CL, Letarte M: Hereditary haemorrhagic telangiectasia and pulmonary arteriovenous malformations: Issues in clinical management and review of pathogenic mechanisms. *Thorax* 54:714-729, 1999.

102. Kjeldsen AD, Oxhoj H, Andersen PE, et al: Pulmonary arteriovenous malformations: Screening procedures and pulmonary angiography in patients with hereditary hemorrhagic telangiectasia. *Chest* 116:432-439, 1999.

103. Cottin V, Plauchu H, Bayle JY, et al: Pulmonary arteriovenous malformations in patients with hereditary hemorrhagic telangiectasia. *Am J Respir Crit Care Med* 169:994-1000, 2004.

104. Dutton JA, Jackson JE, Hughes JM, et al: Pulmonary arteriovenous malformations: Results of treatment with coil embolization in 53 patients. *AJR Am J Roentgenol* 165:1119-1125, 1995.

105. Chilvers ER, Whyte MK, Jackson JE, et al: Effect of percutaneous transcatheter embolization on pulmonary function, right-to-left shunt, and arterial oxygenation in patients with pulmonary arteriovenous malformations. *Am Rev Respir Dis* 142:420-425, 1990.

106. Mager JJ, Zanen P, Verzijlbergen F, et al: Quantification of right-to-left shunt with (99m) Tc-labelled albumin macroaggregates and 100 percent oxygen in patients with hereditary haemorrhagic telangiectasia. *Clin Sci (London)* 102:127-134, 2002.

107. Lee WL, Graham AF, Pugash RA, et al: Contrast echocardiography remains positive after treatment of pulmonary arteriovenous malformations. *Chest* 123:351-358, 2003.

108. Chung CW, Doherty JU, Kotler R, et al: Pulmonary artery aneurysm presenting as a lung mass. *Chest* 108:1164-1166, 1995.

109. Veldtman GR, Dearani JA, Warnes CA: Low pressure giant pulmonary artery aneurysms in the adult: Natural history and management strategies. *Heart* 89:1067-1070, 2003.

110. Fernandes V, Kaluza GL, Zymek PT, et al: Successful balloon valvuloplasty in an adult patient with severe pulmonic stenosis and aneurysmal poststenotic dilatation. *Catheter Cardiovasc Interv* 55:376-380, 2002.

111. Tami LF, McElderry MW: Pulmonary artery aneurysm due to severe congenital pulmonic stenosis. Case report and literature review. *Angiology* 45:383-390, 1994.

112. Deterling RA, Claggett T: Aneurysm of the pulmonary artery: Review of the literature and report of a case. *Am Heart J* 34:471-499, 1947.

113. van Rens MT, Westermann CJ, Postmus PE, et al: Untreated idiopathic aneurysm of the pulmonary artery long-term follow-up. *Respir Med* 94:404-405, 2000.

114. Brown M, Pysher T, Coffin CM: Lymphangioma and congenital pulmonary lymphangiectasis: A histologic, immunohistochemical, and clinicopathologic comparison. *Mod Pathol* 12:569-575, 1999.

115. Levine C: Primary disorders of the lymphatic vessels—a unified concept. *J Pediatr Surg* 24:233-240, 1989.

116. Faul JL, Berry GJ, Colby TV, et al: Thoracic lymphangiomas, lymphangiectasis, lymphangiomatosis, and lymphatic dysplasia syndrome. *Am J Respir Crit Care Med* 161:1037-1046, 2000.

117. Parker RJ, Cadman PJ, Wathen CG: Lymphangioma: A rare cause of a mediastinal mass. *Thorax* 59:820, 2004.

118. Pilla TJ, Wolverson MK, Sundaram M, et al: CT evaluation of cystic lymphangiomas of the mediastinum. *Radiology* 144:841-842, 1982.

119. Brown LR, Reiman HM, Rosenow EC, III, et al: Intrathoracic lymphangioma. *Mayo Clin Proc* 61:882-892, 1986.

120. Maria A, Aggarwal R: Lymphomatous malformation of the chest wall. *Indian Pediatr* 41:742, 2004.

121. Telander RL, Kaufman BH, Gloviczki P, et al: Prognosis and management of lesions of the trunk in children with Klippel-Trenaunay syndrome. *J Pediatr Surg* 19:417-422, 1984.

122. Wagenaar SS, Swierenga J, Wagenvoort CA: Late presentation of primary pulmonary lymphangiectasis. *Thorax* 33:791-795, 1978.

123. Yamagishi S, Koizumi K, Hirata T, et al: Experience of thoracoscopic extirpation of intrapulmonary lymphangioma. *Jpn J Thorac Cardiovasc Surg* 53:313-316, 2005.

124. Chikkamuniyappa S, Heim-Hall J, Jagirdar J: Solitary endobronchial lymphangioma: A case report and review of literature. *Scientific World J* 5:103-108, 2005.

125. Lee CH, Kim YD, Kim KI, et al: Intrapulmonary cystic lymphangioma in a 2-month-old infant. *J Korean Med Sci* 19:458-461, 2004.

126. Nagayasu T, Hayashi T, Ashizawa K, et al: A case of solitary pulmonary lymphangioma. *J Clin Pathol* 56:396-398, 2003.

127. Daya SK, Gowda RM, Gowda MR, et al: Thoracic cystic lymphangioma (cystic hygroma): A chest pain syndrome—a case report. *Angiology* 55:561-564, 2004.

128. Handa R, Kale R, Upadhyay KK: Isolated mediastinal lymphangioma herniating through the intercostal space. *Asian J Surg* 27:241-242, 2004.

129. Rostom AY: Treatment of thoracic lymphangiomatosis. *Arch Dis Child* 83:138-139, 2000.

130. Hirunwiwatkul P: Radiofrequency tissue volume reduction: Suggested treatment for lymphatic malformation. *J Med Assoc Thai* 87:834-838, 2004.

131. Cutillo DP, Swayne LC, Cucco J, et al: CT and MR imaging in cystic abdominal lymphangiomatosis. *J Comput Assist Tomogr* 13:534-536, 1989.

132. Goh BK, Tan YM, Ong HS, et al: Intra-abdominal and retroperitoneal lymphangiomas in pediatric and adult patients. *World J Surg* 2005.

133. Alvarez OA, Kjellin I, Zuppan CW: Thoracic lymphangiomatosis in a child. *J Pediatr Hematol Oncol* 26:136-141, 2004.

134. Bouchard S, Di Lorenzo M, Youssef S, et al: Pulmonary lymphangiectasia revisited. *J Pediatr Surg* 35:796-800, 2000.

135. Hirano H, Nishigami T, Okimura A, et al: Autopsy case of congenital pulmonary lymphangiectasis. *Pathol Int* 54:532-536, 2004.

136. Barker PM, Esther CR, Jr, Fordham LA, et al: Primary pulmonary lymphangiectasia in infancy and childhood. *Eur Respir J* 24:413-419, 2004.

137. Esther CR, Jr, Barker PM: Pulmonary lymphangiectasia: Diagnosis and clinical course. *Pediatr Pulmonol* 38:308-313, 2004.

138. Alfano V, Tritto G, Alfonsi L, et al: Stable reversal of pathologic signs of primitive intestinal lymphangiectasia with a hypolipidic, MCT-enriched diet. *Nutrition* 16:303-304, 2000.

139. Ballinger AB, Farthing MJ: Octreotide in the treatment of intestinal lymphangiectasia. *Eur J Gastroenterol Hepatol* 10:699-702, 1998.

140. Marks R, Ellis JP: Yellow nails. A report of six cases. *Arch Dermatol* 102:619-623, 1970.

141. D'Alessandro A, Muzi G, Monaco A, et al: Yellow nail syndrome: Does protein leakage play a role? *Eur Respir J* 17:149-152, 2001.

142. Bokszczanin A, Levinson AI: Coexistent yellow nail syndrome and selective antibody deficiency. *Ann Allergy Asthma Immunol* 91:496-500, 2003.

143. Tanaka E, Matsumoto K, Shindo T, et al: Implantation of a pleurovenous shunt for massive chylothorax in a patient with yellow nail syndrome. *Thorax* 60:254-255, 2005.

144. Pietra CG, Capron F, Stewart S, et al: Pathologic assessment of vasculopathies in pulmonary hypertension. *J Am Coll Cardiol* 43:25S-32S, 2004.

145. Case records of the Massachusetts General Hospital. Weekly clinicopathological exercises. Case 25-2000: A 69-year-old woman with pleuritic pain and a pulmonary arterial obstruction. *N Engl J Med* 343:493-500, 2000.

146. Markowitz DH, Mark EJ: Case records of the Massachusetts General Hospital. Weekly clinicopathological exercises. Case 13-2002: A 43-year-old man with renal carcinoma and worsening dyspnea. *N Engl J Med* 46:1309-1317, 2002.

Chapter 15

Pulmonary Vasculitis

Dayna J. Groskreutz, MD,

Jess Mandel, MD

The vasculitides are diverse diseases characterized by inflammation within and around blood vessel walls.[1] The initial clinical presentation reflects involvement of individual or multiple organs, including the lungs. Certain systemic signs and symptoms should alert the clinician to the possibility of vasculitis, including fatigue, fever, weight loss, palpable purpura, mononeuritis multiplex, arthralgias, abdominal pain, and renal insufficiency. Specific pulmonary manifestations such as hemoptysis, stridor, cough, and dyspnea should also make the clinician suspicious of an underlying vasculitis. This chapter will provide an overview of the vasculitides with a propensity for pulmonary involvement.[2]

Although all vasculitides can become apparent with systemic symptoms such as fatigue, fever, or abnormalities of the skin, respiratory complaints are frequently the predominant clinical feature of vasculitides that involve the lung. Hemoptysis is a common and often life-threatening initial symptom of vasculitis. In some disease entities such as Behçet syndrome, hemoptysis can result from rupture of the pulmonary artery and lead rapidly to death. More often, hemoptysis from vasculitis is associated with diffuse alveolar hemorrhage and the histopathologic finding of pulmonary capillaritis. In association with dyspnea and cough, upper airway problems, including symptoms of sinusitis or epistaxis, can be important clues to an underlying vasculitis such as Wegener granulomatosis. Progressive symptoms in a patient with asthma might suggest Churg-Strauss syndrome.

Vasculitis can be primary or secondary, systemic or isolated to one organ, and infectious or noninfectious in etiology. Classification of these disorders into groups and even distinguishing among these conditions is sometimes difficult. In 1993, the Chapel Hill Consensus Conference proposed a classification guideline based upon the predominant size of the blood vessel affected by vasculitis. According to those guidelines, the large vessel vasculitides include giant cell arteritis and Takayasu arteritis. The medium-sized vessel vasculitides are polyarteritis nodosa, Kawasaki disease, and isolated central nervous system vasculitis, while the small vessel vasculitides include Wegener granulomatosis, Churg-Strauss syndrome, microscopic polyangiitis, Henoch-Schönlein purpura, essential cryoglobulinemic vasculitis, cutaneous leukocytoclastic vasculitis, hypersensitivity vasculitis, vasculitis secondary to connective tissue disorders, and vasculitis secondary to viral infection.

Another manner in which the vasculitides are classified is by antineutrophil cytoplasmic antibody (ANCA) positivity. The ANCA-associated vasculitides include Wegener granulomatosis, microscopic polyangiitis, and Churg-Strauss syndrome. ANCA was first reported in association with segmental necrotizing glomerulonephritis in the 1980s.[3,4] In 1985, van der Woude reported diffuse cytoplasmic staining of neutrophils, and this pattern has become known as cytoplasmic ANCA (c-ANCA).[5] The c-ANCA is directed specifically against proteinase 3 (PR3), a 29-kDa serine proteinase found in the azurophilic granules of neutrophils and the peroxidase-positive lysosomes of monocytes. In contrast, a perinuclear fluorescence of alcohol-fixed neutro phils is known as perinuclear ANCA (p-ANCA).[6] The p-ANCA is due to antibodies directed against myeloperoxidase, a 140-kDa covalently linked dimer found in the same cellular location as PR3; the different localization of staining is largely an artifact of preparation.[7] ANCA can be detected with immunofluorescence, enzyme-linked immunosorbent assay, and radioimmunoassay.

The presence of ANCA antibodies can be used to support the diagnosis of individual ANCA-associated vasculitides, but in most cases they do not eliminate the need for a tissue biopsy confirming the diagnosis. c-ANCA has a sensitivity of 90 percent in patients with active classic Wegener granulomatosis, whereas in limited Wegener granulomatosis (Wegener granulomatosis without kidney involvement), the sensitivity ranges from 43 to 70 percent.[8] p-ANCA typically is associated with Churg-Strauss syndrome, microscopic polyangiitis, and idiopathic necrotizing and crescentic glomerulonephritis. The positive predictive value of p-ANCA in one study was only 57 percent by immunofluorescence and 71 percent by enzyme immunoassay.[9]

Giant Cell Arteritis

Giant cell arteritis, also known as temporal arteritis, is a systemic vasculitis predominantly involving medium and large arteries in the head and neck. In 1932, Horton described giant cell arteritis as polymyalgia rheumatica, headache, and systemic illness (fever, fatigue, weight loss) in an elderly patient.[10] Blindness may result from an anterior ischemic optic neuropathy caused by occlusion of the posterior ciliary artery, a branch of the ophthalmic artery.[11] Other symptoms may include scalp tenderness in the temporal artery distribution, jaw or limb claudication, diplopia, amaurosis fugax, fever of unknown origin, transient ischemic attack, stroke, or acute lingual ischemia.[12] Aortitis may develop and result in aortic aneurysm or dissection.

Mononuclear infiltrates with giant cell formation in the large pulmonary arteries have been documented in patients with giant cell arteritis.[13] Pulmonary symptoms and signs usually occur with other systemic manifestations of giant cell arteritis, and may affect 10 percent of patients.[14] They can include cough, hemoptysis, pharyngitis, pulmonary interstitial infiltrates, pleural effusions, intraalveolar hemorrhage, anterior neck pain, and a sensation of choking.

The cause of giant cell arteritis is unknown. It has been suggested that antigen recognition by T cells and antigen-presenting cells within the adventitia leads to production of cytokines and chemokines resulting in mononuclear cell infiltration. Interferon-γ and tumor necrosis factor from helper T (T_H1) lymphocytes contribute to granuloma formation, while giant cells and macrophages produce platelet-derived growth factor and vascular endothelial growth factor to stimulate neoangiogenesis.[15] The eventual deposition of matrix leads to hyperplasia and obstruction.

To aid in diagnosis of giant cell arteritis, the American College of Rheumatology established five criteria, three of which must be present[16]:

1. Age 50 years or older
2. New-onset localized headache
3. Temporal artery tenderness or decreased temporal artery pulse
4. Erythrocyte sedimentation rate (ESR) of 50mm/hour or higher
5. Abnormal temporal artery biopsy findings demonstrating mononuclear infiltration or granulomatous inflammation

Giant cell arteritis occurs most often in whites, and women are affected twice as often as men.[15] The most common laboratory abnormality in giant cell arteritis is an elevated ESR (average 100mm/hour), and 30 percent of patients also have a mildly elevated alkaline phosphatase value, potentially due to hepatic arteritis.[11]

The gold standard for diagnosis is a temporal artery biopsy displaying characteristic inflammatory findings, such as granulomatous arteritis, with prominent Langerhans giant cells and predominant involvement of the tunica media.[17] Necrosis of vascular smooth muscle and deranged internal elastic membranes may be observed. Predominant inflammatory cells include lymphocytes, plasma cells, and macrophages, but eosinophils and neutrophils also may be present. Giant cell infiltrates within the large pulmonary arteries, as well as pulmonary artery aneurysms have been reported.[13,18]

A wide variety of pulmonary radiographic findings have been described in giant cell arteritis. The chest radiographic findings can be normal, but coarse nodules and diffuse interstitial infiltrates have also been reported.[19]

It is unclear whether giant cell arteritis has any measurable effect on pulmonary function testing. One study attempted to quantify abnormalities in pulmonary function tests of patients with giant cell arteritis.[20] No significant differences were identified between the study group consisting of 17 patients with giant cell arteritis and 9 with polymyalgia rheumatica and no history of tobacco use or known lung disease, versus 26 healthy controls matched for age and sex, although asymptomatic restrictive or obstructive defects were detected in several patients with giant cell arteritis.

No randomized clinical studies have been performed to demonstrate the efficacy of management for giant cell arteritis with pulmonary involvement, but case reports suggest that glucocorticoids given for systemic symptoms leads to improvement of respiratory symptoms.[11] Initial recommended therapy in giant cell arteritis is 40-60 mg of prednisone daily, with tapering after 2 to 4 weeks if symptoms have improved.[21] A number of alternative agents such as methotrexate have been investigated for giant cell arteritis, but none has proved unequivocally superior to prednisone.[22] Because of the risk of irreversible blindness, management should be started as soon as possible after the diagnosis is established, and in some circumstances while the diagnostic evaluation is underway.

Takayasu Arteritis

Takayasu arteritis is an idiopathic, chronic large vessel vasculitis usually affecting the aorta and its proximal branches, and involving the pulmonary artery in 50-80 percent of cases.[23] Isolated pulmonary manifestations of Takayasu arteritis are rare but can include dyspnea, pleurisy, hemoptysis, pleural effusion, interstitial pneumonitis, and respiratory failure.[24,25] Pulmonary hypertension was diagnosed in 27 percent of patients with Takayasu arteritis in one series, although its overall prevalence is unclear.[26]

Takayasu arteritis was first described by Oota in 1940.[27] The inflammatory processes causes thickening of affected arteries, with proximal dilation. Arteries commonly affected include the aorta and the subclavian, carotid, and vertebral arteries.[16] Multiple pathologic features of pulmonary artery involvement have also been described, including intimal fibrosis, thinning of the media with disruption of elastic fibers, bandlike fibrosis of the adventitia, and complete occlusion of the pulmonary artery caused by loose fibrous tissue in the lumen.[28] A unique feature of pulmonary artery involvement in Takayasu arteritis is called stenosis-recanalization, or the "vessel-in-vessel" feature. Grossly it appears to be an organization and recanalization of a thromboembolus, but newly formed arterial channels through the obstructed lumen originate from the vasa vasorum and are branches of the bronchial artery.[28]

Takayasu arteritis occurs throughout the world but appears most prevalent in East Asia. In Japan, approximately 150 new cases are reported per year.[16] The disease usually affects women of reproductive age, and women are afflicted 8-10 times more frequently than men.[25] The etiology of Takayasu arteritis is unknown. Genetic, infectious, and hormonal factors have been suggested, but no clear causality has been established.

Patients with Takayasu arteritis frequently suffer from fatigue, weight loss, and low-grade fever. As the disease progresses, vascular symptoms occur, including cool extremities and arm or leg claudication. On physical examination, patients may display reduced or unequal blood pressure in the extremities, decreased strength of pulses, synovitis, or hypertension caused by narrowing of the renal artery. Subclavian, axillary, and carotid bruits are sometimes present. Other cardiovascular complications include aortic root dilation, aortic insufficiency, dysrhythmias, cardiomyopathy, coronary vasculitis and, rarely, pericarditis and myocarditis. Laboratory findings usually include hypoalbuminemia and a nonspecific elevation of acute-phase reactants such as C-reactive protein and ferritin.

Conventional contrast arteriography historically has been central in the diagnosis of Takayasu arteritis and usually reveals focal areas of smooth-walled tapering or narrowing, with associated areas of dilation and collateral circulation.[16] Luminal irregularities and ectasias or aneurysms of large vessels may be appreciated.[25] Computed tomography (CT), magnetic resonance imaging (MRI), ultrasonography, and positron-emission tomography also have diagnostic utility in assessing lumen size, vessel wall thickness, and progression of disease, and are relied upon increasingly in lieu of conventional angiography for establishing the diagnosis.

The primary treatment of Takayasu arteritis is glucocorticoids. Prednisone at initial doses of 45-60 mg usually alleviates the systemic symptoms and retards progression of inflammation.[21] One-half of patients with Takayasu arteritis attain remission with glucocorticoid therapy, but one-half of responders will relapse when treatment is tapered.[15] Steroid-sparing agents may be useful; in one small study, low-dose methotrexate allowed most patients to discontinue glucocorticoid therapy.[29] Mycophenolate mofetil, cyclophosphamide, and antitumor necrosis factor agents are other alternatives or adjuncts to glucocorticoid therapy. For vessels in which irreversible stenosis has already occurred, angioplasty, intravascular stents, or surgical bypass grafting may be required.

Wegener Granulomatosis

Wegener granulomatosis is a systemic granulomatous disease first described by Klinger in 1931[30] and later by Wegener in 1936.[31] It typically affects the upper and lower airways, as well as the skin and kidneys. Other organs can be involved, including the joints, eyes, nervous system, heart, gastrointestinal tract, thyroid, liver, and breast. The peak incidence is in the fourth through sixth decades of life, and there is no gender predominance.[32]

In 1990 the American College of Rheumatology developed four criteria to aid in the diagnosis of Wegener granulomatosis[33]:

1. Nasal or oral inflammation
2. Abnormal chest radiograph findings
3. Abnormal urinary sediment
4. Granulomatous inflammation on a biopsy specimen (or the presence of hemoptysis if no biopsy specimen is available)

The presence of two or more criteria was reported to have a diagnostic sensitivity of 88 percent and specificity of 92 percent.

The exact etiology of Wegener granulomatosis remains unknown, but multiple factors such as infection, inhalation of silica or grain dust, genetic predisposition, alloantibodies, antigen-antibody complex deposition, and abnormal cell-mediated immunity have been suggested.

Wegener granulomatosis is associated with a multitude of symptoms. Patients often complain of sinus pain, nasal congestion, epistaxis, otitis media, hearing loss, rhinorrhea, or purulent nasal discharge. They may have ocular symptoms of conjunctivitis, episcleritis, or scleritis. They may also report systemic symptoms such as fever, weight loss, arthralgias, and rash. Pulmonary complaints include dyspnea, cough, hemoptysis, and chest pain, and laryngotracheobronchial involvement may result in wheezing, stridor, or a change in voice. Classic Wegener granulomatosis is typically a multisystem disease, whereas limited Wegener granulomatosis can manifest with isolated upper or lower airway symptoms.

Notable laboratory findings include a positive c-ANCA and anti-PR3, which is present in 85-90 percent of patients with systemic disease. Anemia, thrombocytosis, and leukocytosis are also detected frequently. The ESR usually is greater than 70 mm/hour.[34] Occasionally eosinophilia and elevated immunoglobulin E are present. c-ANCA alone is not diagnostic of Wegener granulomatosis, but when combined with two of the above American College of Rheumatology criteria, the diagnosis can be made fairly certainly. Nonetheless, tissue biopsy is required in many cases to confirm or definitively establish the diagnosis.

Chest radiograph and CT typically show cavitating or noncavitating bilateral nodules, infiltrates, and hilar and mediastinal adenopathy. Rarely a reticulonodular interstitial pattern is seen. Air space disease or ground glass opacities may reflect diffuse alveolar hemorrhage. Bronchial wall involvement can result in segmental, lobar, or total lung collapse. Tracheobronchial narrowing may be appreciated with CT.

In patients with Wegener granulomatosis, bronchoscopy may reveal stenosis, ulceration, or airway hemorrhage. In one study, bronchoalveolar lavage (BAL) of patients with the condition showed high levels of neutrophils and eosinophils,[35] and high BAL fluid levels of cytokines such as interleukin (IL)-8 and granulocyte colony-stimulating factor have been reported.[36] If diffuse alveolar hemorrhage is present, BAL may show a progressively bloody infiltrate with successive lavages.

Microscopically, there is typically distortion of the normal lung architecture. Histopathologic findings include granuloma formation by multinucleated giant cells, T cells, histiocytes, plasma cells, neutrophils, and eosinophils, geographic necrosis, and a necrotizing vasculitis of small and medium-sized vessels, with fibrinoid necrosis of the media and involvement of the vessel wall by a mixed inflammatory infiltrate.[37] To be characterized unequivocally as a vasculitis, the inflamed vessels should be located within relatively normal lung parenchymal tissue. Sterile microabscesses of neutrophils also may be observed. If alveolar hemorrhage has occurred, hemosiderin-laden macrophages may be visible.

Management is focused upon immunosuppression. For generalized Wegener granulomatosis, cyclophosphamide (1-2 mg/kg/day) and glucocorticoids (prednisone 1 mg/kg/day) are standard therapies. In the past, this management was continued for 1 year following initiation, but with the potential toxicity of cyclophosphamide, the duration frequently is shortened to 3 to 6 months, followed by maintenance therapy with a less toxic agent. Methotrexate (20-25 mg once a week) and azathioprine (1-3 mg/kg/day) have been employed in this situation. Some small studies suggest that methotrexate and glucocorticoids may be effective both initially and as maintenance therapy for non-life-threatening Wegener granulomatosis, but patients treated in this manner must be monitored closely for evidence of deterioration that would prompt a switch in therapy to cyclophosphamide.

Trimethoprim-sulfamethoxazole has been reported by some investigators to produce a favorable response in patients with indolent or progressive Wegener granulomatosis.[38] The exact mechanism is unknown, but its beneficial effect may be the result of antimicrobial or immunomodulatory effects. Surveillance for pancytopenia is essential when trimethoprim-sulfamethoxazole is used, particularly when used concomitantly with methotrexate. In general, trimethoprim-sulfamethoxazole should not be used as monotherapy, but it may be useful as an adjunctive therapy.

Behçet Disease

Behçet disease, first described in 1937 by Turkish dermatologist, Hulusi Behçet, is a syndrome characterized by oral ulcers, genital ulcers, and uveitis.[39] The disease has been reported worldwide, but the highest incidence appears to be along the ancient Silk Road extending from western China to the Mediterranean basin.[40] The disease affects males and females with similar frequency and usually develops during the second or third decade of life. Recurrent exacerbations and remissions are typical in Behçet disease. Young age of onset and male sex appear to be negative prognostic indicators.

The pathogenesis of Behçet disease is poorly understood, but some speculate that it is associated with infection by *Staphylococcus aureus*, *Prevotella*, *Chlamydia*, or hepatitis C, and human leukocyte antigen (HLA)-B51 positivity.[41-43,44] Some studies suggest that Behçet disease is caused by a T_H1-type immune response, especially during flares of the disease, whereas T_H2 cytokines predominate as the disease remits.[44]

The diagnosis of Behçet disease is made when recurrent oral ulceration is present in association with two other criteria:

- Recurrent genital ulceration
- Anterior or posterior uveitis
- Retinal vasculitis
- Skin lesions (erythema nodosum, pseudofolliculitis, or papulopustular lesions)
- A positive skin pathergy test (a 2-3 mm papule or pustule appearing 24 to 48 hours after a sterile pin prick)

Vascular lesions can develop and may include aortic and pulmonary artery aneurysms, thrombophlebitis of medium-sized vessels particularly in the lower extremities, and venous thrombosis. Pulmonary manifestations of Behçet disease include pulmonary embolism, pulmonary infarction,

cor pulmonale, organizing pneumonia, pleurisy, mediastinal and hilar lymphadenopathy, and pleural effusions.[44]

Pulmonary artery aneurysms caused by vasculitis are rare overall, but Behçet disease is the most common cause, with more than 200 cases reported in the literature[40] (FIGURE 15-1). Pulmonary artery aneurysms in Behçet disease usually affect young males and are often bilateral and multiple.[45] They carry a poor prognosis, as a 30 percent 2-year mortality has been reported.[46] Hemoptysis is the most common initial symptom, and it occurs when the aneurysm erodes and ruptures into a bronchus. They are located most frequently in the right lower lobe arteries, followed by the right and left main pulmonary arteries.[47]

The aneurysms can appear as hilar enlargement or multilobular round opacities on chest radiography, and they can appear as saccular or fusiform dilations with homogenous contrast filling simultaneously with the pulmonary artery using CT angiography.[40] Their contours may be obscured when there is active bleeding, and the aneurysms may be missed if they are occluded by thrombus.

Conventional pulmonary angiography generally should be avoided because of the risk of thrombus and aneurysm development secondary to catheter trauma or bolus injection of contrast media, as well as the danger of precipitating rupture of an existing aneurysm.[48] Conventional chest radiography is used commonly in the initial assessment. CT may be useful in Behçet disease because it can demonstrate many manifestations, including abnormalities of vessel lumen and wall, perivascular tissues, lung parenchyma, pleura, and mediastinal structures.[49] Magnetic resonance

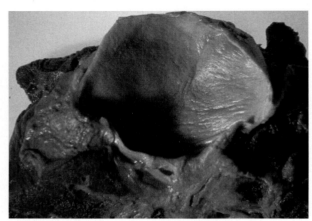

Figure 15-1. Pulmonary Arterial Aneurysm. (Courtesy of Dr. Giuseppe G. Pietra.)

angiography, which does not require radiocontrast, has also been used successfully as a diagnostic procedure.[50]

The histopathology of Behçet disease demonstrates a systemic vasculitis of small, medium, and large vessels of both arterial and venous origin. Inflammatory infiltrates may be neutrophilic, mononuclear, or mixed, and thrombus formation can occur, particularly in vessels with prominent lymphocytic infiltrates.[40] Pulmonary artery aneurysms are characterized by perivascular infiltrates surrounding the vasa vasorum, intimal thickening, degenerative changes in the elastic lamina, thrombotic occlusion, and recanalization.[40] Laboratory tests supporting the diagnosis of Behçet disease include HLA-B51 positivity and a positive prick test for *Streptococcus* antigens.

Management of Behçet disease and the associated pulmonary artery aneurysms consists primarily of immunosuppressive agents. No controlled trials comparing the efficacy of agents exist, but pulse intravenous cyclophosphamide and methylprednisolone are used most frequently.[51] Cyclosporine, azathioprine, and methotrexate have also been employed and appear to be acceptable alternatives to cyclophosphamide.[51,52]

Anticoagulation may be considered in patients with thrombus formation, but it is contraindicated in patients with hemoptysis. Aspirin and dipyridamole have been used under these circumstances.[45] Embolization of pulmonary arterial aneurysms has been undertaken to manage massive bleeding, although the risk of pulmonary infarction is high.[50] Surgical resection may be required in patients with a single pulmonary artery aneurysm who have failed medical management, although there is a risk of recurrent aneurysm development at the anastomotic site.[53]

Microscopic Polyangiitis

Microscopic polyangiitis is an ANCA-associated pauci-immune small-vessel necrotizing vasculitis, affecting capillaries, arterioles, and venules. Microscopic polyangiitis was first described as "microscopic polyarteritis" by Davson in 1948,[54] but the name was altered in 1994 at the Chapel Hill Consensus Conference on the Nomenclature of Systemic Vasculitis, because patients with this entity have involvement of many different types of vessels and some lack arteritis.[55] Microscopic polyangiitis frequently manifests as a pulmonary-renal syndrome because of the concurrent development of crescentic glomerulonephritis and hemorrhagic pulmonary capillaritis.

There is a slight male predominance, and the peak incidence is in the 55-year-old to 74-year-old age group.[56] The etiology is unclear, but associations have been hypothesized with silica and solvent exposure, or medications such as propylthiouracil, hydralazine, and penicillamine.[56] Common initial symptoms and signs include renal failure, alveolar hemorrhage, purpura, peripheral neuropathy, abdominal pain and bleeding, myalgias, and arthralgias. Pulmonary symptoms include cough, chest pain, and shortness of breath. Upper respiratory symptoms can occur, but severe destructive disease of the upper respiratory tract is more suggestive of Wegener granulomatosis. Interstitial fibrosis may develop during the chronic phase of acute hemorrhagic alveolar capillaritis. Pulmonary artery aneurysms occasionally develop.[57]

Chest radiographic findings usually consist of bilateral, patchy air space disease resulting from diffuse alveolar hemorrhage. In one retrospective study of chest CT findings among 62 patients with p-ANCA (antimyeloperoxidase) positivity (51 with microscopic polyangiitis and 11 with Churg-Strauss syndrome), 94 percent demonstrated ground glass attenuation, 78 percent showed signs of consolidation, and 51 percent displayed thickening of the bronchovascular bundles.[58]

Pulmonary function testing may demonstrate an elevated diffusing capacity of carbon monoxide because of binding to extravasated blood in the alveoli. BAL often reveals blood or hemosiderin-laden macrophages.

Microscopic polyangiitis, like Wegener granulomatosis and Churg-Strauss syndrome, is associated with circulating ANCA, found in approximately 75 percent of patients.[59] Patients most commonly are positive for p-ANCA (antimyeloperoxidase), although a significant proportion display a c-ANCA (anti-PR3) pattern.[55]

Pathologic specimens in microscopic polyangiitis demonstrate a necrotizing vasculitis with few or no immune deposits. The three key histopathologic features include segmental distribution of vascular injury, infiltration with neutrophils, and fibrinoid necrosis.[60] There should not be evidence of granulomatous inflammation, and the finding of such inflammation supports a diagnosis of Wegener granulomatosis or Churg-Strauss syndrome, rather than microscopic polyangiitis. Early in the disease during the acute phase, infiltrates contain neutrophils, often with leukocytoclasia (degranulation and fragmentation of neutrophils). Later in the disease, monocytes, macrophages, and lymphocytes predominate, with only scattered neutrophils and eosinophils observed.[55] Hemosiderin-laden macrophages may be seen in BAL fluid if there has been active alveolar hemorrhage. Thrombosis may be seen, as well. Late in the disease, sclerotic vascular lesions may develop at sites of previous vasculitis.

Management of microscopic polyangiitis is similar to that of Wegener granulomatosis, including oral cyclophosphamide (2.0-2.5 mg/kg/day) and prednisone 1 mg/kg/day oral combination therapy.[56] Due to the significant side effects of cyclophosphamide, some advocate limiting its use to only 1 year or less and switching to azathioprine or methotrexate as early as 3 months into management.[61] Adjunctive and alternative therapies such as plasma exchange, mycophenolate mofetil, intravenous immunoglobulin, B-cell and T-cell depletion, and anti-tumor necrosis factor remain under investigation.

Churg-Strauss Syndrome

Churg-Strauss syndrome is a systemic disease first described in 1951 as an "allergic angiitis and granulomatosis."[62] The syndrome consists of a systemic, small vessel necrotizing vasculitis of arteries and veins, extravascular granulomas, and eosinophilia, usually occurring in patients with a history of asthma or allergic features.[63]

Clinically, the disease consists of three phases:

1. A prodromal phase of asthma and allergic rhinitis
2. An eosinophilic phase characterized by peripheral eosinophilia and eosinophilic tissue infiltrates
3. A vasculitic phase with a life-threatening systemic vasculitis of medium and small vessels, associated with vascular and extravascular granulomatosis

The vasculitic phase emerges within approximately 9 years after the onset of asthma, and a shorter duration of asthma before the emergence of the vasculitis is associated with a poorer prognosis.[64] In one study, the mean age of Churg-Strauss syndrome at diagnosis was 48 years, and the male-to-female ratio was approximately 1:1.[65]

The typical patient has allergic rhinitis, asthma, pulmonary infiltrates, and peripheral eosinophilia; however, individual manifestations may occur in isolation, and some features of the disease exist for years before systemic vasculitis develops.[66] Pulmonary involvement with glucocorticoid-requiring asthma or eosinophilic infiltrates is almost always present. Other manifestations include peripheral neuropathies, abdominal pain, diarrhea, cardiomyopathy, purpuric rash, bowel obstruction, bowel perforation, glomerulonephritis, pleural effusions, and arthralgias.[65,67] Central nervous system vasculitis can result in stroke and epilepsy, while cardiac involvement can result in congestive heart failure. Neurologic and cardiac complications are significant causes of mortality.

In 1990, the American College of Rheumatology proposed a set of classification criteria to aid in the diagnosis of Churg-Strauss syndrome.[68] The presence of four of the following criteria reportedly yields a sensitivity of 85 percent and a specificity of 99.7 percent for the diagnosis:

- Asthma
- Eosinophilia greater than 10 percent
- Mononeuropathy or polyneuropathy
- Migratory pulmonary infiltrates
- Paranasal sinus abnormalities
- Biopsy-proven accumulation of eosinophils in an extravascular location

Previously used criteria include asthma, blood eosinophil count greater than $1,500/mm^3$, and symptoms of systemic vasculitis involving at least two extrapulmonary sites.[69]

The etiology of Churg-Strauss is unknown, but various drugs have been implicated in case reports including chlorothiazide, allopurinol, glibenclamide, phenytoin, carbamazepine, quinine, mesalamine, macrolides, and cocaine.[70,71] A Churg-Strauss-like syndrome (Wechsler syndrome) has been reported in glucocorticoid-dependent asthmatics treated with leukotriene receptor antagonists such as zafirlukast and montelukast, with concurrent reduction in glucocorticoid dosage.[72] It is believed that this complication is related to glucocorticoid withdrawal unmasking preexisting Churg-Strauss syndrome rather than a reaction to the leukotriene receptor antagonists, themselves, but a direct effect of the medications cannot be excluded entirely.

Radiographic findings are variable. Typical are transient, migratory, and patchy infiltrates in an alveolar pattern. A retrospective review of nine patients with biopsy-proven Churg-Strauss syndrome demonstrated the following findings on chest radiograph: bilateral, nonsegmental consolidation in five patients, reticulonodular opacities in three patients, bronchial wall thickening in three patients, and multiple nodules in one patient.[63] High-resolution CT findings included ground glass opacities in all nine patients, subpleural airspace consolidation in five patients, centrilobular nodules in eight patients, bronchial wall thickening in seven patients, and increased vessel caliber in five patients.[63]

Approximately 50-70 percent of patients have p-ANCA (antimyeloperoxidase) antibodies. Titers may correlate with disease activity, with high levels during remission associated with relapses.[64] BAL demonstrates an increased number of eosinophils.

The pulmonary histologic findings in Churg-Strauss syndrome typically include necrotizing vasculitis affecting both arteries and veins, and areas resembling eosinophilic pneumonia.[64] Vasculitic lesions may be granulomatous or non-granulomatous, and granulomas can measure more than 1.0 millimeter in diameter.[64]

Glucocorticoids generally are effective for Churg-Strauss syndrome management. Patients typically are treated with 1.0 mg/kg/day of oral prednisone or, in severe cases, with methylprednisolone 1.0 gram intravenously every day for 3-5 days. After symptoms improve and laboratory values such as eosinophilia and ESR normalize, glucocorticoids can be tapered, usually within 1 month. In patients with poor prognostic factors such as cardiomyopathy, central nervous system involvement, gastrointestinal tract involvement, or renal insufficiency, or in patients in whom glucocorticoid management has failed, cyclophosphamide or azathioprine may be added. Plasma exchange and intravenous immune globulin have been used in patients with fulminant disease or if conventional therapy has failed.[73]

Pulmonary Capillaritis

Pulmonary capillaritis is a histopathologic entity characterized by neutrophilic infiltration of the alveolar interstitium, occlusion of pulmonary capillaries by fibrinous thrombi, and fibrinoid necrosis of alveolar walls[2] (FIGURE 15-2). These changes result in disruption of the alveolar-capillary interface and release of plasma and formed blood elements into the alveoli. Hemosiderin-laden macrophages indicate previous destruction of extravasated red blood cells (FIGURE 15-3). Iron deposition (siderosis) in the pulmonary vasculature may be appreciated (FIGURE 15-4). Another frequent finding is leukocytoclasia, which refers to

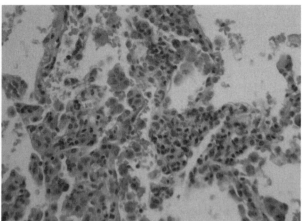

Figure 15-2. Medium-power photomicrograph showing capillaritis and hemorrhage in a patient with systemic lupus erythematosus. The inflammatory infiltrate consists primarily of neutrophils. (Hematoxylin and eosin stain.) (Courtesy of Dr. Giuseppe G. Pietra.) (See Color Plate 11).

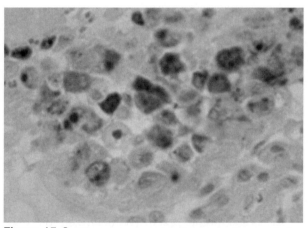

Figure 15-3. Photomicrograph showing hemosiderin-laden macrophages (staining blue due to their iron content) in a patient with Goodpasture syndrome. (Prussian blue stain.) (Courtesy of Dr. Giuseppe G. Pietra.) (See Color Plate 11).

pyknotic cells and nuclear fragments resulting from neutrophils undergoing apoptosis.[74]

Pulmonary capillaritis is seen most frequently in association with the small vessel vasculitides, particularly with the ANCA-associated vasculitides, such as Wegener granulomatosis, Churg-Strauss syndrome, and microscopic polyangiitis. It has also been reported with Behçet disease, Henoch-Schönlein purpura, isolated pauci-immune pulmonary capillaritis, and in other vasculitides.[74]

Pulmonary capillaritis can be a cause of diffuse alveolar hemorrhage (other causes are discussed

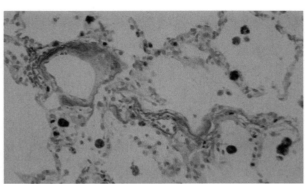

Figure 15-4. Photomicrograph showing blue areas of siderosis of a pulmonary vein and alveolar capillary in a patient with Goodpasture syndrome. (Prussian blue stain.) (Courtesy of Dr. Giuseppe G. Pietra.) (See Color Plate 11).

later). Bland pulmonary hemorrhage can occur with pulmonary capillaritis and is characterized by bleeding into the alveolar spaces without underlying inflammation.[75]

Patients with pulmonary capillaritis typically seek treatment for hemoptysis, although that complaint is not universal. Fatigue, cough, and dyspnea are other common symptoms. Chest radiography typically shows patchy alveolar infiltrates, and laboratory analysis may reveal anemia, depending upon the severity and chronicity of the capillaritis. Pulmonary function testing may reveal an increased diffusing capacity for carbon monoxide due to the increased uptake by hemoglobin in red blood cells within the alveoli.

Management of pulmonary capillaritis must be prompt to avoid life-threatening complication of hemoptysis. Typically, high-dose glucocorticoid therapy consisting of intravenous methylprednisolon 1.0 gram/day for 3 days, is given. Plasma exchange is also frequently employed, particularly if Goodpasture syndrome or an ANCA-associated vasculitis is suspected. Eventual management with oral cyclophosphamide is considered depending upon the etiology of the disease underlying the pulmonary capillaritis.

Diffuse Alveolar Hemorrhage

Diffuse alveolar hemorrhage results from the accumulation of red blood cells within the alveolar spaces. Pulmonary capillaritis, as discussed above, is one cause of diffuse alveolar hemorrhage, which can also result from coagulopathy, infections (e.g., endocarditis, human immunodeficiency virus),

mitral stenosis, neoplasms, drugs and inhaled toxins, other autoimmune diseases, and pulmonary veno-occlusive disease. Diffuse alveolar damage, the pathologic lesion associated with acute respiratory distress syndrome, can also cause diffuse alveolar hemorrhage.[75]

Diffuse alveolar hemorrhage can be life threatening. When it is suspected, the patient should be monitored closely, the respiratory status supported, and prompt evaluation and treatment initiated. Patients with diffuse alveolar hemorrhage frequently complain of dyspnea, fever, and cough. Hemoptysis may be noted, but it may be absent in up to one-third of patients.[76] Bilateral diffuse alveolar infiltrates typically are seen on chest radiograph, and this finding should always prompt consideration of the diagnosis. In cases of profound acute bleeding or chronic hemorrhage, an iron deficiency anemia may be detected. BAL often is recommended to eliminate infection as a possible cause of diffuse alveolar hemorrhage. The BAL in diffuse alveolar hemorrhage has been described as showing a progressively bloody return with successive lavages, but the sensitivity and specificity of such a finding is unclear. One study examined the frequency of hemosiderin-laden macrophages in BAL fluid of immunocompromised patients and found that the number of these cells correlated closely with the degree of hemorrhage seen in corresponding histologic specimens obtained from the same patients by open lung biopsy or during autopsy.[77]

The histopathologic findings in diffuse alveolar hemorrhage are variable and include pulmonary capillaritis, diffuse alveolar damage, and a bland hemorrhagic pattern without associated inflammation. Pulmonary capillaritis is seen with diffuse alveolar hemorrhage associated with Wegener granulomatosis, microscopic polyangiitis, lupus, polymyositis, antiphospholipid antibody syndrome, and medications. Pulmonary capillaritis and drug-induced vasculitis are discussed elsewhere in this chapter. Diffuse alveolar damage can been seen in diffuse alveolar hemorrhage due to lupus, crack cocaine inhalation, bone marrow transplantation, and radiation therapy, while bland pulmonary hemorrhage can be seen with coagulation disorders, inhaled toxins, mitral stenosis, and idiopathic pulmonary hemosiderosis.[78] Of note, transbronchial lung biopsies generally are not helpful in determining the cause of diffuse alveolar hemorrhage, because the areas of involvement are often patchy.[79] Surgical lung biopsy should be obtained if the diagnosis cannot be made by tissue biopsy in a less invasive manner from sites such as the kidney or nasal mucosa.

Finding the cause of diffuse alveolar hemorrhage and initiating prompt management can influence outcome favorably, particularly when there is renal insufficiency, because this is more likely to be irreversible than is respiratory failure.[80] A detailed medical history and physical examination should be performed, with particular focus on the causes discussed above. In addition, a complete blood count, urinalysis with microscopy, creatinine, and coagulation studies should be obtained. Serologic tests such as ANCA, antinuclear antibodies, rheumatoid factor, and antibodies to the glomerular basement membrane, phospholipids, and double stranded-deoxyribonucleic acid should be obtained.

Management must be initiated rapidly if the clinician is suspicious of an immune-mediated cause for diffuse alveolar hemorrhage and infection has been ruled out. In most causes, management involves immunosuppression, starting with high-dose glucocorticoids (1.0 gram of intravenous methylprednisolone every day for 3 days). In cases of ANCA-associated vasculitis, Goodpasture syndrome, and antiphospholipid antibody syndrome, plasma exchange should be considered, as well.[81] In many cases of diffuse alveolar hemorrhage caused by systemic autoimmune processes, cyclophosphamide is indicated as part of the initial therapy and can be given either orally or intravenously. High-dose acute management with cyclophosphamide should be undertaken with extreme care and with a high index of suspicion for nosocomial infection or hemorrhagic cystitis. Trimethoprim-sulfamethoxazole for prophylaxis of *Pneumocystis jiroveci (carinii)* pneumonia and mercaptoethane sulfonate (mesna) to reduce bladder toxicity should be considered when intravenous cyclophosphamide is employed.

Idiopathic Pulmonary Hemosiderosis

The term "idiopathic pulmonary hemosiderosis" is used to describe repeated episodes of diffuse alveolar hemorrhage with no known underlying cause. It is a condition characterized by chronic alveolar hemorrhage with consequent accumulation of hemosiderin and iron in the lung, and thickening of the alveolar basement membrane, resulting in progressive fibrosis.[82,83] Since first described as "brown lung induration" by Virchow in 1864,[84] the pathogenesis has been attributed to a defect in the pulmonary basement membrane,[85] abnormal acid mucopolysaccharide in elastic fibers of the lung,[86] milk allergy,[87] celiac disease,[88] and genetic factors.[89]

Most cases of idiopathic pulmonary hemosiderosis occur in children or adults under the age of 30. A male predominance in adults has been noted.[90] The incidence in adults is unknown, but one Swedish study suggested an annual pediatric incidence of 0.24 cases per million children.[91]

The pathogenesis of idiopathic pulmonary hemosiderosis is unclear, but there is likely a defect in either the alveolar basement membrane or the endothelial cell.[92] Given the high frequency of other autoimmune diseases in patients with idiopathic pulmonary hemosiderosis, the possibility of an immune disorder has been suggested, but immunohistochemical analysis of lung tissue has not supported such a mechanism.[90]

The clinical triad of idiopathic hemoptysis, pulmonary infiltrates, and iron deficiency anemia defines idiopathic pulmonary hemosiderosis. Symptoms often include dyspnea, cough, and fatigue. Death due to massive hemoptysis has been reported.[90]

The chest radiograph frequently shows bilateral, diffuse alveolar infiltrates, and patients with long-standing disease can show evidence of fibrosis. Chest CT usually shows diffuse alveolar opacifications, primarily in the lower lobes, and can also show ground glass areas.[93]

Laboratory studies usually reveal anemia, and fecal occult blood tests may be positive from swallowing of bloody sputum, leading to a fruitless evaluation for gastrointestinal blood loss. Pulmonary function tests may show an elevated diffusing capacity for carbon monoxide (DL_{CO}), because the hemoglobin within extravasated red blood cells within the alveoli avidly binds carbon monoxide.[90] If fibrosis has developed in advanced idiopathic pulmonary hemosiderosis, restrictive pulmonary function test results may be observed. Bronchoscopy with BAL frequently shows a grossly bloody return.

Lung biopsy classically demonstrates hemosiderosis without evidence of vasculitis, capillaritis, infection, inflammation, granulomas, or deposition of immunoglobulin in a specific pattern. A combination of acute intraalveolar hemorrhage and hemosiderin-laden macrophages are seen. The hemosiderin iron is trapped in the alveolar macrophages and stimulates them to produce ferritin, resulting in an elevated serum ferritin even in the presence of iron deficiency anemia. Alveolar walls may be thickened, and Type II pneumocytes are typically increased in number.

Treatment is usually supportive, although high-dose glucocorticoids are often prescribed. There are no large prospective controlled studies to validate their efficacy. One retrospective series of glucocorticoid therapy in 23 patients found that in those initially treated with methylprednisolone 2 mg/kg/day followed by low-dose glucocorticoids, there was one death, seven patients lost to follow-up, seven patients eventually weaned from glucocorticoids, and eight patients remaining on low-dose glucocorticoids but alive 8 years later.[94] The mean survival of patients with idiopathic pulmonary hemosiderosis has been reported to be 2.5-3.0 years,[82] suggesting but not proving some benefit to treatment. However, another more recent retrospective study of 17 children treated with immunosuppression showed a survival of 86 percent after 5 years.[95]

Recommendations include methylprednisolone at 0.5-0.75 mg/kg/day, with induction continuing until clinical improvement occurs, usually approximately 1-2 months.[93] Inhaled flunisolide has been administered successfully to maintain stable symptoms in patients initially treated with systemic steroids.[96] Azathioprine may also be effective in some patients.[97] and other agents such as hydroxychloroquine, cyclophosphamide, and methotrexate have been prescribed when glucocorticoids have proven ineffective. Lung transplantation has been performed for idiopathic pulmonary hemosiderosis, although recurrence in the allograft may occur.[98]

Eosinophilia-Myalgia Syndrome

Eosinophilia-myalgia syndrome was identified in New Mexico in 1989 when three women developed severe myalgias and peripheral blood eosinophilia. All had consumed L-tryptophan, an essential amino acid used as a supplement to treat insomnia, depression, and obesity in the 1980s. The Centers for Disease Control (CDC) soon established three criteria for eosinophilia-myalgia syndrome:

1. Peripheral eosinophil count greater than or equal to 1,000 cells/mm^3
2. Severe myalgias that limit daily activities
3. Exclusion of infectious, neoplastic, or other illnesses that may account for the first two findings

By August 1990, 1,536 cases of eosinophilia-myalgia syndrome had been identified by the CDC, and nearly all affected patients had ingested tryptophan.[99]

The pathophysiology of eosinophilia-myalgia syndrome is poorly understood. Nonspecific constitutional symptoms probably are caused by immunologic and inflammatory events during the acute phase of the disease. Serum levels of cytokines such as IL-5, interferon-γ, IL-2, and IL-4 may be elevated, especially during the acute phase and in patients with fasciitis and eosinophilia.[100]

The signs and symptoms of eosinophilia-myalgia syndrome are variable, but many patients complain of flu-like constitutional symptoms such as fever, weight loss, and fatigue. Pulmonary symptoms include nonproductive cough and dyspnea in 30-80 percent during the acute phase.[101] Of the original 1,500 cases identified by 1990, 611 (59 percent) reported cough or dyspnea.[102] Interviews of 16 patients meeting CDC criteria for eosinophilia-myalgia syndrome were performed in another study, and pulmonary symptoms appeared more prevalent: 14 (87 percent) reported dyspnea, 10 (62 percent) complained of chest tightness, 7 (44 percent) had chest pain, 7 (44 percent) reported wheezing, and 5 (31 percent) complained of a nonproductive cough.[103]

Eosinophilia-myalgia syndrome generally is characterized as having two phases: acute and chronic. The acute phase includes myalgias, fevers, rash, arthralgias, weight gain, edema, and dyspnea, while the chronic phase includes muscle cramps and pain, weakness, weight loss, fatigue, neuropathy, and scleroderma-like skin changes.

Chest radiograph findings are variable. A retrospective study reviewed the chest radiographs of 18 patients identified by state epidemiologists as meeting criteria for eosinophilia-myalgia syndrome. Of the 18 patients, 9 had normal results. Three radiographs demonstrated fine, irregular linear opacities most prominent at the bases, while three exhibited fine, irregular linear opacities and pleural effusions, and three others showed pleural effusions and confluent opacities.[104]

Common histologic abnormalities found on open lung biopsy include small to medium vessel vasculitis, with a mixed inflammatory cell infiltrate of lymphocytes and eosinophils involving both arteries and veins, as well as interstitial pneumonitis with thickening of the alveolar septae by infiltration of eosinophils and lymphocytes and alveolar exudates of histiocytes and eosinophils.[105]

Pulmonary function tests can reveal an impaired DL_{CO}. In one study of 16 patients meeting the CDC criteria for eosinophilia-myalgia syndrome, 12 (75 percent) had a decreased DL_{CO}, and the mean DL_{CO} for the entire group fell below normal (70 ± 6 percent of predicted).[103] Another study of 15 patients reported a decreased DL_{CO} in 77 percent.[106]

Pulmonary arterial hypertension can develop in patients with eosinophilia-myalgia syndrome. In five patients presented in a 1990 case series, three had clinical or histologic evidence of pulmonary arterial hypertension, although all were selected for the study because of pulmonary symptoms.[107] In a different case series, only 1 of 20 patients with eosinophilia-myalgia syndrome had evidence of pulmonary arterial hypertension.[108] The true incidence remains unknown.

Drug-Induced Vasculitis

A number of drugs have been associated with small to medium vessel vasculitis and diffuse alveolar hemorrhage. Propylthiouracil, D-penicillamine, hydralazine, sulfasalazine, minocycline, and allopurinol have been reported to cause an ANCA-associated pulmonary vasculitis.[74] Diffuse alveolar hemorrhage has been reported as a result of propylthiouracil, D-penicillamine, allopurinol, phenytoin, minocycline, leukotriene antagonists, cocaine, and all-trans-retinoic acid. Diffuse alveolar hemorrhage can develop from one of three mechanisms[80]:

- Immune or hypersensitivity reaction
- Direct injury to the alveolar capillary basement membrane
- Coagulation defect induced by the medication

The clinical picture is indistinguishable from that of diffuse alveolar hemorrhage of other causes, and the possibility of drug-induced vasculitis is often suspected only after a thorough review of the medication list. As in other cases of diffuse alveolar hemorrhage, dyspnea, cough, and fever accompanied by patchy alveolar infiltrates on chest radiograph, anemia and, progressively, blood return on BAL support the diagnosis.

Histologic findings are variable in drug-induced diffuse alveolar hemorrhage. Pulmonary capillaritis, pulmonary veno-occlusive disease, Wegener-like vasculitis, diffuse alveolar damage, and bland pulmonary hemorrhage have all been reported.[80]

Management involves removal of the suspected causative drug and immunosuppression as appropriate for ANCA-associated vasculitis as discussed earlier.[74] A notable exception is pulmonary capillaritis due to all-trans-retinoic acid, in which the drug should be discontinued if possible and high-dose intravenous glucocorticoid therapy should be added.[80] Later reintroduction of all-trans-retinoic acid may be possible when the syndrome has resolved.

Hughes-Stovin Syndrome

Hughes-Stovin syndrome, described in 1959, is a rare disease characterized by multiple pulmonary artery aneurysms and peripheral venous thrombosis.[109] The similar findings of venous thrombosis and aneurysms of the pulmonary arteries in both Hughes-Stovin syndrome and Behçet disease suggest that the two disorders are related. Right external carotid artery aneurysms,[110] bronchial artery aneurysms, and left hepatic artery aneurysms have all been reported with Hughes-Stovin syndrome.[111]

Symptoms typically include fevers, chills, hemoptysis, and cough. Hemoptysis can be massive and a terminal event when caused by rupture of a pulmonary or bronchial artery aneurysm. Hughes-Stovin syndrome is not characterized by the oral and genital ulcers, iritis, or arthralgias seen in Behçet disease. The syndrome typically affects young adult men, but there are also rare case reports of women with the syndrome.[112]

Radiographic findings include bilateral hilar enlargement on chest radiograph and aneurysms of the pulmonary artery on contrast chest CT.[113] Magnetic resonance angiography also may be useful in documenting pulmonary arterial aneurysms.[114]

Histologic findings in Hughes-Stovin syndrome are similar to those of Behçet disease and demonstrate destruction of the pulmonary arteries and perivascular inflammation.[115] Histologic samples in one study demonstrated pulmonary vasculitis involving all layers of the pulmonary arteries and veins.[46]

Hughes-Stovin syndrome is rare, so there are no controlled studies to determine effective management. Glucocorticoids and immunosuppressive therapy have been prescribed, but the effectiveness is questionable because of the fulminant and fatal course of most cases despite this management.[111]

Necrotizing Sarcoid Granulomatosis

Necrotizing sarcoid granulomatosis, described by Liebow in 1973,[116] consists of three pathologic findings: coalescent sarcoid-like granulomas, granulomatous vasculitis, and necrosis. The etiology is unknown and the relationship to classical sarcoidosis is not entirely clear. Necrotizing sarcoid granulmatosis usually affects individuals between the ages of 40 and 50.[117] There appears to be a female predominance.

Pulmonary symptoms include cough, dyspnea, and chest pain. Systemic symptoms include fever, weight loss, and weakness. Extrapulmonary involvement of the eye,[118] heart,[119] and nervous sytem[120] have been reported.

Radiographic findings frequently include multiple or single pulmonary nodules with or without hilar adenopathy.[121] One retrospective study of seven patients with necrotizing sarcoid granulomatosis and an initial complaint of pleuritic chest pain revealed pleural involvement in six and mediastinal adenopathy in five, as well as several patients with solitary pulmonary nodules, multiple pulmonary nodules, and lower lobe pulmonary infiltrates.[122]

There is no specific laboratory test used to diagnose necrotizing sarcoid granulomatosis, but an elevated ESR may be seen. Tissue biopsy typically shows coalescent sarcoid granulomas containing areas of necrosis and a prominent granulomatous vasculitis usually involving the intima, media, and adventitia of vessels. Pulmonary function tests show a restrictive pattern,[123] and a reduced diffusing capacity has been reported.[122]

Whether necrotizing sarcoid granulomatosis is a distinct clinical entity or a subset of sarcoidosis is a controversial. Biopsy in sarcoidosis generally shows less vasculitis and necrosis, with infrequent cavitation and pleural involvement.[124] Hilar lymphadenopathy and extrapulmonary manifestations are more frequent in sarcoidosis, although they have been reported in necrotizing sarcoid granulomatosis. Elevated plasma angiotensin-converting enzyme level and positive immunohistochemical staining of angiotensin-converting enzyme in tissue are associated with sarcoidosis, but not with necrotizing sarcoid granulomatosis.[124]

Necrotizing sarcoid granulomatosis is unusual in that remission without management or following glucocorticoid therapy is frequent. However, progressive disease can develop in some cases, culminating in respiratory failure and cor pulmonale.[124]

References

1. Rubin L: *Pulmonary vasculitis and pulmonary hypertension,* ed 3, Philadelphia, 2000, Saunders.
2. Sullivan EJ, Hoffman, GS: Thoracic manifestations of systemic autoimmune disease. *Clin Chest Med* 19:759-776, 1998.
3. Andrassy K, Koderisch J, Rufer M, et al: Detection and clinical implication of anti-neutrophil cytoplasm antibodies in Wegener's granulomatosis and rapidly progressive glomerulonephritis. *Clin Nephrol* 32:159-167, 1989.
4. Savige JA, Yeung SP, Gallicchio M, et al: Two ELISAs to detect anti-neutrophil cytoplasm antibodies (ANCA) in various vasculitides. *Pathology* 21: 282 287, 1989.
5. van der Woude FJ, Rasmussen N, Lobatto S, et al: Autoantibodies against neutrophils and monocytes: Tool for diagnosis and marker of disease activity in Wegener's granulomatosis. *Lancet* 1:425-429, 1985.
6. Falk RJ, Jennette JC: Anti-neutrophil cytoplasmic autoantibodies with specificity for myeloperoxidase in patients with systemic vasculitis and idiopathic necrotizing and crescentic glomerulonephritis. *N Engl J Med* 318:1651-1657, 1988.
7. Seo P, Stone JH: The antineutrophil cytoplasmic antibody-associated vasculitides. *Am J Med* 117:39-50, 2004.
8. Burns A: Pulmonary vasculitis. *Br J Hosp Med* 58:389-392, 1997.
9. Boomsma MM, Stegeman CA, van der Leij MJ, et al: Prediction of relapses in Wegener's granulomatosis by measurement of antineutrophil cytoplasmic antibody levels: A prospective study. *Arthritis Rheum* 43:2025-2033, 2000.
10. Horton BT, Magath BT, Brown GE: An undescribed form of arteritis of the temporal vessels. *Proc Staff Meet Mayo Clin* 7:700-701, 1932.
11. Hellmann DB: Temporal arteritis: A cough, tooth ache, and tongue infarction. *JAMA* 287:2996-3000, 2002.
12. Gur H, Ehrenfeld M, Izsak E: Pleural effusion as a presenting manifestation of giant cell arteritis. *Clin Rheumatol* 15:200-203, 1996.
13. Wagenaar SS, Westermann CJ, Corrin B: Giant cell arteritis limited to large elastic pulmonary arteries. *Thorax* 36:876-877, 1981.
14. Larson TS, Hall S, Hepper NG, et al: Respiratory tract symptoms as a clue to giant cell arteritis. *Ann Intern Med* 101:594-597, 1984.
15. Maksimowicz-McKinnon K, Hoffman GS: Large-vessel vasculitis. *Semin Respir Crit Care Med* 25:569-679, 2004.
16. Hunder GG, Bloch DA, Michel BA, et al: The American College of Rheumatology 1990 criteria for the classification of giant cell arteritis. *Arthritis Rheum* 33:1122-1128, 1990.
17. Karam GH, Fulmer JD: Giant cell arteritis presenting as interstitial lung disease. *Chest* 82:781-784, 1982.
18. Dennison AR, Watkins RM, Gunning AJ: Simultaneous aortic and pulmonary artery aneurysms due to giant cell arteritis. *Thorax* 40:156-157, 1985.

19. Kramer MR, Melzer E, Nesher G, et al: Pulmonary manifestations of temporal arteritis. *Eur J Respir Dis* 71:430-433, 1987.

20. Acritidis NC, Andonopoulos AP, Galanopoulou V, et al: Pulmonary function of nonsmoking patients with giant cell arteritis and/or polymyalgia rheumatica a controlled study. *Clin Rheumatol* 7:231-236, 1988.

21. Hunder GG: Takayasu's arteritis. In: Rose BD, editor: *UpToDate,* Wellesley, MA, v13.3, UpToDate.

22. Spiera RF, Mitnick HJ, Kupersmith M, et al: A prospective, double-blind, randomized, placebo controlled trial of methotrexate in the treatment of giant cell arteritis (GCA). *Clin Exp Rheumatol* 19:495-501, 2001.

23. Weatherall DJ, Ledingham JGG, Warrell DA: *Takayasu's disease,* ed 3, Oxford, 1996, Oxford University Press.

24. Cilli A, Ozdemir T, Ogus C: Takayasu's arteritis presenting with bilateral parenchymal consolidations and severe respiratory failure. *Respiration* 68:628-630, 2001.

25. Savage BJ, Gupta RK, Angle J, et al: Takayasu arteritis presenting as a pulmonary-renal syndrome. *Am J Med Sci* 325:275-281, 2003.

26. Kawai C IK, Kato M: "Pulmonary pulseless disease": Pulmonary involvement in so-called Takayasu's disease. *Chest* 73:651-657, 1978.

27. Oota K: Ein Seltener Fall von beiderseitigem Carotis-Subclaviaverschluss. *Trans Soc Path Jpn* 30:680-690, 1940.

28. Matsubara O, Yoshimura N, Tamura A, et al: Pathological features of the pulmonary artery in Takayasu arteritis. *Heart Vessels Suppl* 7:18-25, 1992.

29. Hoffman GS, Leavitt RY, Kerr GS, et al: Treatment of glucocorticoid-resistant or relapsing Takayasu arteritis with methotrexate. *Arthritis Rheum* 37:578-582, 1994.

30. Klinger H: Grenzformen der Periarteritis Nodosa. *Pathology* 42:455-480, 1931.

31. Wegener F: Uber generalisierte septische Gefa Berkrankungen. *Verh Dtsch Ges Pathol* 29:202-210, 1936.

32. Lynch JP, White E, Tazelaar H, et al: Wegener's granulomatosis: Evolving concepts in treatment. *Semin Respir Crit Care Med* 25:491-521, 2004.

33. Leavitt RY, Fauci AS, Bloch DA, et al: The American College of Rheumatology 1990 criteria for the classification of Wegener's granulomatosis. *Arthritis Rheum* 33:1101-1107, 1990.

34. Radice A, Sinico RA: Antineutrophil cytoplasmic antibodies (ANCA). *Autoimmunity* 38:93-103, 2005.

35. Hoffman GS, Sechler JM, Gallin JI, et al: Bronchoalveolar lavage analysis in Wegener's granulomatosis. A method to study disease pathogenesis. *Am Rev Respir Dis* 143:401-407, 1991.

36. Mukae H, Matsumoto N, Ashitani J, et al: Neutrophil-related cytokines and neutrophil products in bronchoalveolar lavage fluid of a patient with ANCA negative Wegener's granulomatosis. *Eur Respir J* 9:1950-1954, 1996.

37. Fraser RS, Muller NL, Colman N, et al: *Vasculitis,* Philadelphia, 1999, WB Saunders.

38. DeRemee RA, McDonald TJ, Weiland LH: Wegener's granulomatosis: Observations on treatment with antimicrobial agents. *Mayo Clin Proc* 60:27-32, 1985.

39. Behçet H: Uber rezidivierende, aphtose, durch ein Virus verursachte Geschwure am Mund, am Auge und an den Genitalien. *Dermatol Wochenschr* 105:1152-1157, 1937.

40. Erkan F, Gul A, Tasali E: Pulmonary manifestations of Behçet's disease. *Thorax* 56:572-578, 2001.

41. Hatemi G, Bahar H, Uysal S, et al: The pustular skin lesions in Behçet's syndrome are not sterile. *Ann Rheum Dis* 63:1450-1452, 2004.

42. Ayaslioglu E, Duzgun N, Erkek E, et al: Evidence of chronic *Chlamydia pneumoniae* infection in patients with Behçet's disease. *Scand J Infect Dis* 36:428-430, 2004.

43. Sonmezoglu M, Dervis E, Badur S, et al: Examination of the relationship between the hepatitis C virus and Behçet's disease. *J Dermatol* 31:442-443, 2004.

44. Kurokawa MS, Yoshikawa H, Suzuki N: Behçet's disease. *Thorax* 56:572-578, 2004.

45. Mahendran C, Singh P, Mani NB, et al: Successful treatment of pulmonary artery aneurysms secondary to possible Behçet's disease. *Respiration* 69:355-358, 2002.

46. Hamuryudan V, Yurdakul S, Moral F, et al: Pulmonary arterial aneurysms in Behçet's syndrome: A report of 24 cases. *Br J Rheumatol* 33:48-51, 1994.

47. Tunaci M, Ozkorkmaz B, Tunaci A, et al: CT findings of pulmonary artery aneurysms during treament for Behçet's disease. *AJR Am J Roentgenol* 172:729-733, 1999.

48. Aktogu S, Erer OF, Urpek G, et al: Multiple pulmonary arterial aneurysms in Behçet's disease: Clinical and radiologic remission after cyclophosphamide and corticosteroid therapy. *Respiration* 69:178-181, 2002.

49. Hiller N, Lieberman S, Chajek-Shaul T, et al: Thoracic manifestations of Behçet disease at CT. *Radiographics* 24:801-808, 2004.

50. Mouas H, Lortholary O, Lacombe P, et al: Embolization of multiple pulmonary arterial

aneurysms in Behçet's disease. *Scand J Rheumatol* 25:58-60, 1996.

51. Acican T, Gurkan OU: Azathioprine-steroid combination therapy for pulmonary arterial aneurysms in Behçet's disease. *Rheumatol Int* 20:171-174, 2001.

52. Vansteenkiste JF, Peene P, Verschakelen JA, et al: Cyclosporin treatment in rapidly progressive pulmonary thromboembolic Behçet's disease. *Thorax* 45:295-296, 1990.

53. Tuzun H, Hamuryudan V, Yildirim S, et al: Surgical therapy of pulmonary arterial aneurysms in Behçet's syndrome. *Ann Thorac Surg* 61:733-735, 1996.

54. Davson BJ, Plat R: The kidney in periarteritis nodosa. *Q J Med* 67:175-202, 1948.

55. Jennette JC, Falk RJ, Andrassy K, et al: Nomenclature of systemic vasculitides. Proposal of an international consensus conference. *Arthritis Rheum* 37:187-192, 1994.

56. Smyth L, Gaskin G, Pusey CD: Microscopic polyangiitis. *Semin Respir Crit Care Med* 25:523-533, 2004.

57. Ortiz-Santamaria V, Olive A, Holgado S, et al: Pulmonary aneurysms in microscopic polyangiitis. *Clin Rheumatol* 22:498-499, 2003.

58. Ando Y, Okada F, Matsumoto S, et al: Thoracic manifestation of myeloperoxidase-antineutrophil cytoplasmic antibody (MPO-ANCA)-related disease: CT findings in 51 patients. *J Comput Assist Tomogr* 28:710-716, 2004.

59. Guillevin L, Durand-Gasselin B, Cevallos R, et al: Microscopic polyangiitis: Clinical and laboratory findings in eighty-five patients. *Arthritis Rheum* 42:421-430, 1999.

60. Eschun GM, Mink SN, Sharma S: Pulmonary interstitial fibrosis as a presenting manifestation in perinuclear antineutrophilic cytoplasmic antibody microscopic polyangiitis. *Chest* 123:297-301, 2003.

61. Jayne D, Rasmussen N, Andrassy K, et al: A randomized trial of maintenance therapy for vasculitis associated with antineutrophil cytoplasmic autoantibodies. *N Engl J Med* 349:36-44, 2003.

62. Churg J, Strauss L: Allergic granulomatosis, allergic angiitis, and periarteritis nodosa. *Am J Pathol* 27:277-301, 1951.

63. Choi YH, Im JG, Han BK, et al: Thoracic manifestation of Churg-Strauss syndrome: Radiologic and clinical findings. *Chest* 117:117-124, 2000.

64. Guillevin L, Pagnoux C, Mouthon L: Churg-Strauss Syndrome. *Semin Respir Crit Care Med* 25:535-545, 2005.

65. Guillevin L, Cohen P, Gayraud M, et al: Churg-Strauss syndrome. Clinical study and long-term follow-up of 96 patients. *Medicine (Baltimore)* 78:26-37, 1999.

66. King TE, Jr: Churg-Strauss syndrome (allergic granulomatosis and angiitis). In: Rose BD, editor: *UpToDate*, Wellesley, MA, v13.3, 2006, UpToDate.

67. Boccagni C, Tesser F, Mittino D, et al: Churg-Strauss syndrome associated with the leukotriene antagonist montelukast. *Neurol Sci* 25:21-22, 2004.

68. Masi AT, Hunder GG, Lie JT, et al: The American College of Rheumatology 1990 criteria for the classification of Churg-Strauss syndrome (allergic granulomatosis and angiitis). *Arthritis Rheum* 33:1094-1100, 1990.

69. Lanham JG, Elkon KB, Pusey CD, et al: Systemic vasculitis with asthma and eosinophilia: A clinical approach to the Churg-Strauss syndrome. *Medicine (Baltimore)* 63:65-81, 1984.

70. Martin RM, Wilton LV, Mann RD: Prevalence of Churg-Strauss syndrome, vasculitis, eosinophilia and associated conditions: Retrospective analysis of 58 prescription-event monitoring cohort studies. *Pharmacoepidemiol Drug Saf* 8:179-189, 1999.

71. Orriols R, Munoz X, Ferrer J, et al: Cocaine-induced Churg-Strauss vasculitis. *Eur Respir J* 9:175-177, 1996.

72. Wechsler ME, Garpestad E, Flier SR, et al: Pulmonary infiltrates, eosinophilia, and cardiomyopathy following corticosteroid withdrawal in patients with asthma receiving zafirlukast. *JAMA* 279:455-457, 1998.

73. Jayne DR, Lockwood CM: Intravenous immunoglobulin as sole therapy for systemic vasculitis. *Br J Rheumatol* 35:1150-1153, 1996.

74. Lee AS, Specks U: Pulmonary capillaritis. *Semin Respir Crit Care Med* 25:547-555, 2004.

75. Schwarz MI: The diffuse alveolar hemorrhage syndromes. In: Rose BD, editor: *UpToDate*, Wellesley, MA, v13.3, 2006, UpToDate.

76. Zamora MR, Warner ML, Tuder R, et al: Diffuse alveolar hemorrhage and systemic lupus erythematosus. Clinical presentation, histology, survival, and outcome. *Medicine (Baltimore)* 76:192-202, 1997.

77. Kahn FW, Jones JM, England DM: Diagnosis of pulmonary hemorrhage in the immunocompromised host. *Am Rev Respir Dis* 136:155-160, 1987.

78. Specks U: Diffuse alveolar hemorrhage syndromes. *Curr Opin Rheumatol* 13:12-17, 2001.

79. Schnabel A, Holl-Ulrich K, Dalhoff K, et al: Efficacy of transbronchial biopsy in pulmonary vasculitides. *Eur Respir J* 10:2738-2743, 1997.

80. Schwarz MI, Fontenot AP: Drug-induced diffuse alveolar hemorrhage syndromes and vasculitis. *Clin Chest Med* 25:133-140, 2004.

81. Klemmer PJ, Chalermskulrat W, Reif MS, et al: Plasmapheresis therapy for diffuse alveolar hemor-

rhage in patients with small-vessel vasculitis. *Am J Kidney Dis* 42:1149-1153, 2003.

82. Soergel KH, Sommers SC: Idiopathic pulmonary hemosiderosis and related syndromes. *Am J Med* 32:499-507, 1962.

83. Cohen S: Idiopathic pulmonary hemosiderosis. *Am J Med Sci* 317:67-74, 1999.

84. Virchow R: *Die Krankhaften Geschwulste,* Berlin, 1864, August Hirschwald.

85. Ceelen W: Die Krieslau Ferstrongen der Lung. In: *Handbuch der speziellen Pathologischen and Anatokie und Histologie,* Berlin, 1931, Springer Verlag, pp 1-163.

86. Probst A: Morphologie und Pathogenes der esentieller Lungenhamosiderose. *Virchows Arch* 326:633, 1955.

87. Heiner DC, Sears JW, Kniker WT: Multiple precipitins to cow's milk in chronic respiratory disease. A syndrome including poor growth, gastrointestinal symptoms, evidence of allergy, iron deficiency anemia, and pulmonary hemosiderosis. *Am J Dis Child* 103:634-654, 1962.

88. Wright PH, Menzies IS, Pounder RE, et al: Adult idiopathic pulmonary haemosiderosis and coeliac disease. *Q J Med* 50:95-102, 1981.

89. Beckerman RC, Taussig LM, Pinnas JL: Familial idiopathic pulmonary hemosiderosis. *Am J Dis Child* 133:609-611, 1979.

90. Milman N, Pedersen FM: Idiopathic pulmonary haemosiderosis. Epidemiology, pathogenic aspects and diagnosis. *Respir Med* 92:902-907, 1998.

91. Kjellman B, Elinder G, Garwicz S, et al: Idiopathic pulmonary haemosiderosis in Swedish children. *Acta Paediatr Scand* 73:584-588, 1984.

92. Corrin B, Jagusch M, Dewar A, et al: Fine structural changes in idiopathic pulmonary haemosiderosis. *J Pathol* 153:249-256, 1987.

93. Milman NP: Idiopathic pulmonary hemosiderosis. In: Rose BD, ed. *UpToDate,* Wellesley, MA, v13.3, 2006, UpToDate.

94. Kiper N, Gocmen A, Ozcelik U, et al: Long-term clinical course of patients with idiopathic pulmonary hemosiderosis (1979-1994): Prolonged survival with low-dose corticosteroid therapy. *Pediatr Pulmonol* 27:180-184, 1999.

95. Saeed MM, Woo MS, MacLaughlin EF, et al: Prognosis in pediatric idiopathic pulmonary hemosiderosis. *Chest* 116:721-725, 1999.

96. Tutor JD, Eid NS: Treatment of idiopathic pulmonary hemosiderosis with inhaled flunisolide. *South Med J* 88:984-986, 1995.

97. Rossi GA, Balzano E, Battistini E, et al: Long-term prednisone and azathioprine treatment of a patient with idiopathic pulmonary hemosiderosis. *Pediatr Pulmonol* 13:176-180, 1992.

98. Wroblewski BM, Stefanovic CR, McDonough VM, et al: The challenges of idiopathic pulmonary hemosiderosis and lung transplantation. *Crit Care Nurse* 17:39-44, 1997.

99. Update: Eosinophilia-myalgia syndrome associated with ingestion of L-tryptophan—United States, through August 24, 1990. *MMWR Morb Mortal Wkly Rep* 39:587-589, 1990.

100. Silver R: Pathophysiology of the eosinophilia-myalgia syndrome. *J Rheumatol Suppl* 46:26-36, 1993.

101. Kaufman LD, Philen RM: Tryptophan. Current status and future trends for oral administration. *Drug Saf* 8:89-98, 1993.

102. Swygert LA, Maes EF, Sewell LE, et al: Eosinophilia-myalgia syndrome. Results of national surveillance. *JAMA* 264:1698-1703, 1990.

103. Read CA, Clauw D, Weir C, et al: Dyspnea and pulmonary function in the L-tryptophan-associated eosinophilia-myalgia syndrome. *Chest* 101: 1282-1286, 1992.

104. Williamson MR, Eidson M, Rosenberg RD, et al: Eosinophilia-myalgia syndrome: Findings on chest radiographs in 18 patients. *Radiology* 180: 849-852, 1991.

105. Strumpf IJ, Drucker RD, Anders KH, et al: Acute eosinophilic pulmonary disease associated with the ingestion of L-tryptophan-containing products. *Chest* 99:8-13, 1991.

106. Varga J, Heiman-Patterson TD, Emery DL, et al: Clinical spectrum of the systemic manifestations of the eosinophilia-myalgia syndrome. *Semin Arthritis Rheum* 19:313-328, 1990.

107. Tazelaar HD, Myers JL, Drage CW, et al: Pulmonary disease associated with L-tryptophan-induced eosinophilic myalgia syndrome. Clinical and pathologic features. *Chest* 97:1032-1036, 1990.

108. Martin RW, Duffy J, Engel AG, et al: The clinical spectrum of the eosinophilia-myalgia syndrome associated with L-tryptophan ingestion. Clinical features in 20 patients and aspects of pathophysiology. *Ann Intern Med* 113:124-134, 1990.

109. Hughes J, Stovïn PGJ: Segmental pulmonary artery aneurysm with peripheral venous thrombosis. *Br J Dis Chest* 53:19-27, 1959.

110. Kirk GM, Seal RM: False aneurysm of the pulmonary artery with peripheral venous thrombosis. *Thorax* 19:449-453, 1964.

111. Herb S, Hetzel M, Hetzel J, et al: An unusual case of Hughes-Stovin syndrome. *Eur Respir J* 11:1191-1193, 1998.

112. Kindermann M, Wilkens H, Hartmann W, et al: Images in cardiovascular medicine. Hughes-Stovin syndrome. *Circulation* 108:e156, 2003.

113. Ali-Munive A, Varon H, Maldonado D, et al: [Giant aneurysms of the pulmonary artery and peripheral

venous thrombosis (Hughes-Stovin syndrome): Regression with immunosuppressant therapy.] *Arch Bronconeumol* 37:508-510, 2001.

114. Balci NC, Semelka RC, Noone TC, et al: Multiple pulmonary aneurysms secondary to Hughes-Stovin syndrome: Demonstration by MR angiography. *J Magn Reson Imaging* 8:1323-1325, 1998.

115. Durieux P, Bletry O, Huchon G, et al: Multiple pulmonary arterial aneurysms in Behçet's disease and Hughes-Stovin syndrome. *Am J Med* 71:736-741, 1981.

116. Liebow AA: The J. Burns Amberson lecture—pulmonary angiitis and granulomatosis. *Am Rev Respir Dis* 108:1-18, 1973.

117. Le Gall F, Loeuillet L, Delaval P, et al: Necrotizing sarcoid granulomatosis with and without extrapulmonary involvement. *Pathol Res Pract* 192:306-313; discussion 314, 1996.

118. Bouman KP, Slabbynck H, Cuykens JJ, et al: Necrotizing sarcoid granulomatosis with uveitis: A variant of sarcoidosis? *Acta Clin Belg* 52:367-370, 1997.

119. Gibbs AR, Williams WJ, Kelland D: Necrotising sarcoidal granulomatosis: A problem of identity. A study of seven cases. *Sarcoidosis* 4:94-100, 1987.

120. Strickland-Marmol LB, Fessler RG, Rojiani AM: Necrotizing sarcoid granulomatosis mimicking an intracranial neoplasm: Clinicopathologic features and review of the literature. *Mod Pathol* 13:909-913, 2000.

121. Niimi H, Hartman TE, Muller NL: Necrotizing sarcoid granulomatosis: Computed tomography and pathologic findings. *J Comput Assist Tomogr* 19:920-923, 1995.

122. Chittock DR, Joseph MG, Paterson NA, et al: Necrotizing sarcoid granulomatosis with pleural involvement. Clinical and radiographic features. *Chest* 106:672-676, 1994.

123. Tauber E, Wojnarowski C, Horcher E, et al: Necrotizing sarcoid granulomatosis in a 14-yr-old female. *Eur Respir J* 13:703-705, 1999.

124. Heinrich D, Gordjani N, Trusen A, et al: Necrotizing sarcoid granulomatosis: A rarity in childhood. *Pediatr Pulmonol* 35:407-411, 2003.

Management of the Acutely Ill Patient with Pulmonary Arterial Hypertension

Maren E. Jeffery, MD,

Darren B. Taichman, MD, PhD

Introduction

Patients with pulmonary arterial hypertension (PAH) can require admission to the intensive care unit (ICU) in a number of situations involving either acute hemodynamic instability or respiratory failure (TABLE 16-1). A late diagnosis or acute recognition of advanced PAH and associated cor pulmonale is, unfortunately, a common cause of ICU admission for patients with severe PAH. As an example, such patients may seek medical attention following a syncopal episode with hypotension, or with other manifestations of shock and end-organ dysfunction. In addition, previously diagnosed patients can suffer complications of PAH-directed therapies, including the interruption of continuously infused vasodilator therapy resulting in sudden hemodynamic collapse. Intolerance of recently instituted therapies such as calcium channel antagonists can precipitate hypotension. Dietary or medical noncompliance can lead to fluid retention and decompensated cor pulmonale. Additionally, severe sepsis is a persistent threat in patients requiring indwelling catheters for continuously infused therapies. In each case, acute illness can convert what was a tenuous but nonetheless compensated state of cor pulmonale into a hemodynamically unstable emergency.

This chapter discusses issues to consider when caring for patients with PAH in the ICU. It is important to emphasize that little is known regarding appropriate pharmacologic interventions for acute hypotension or hypoxemia in patients whose predominant underlying medical issue is severe PAH. Prospective and controlled studies are lacking in this population, and care often must be based on information extrapolated from other populations or settings. Data from clinical trials assessing the acute hemodynamic response to various vasodilators, for example, might not reflect the response of an acutely ill patient. Vasodilator trials in published series typically have been performed on an elective basis. Although the participants often are chronically ill, they are nonetheless hemodynamically stable at the initiation of the trial. Similarly, studies assessing the effect of pharmacologic agents on patients suffering acute right-sided heart failure after cardiac surgery might not be fully applicable to patients with chronic pulmonary vascular derangements. Therefore, although useful (and often all that are available), the results of such studies must be interpreted with caution when applied to the acutely ill patient with underlying severe PAH.

Pathophysiologic Considerations— A Vicious Cycle

Patients with severe PAH requiring acute management in an ICU typically suffer from a combination of hypoxemia and systemic hypotension. In such patients, hemodynamic instability often ensues from acute decompensation of an already stressed right ventricle (RV). For this reason, the ability to recognize and understand the pathophysiology of right-sided heart failure is crucial for critical care physicians.

The importance of the RV often is underestimated in clinical practice. This is, perhaps, in part because of the prevalence of ischemic and hyper-

TABLE 16-1

Causes of Acute Hemodynamic Instability in Patients with PAH

Acute Recognition or Late Symptom Onset

Syncope
Shock
Renal failure
Ascites

Acute Medication Failure

Medical noncompliance, interrupted infusions
Intolerance (calcium channel antagonist)

Dietary Indiscretion or Fluid Retention

Increased Metabolic Demands

Infection (e.g., sepsis in patients with central venous catheters for continuously infused therapy)
Fever
Environmental heat

Venous Thromboembolism

Medical and Surgical Procedures, Anesthesia

Pregnancy

PAH, *pulmonary arterial hypertension.*

tensive heart disease, which manifest primarily as left-sided heart dysfunction. Additionally, the RV has been viewed traditionally as a passive conduit between the systemic veins and the pulmonary arteries. This view was based largely on the observation in animal experiments that little hemodynamic compromise followed extensive destruction of the RV free wall,[1] as well as the success of the Fontan procedure (used for management of tricuspid atresia) in which a caval-to-pulmonary artery anastomosis is created and the RV bypassed completely. Both of these observations, however, are predicated on the assumption that RV afterload is normal, which of course is not the case in patients with severe pulmonary hypertension. Subsequent *in vitro* studies in animals[2] and *in vivo* studies in humans[3] have countered the idea of a passive RV, demonstrating that the RV does follow the classic model of left ventricular performance as defined by the end-systolic pressure-volume relation.

Several characteristics of the RV predispose it to dysfunction or failure in patients with severe pulmonary hypertension. Compared with the left ventricle (LV), the normal RV is a smaller, relatively thin-walled, irregularly shaped structure. Despite this, the RV generates an output identical to that of the systemic LV, a feat it is able to accomplish in large part because it ejects into the low-pressure pulmonary circuit with a vascular resistance approximately one-tenth that of the systemic vascular resistance (SVR).[4]

As with the LV, changes in RV output are governed by the Frank-Starling relationship such that RV stroke volume is directly proportional to RV end-diastolic volume, and inversely proportional to an afterload determined by the status of the pulmonic valve and the pulmonary vasculature. Under most circumstances, RV afterload is proportionate to the pulmonary vascular resistance (PVR) or the pulmonary arterial pressure[5] (FIGURE 16-1). The RV, because of its thin walls, is a highly compliant and distensible structure. In response to increased demand, it can increase in size substantially without significant changes in intracavitary filling pressures, and thereby increase its stroke volume. Unlike the LV, however, the RV has relatively poor muscular reserve. Thus, even small increases in right-sided afterload can result in a dramatic decrease in RV output. For example, in response to even mild pulmonary hypertension, the increased RV afterload often is associated with a decrease in the RV ejection fraction. The RV dilates slightly and eventually hypertrophies in response, thereby maintaining its stroke volume, even though the ejection fraction is decreased.[4]

The degree to which PAH impacts RV function depends on its severity and speed of onset. In patients with severe PAH, or in whom the RV

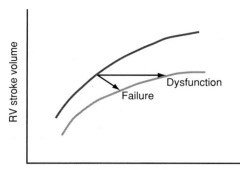

Figure 16-1. Relationship Between Right Ventricular (RV) End-Diastolic Volume and Stroke Volume in RV Dysfunction and RV Failure. In RV dysfunction, the ventricular size increases but stroke volume is maintained so that only the ejection fraction falls. In RV failure both the ejection fraction and stroke volume fall. (Adapted with permission from Vincent JL: Pharmacological management of the pulmonary circulation in critically ill patients. In: Peacock AJ, Rubin LJ, editors: *Pulmonary circulation: Diseases and their treatment,* London, 2004, Arnold, pp 532-537.)

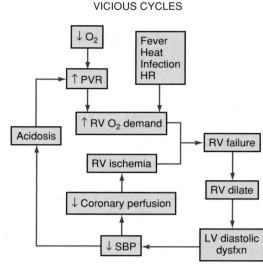

Figure 16-2. Interacting Effects of Hypoxia, Systemic Hypotension, and Metabolic Demands Leading to Further Impairment of Right Ventricular Function. These effects are encountered frequently in the acutely critically ill patient with significant pulmonary hypertension, to result in acute hemodynamic or respiratory compromise, or both.

contractility is reduced by other contributing factors (e.g., sepsis, ischemia, or infarction), the compensatory mechanisms described above may fail, leading to a fall in RV output and, hence, LV output.[5]

Another important characteristic of the RV is that it is perfused throughout the cardiac cycle. Perfusion pressure is equivalent to aortic pressure minus the RV intracavitary pressure. This is important in patients with severe PAH, because their RV intracavitary pressures are already significantly elevated from increased afterload. Systemic hypotension, as can occur with critical illness, further decreases the RV perfusion gradient, making the RV particularly susceptible to ischemia.[4]

A final physiologic characteristic of the RV that can have significant hemodynamic consequences in patients with PAH in the ICU is ventricular interdependence: that proper functioning or malfunctioning of each ventricle affects the other. Maintenance of RV function is important to ensure proper LV function, because the RV delivers the preload necessary for systemic cardiac output. As outlined above, the RV responds to increased cardiac demand and elevated PVR by dilating, which serves to minimize a decrease in stroke volume. The pericardium sets the limits for such dilation. Intrapericardial pressure increases as the RV dilates further, thereby decreasing LV distensibility. Likewise, RV dilation causes a leftward shift of the interventricular septum, which further impinges upon LV filling. This leads to a decrease in systemic cardiac output and, in some cases, systemic

hypotension that can impair the RV perfusion pressure. When RV afterload is fixed, the right ventricular end-diastolic pressure also rises, increasing the oxygen demand of an already stressed heart and further compromising the RV perfusion pressure. Together, these dangers can lead to RV ischemia and a decrease in RV contractility, thus creating a cyclic decline in LV filling and cardiac output.[4]

Further compounding this problem is that many patients with PAH arrive in the ICU with worsening hypoxia. Such hypoxia can cause acute pulmonary vasoconstriction with a resultant increase in PVR, once again increasing the work and oxygen demand of an already stressed right heart. Additional causes of increased oxygen consumption in the ICU can include hyperthermia, infection, hyperthyroidism, and tachycardia of any cause. Acidemia resulting from systemic hypotension and hypoperfusion of multiple organs can augment the vasoconstrictive response to hypoxia, thus completing the vicious cycle of hypoxemia and hemodynamic failure (FIGURE 16-2).

Diagnosis of Right Ventricular Failure in the Intensive Care Unit

For patients with underlying severe pulmonary hypertension, physicians in the ICU should maintain a high index of suspicion that shock may represent a new, potentially minor insult to an already compromised right heart that may lead to acute right-sided heart failure. Clinical clues to right-sided heart dysfunction include elevated internal jugular venous pulsations, a pulsatile liver, peripheral edema out of proportion to pulmonary edema, a right-sided third heart sound, or a tricuspid regurgitation murmur. However, in a patient with systemic hypotension or hypoxia requiring mechanical ventilation, physical examination alone may be of limited utility, and other modalities for assessment of RV function are often required.

Chest radiographs showing enlarged pulmonary arteries or RV are suggestive of significant pulmonary hypertension, but are not diagnostic of right-sided heart failure. The electrocardiogram can provide evidence of pulmonary hypertension and right heart strain, including right axis deviation, right atrial enlargement, right ventricular hypertrophy, right bundle branch block, and the $S_1Q_3T_3$ pattern. None of these, however, is a sensitive or specific marker of pulmonary hypertension or right heart dysfunction.[6]

Two-dimensional echocardiography and right heart catheterization are invaluable tools for diagnosis and management of right-sided heart failure. Right heart catheterization can give direct measurements of the right atrial, right ventricular, pulmonary artery, and pulmonary capillary wedge pressures, as well as facilitate calculation of the SVR, PVR, and cardiac output and index. These values can be helpful in determining a patient's intravascular volume status, as well as ascertaining the etiology of hypotension and monitoring the response to therapy. Likewise, the right ventricular stroke volume and ejection fraction can be monitored using the thermodilution technique with reasonable accuracy and reproducibility. This is performed by injecting a bolus of cold saline into the right atrium, while the temperature in the pulmonary artery is recorded by a rapidly responding thermistor mounted in the catheter.[7-9] Rising pulmonary artery and RV end-diastolic pressures with concomitant fall in RV stroke volume and cardiac output signifies progressive right-sided heart failure with hemodynamic compromise. When significant tricuspid regurgitation complicates severe pulmonary hypertension, however, the thermodilution technique can be misleading in the estimation of RV stroke volume. In this situation, the Fick method may provide a more accurate assessment of cardiac output, although its accuracy may be limited if oxygen consumption is not measured directly. Oxygen consumption in critical illness may be quite different from values reported on nomograms derived under stable, resting conditions. Given these potential inaccuracies in both the thermodilution and Fick methods, it is important to interpret results with caution, with emphasis more on trends in response to therapeutic interventions rather than on absolute values of cardiac output.

Echocardiography can provide complementary information in the assessment of right heart function. Studies evaluating echocardiographic findings of acute-on-chronic right-sided heart failure are limited; however, several investigations have demonstrated relevant findings of acute cor pulmonale in patients with massive pulmonary embolism or acute respiratory distress syndrome (ARDS).[9-13] These include septal dyskinesia (indicating systolic pressure overload), as well as RV hypertrophy and enlargement (characterizing diastolic pressure and volume overload). RV hypertrophy is characteristically seen with chronic but not acute elevations in pulmonary arterial pressures. This can be helpful in evaluating the chronicity of pulmonary hypertension and the likely cause of acute deterioration when little patient history is known. Ventricular dilation and hypokinesis can occur with either acute or chronic elevations in pulmonary pressures.

Echocardiographic changes seen in right-sided heart failure underscore the normal interdependence of the ventricles. In the normal patient, the left and right ventricles begin and end contraction at approximately the same time. However, with increased RV afterload, the right ventricular systole is prolonged, so that the RV continues to contract after LV systole has ended. At this time, the pressure in the RV cavity may exceed that of the LV, and reversal of the trans-septal pressure gradient causes leftward displacement of the septal wall best seen in the parasternal short-axis view (FIGURE 16-3).[10] RV pressure overload may also manifest as RV hypertrophy on echocardiography, although it is difficult to extrapolate information regarding RV function from the observation of RV hypertrophy alone.

Echocardiography can also demonstrate RV enlargement. Because the pulmonary and systemic cardiac outputs are equal (assuming no intracardiac shunt is present), a normal RV has an end-diastolic volume similar to that of the LV. Although LV volume can be assessed relatively easily by echocardiography (normal LV volume is approximately 70 cm^3), the RV volume cannot because of its irregular shape. However, determination of RV volume is not as important as the accurate diagnosis of RV dilation. Right ventricular diastolic

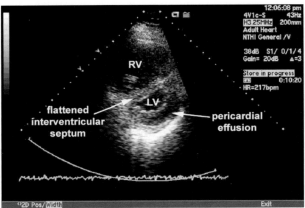

Figure 16-3. Echocardiographic findings of right-sided heart failure frequently seen in those with pulmonary hypertension. Short-axis echocardiographic view of the right (RV) and left (LV) ventricles in a 57-year-old man with pulmonary arterial hypertension (PAH). Note the flattening of the interventricular septum which forms a "D-shaped" configuration with the LV, indicative of RV pressure overload. Also noted is a pericardial effusion, a poor prognostic sign in patients with PAH. (Courtesy of Richard L. Weiss, MD.)

dimensions can be obtained by measuring RV end-diastolic area in the long-axis from an apical four-chamber view, or by a transesophageal approach. Vieillard-Baron and colleagues suggest that because pericardial constraint necessarily results in LV restriction when the RV dilates acutely, the best way to quantify RV dilation is to measure the ratio between the RV and LV end-diastolic areas. Normal values in 50 healthy volunteers are 0.48 ± 0.12,[12] with moderate RV dilation defined as a diastolic ventricular ratio greater than 0.6, and severe RV dilation as a ratio greater than 1.0 in patients with acute cor pulmonale.[14] There are limitations, however, in the application of this principle, because RV cavity enlargement may also be observed in more than 50 percent of patients with RV infarction (although the presence of LV posterior or inferior free wall abnormalities in a heart with RV infarction often helps to distinguish this from cor pulmonale). Likewise, chronic LV dilation, as seen with valvular disease or dilated cardiomyopathies, can invalidate this ratio.[10]

Echocardiographic findings frequently associated with right ventricular enlargement include right atrial enlargement, inferior vena caval dilation, and tricuspid regurgitation. Measurement of the maximal velocity of regurgitant flow through the tricuspid valve allows an estimation of the pulmonary arterial pressure.[10]

Demonstration of cor pulmonale by echocardiography should prompt the physician to investigate and manage the precipitating causes of worsening RV function. These principles of management are discussed further in the following section. Unfortunately, the role of echocardiography in monitoring improvement in RV function in patients with chronic pulmonary hypertension is not well defined. Studies of patients with acute cor pulmonale secondary to massive pulmonary embolism suggest that in most patients, both septal dyskinesia and the ratio of RV-to-LV end-diastolic areas are improved significantly within 10-15 days of management for pulmonary embolism (regardless of whether patients received heparin or thrombolytics).[12] Whether these variables can or should be followed similarly in patients with chronic PAH to determine the success of efforts to improve acutely worsened RV function is not clear, because data regarding the role of serial echocardiography in this situation are lacking.

Management of Hypotension

The factors governing RV stroke volume are identical to those for the LV: preload, myocardial contractility, and afterload. Treatment of the hemodynamically unstable patient with underlying severe PAH should therefore be targeted at one or more of these aspects. Management of hypoxia and systemic hypotension are likewise important, because they can contribute to RV ischemia.

Preload

As in most situations, systemic hypotension is appropriately first approached with the administration of intravenous fluids. Indeed, patients with cor pulmonale can require higher than normal right atrial ("filling") pressures to maintain cardiac output. It must be recognized, however, that in many acutely hypotensive patients with severe PAH there has already been an increase over chronic right ventricular dilation. RV distention may be the cause of hypotension (as described above), and fluid removal may therefore be required for improvement. As such, the aggressive administration of additional fluid may not be helpful and may actually worsen cardiac function. Thus, although an initial fluid challenge is reasonable in the hypotensive patient, it must be performed with caution. In the absence of apparent benefit, it is often appropriate to discontinue fluid administration and use vasoactive drugs for hemodynamic support earlier than in other hypotensive patients. With such hemodynamic support, diuresis (if required) might be accomplished to reestablish more favorable ventricular filling pressures.

Contractility

When evidence of severe RV failure exists, intravenous inotropic agents may be employed in an attempt to increase RV contractility. Although no agent has been clearly established as superior in studies of hemodynamically unstable patients with PAH, dobutamine often is used initially for its inotropic effects. In addition, some investigations have noted a reduction in PVR with dobutamine. Bradford and others, for example, demonstrated that in anesthetized, mechanically ventilated rabbits with pulmonary hypertension induced by U46619 (a thromboxane analog), dobutamine produced dosage-dependent decreases in PVR and mean arterial pressure, as well as increases in cardiac output.[15] This finding was corroborated in a study of 66 patients undergoing cardiac transplant evaluation.[16] Dobutamine use, however, frequently is limited by systemic hypotension caused by peripheral vasodilation.

Phosphodiesterase inhibitors such as milrinone have also been used successfully in this population, although milrinone has similar limitations in that it, too, can cause peripheral vasodilation and hypotension. Its longer half-life may be problematic for titrating therapy in highly unstable patients. In a similar study on rabbits with U46619-induced pulmonary hypertension, an infusion of milrinone decreased PAP, PVR, mean arterial pressure, and SVR while increasing CO in a dosage-dependent fashion.[17] Similar improvements in PVR, pulmonary blood flow, and RV contractility were seen in dogs with monocrotaline pyrrole-induced PAH.[18,19] Milrinone likewise produces beneficial inotropic and peripheral vasodilator effects and can reduce PVR in patients with heart failure and severe pulmonary hypertension.[20,21]

Systemic Hypotension

As with the inotropic agents above, no pressor agent is clearly superior for managing hypotension in these patients. The ideal drug, of course, would be one that increases systolic blood pressure (and thereby RV perfusion pressure) without increasing PVR. Norepinephrine frequently is viewed as the pressor of choice, with both inotropic and peripheral vasoconstricting effects. Although the reported effects on PVR have varied,[22-24] norepinephrine does not appear to induce significant increases in pulmonary arterial pressures. Dopamine[25] or isoproterenol[22] can also be considered for systemic hypotension management, watching closely for problematic tachycardia with either agent or hypotension with isoproterenol due to its β-2 (vasodilatory) effects. In rare cases of severe LV dysfunction with cardiogenic shock, LV assist devices may be employed to improve cardiac output and RV perfusion.[26]

Afterload Reduction

Pulmonary vasodilation is required frequently to improve RV function and reverse shock. Several agents can effectively reduce PVR. These include nitrates,[27-29] hydralazine,[30] and nitroprusside[30,31] administered intravenously, as well as calcium channel antagonists given orally.[32-36] All of these agents can decrease PVR and result in improvement in cardiac output and oxygenation. Adenosine also has been used to induce pulmonary vasodilation and improve hemodynamics in a study of 10 patients with PAH after cardiac surgery.[37] Intravenous epoprostenol (prostacyclin, PGI_2, Flolan) can likewise be used to reduce PVR.[38-41] Although metabolism within the pulmonary vasculature limits the effect of these agents on the systemic circulation, they nonetheless can cause peripheral vasodilation and hypotension. Furthermore, nonspecific pulmonary vasodilation caused by these agents when given systemically can result in worsened ventilation-perfusion mismatch by preventing hypoxic vasoconstriction from occurring as it should in poorly ventilated areas. This can occur, for example, with their use in patients with significant atelectasis or pneumonia and cause worsened hypoxemia. For these reasons, the use of inhaled pulmonary vasodilators is often preferable in the acute setting.

The relative safety of inhaled vasodilator therapy in patients with severe PAH has been demonstrated in several situations.[31,42,46] In one study of eight patients with severe idiopathic PAH, both intravenous prostacyclin and inhaled nitric oxide brought about significant reductions in PVR (from an approximate mean of 15 to 10 Wood units) (FIGURE 16-4). In contrast, whereas inhaled nitric oxide had no significant effect on SVR, there was a

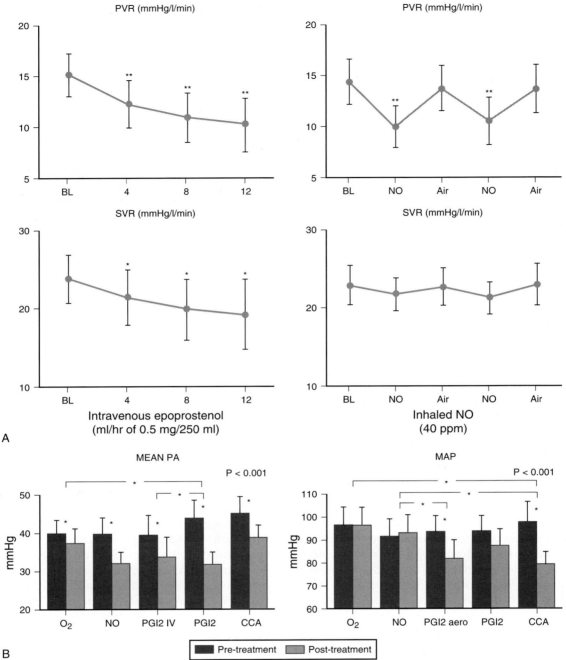

Figure 16-4. Hemodynamic Effects of Oral, Intravenous, and Inhaled Vasodilators in Patients With Pulmonary Arterial Hypertension. **A.** Comparison of effects on pulmonary (PVR) and systemic (SVR) vascular resistance of intravenous epoprostenol and inhaled nitric oxide in eight patients with idiopathic pulmonary arterial hypertension. Escalating doses of epoprostenol were administered as indicated and compared with baseline (BL) hemodynamic values before infusion ($^*P < .05$; nitric oxide administration was alternated and compared with hemodynamics while breathing air ($^{**}P < .01$). Note that although PVR was decreased by both infused epoprostenol and inhaled nitric oxide, SVR was lowered by infused but not by inhaled therapy. (Adapted with permission from Pepke-Zaba J H, Dinh-Xuan AT, Stone D, et al: Inhaled nitric oxide as a cause of selective pulmonary vasodilation in pulmonary hypertension. *Lancet* 338(8776):1173-1174, 1991.) **B.** Acute effects of oxygen, nitric oxide, intravenous (i.v.) or aerosolized (aero) prostacyclin (*PGI2*) or oral calcium channel antagonists (*CCA*) on mean pulmonary artery (*PA*) and mean arterial (*MAP*) pressures in eight patients with pulmonary arterial hypertension associated with fibrotic lung disease. Note that although all agents lowered pulmonary artery pressures, MAP was lowered by intravenous or oral vasodilators, but not by inhaled or aerosolized agents. $^*P < .05$ for comparison of pre-drug and post-drug administration for each agent. (Reproduced with permission from Olschewski H, Ghofrani HA, Walmrath D, et al: Inhaled prostacyclin and iloprost in severe pulmonary hypertension secondary to lung fibrosis. *Am J Respir Crit Care Med* 160(2):600-607, 1999.)

significant reduction in SVR with intravenous prostacyclin.[47] Similarly, in a study of eight patients with PAH caused by fibrotic lung disease, the administration of inhaled nitric oxide, aerosolized or intravenous prostacyclin, or oral calcium channel antagonists resulted in significant reductions in PVR. The systemic vasodilatory effects of intravenous prostacyclin or oral calcium antagonists, however, brought about significant reductions in systemic blood pressure. This was not seen with either inhaled nitric oxide or inhaled prostacyclin[48] (see FIGURE 16-4). Thus, inhalational therapy may be a safer means of reducing PVR by avoiding systemic dilation and hypotension. In a single study of 35 patients with idiopathic PAH, inhaled iloprost was more effective than inhaled nitric oxide in promoting pulmonary vasodilation and increasing cardiac output.[49] The choice of inhaled agent may be dictated by institutional availability. Significant differences in the cost of acquisition have resulted in a preference for inhaled prostacyclin over inhaled nitric oxide at some centers.[50]

Regardless of the agent, inhaled vasodilators can be used to help stabilize an acutely ill patient and serve as a bridge toward the institution of long-term vasodilatory therapies. The phosphodiesterase 5 inhibitor, sildenafil, has been shown to decrease PVR in some patients with PAH. Small cases series have demonstrated significant reduction in PVR and increased cardiac output in response to orally administered sildenafil alone or in combination with either inhaled iloprost or nitric oxide, without an adverse effect on systemic blood pressure.[51-53] Not all patients responded, however, and it must be emphasized that these trials were performed in stable patients on an elective basis. The safety and efficacy of such oral therapy in those with acute illness has not been established.

Management of Hypoxemia

As for all other patients, the goals of supportive care are to decrease the demand for oxygen while simultaneously improving its delivery. Administration of supplemental oxygen is the vital first intervention for hypoxemia. Oxygen is an important pulmonary vasodilator and can help reduce PVR and improve cardiac output.[54] Although an oxyhemoglobin saturation of at least 90 percent often is considered sufficient for treatment of patients with ARDS or other types of hypoxemic respiratory failure, this may not be

sufficient for those with significant PAH. Higher oxyhemoglobin saturations (e.g., 95-96 percent) may be required to fully prevent hypoxic pulmonary vasoconstriction.[6] Unfortunately, achieving such goals may not be possible in many patients, such as those with significant right-to-left shunting of blood across a patent foramen ovale or an atrial septal defect.

Many patients will require mechanical ventilatory support. As in other patients, mechanical ventilation can improve oxygenation and decrease the work of breathing and oxygen consumption. There are, however, potential consequences of positive-pressure ventilation on the pulmonary vasculature that warrant special consideration in the patient with significant underlying PAH.

The pulmonary vasculature can be simplistically divided into intra-alveolar and extra-alveolar vessels (see Chapter 1). These vessels are affected differently at high and low lung volumes (FIGURE 16-5). With positive pressure ventilation,

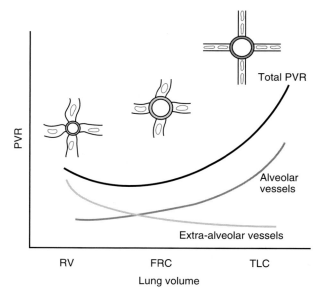

Figure 16-5. Effect of Lung Volumes on Pulmonary Vascular Resistance (PVR). At low lung volumes, PVR rises due to compression of extra-alveolar vessels. At high lung volumes, alveolar vessels (capillaries) are stretched and their caliber reduced, resulting in increased vascular resistance. (Adapted with permission from West JB: *Respiratory physiology. The essentials,* ed 6, Baltimore, 2000, Lippincott Williams & Wilkins; and Pinsky MR: Effects of mechanical ventilation on the pulmonary circulation. In: Peacock AJ, Rubin LJ, editors: *Pulmonary circulation: Diseases and their treatment,* London, 2004, Arnold, pp 497-517.)

intra-alveolar vessels may be compressed as alveolar pressures increase at high lung volumes. As a result, there is an increase in the resistance of these vessels. At lower lung volumes extra-alveolar vessels can be compressed with the collapse of alveolar units and subsequent atelectasis. These effects can result in a rise in PVR both at low and high lung volumes. Thus, in approaching mechanical ventilation in the patient with an underlying abnormality in PVR, it is particularly important to attempt to avoid hyperinflation, as well as alveolar closure at lower lung volumes.

Positive end expiratory pressure (PEEP) is used frequently in patients requiring mechanical ventilation to minimize atelectasis and improve oxygenation. This is appropriate, as well, in patients with PAH with the aim of preventing extra-alveolar vessel collapse and a resultant increase in vascular resistance. PEEP serves to promote opening of closed alveolar units and to prevent "derecruitment" of opened alveoli. Progressively increased levels of PEEP often are added in an attempt to improve oxygenation. Although a reasonable maneuver in hypoxemic patients, including those with severe PAH, PEEP must be used with particular caution in such patients. It is important to remember that high levels of PEEP can compress intra-alveolar capillaries, thus increasing vascular resistance and, ultimately, RV pressures. This can eventually decrease cardiac output as described above. Further, a rise in right ventricular pressure might increase preexisting right-to-left shunting across a patent foramen ovale. In this way, efforts aimed at improving hypoxemia may actually contribute to further worsening of oxygenation in some patients with severe PAH.

The use of permissive hypercapnia can also be problematic when applied to patients with severe PAH. Reduced tidal volumes are employed appropriately in an attempt to minimize alveolar damage induced by mechanical ventilation, often necessitating the development of hypercapnia. Such elevations of PCO_2, however, can increase pulmonary artery pressures. In one study of 15 patients with ARDS, a reduction in tidal volume from 12 to 6 cc/kg led to an increase in $PaCO_2$ from 38 to 49 mmHg. This was associated with a modest increase in mean pulmonary artery pressures (from 23 to 30 mmHg).[55] Although likely inconsequential in most patients, such an incremental increase in mean pulmonary artery pressures might be hemodynamically significant in one with underlying severe PAH.

Hypoxic pulmonary vasoconstriction is augmented in hypercarbic conditions. Whether this is due to the hypercapnia itself or resultant acidosis has been the subject of longstanding debate.[56] In contrast, hyperventilation can be used to induce a mild respiratory alkalosis and promote pulmonary vasodilation. This maneuver has been employed with some success in mechanically ventilated patients with PAH. Hyperventilation, however, should be used cautiously to avoid air trapping. Rapid respiratory rates with air trapping can cause hyperinflation and an increase in PVR from alveolar compression, as described previously.

Other notable causes of increased PVR in mechanically ventilated patients, including bronchospasm, stress, and agitation, should be managed aggressively. In one study of pediatric patients, for example, endotracheal suctioning was associated with a marked increase in heart rate, mean pulmonary artery pressure, and a greater than 150 percent increase in PVR. In this study, these deleterious effects were prevented with careful use of a narcotic analgesic (fentanyl) given before endotracheal suctioning.[57]

Cardiac Arrest

Cardiac arrest occurs frequently in critically ill patients with severe PAH. In one retrospective study involving 3,130 patients with PAH at 17 centers over 4 years, 513 cases of cardiac arrest were identified.[58] Cardiopulmonary resuscitation was attempted in 26 percent and was unsuccessful in almost 80 percent of cases. Survival 90 days post-cardiac arrest was only 6 percent in these patients, despite CPR being initiated in less than 1 minute in nearly three-quarters of cases, and 63 percent occurring in ICUs. Of note, there were no persistent neurologic deficits in the eight patients who did survive beyond 7 days after cardiac arrest.

Future Directions

Improvements in the care of patients with severe PAH and acute hemodynamic instability or respiratory failure will require specific studies of this population. Controlled studies of management with vasodilators and inotropic agents in those with hemodynamic instability, however, are extremely difficult to perform. Improvements in invasive and noninvasive means of monitoring may also help to improve outcomes. Ultimately, progress toward earlier diagnosis and more effective long-term treatment of patients with PAH should hopefully result in a reduction in the number of patients requiring such acute critical interventions.

References

1. Starr I, Jeffers WA, Meade RH: The absence of conspicuous increments of venous pressure after severe damage to the right ventricle of the dog, with a discussion of the relation between clinical congestive failure and heart disease. *Am Heart J* 26:291-300, 1943.

2. Maughan WL, Shoukas AA, Sagawa K, et al: Instantaneous pressure-volume relationship of the canine right ventricle. *Circ Res* 44:309-315, 1979.

3. Dell'Italia LJ, Walsh RA: Application of a time varying elastance model to right ventricular performance in man. *Cardiovasc Res* 22:864-874, 1988.

4. Doyle AR, Dhir AK, Moors AH, et al: Treatment of perioperative low cardiac output syndrome. *Ann Thorac Surg* 59:S3-S11, 1995.

5. Vincent JL: Pharmacological management of the pulmonary circulation in critically ill patients. In: Peacock AJ, Rubin LJ, editors: *Pulmonary circulation: Diseases and their treatment,* London, 2004, Arnold, pp 532-537.

6. Schmidt GA, Wood LDH: Acute right heart syndromes. In: Hall JB, Schmidt GA, Wood LDH, editors: *Principles of critical care,* New York, 1992, McGraw-Hill.

7. Voelker W, Gruber HP, Ickrath O, et al: Determination of right ventricular ejection fraction by thermodilution technique—a comparison to biplane cineventriculography. *Intensive Care Med* 14:461-466, 1988.

8. Spinale FG, Smith AC, Carabello BA, et al: Right ventricular function computed by thermodilution and ventriculography. A comparison of methods. *J Thorac Cardiovasc Surg* 99:141-152, 1990.

9. Jardin F, Brun-Ney D, Hardy A, et al: Combined thermodilution and two-dimensional echocardiographic evaluation of right ventricular function during respiratory support with PEEP. *Chest* 99:162-168, 1991.

10. Vieillard-Baron A, Prin S, Chergui K, et al: Echo-Doppler demonstration of acute cor pulmonale at the bedside in the medical intensive care unit. *Am J Respir Crit Care Med* 166:1310-1319, 2002.

11. Hamel E, Pacouret G, Vincentelli D, et al: Thrombolysis or heparin therapy in massive

12. pulmonary embolism with right ventricular dilation: Results from a 128-patient monocenter registry. *Chest* 120:120-125, 2001.

12. Vieillard-Baron A, Page B, Augarde R, et al: Acute cor pulmonale in massive pulmonary embolism: Incidence, echocardiographic pattern, clinical implications and recovery rate. *Intensive Care Med* 27:1481-1486, 2001.

13. Goldhaber SZ, Visani L, De Rosa M: Acute pulmonary embolism: Clinical outcomes in the International Cooperative Pulmonary Embolism Registry (ICOPER). *Lancet* 353:1386-1389, 1999.

14. Jardin F, Dubourg O, Bourdarias JP: Echocardiographic pattern of acute cor pulmonale. *Chest* 111: 209-217, 1997.

15. Bradford KK, Deb B, Pearl RG: Combination therapy with inhaled nitric oxide and intravenous dobutamine during pulmonary hypertension in the rabbit. *J Cardiovasc Pharmacol* 36:146-151, 2000.

16. Murali S, Uretsky BF, Reddy PS, et al: Reversibility of pulmonary hypertension in congestive heart failure patients evaluated for cardiac transplantation: Comparative effects of various pharmacologic agents. *Am Heart J* 122:1375-1381, 1991.

17. Deb B, Bradford K, Pearl RG: Additive effects of inhaled nitric oxide and intravenous milrinone in experimental pulmonary hypertension. *Crit Care Med* 28:795-799, 2000.

18. Chen EP, Bittner HB, Davis RD, et al: Right ventricular failure—insights provided by a new model of chronic pulmonary hypertension. *Transplantation* 63:209-216, 1997.

19. Chen EP, Bittner HB, Davis RD Jr, et al: Milrinone improves pulmonary hemodynamics and right ventricular function in chronic pulmonary hypertension. *Ann Thorac Surg* 63:814-821, 1997.

20. Pamboukian SV, Carere RG, Webb JG, et al: The use of milrinone in pre-transplant assessment of patients with congestive heart failure and pulmonary hypertension. *J Heart Lung Transplant* 18: 367-371, 1999.

21. Givertz MM, Hare JM, Loh E, et al: Effect of bolus milrinone on hemodynamic variables and pulmonary vascular resistance in patients with severe left ventricular dysfunction: A rapid test for reversibility of pulmonary hypertension. *J Am Coll Cardiol* 28:1775-1780, 1996.

22. Kwak YL, Lee CS, Park YH, et al: The effect of phenylephrine and norepinephrine in patients with chronic pulmonary hypertension. *Anaesthesia* 57:9-14, 2002.

23. Jaillard S, Elbaz F, Bresson-Just S, et al: Pulmonary vasodilator effects of norepinephrine during the development of chronic pulmonary hypertension in neonatal lambs. *Br J Anaesth* 93:818-824, 2004.

24. Kerbaul F, Rondelet B, Motte S, et al: Effects of norepinephrine and dobutamine on pressure load-induced right ventricular failure. *Crit Care Med* 32:1035-1040, 2004.

25. Holloway EL, Polumbo RA, Harrison DC: Acute circulatory effects of dopamine in patients with pulmonary hypertension. *Br Heart J* 37:482-485, 1975.

26. Martin J, Siegenthaler MP, Friesewinkel O, et al: Implantable left ventricular assist device for treatment of pulmonary hypertension in candidates for orthotopic heart transplantation—a preliminary study. *Eur J Cardiothorac Surg* 25:971-977, 2004.

27. Rasch DK, Lancaster L: Successful use of nitroglycerin to treat postoperative pulmonary hypertension. *Crit Care Med* 15:616-617, 1987.

28. Sibbald WJ, Short AI, Driedger AA, et al: The immediate effects of isosorbide dinitrate on right ventricular function in patients with acute hypoxemic respiratory failure. A combined invasive and radionuclide study. *Am Rev Respir Dis* 131:862-868, 1985.

29. Pearl RG, Rosenthal MH, Schroeder JS, et al: Acute hemodynamic effects of nitroglycer in pulmonary hypertension. *Ann Intern Med* 99:9-13, 1983.

30. Brent BN, Berger HJ, Matthay RA, et al: Contrasting acute effects of vasodilators (nitroglycerin, nitroprusside, and hydralazine) on right ventricular performance in patients with chronic obstructive pulmonary disease and pulmonary hypertension: A combined radionuclide-hemodynamic study. *Am J Cardiol* 51:1682-1689, 1983.

31. Cockrill BA, Kacmarek RM, Fifer MA, et al: Comparison of the effects of nitric oxide, nitroprusside, and nifedipine on hemodynamics and right ventricular contractility in patients with chronic pulmonary hypertension. *Chest* 119:128-136, 2001.

32. Packer M: Therapeutic application of calcium-channel antagonists for pulmonary hypertension. *Am J Cardiol* 55:196B-201B, 1985.

33. Phillips BG, Bauman JL, Schoen MD, et al: Serum nifedipine concentrations and response of patients with pulmonary hypertension. *Am J Cardiol* 77:996-999, 1996.

34. Woodmansey PA, O'Toole L, Channer KS, et al: Acute pulmonary vasodilatory properties of amlodipine in humans with pulmonary hypertension. *Heart* 75:171-173, 1996.

35. Malik AS, Warshafsky S, Lehrman S: Meta-analysis of the long-term effect of nifedipine for pulmonary hypertension. *Arch Intern Med* 157:621-625, 1997.

36. Sajkov D, Wang T, Frith PA, et al: A comparison of two long-acting vasoselective calcium antagonists in pulmonary hypertension secondary to COPD. *Chest* 111:1622-1630, 1997.

37. Fullerton DA, Jones SD, Grover FL, et al: Adenosine effectively controls pulmonary hypertension after cardiac operations. *Ann Thorac Surg* 61:1118-1123; discussion 1123-1124, 1996.

38. Kuhn KP, Byrne DW, Arbogast PG, et al: Outcome in 91 consecutive patients with pulmonary arterial hypertension receiving epoprostenol. *Am J Respir Crit Care Med* 167:580-586, 2003.

39. Barst RJ, Rubin LJ, Long WA, et al: A comparison of continuous intravenous epoprostenol (prostacyclin) with conventional therapy for primary pulmonary hypertension. The Primary Pulmonary Hypertension Study Group. *N Engl J Med* 334:296-302, 1996.

40. Higenbottam T, Butt AY, McMahon A, et al: Long-term intravenous prostaglandin (epoprostenol or iloprost) for treatment of severe pulmonary hypertension. *Heart* 80:151-155, 1998.

41. Nagaya N, Sasaki N, Ando M, et al: Prostacyclin therapy before pulmonary thromboendarterectomy in patients with chronic thromboembolic pulmonary hypertension. *Chest* 123:338-343, 2003.

42. Ichinose F, Roberts JD, Jr, Zapol WM: Inhaled nitric oxide: A selective pulmonary vasodilator: Current uses and therapeutic potential. *Circulation* 109:3106-3111, 2004.

43. Cuthbertson BH, Dellinger P, Dyar OJ, et al: UK guidelines for the use of inhaled nitric oxide therapy in adult ICUs. American-European Consensus Conference on ALI/ARDS. *Intensive Care Med* 23:1212-1218, 1997.

44. Olschewski H, Walmrath D, Schermuly R, et al: Aerosolized prostacyclin and iloprost in severe pulmonary hypertension. *Ann Intern Med* 124:820-824, 1996.

45. Haraldsson A, Kieler-Jensen N, Nathorst-Westfelt U, et al: Comparison of inhaled nitric oxide and inhaled aerosolized prostacyclin in the evaluation of heart transplant candidates with elevated pulmonary vascular resistance. *Chest* 114:780-786, 1998.

46. Girard C, Lehot JJ, Pannetier JC, et al: Inhaled nitric oxide after mitral valve replacement in patients with chronic pulmonary artery hypertension. *Anesthesiology* 77:880-883, 1992.

47. Pepke-Zaba J H, Dinh-Xuan AT, Stone D, et al: Inhaled nitric oxide as a cause of selective pulmonary vasodilatation in pulmonary hypertension. *Lancet* 338:1173-1174, 1991.

48. Olschewski H, Ghofrani HA, Walmrath D, et al: Inhaled prostacyclin and iloprost in severe pulmonary hypertension secondary to lung fibrosis. *Am J Respir Crit Care Med* 160:600-607, 1999.

49. Hoeper MM, Olschewski H, Ghofrani HA, et al: A comparison of the acute hemodynamic effects

of inhaled nitric oxide and aerosolized iloprost in primary pulmonary hypertension. German PPH study group. *J Am Coll Cardiol* 35:176-182, 2000.

50. Reily D, Moore D, Hanson CW, et al: Implementation and cost savings of a hospital wide drug substitution program using inhaled prostacyclin to eliminate inhaled nitric oxide. *Am J Respir Crit Care Med* 167:A38, 2004.

51. Leuchte HH, Schwaiblmair M, Baumgartner RA, et al: Hemodynamic response to sildenafil, nitric oxide, and iloprost in primary pulmonary hypertension. *Chest* 125:580-586, 2004.

52. Ghofrani HA, Wiedemann R, Rose F, et al: Combination therapy with oral sildenafil and inhaled iloprost for severe pulmonary hypertension. *Ann Intern Med* 136:515-522, 2002.

53. Michelakis E, Tymchak W, Lien D, et al: Oral sildenafil is an effective and specific pulmonary vasodilator in patients with pulmonary arterial hypertension: Comparison with inhaled nitric oxide. *Circulation* 105:2398-2403, 2002.

54. Roberts DH, Lepore JJ, Maroo A, et al: Oxygen therapy improves cardiac index and pulmonary vascular resistance in patients with pulmonary hypertension. *Chest* 120:1547-1555, 2001.

55. Amato MB, Barbas CS, Medeiros DM, et al: Beneficial effects of the "open lung approach" with low distending pressures in acute respiratory distress syndrome. A prospective randomized study on mechanical ventilation. *Am J Respir Crit Care Med* 152:1835-1846, 1995.

56. Fishman AP: The enigma of hypoxic pulmonary vasoconstriction. In: Fishman AP, editor: *The pulmonary circulation: Normal and abnormal,* Philadelphia, 1990, University of Pennsylvania Press.

57. Hickey PR, Hansen DD, Wessel DL, et al: Pulmonary and systemic hemodynamic responses to fentanyl in infants. *Anesth Analg* 64:483-486, 1985.

58. Hoeper MM, Galie N, Murali S, et al: Outcome after cardiopulmonary resuscitation in patients with pulmonary arterial hypertension. *Am J Respir Crit Care Med* 165:341-344, 2002.

17 Chapter

Pregnancy and Pulmonary Hypertension

Jess Mandel, MD

Pregnancy normally is marked by a number of physiologic adaptations involving multiple organ systems, and patients with pulmonary hypertension are particularly prone to difficulties in responding to the cardiopulmonary demands of the pregnant state. This section will focus on pregnancy in patients with pulmonary hypertension, particularly the group of disorders that comprise the spectrum of pulmonary arterial hypertension (PAH) (TABLE 17-1). Because of the impairments of cardiovascular function that characterize PAH and the distinctive medications that frequently are used to manage the condition, pregnancy in patients with pulmonary hypertension presents unique challenges.

Normal Physiologic Changes During Pregnancy

A myriad of maternal physiologic changes take place during pregnancy, encompassing nearly all organ systems in the body. Of greatest significance to the patient with PAH are changes that affect cardiac performance and vascular properties, including alterations in blood volume, cardiac output, pulmonary and systemic vascular resistance, and coagulability.

Blood Volume

Expansion of maternal blood volume is detectable as early as the fourth week of pregnancy. The blood volume continues to expand until approximately 28-34 weeks of gestation, after which it plateaus until delivery. Most of this expansion is the result of changes in plasma volume, which increases to values 30 to 50 percent above the nonpregnant state by the end of pregnancy. In addtion, there is

an increase in red blood cell mass beginning at 8-10 weeks of gestation, to approximately 25 pecent over nonpregnant values by delivery, provided that iron intake is adequate. Because plasma volume expansion exceeds the increase in red blood cell mass, "physiologic anemia" with a decreased hematocrit generally develops most prominently during the third trimester, although oxygen carrying capacity is increased over that of the nonpregnant state.[1-4]

Cardiac Output

Cardiac output increases by approximately 50 percent over the course of pregnancy. This is caused mostly by a progressive diminution in systemic vascular resistance that begins around the fifth week of pregnancy (due to both systemic vasodilation and the development of the low-resistance uteroplacental circulation), increased preload from enlarged circulatory volume, and an increase in heart rate.[5-7] Labor and delivery introduce anxiety, pain, and fluctuations in venous return caused by Valsalva maneuvers, uterine contractions, and uterine involution. Cardiac output may increase 25-50 percent over prelabor values in active and second stage labor, and as high as 80 percent over prelabor values during the immediate postpartum period as the patient's blood is returned from the uterus to the central circulation.[4,8] The increase in cardiac output associated with labor and delivery is blunted significantly by general anesthesia and, to a lesser degree, by epidural anesthesia. These effects usually are well tolerated by the healthy mother, but they may be deleterious in mothers with pulmonary hypertension.[9,10]

A degree of hypertrophy and cardiac enlargement normally occurs during pregnancy and may

TABLE 17-1

Classification and Causes of Pulmonary Hypertension

1. Pulmonary Arterial Hypertension (PAH)
   1.1. Idiopathic (IPAH)
   1.2. Familial (FPAH)
   1.3. Associated with (APAH):
       1.3.1. Collagen vascular disease
       1.3.2. Congenital systemic-to-pulmonary shunts
       1.3.3. Portal hypertension
       1.3.4. HIV infection
       1.3.5. Drugs and toxins
       1.3.6. Other (thyroid disorders, glycogen storage disease, Gaucher disease, hereditary hemorrhagic telangiectasia, hemoglobinopathies, myeloproliferative disorders, splenectomy)
   1.4. Associated with significant venous or capillary involvement
       1.4.1. Pulmonary veno-occlusive disease (PVOD)
       1.4.2. Pulmonary capillary hemangiomatosis (PCH)
   1.5. Persistent pulmonary hypertension of the newborn
2. Pulmonary hypertension with left-sided heart disease
   2.1. Left-sided atrial or ventricular heart disease
   2.2. Left-sided valvular heart disease
3. Pulmonary hypertension associated with lung diseases or hypoxemia
   3.1. Chronic obstructive pulmonary disease
   3.2. Interstitial lung disease
   3.3. Sleep-disordered breathing
   3.4. Alveolar hypoventilation disorders
   3.5. Long-term exposure to high altitude
   3.6. Developmental abnormalities
4. Pulmonary hypertension due to chronic thrombotic or embolic disease
   4.1. Thromboembolic obstruction of proximal pulmonary arteries
   4.2. Thromboembolic obstruction of distal pulmonary arteries
   4.3. Nonthrombotic pulmonary embolism (tumor, parasites, foreign material)
5. Miscellaneous (sarcoidosis, histiocytosis X, lymphangiomatosis, compression of pulmonary vessels [adenopathy, tumor, fibrosing mediastinitis])

HIV, *human immunodeficiency virus.*
Adapted from Rubin LJ: Diagnosis and management of pulmonary arterial hypertension: ACCP evidence-based clinical practice guidelines. Chest 126:7S-10S, 2004.

be accompanied by multivalvular regurgitation; such changes normally regress during the postpartum period.[11,12] Likewise, heart rate, systemic vascular resistance, and cardiac output begin to return to prepregnant values within hours of delivery, although they may not normalize fully for up to 6-12 months.[13,14]

Pulmonary Vascular Resistance

The increased pulmonary blood flow that is obligated by an increased cardiac output results in recruitment of additional, previously unutilized capillaries from Zones 1 and 2 in the West model (see Chapter 1). This recruitment, along with distention of previously recruited, high-compliance blood vessels, results in a fall in pulmonary vascular resistance with normal pregnancy, while pulmonary artery pressures are generally without net change.[15]

Thrombophilia

Pregnancy, particularly during the third trimester and postpartum periods, is a hypercoagulable state, marked by a relative resistance to activated protein C, decreased serum levels of protein S, and increased levels of factors I, II, V, VII, VIII, X, and XII.[16-18] This likely represents an adaptation to reduce the volume of hemorrhage at the time of delivery, but it also influences the risk for venous thromboembolism. In addition, hypercoagulability may play a role in accelerating the progression of pulmonary hypertension of any cause.[19]

Impact of Pulmonary Vascular Disease

As is clear from the preceding discussion, significant plasticity of the cardiovascular system normally is required during pregnancy, delivery, and the postpartum period. Patients with pulmonary vascular disease may be incapable of navigating the adaptations that are required for successful maternal and fetal outcomes, and they may first develop symptoms as a result of the physiologic stresses of pregnancy. For these reasons, maternal mortality rates among pregnant women with pulmonary hypertension remain significant, despite improvements in obstetrical care, anesthesia, and medical therapy for PAH over the past several decades.

Difficulties with cardiovascular adaptation are primarily a consequence of baseline pulmonary vascular and cardiac abnormalities. The decreased compliance and decreased recruitability of the diseased pulmonary vascular bed complicates the normal ability to reduce pulmonary vascular resistance in response to the increased circulatory demands of pregnancy, particularly with exertion. As a result, pulmonary artery pressures rise more linearly with cardiac output, dramatically increasing right ventricular afterload. This additional stress on the right ventricle occurs along with limited cardiovascular reserve, and symptoms and signs of decompensated cor pulmonale can develop, including dyspnea, peripheral edema, cough, and hepatic congestion. Symptoms usually are noted initially with exertion and then variably progress to occur at rest during pregnancy and delivery, depending upon the severity of the underlying condition and the effectiveness of management. The inability to augment cardiac output during delivery is particularly problematic, because tissue metabolic demands are high and significant blood loss frequently occurs. Progressive symptoms of cor pulmonale, right ventricular failure, and cardiogenic shock may ensue. Pregnant patients with PAH are also at risk for sudden death from malignant dysrhythmias or pulmonary thromboembolism, as well as stroke if intracardiac shunting is present from Eisenmenger syndrome or a patent foramen ovale.[8,20,21]

If PAH has not been diagnosed before pregnancy, dyspnea usually is attributed to other causes initially. Dyspnea may occur at some point in up to 70 percent of pregnancies, most commonly during the first or second trimesters.[22] Most cases are attributed to "dyspnea of pregnancy," a condition that is not entirely understood but appears to relate to an increased respiratory drive secondary to increased plasma progesterone concentrations. Venous thromboembolic disease is the most common pulmonary vascular disease to complicate pregnancy and should be considered in any pregnant patient with dyspnea.[23-25] Asthma,

which may either worsen or remit during pregnancy, and peripartum cardiomyopathy frequently are considered before the diagnosis of PAH is established.[26]

Pregnancy has not been clearly established as a risk factor for PAH. In reports of PAH diagnosed in association with pregnancy, it has been difficult to discern whether pregnancy precipitated PAH, or if the increased cardiovascular demands of pregnancy unmasked previously asymptomatic pulmonary vascular disease.[27] No association between either pregnancy or the use of oral contraceptives and IPAH was found in the National Institutes of Health Registry for the Characterization of Primary Pulmonary Hypertension.[28]

Maternal and Fetal Outcomes

Because of the difficulties in achieving effective cardiovascular adaptation during pregnancy, maternal and fetal risk is significant when PAH is present. A landmark 1964 review described the outcome of 23 pregnancies occurring in 16 patients.[8] Nine patients (39 percent) died during pregnancy (including a patient who had felt that her pulmonary status improved during her previous four pregnancies before dying during the fifth), two patients deteriorated but had nonfatal outcomes during pregnancy, four were unchanged, and one improved. Symptoms were noted initially during pregnancy in 3 of 23 pregnancies, and there did not appear to be a correlation between the duration of symptoms and outcome. Seven of the nine deaths occurred "suddenly from circulatory collapse," and six occurred during the last 2 months of pregnancy or during the puerperium.

A 1979 review examined 70 pregnancies in 44 women with Eisenmenger syndrome and found a maternal mortality rate of 52 percent.[29] Labor, delivery, and the postpartum period were again noted to be the most dangerous times. Fifty-five percent of deliveries occurred prematurely, and approximately one-third of infants exhibited intrauterine growth retardation. A perinatal infant mortality of 28 percent was observed, primarily associated with complications of prematurity. A literature review examining published cases between 1978 and 1996 described a maternal mortality rate of 36 percent in Eisenmenger syndrome, 30 percent in IPAH, and 56 percent in pulmonary hypertension from other causes, including anorectic drug use, liver disease, connective tissue diseases, and chronic thromboembolic disease.[30] The first month after delivery again constituted the interval of greatest risk for maternal death. Finally, a 1995 single-center series of 13 pregnancies in 12 women with Eisenmenger syndrome reported three spontaneous abortions, one premature labor at 23 weeks, and three maternal deaths.[31]

It should be noted that most of these series predate the availability of epoprostenol and other modern treatment modalities that have improved long-term outcomes in patients with PAH. In addition, it is likely that more patients with less severe PAH are diagnosed than was the case when these series were being compiled. Although it is speculated that pregnancy in the context of less severe disease and with current PAH management may result in less dire outcomes, this hypothesis has not been well supported, and series with state-of-the-art management of PAH continue to report unacceptably poor maternal and fetal outcomes.[32]

Contraception and Pregnancy Termination

Although some authors have asserted that pregnancy may be a reasonable option after at least 1 year of therapy that has resulted in near-normal right ventricular function, most practitioners strongly advise women with significant, symptomatic pulmonary hypertension to avoid pregnancy.[15,33] Surgical sterilization of the male partner is the safest and most effective method of contraception for the woman with PAH, although barrier methods and hormonal methods and are widely used and are acceptable provided no contraindications such as venous thromboembolism are present. Of note, the effectiveness of hormonal contraceptives may be diminished by certain medications used for PAH, such as bosentan.

Should pregnancy occur, counseling regarding the risks of continuing the pregnancy should be undertaken, and the option of pregnancy termination should be offered.[34] This is a particularly relevant issue if the patient becomes pregnant while receiving bosentan, sitaxsentan, or other endothelin-1 receptor antagonists, all of which are potent teratogens and are contraindicated in pregnancy.[35] Nonetheless, termination of pregnancy is not without significant risk in women with PAH, and fatalities and near fatalities have occurred during this procedure.[29,36]

Management of PAH During Pregnancy

Should the patient elect to continue the pregnancy to term, her management should include input from specialists with expertise in high-risk obstetrics, pulmonary hypertension and, if applicable, adult congenital heart disease. Essentially, there are no controlled trials to guide therapy in this situation, and management is based on clinical experience and judgment, extrapolation of data from nonpregnant patients, and imputed biologic and physiologic plausibility.

Limitation of Activity

Patients with PAH are under significant physiologic stress by virtue of changes that normally accompany pregnancy, and therefore they should minimize additional cardiac demands. Care should be taken to lie in the left lateral decubitus position to avoid inferior vena caval compression and diminution of venous return. Hospital admission during the second trimester should be considered because of the high frequency of preterm labor and the tenuous cardiovascular status of the mother.[34,37]

Supplemental Oxygen

Supplemental oxygen should be used as necessary to maintain maternal PaO_2 over 70 mmHg. Although this value is higher than the threshold generally used to determine the need for long-term oxygen therapy, maternal PaO_2 is generally in excess of 100 mmHg during normal pregnancies (primarily because of normal increases in alveolar ventilation), and maternal PaO_2 values less than 70mmHg in women who live at high altitudes have been associated with intrauterine growth retardation.[38,39]

Diuretics

Diuretics have traditionally been avoided during pregnancy because of concerns that excessive reductions in maternal blood volume may impair fetal nutrition, oxygenation, and growth. Nonetheless, many pregnant women with PAH require diuretics in order to prevent or manage deleterious hypervolemia.[40] Torsemide generally is preferred if a loop diuretic is required because it is classified as Food and Drug Administration pregnancy risk category B, whereas furosemide and bumetanide are in risk category C. Ethacrynic acid is used rarely because of concerns regarding ototoxicity. Spironolactone should be avoided because of concerns that its antiandrogenic activity may feminize male fetuses.[41]

Anticoagulation

The risk of venous thromboembolism is increased 6-fold to 10-fold during pregnancy.[42,43] Patients with PAH already have limited cardiopulmonary reserve and thus can be expected to tolerate pulmonary emboli poorly. In addition, patients with Eisenmenger syndrome or a patent foramen ovale are at risk for paradoxical emboli.

For these reasons, anticoagulation generally is recommended, although consensus on this point is incomplete and there is a risk of worsening hemorrhage during delivery, which is poorly tolerated.[15,34,44] Because of its ease of administration and absence of documented adverse fetal effects, low-molecular-weight heparin generally is used during pregnancy.[45] Centers vary in the dosage of heparin employed, with some favoring full-dosage anticoagulation and others opting for prophylactic dosages unless venous thromboembolism is documented.[46] In contrast to its use in nonpregnant patients, some authors recommend that pregnant patients undergo periodic measurement of anti-factor Xa levels 4 hours after injection, with titration of the dosage to achieve a level of 0.5-1.2 units/mL.[47]

Tight control of anticoagulation around the time of delivery is critical to minimize the risk of excessive vaginal or operative bleeding that could precipitate cardiac decompensation, and to reduce the risk of spinal or epidural hematoma if neuraxial anesthesia is used.[48] For this reason, transition from low-molecular-weight to unfractionated heparin is recommended several weeks before delivery is anticipated.

Following delivery, warfarin can be initiated safely and does not preclude breast-feeding in the absence of other contraindications, because the active drug is excreted minimally in breast milk. Because of the well-documented risk of maternal deterioration and death during the postpartum period and the belief that at least some of these adverse events are due to pulmonary thromboembolism, anticoagulation should be continued for at least 2-6 months after delivery. Continued anticoagulation thereafter may be appropriate for PAH management, depending on its severity.[49]

Pulmonary Vasodilators and Remodeling Agents

The basic principles of employing pulmonary vasodilators and agents that induce pulmonary vascular remodeling are described elsewhere (see Chapter 7). The treatment selected for the pregnant patient must be as safe as possible for the developing fetus and also be sufficiently efficacious to control the patient's pulmonary hypertension despite the physiologic challenges posed by pregnancy, parturition, and the puerperium. Except for the rare woman with documented normalization of pulmonary hemodynamics on oral calcium channel antagonists, continuous intravenous epoprostenol (prostacyclin [Flolan]) is generally the drug of choice for patients with disease of more than very mild severity, because it has both the best evidence of efficacy in nonpregnant patients and the best record of safety in pregnant patients (although this record is admittedly small)[33,50-52] (TABLE 17-2).

Treprostinil (Remodulin) delivered continuously by the intravenous or subcutaneous routes has not shown definitive adverse effects in this situation, although clinical experience is more limited than with epoprostenol. Inhaled iloprost (Ventavis) has been used successfully in some cases, but systemic distribution of the drug occurs despite its route of administration, and the drug has shown adverse fetal effects in some, but not all, studies.[46]

Among oral agents, bosentan (Tracleer) is *absolutely* contraindicated in pregnancy because of its potent teratogenic effects and should be discontinued immediately in patients who become pregnant. Other endothelin-1 receptor antagonists that are under development, such as sitaxsentan (Thelin) and ambrisentan, are likewise contraindicated during pregnancy. In contrast, sildenafil (Revatio, Viagra) appears to be safe during pregnancy, although this conclusion is drawn primarily from animal studies, and experience with its safety and efficacy in pregnant patients is relatively limited.[53,54] Sildenafil may be a reasonable therapeutic option in pregnant patients with asymptomatic or mildly symptomatic and hemodynamically minor pulmonary hypertension.

Management During Labor, Delivery, and the Postpartum Period

In most cases in which PAH is significant, bedrest is prescribed beginning in the second trimester, with a low threshold for hospital admission for close

TABLE 17-2

Pregnancy Risk Factors of Agents for Pulmonary Hypertension

Medication	FDA Pregnancy Risk Factor*
Epoprostenol (prostacyclin [Flolan])	B
Treprostinil (Remodulin)	B
Iloprost (Ventavis)	C
Bosentan (Tracleer)	X
Sildenafil (Revatio, Viagra)	B
Nitric oxide	C

*Category A: Controlled studies show no risk: Adequate, well-controlled studies in pregnant women have failed to demonstrate risk to the fetus.
Category B: No evidence of risk in humans: Either animal studies showed risk (but human findings do not) or, if no adequate human studies have been performed, animal findings are negative.
Category C: Risk cannot be ruled out: Human studies are lacking and animal studies are either positive for fetal risk or lacking as well. However, potential benefits may justify the potential risks.
Category D: Positive evidence of risk: Investigational or postmarketing data show risk to the fetus. Nevertheless, potential benefits may outweigh the risk.
Category X: Contraindicated in pregnancy: Studies in animals or humans, or investigational or postmarketing reports have shown fetal risk which clearly outweighs any possible benefit to the patient.
FDA, Food and Drug Administration.

observation and further management at any time during the pregnancy should clinical deterioration or uterine contractions develop. Because of the unique hemodynamic challenges of labor and delivery, pregnant patients with PAH require vigilant monitoring, frequently necessitating arterial and central venous catheterization as labor begins. Pulmonary arterial catheterization is more controversial and some have argued against its use.[30] The risk of abrupt hemodynamic collapse and death at this time necessitates an inpatient multidisciplinary care team with expertise in high-risk obstetrics, pulmonary hypertension, critical care, anesthesia, and neonatology. Intensification of PAH therapy with intravenous or inhaled epoprostenol or inhaled nitric oxide sometimes is required, and intravascular fluid shifts associated with both hemorrhage or overzealous intravenous fluid administration should be minimized.[51,55-59]

There is no clear consensus regarding the optimal mode of delivery. Cesarian delivery avoids the risks of a prolonged second stage of labor, uncontrolled hemorrhage, and the hemodynamic stress of bearing down but is associated with an increased anesthetic risk. Assisted vaginal delivery with shortening of the second stage of labor with low forceps delivery is preferred in some centers and has shown a lower mortality rate in some uncontrolled series, particularly in the Eisenmenger syndrome population.[37] In either event, neuraxial or general anesthesia should be performed carefully to minimize peripheral vasodilation and potential hemodynamic deterioration.[60] Anesthetic goals include prevention of increases in pulmonary vascular resistance by treatment of pain, anxiety, acidemia, hypercarbia, and hypoxemia; maintenance of mild elevations of intravascular volume and cardiac filling pressures; prevention of large or sudden decreases in systemic blood pressure; and prevention of myocardial depression during general anesthesia.[34,61]

In-hospital monitoring usually is continued for at least 2 weeks after delivery.[34] Heparin should be restarted when bleeding has abated, and warfarin initiated and continued for an additional 2-6 months.[32] In general, pulmonary vasodilator-remodeling agents should not be weaned for at least 3-6 months after delivery. Because of the paucity of data on the excretion of these medications in breast milk, breast-feeding generally is discouraged. Physical therapy may be required to help reverse deconditioning that has developed as a result of bedrest and must be monitored closely to prevent excessive stress on the cardiovascular system.

Conclusions

The diagnosis of previously undetected PAH during pregnancy is challenging because of the nonspecific nature of its clinical picture and the high frequency of dyspnea and edema in the general pregnant population. Pregnancy is a profoundly dangerous condition for patients with PAH, with a historical maternal mortality rate of 30-50 percent, and it is not clear that this has been reduced decisively by current management techniques. Pregnancy should be avoided in this population whenever possible, and termination of pregnancy in patients with significant PAH should be considered.

Should pregnancy be continued, the importance of a multidisciplinary care team cannot be overstated. Continuous intravenous epoprostenol, in conjunction with oxygen, anticoagulation, and diuretics, remains the medication of choice in this situation because of the greater clinical experience with its safety and efficacy. Oral sildenafil may be a reasonable option in patients with borderline or mild disease, whereas bosentan and other endothelin receptor antagonists are absolutely contraindicated because of their teratogenic potential. Most maternal deaths have occurred during the third trimester or the puerperium, and close monitoring and aggressive therapy is particularly critical during these periods.

References

1. Ueland K: Maternal cardiovascular dynamics. VII. Intrapartum blood volume changes. *Am J Obstet Gynecol* 126:671-677, 1976.
2. Pritchard J: Changes in the blood volume during pregnancy and delivery. *Anesthesiology* 26:393-399, 1965.
3. Lund C, Donovan J: Blood volume during pregnancy. Significance of plasma and red cell volumes. *Am J Obstet Gynecol* 98:394-403, 1967.
4. Foley M: Maternal cardiovascular adaptation to pregnancy. In: Rose B, editor: *UpToDate,* vol 13.2, Wellesley, MA, 2005, UpToDate.
5. Robson S, Hunter S, Boys R, et al: Serial study of factors influencing changes in cardiac output during human pregnancy. *Am J Physiol* 256:H1060-H1065, 1989.
6. Capeless E, Clapp J: Cardiovascular changes in early phase of pregnancy. *Am J Obstet Gynecol* 161: 1449-1453, 1989.
7. Duvekot J, Peeters L: Maternal cardiovascular hemodynamic adaptations to pregnancy. *Obstet Gynecol Surv* 49:S1-S14, 1994.
8. McCaffrey R, Dunn L: Primary pulmonary hypertension in pregnancy. *Obstet Gynecol Surv* 19:567-591, 1964.
9. Robson S, Dunlop W, Boys R, et al: Cardiac output during labor. *Br Med J (Clin Res Ed)* 295:1169-1172, 1987.
10. Slomka F, Salmeron S, Zetlaoui P, et al: Primary pulmonary hypertension and pregnancy: Anesthetic management for delivery. *Anesthesiology* 69:959-961, 1988.
11. van Oppen A, Stigter R, Bruinse H: Cardiac output in normal pregnancy: A critical review. *Obstet Gynecol* 87:310-318, 1996.
12. Mone S, Sanders S, Colan S: Control mechanisms for physiologic hypertrophy of pregnancy. *Circulation* 94:667-672, 1996.
13. Clapp JF, III, Capeless E: Cardiovascular function before, during, and after the first and subsequent pregnancies. *Am J Cardiol* 80:1469-1473, 1997.
14. Robson S, Hunter S, Moore M, et al: Haemodynamic changes during the puerperium: A Doppler and M-mode echocardiographic study. *Br J Obstet Gynaecol* 94:1028-1039, 1987.
15. Weiss B, Hess O: Pulmonary vascular disease and pregnancy: Current controversies, management strategies, and perspectives. *Eur Heart J* 21:104-115, 2000.
16. Pechet L, Alexander B: Clotting factors in pregnancy. *N Engl J Med* 265:1093-1097, 1961.
17. Walker M, Garner P, Keely E, et al: Changes in activated protein C resistance during normal pregnancy. *Am J Obstet Gynecol* 177:162-169, 1997.
18. Hellgren M, Blomback M: Studies on blood coagulation and fibrinolysis in pregnancy, during delivery and in the puerperium. I. Normal condition. *Gynecol Obstet Invest* 12:141-154, 1981.
19. Rich S, Kaufmann E, Levy P: The effect of high dose calcium channel blockers on survival in primary pulmonary hypertension. *N Engl J Med* 327:76-81, 1992.
20. Daliento L, Somerville J, Presbitero P, et al: Eisenmenger syndrome. Factors relating to deterioration and death. *Eur Heart J* 19:1845-1855, 1998.
21. Jaigobin C, Silver F: Stroke and pregnancy. *Stroke* 31:2948-2951, 2000.
22. Prowse C, Gaensler E: Respiratory and acid-base changes during pregnancy. *Anesthesiology* 26: 381-392, 1965.
23. McPhedran P: Venous thromboembolism during pregnancy. In: Burrow G, Duffy T, Copel J, editors: *Medical complications during pregnancy,* Philadelphia, 2004, Elsevier Saunders, pp 87-102.
24. Greer I: Prevention and management of venous thromboembolism in pregnancy. *Clin Chest Med* 24:123-137, 2003.
25. Phillips O: Venous thromboembolism in the pregnant woman. *J Reprod Med* 48:921-929, 2003.
26. Zeldis S: Dyspnea during pregnancy. Distinguishing cardiac from pulmonary causes. *Clin Chest Med* 13:567-585, 1992.
27. Dawkins K: Primary pulmonary hypertension and pregnancy. *Chest* 89:383-388, 1986.
28. Rich S, Dantzker D, Ayres S, et al: Primary pulmonary hypertension. A national prospective study. *Ann Intern Med* 107:216-223, 1987.
29. Gleicher N, Midwall J, Hochberger D: Eisenmenger's syndrome and pregnancy. *Obstet Gynecol* 34:721-741, 1979.
30. Weiss B, Zemp L, Seifert B, et al: Outcome of pulmonary vascular disease in pregnancy: A systematic overview from 1978 through 1996. *J Am Coll Cardiol* 31:1650-1657, 1998.

31. Avila W, Grinberg M, Snitcowsky R, et al: Maternal and fetal outcome in pregnant women with Eisenmenger's syndrome. *Eur Heart J* 16:460-464, 1995.

32. Bonnin M, Mercier F, Sitbon O, et al: Severe pulmonary hypertension during pregnancy: Mode of delivery and anesthetic management of 15 consecutive cases. *Anesthesiology* 102:1133-1137, 2005.

33. Easterling T, Ralph D, Schmucker B: Pulmonary hypertension in pregnancy: Treatment with pulmonary vasodilators. *Obstet Gynecol* 93:494-498, 1999.

34. Warnes C: Pregnancy and pulmonary hypertension. *Int J Cardiol* 97:11-13, 2004.

35. Clouthier D, Williams S, Hammer R, et al: Cell-autonomous and nonautonomous actions of endothelin-A receptor signaling in craniofacial and cardiovascular development. *Dev Biol* 261:506-519, 2003.

36. Satoh H, Masuda Y, Izuta S, et al: Pregnant patient with primary pulmonary hypertension: General anesthesia and extracorporeal membrane oxygenation support for termination of pregnancy. *Anesthesiology* 97:1638-1640, 2002.

37. Vongpatanasin W, Brickner M, Hillis L, et al: The Eisenmenger syndrome in adults. *Ann Intern Med* 128:745-755, 1998.

38. Moore L, Rounds S, Jahnigen D, et al: Infant birth weight is related to maternal arterial oxygenation at high altitude. *J Appl Physiol* 52:695-699, 1982.

39. Mandel J, Weinberger S. Pulmonary diseases. In: Burrow G, Duffy T, Copel J, editors: *Medical complications during pregnancy*, Philadelphia, 2004, Elsevier Saunders.

40. Al-Mobeireek A, Almutawa J, Alsatli R: The nineteenth pregnancy in a patient with cor pulmonale and severe pulmonary hypertension: A management challenge. *Acta Obstet Gynecol Scand* 82:676-678, 2003.

41. Hecker A, Hasan S, Neumann F: Disturbances in sexual differentiation of rat foetuses following spironolactone treatment. *Acta Endocrinol (Copenh)* 95:540-545, 1980.

42. Martinelli I: Risk factors in venous thromboembolism. *Thromb Haemost* 86:395-403, 2001.

43. Eldor A: Thrombophilia, thrombosis and pregnancy. *Thromb Haemost* 86:104-111, 2001.

44. Pitts J, Crosby W, Basta L: Eisenmenger's syndrome in pregnancy: Does heparin prophylaxis improve the maternal mortality rate? *Am Heart J* 91:321-326, 1977.

45. ACOG committee opinion: Safety of Lovenox in pregnancy. *Obstet Gynecol* 100:845-846, 2002.

46. Elliot C, Stewart P, Webster V, et al: The use of iloprost in early pregnancy in patients with pulmonary arterial hypertension. *Eur Respir J* 26:168-173, 2005.

47. Bates S, Greer I, Hirsh J, et al: Use of antithrombotic agents in pregnancy: The Seventh ACCP Conference on Antithrombotic and Thrombolytic Therapy. *Chest* 126(3 Suppl):627S-644S, 2004.

48. Lumpkin M: FDA public health advisory. *Anesthesiology* 88:27A-28A, 1998.

49. Badesch D, Abman S, Ahearn G, et al: Medical therapy for pulmonary arterial hypertension: ACCP evidence-based clinical practice guidelines. *Chest* 126:35S-62S, 2004.

50. Geohas C, McLaughlin V: Successful management of pregnancy in a patient with Eisenmenger syndrome with epoprostenol. *Chest* 124:1170-1173, 2003.

51. Badalian S, Silverman R, Aubry R, et al: Twin pregnancy in a woman on long-term epoprostenol therapy for primary pulmonary hypertension. A case report. *J Reprod Med* 45:149-152, 2000.

52. Stewart R, Tuazon D, Olson G, et al: Pregnancy and primary pulmonary hypertension: Successful outcome with epoprostenol therapy. *Chest* 119:973-975, 2001.

53. Lacassie H, Germain A, Valdes G, et al: Management of Eisenmenger syndrome in pregnancy with sildenafil and L-arginine. *Obstet Gynecol* 103:1118-1120, 2004.

54. Molelekwa V, Ahkter P, McKenna P, et al: Eisenmenger's syndrome in a 27 week pregnancy—management with bosentan and sildenafil. *Ir Med J* 98:87-88, 2005.

55. Goodwin T, Gherman R, Hameed A, et al: Favorable response of Eisenmenger syndrome to inhaled nitric oxide during pregnancy. *Am J Obstet Gynecol* 180:64-67, 1999.

56. Hill L, De Wet C, Jacobsohn E, et al: Peripartum substitution of inhaled for intravenous prostacyclin in a patient with primary pulmonary hypertension. *Anesthesiology* 100:1603-1605, 2004.

57. Monnery L, Nanson J, Charlton G: Primary pulmonary hypertension in pregnancy: A role for novel vasodilators. *Br J Anaesth* 87:295-298, 2001.

58. Lam G, Stafford R, Thorp J, et al: Inhaled nitric oxide for primary pulmonary hypertension in pregnancy. *Obstet Gynecol* 98:895-898, 2001.

59. Lust K, Boots R, Dooris M, et al: Management of labor in Eisenmenger syndrome with inhaled nitric oxide. *Am J Obstet Gynecol* 181:419-423, 1999.

60. Midwall J, Jaffin H, Herman M, et al: Shunt flow and pulmonary hemodynamics during labor and delivery in the Eisenmenger syndrome. *Am J Cardiol* 42:299-303, 1978.

61. Mushlin P, Davidson K: Cardiovascular disease during pregnancy. In: Datta S, editor: *Anesthetic and obstetric management of high-risk pregnancy*, New York, 1996, Springer.

Pulmonary Hypertension in Children

Asrar Rashid, MBChB, MRCP, MRCPCH, DTM&H

D. Dunbar Ivy, MD

Pulmonary hypertension in children previously carried a very poor prognosis. In a 1965 series of 35 patients with idiopathic ("primary") pulmonary arterial hypertension (IPAH), 22 patients died within 1 year of the onset of symptoms and none survived longer than 7 years.[1] In 1995, the prognosis was still poor, with the median survival in a series of 18 children with IPAH being 4.12 years.[2] Since then, advances in understanding the biology of the normal and hypertensive pulmonary circulations have led to a broader pharmacologic arsenal and improved prognosis of children with pulmonary hypertension. For example, in one 2004 series, children with severe IPAH and acute pulmonary vasoreactivity treated with calcium channel blockers displayed survival after 1, 5, and 10 years of 97 percent, 97 percent, and 81 percent, respectively.[3] Survival of children treated with epoprostenol (n = 35) after 1, 5, and 10 years was 94 percent, 81 percent, and 61 percent, respectively.[3]

Pulmonary hypertension may be an idiopathic or primary phenomenon (i.e., without an underlying cause) or secondary to or associated with other disease processes. IPAH is a rare and poorly understood situation diagnosed by excluding conditions known to be associated with or to cause pulmonary hypertension. Without appropriate management, IPAH is progressive and fatal. In contrast, the natural history of pulmonary arterial hypertension from congenital heart disease has a broad range of survival, from months to decades.

This chapter will discuss the diagnosis and treatment of children with pulmonary arterial hypertension. The selection of appropriate therapies is complex, requiring familiarity with the underlying disease process, complicated delivery systems and dosing regimens, and medication complications.

Definition

Pulmonary hypertension is defined as a mean pulmonary artery pressure greater than 25 mmHg at rest, or greater than 30 mmHg during exercise.[4] In 1998 the World Health Organization proposed a new classification of pulmonary hypertension, and this was updated in 2003. This classification is appropriate to both the pediatric and adult age groups and is elaborated in Chapter 5.

Diagnostic Evaluation

The most successful strategy for managing moderate to severe pulmonary hypertension is to manage its underlying cause. Evaluation, therefore, involves a complete history and examination (TABLE 18-1) and extensive evaluation (TABLE 18-2) aiming at differentiating among known causes.[5-7] Symptoms may include exertional dyspnea, reduced exercise tolerance, orthopnea, atypical chest pain, hemoptysis, feeding intolerance, or growth failure. Syncope may be indicative of end-stage disease.

Special situations may predispose children to pulmonary arterial hypertension. As an example, children living at altitude and coming to medical attention with high altitude pulmonary edema should be screened for pulmonary hypertension.[8] In addition, children with biliary atresia, cavernous transformation of the portal vein, primary sclerosing cholangitis, or cryptogenic cirrhosis may have portopulmonary hypertension with an associated high mortality.[9] Some medications, such as phenyl-

TABLE 18-1

History and Examination

History

Diet pill, contraceptive pill, methamphetamine use
Onset and duration of pulmonary hypertension
Family history of pulmonary hypertension
Prior cardiac and other surgeries
Residence at high altitude

Symptoms

Chest pain, dyspnea, shortness of breath, syncope

Physical Examination

Loud second heart sound, systolic murmur of tricuspid regurgitation or diastolic murmur of pulmonary insufficiency, palpable second heart sound, peripheral edema, jugular venous distention

TABLE 18-2

Diagnostic Evaluation of Pulmonary Hypertension

Chest radiograph (signs of cardiomegaly and enlarged pulmonary arteries)
ECG (right ventricular hypertrophy and ST-T changes)
Echocardiogram (right ventricular hypertrophy, exclude congenital heart disease, quantify right ventricular systolic pressures)
Cardiac catheterization with acute vasodilator testing (evaluate pulmonary artery pressure and resistance and degree of pulmonary reactivity)
Liver evaluation
Hepatic function tests
Abdominal ultrasonography (portopulmonary hypertension)
Hepatitis profile
Complete blood count, urinalysis
Thrombophilia evaluation
DIC screen
Factor V Leiden
Antithrombin III
Prothrombin mutation 22010
Protein C
Protein S
Anticardiolipin IgG or IgM
Russell viper venom test
Evaluation of possible collagen vascular disease
Antinuclear antibody with profile (DNA, Smith, RNP, SSA. SSB, centromere, SCL-70)
Rheumatoid factor
Erythrocyte sedimentation rate
Complement
Evaluation of possible chronic lung disease
Pulmonary function tests with DL_{CO} or bronchodilators (to exclude obstructive/restrictive disease)
Sleep study and pulse oximetry (degree of hypoxia or diminished ventilatory drive)
CT or MRI scan of chest (evaluation of thromboembolic disease or interstitial lung disease)
Ventilation-perfusion test
Lung biopsy
Six-minute walk test or cycle ergometry
HIV test
Thyroid function tests
Toxicology screen (cocaine, methamphetamine, and HIV testing)

CT, *computed tomography;* DIC, *disseminated intravascular coagulation;* DL_{CO}, *diffusing capacity for carbon monoxide;* DNA, *deoxyribonucleic acid;* ECG, *electrocardiogram;* HIV, *human immunodeficiency virus;* IgG, *immunoglobulin G;* IgM, *immunoglobulin M;* MRI, *magnetic resonance imaging;* RNP, *ribonucleoprotein;* SCL-70, *scleroderma-70;* SSA, *Sjögren's syndrome A;* SSB, *Sjögren's syndrome B.*

TABLE 18-3

Exercise Parameters Associated With Adverse Outcomes (Death or the Initiation of Epoprostenol Therapy) Among 40 Pediatric Patients With Pulmonary Arterial Hypertension

Variable	Adverse Outcome	No Adverse Outcome	P
Age	11.5 ± 0.7	11.5 ± 3.5	NS
Peak $\mathring{V}O_2$	14.6 ± 3.9	26.8 ± 7.2	<.0001
Percent peak $\mathring{V}O_2$	33 ± 8	60 ± 4	<.0001
$\mathring{V}_E/\mathring{V}CO_2$	55 ± 11	39 ± 8	<.0001
Percent $\mathring{V}_E/\mathring{V}CO_2$	170 ± 32	126 ± 20	<.0001
Percent O_2 pulse	40 percent	66 percent	0.04

NS, *nonsignificant*
From Yetman AT, Taylor AL, Doran A, et al: Utility of cardiopulmonary stress testing in assessing disease severity in children with pulmonary arterial hypertension. Am J Cardiol 95(5):697-699, 2005.

propanolamine, may predispose to severe pulmonary hypertension.[10]

Noninvasive testing can be useful for screening and assessing prognosis (see TABLE 18-2). Echocardiography is important in estimating pulmonary pressures and evaluating for structural abnormalities. Cardiopulmonary exercise testing also may be helpful provided severe disease is not present. In one study of 40 children with pulmonary arterial hypertension and a healthy control population, peak oxygen consumption correlated strongly with pulmonary vascular resistance measured by cardiac catheterization. A peak oxygen consumption of less than 15 mL/kg/min predicted a worse outcome or the need for additional therapy (TABLE 18-3).[11] Because respiratory disease is an important cause of pulmonary hypertension, radiographic and physiologic evaluation of the lung should be undertaken to exclude parenchymal lung disease. Cardiac catheterization is important to evaluate pulmonary artery pressures and resistance, as well as to determine acute reactivity of the pulmonary vasculature.

Congenital Heart Disease

A variety of congenital cardiac lesions can cause pulmonary hypertension[12] (TABLE 18-4). The age at which these lesions produce irreversible pulmonary vascular disease varies. In general, patients with a ventricular septal defect or patent ductus arteriosus do not develop irreversible pulmonary vascular changes before 2 years of age. Children with Down syndrome may have an increased risk of pulmonary hypertension if congenital cardiac lesions are present. Similarly,

infants with atrial or ventricular septal defects with concomitant chronic lung disease are at increased risk for the early development of severe pulmonary vascular disease. In one study of infants with bronchopulmonary dysplasia who underwent cardiac surgery for the repair of congenital heart disease, 25 percent of those who died had pulmonary arterial hypertension.[13]

Patients with cyanotic congenital cardiac lesions such as transposition of the great arteries, truncus arteriosus, and univentricular heart with high flow also may develop pulmonary hypertension. Palliative shunting operations for certain cardiac anomalies designed to increase pulmonary blood flow also may lead to pulmonary hypertension. Hypoxia with increased shunting is believed to be a potent stimulus for the rapid development of pulmonary vascular disease. Total correction of many cardiac lesions during the first months of life may prevent the later development of pulmonary hypertension.

Eisenmenger Syndrome

Eisenmenger syndrome is characterized by pulmonary hypertension with a reversed central shunt.[14] In general, the term is used for shunts distal to the tricuspid valve. Patients have elevated pulmonary vascular resistance and bidirectional or right-to-left shunting through a systemic-to-pulmonary connection, such as a ventricular septal defect, patent ductus arteriosus, univentricular heart, or aortopulmonary window. The shunt is initially left to right, but as the underlying condition continues to increase pulmonary vascular resistance, there is a reversal of the shunt to a right-to-left

TABLE 18-4

Cardiac Lesions Associated with Pulmonary Hypertension

Left-to-right Shunts

Ventricular septal defect
Atrioventricular septal (canal) defect
Patent ductus arteriosus
Atrial septal defect
Aortopulmonary window

Increased Pulmonary Venous Pressure

Cardiomyopathy
Coarctation of the aorta (left ventricular diastolic dysfunction)
Hypoplastic left heart syndrome
Shone complex
Mitral stenosis
Supravalvular mitral ring
Cor triatriatum
Pulmonary vein stenosis or veno-occlusive disease
Total anomalous pulmonary venous return

Cyanotic Heart Disease

Transposition of the great arteries
Truncus arteriosus
Tetralogy of Fallot (pulmonary atresia, ventricular septal defect)
Univentricular heart (high-flow ± restrictive atrial septum)

Anomalies of the Pulmonary Artery or Pulmonary Vein

Origin of a pulmonary artery from the aorta
Unilateral "absence" of a pulmonary artery
Scimitar syndrome

Palliative Shunting Operations

Waterston anastomosis
Potts anastomosis
Blalock-Taussig anastomosis

configuration, leading to cyanosis and erythrocytosis. In general, the prognosis of patients with Eisenmenger syndrome is much better than for patients with IPAH, but syncope, right-sided heart failure, and severe hypoxemia are similarly associated with a poor prognosis. Phlebotomy may be used in those with Eisenmenger syndrome to provide temporary relief of hyperviscosity symptoms or to improve perioperative hemostasis but should not be routinely recommended.[15] Noncardiac surgery is associated with a high mortality rate and should be managed by a multidisciplinary team experienced in the care of patients with this condition.

Idiopathic Pulmonary Arterial Hypertension

IPAH is a rare disease that occurs most frequently in young adult females.[16] IPAH is characterized by progressive and sustained elevations of pulmonary artery pressure without a defined etiology. Although generally developing in the adult population, pediatric IPAH is well reported and carried a dismal prognosis in the National Institutes of Health cohort, with a median survival of only 10 months in individuals less than 16 years old.[16a] Evaluation for possible IPAH in the pediatric age group is similar to that outlined for adults (see Chapter 6), but increased scrutiny for congenital cardiac disease is appropriate, and acute pulmonary vasoreactivity may be more common in this age group.[3] Obstructive sleep apnea and chronic thromboembolic disease are less commonly encountered in the pediatric age group, but they still require exclusion.

The clinical picture of IPAH in older children is similar to that in adults, with dyspnea on exertion, syncope, and chest pain as prominent findings. However, symptoms in infants and young children may be subtle and may include such nonspecific findings as poor appetite, failure to thrive, lethargy, tachycardia, vomiting, and irritability.

Familial Pulmonary Arterial Hypertension

Between 6 and 12 percent of cases of IPAH may be familial in origin with an autosomal dominant pattern of inheritance, and the disease manifests at younger ages with subsequent generations (termed "genetic anticipation").[17] The cause in childhood appears heterogeneous in nature, with genetic defects of transforming growth factor-β receptors playing an important role.[18] Diverse germline heterozygous mutations in the gene that encodes for the bone morphogenetic protein receptor-II (BMPR2) on chromosome 2q33 cause familial pulmonary arterial hypertension.[19] These mutations appear to cause uncontrolled proliferation of vascular smooth muscle.[22,23] More than 50 disease-causing defects in the *BMPR2* gene have been reported, although many have been identified in patients with no family history of pulmonary arterial hypertension, implying either a low disease penetrance or spontaneous mutations.[19-21, 24,25]

BMPR2 is a type 2 receptor of the transforming growth factor-β superfamily of cytokines, members of which are essential for the cellular proliferation, differentiation, and apoptosis. However, the role of *BMPR2* mutations in children remains less well understood. *BMPR2* mutations were not found in 13 children with IPAH[26] and have been found in only 6 percent of a mixed cohort of adults and children with pulmonary arterial hypertension associated with congenital heart defects.[27] One study evaluated genes encoding receptor members of the transforming growth factor-β cell-signaling pathway in 18 children with PAH (16 with IPAH and 2 with congenital heart defects). Germline mutations were observed in four patients (22 percent), all of whom had idiopathic PAH. Two of the mutations observed occurred in *BMPR2*. Mutations of the type 1 receptor activin receptor-like kinase (ALK)-1 may rarely cause pulmonary hypertension,[28] and a missense mutation of ALK-1 and a branch-site mutation of endoglin were also detected. Initial clinical features or progression of pulmonary hypertension did not distinguish between patients with or without mutations in the various genes.[28a]

Other genetic loci may also play important roles. Studies have suggested an impact by the serotonin transporter gene in some adults with PAH, and a study in children found that homozygosity for the long variant of the serotonin transporter gene was highly associated with idiopathic pulmonary hypertension in children.[29]

Clinical and genetic screening of first-degree relatives may be considered for early identification of at-risk individuals. Genetic screening involves analysis for *BMPR2* mutations, although failure to detect a mutation does not exclude development of IPAH in the future.[23] Clinical screening includes a chest radiograph, electrocardiogram, echocardiogram, and possibly a cardiopulmonary exercise test.

Respiratory Disease

Parenchymal lung disease is an important cause of pulmonary hypertension in many patients. Complications include hypoxic pulmonary vasoconstriction causing increased pulmonary artery pressures and can lead to right ventricular hypertrophy and failure. Right ventricular function usually is preserved until disease is advanced. In most cases, correction of hypoxia can lead to reversal of pulmonary hypertension. However, the development of cor pulmonale carries a poorer prognosis for reversibility.

Management of cor pulmonale depends on the precise etiology of lung disease, as well as disease severity. Nocturnal oxygen administration may alleviate hypoxia, typically without causing hypercapnia. In patients with cystic fibrosis, calcium channel blockers have not been proven effective and may worsen oxygenation when cor pulmonale is present.[30,31] For patients with end-stage lung disease from cystic fibrosis, lung transplantation may represent the most attractive option, although long-term outcomes remain disappointing.

Disorders of respiratory mechanics may also lead to hypoxia and pulmonary hypertension, as can bronchopulmonary dysplasia.[32-32a] More recent studies have suggested that abnormalities of the pulmonary vasculature may be a primary rather than secondary cause of abnormal alveolarization in bronchopulmonary dysplasia.[33] Patients with congenital diaphragmatic hernia are at risk for pulmonary hypertension, which can develop during any phase of the disease. In addition to lung hypoplasia, patients with congenital diaphragmatic hernia may develop pulmonary artery or pulmonary vein stenosis.[34]

Thromboembolic Disease

Chronic thromboembolic disease as a cause of pulmonary hypertension in children is uncommon.

However, the condition can occur rarely, and an accurate diagnosis is essential for management.[35] Predisposing factors include collagen vascular diseases, thrombophilia, bacterial endocarditis, and ventriculoatrial shunt for hydrocephalus. Likewise, oral contraceptive agents may cause hypercoagulability, leading to pulmonary thromboembolic phenomena.

Diagnosis of chronic thromboembolic pulmonary hypertension in children requires a high index of suspicion, as well as evaluation by ventilation-perfusion scintigraphy, computed tomography scanning, or angiography. In adults with chronic thromboembolic pulmonary hypertension, surgically accessible disease, and no severe comorbidities, pulmonary thromboendarterectomy has been demonstrated to improve survival and quality of life in adult patients. A similar approach should be considered for children who develop this condition despite the relative paucity of data in the pediatric age group (see Chapter 13).

Therapeutic Considerations

General Principles

Most children with mild pulmonary hypertension do not require treatment other than therapy directed toward the underlying cause of the condition. Therefore, a complete evaluation to determine all causes is imperative. Other general principles include avoidance of pregnancy, which is associated with significant maternal and fetal risk from the cardio- pulmonary demands of normal pregnancy. Oral contraceptive use is a risk factor for venous thromboembolism, which may be poorly tolerated in this population (see Chapter 17)

Vasodilator Therapy

Without therapy, and sometimes despite appropriate surgical correction of congenital cardiac lesions, pulmonary arterial hypertension progresses at a variable rate. Because vasoconstriction is an important component of medial hypertrophy, vasodilators frequently are used to decrease pulmonary artery pressure, improve cardiac output, and potentially reverse some of the pulmonary vascular changes noted in the lung. Our long-term strategy for pulmonary hypertension management in children is shown (FIGURE 18-1).

Before starting vasodilator therapy, vasodilator responsiveness should be assessed in a controlled

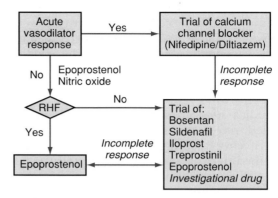

LONG-TERM PAH TREATMENT STRATEGY: 2006

Consider: atrial septostomy/lung transplantation

Figure 18-1. Algorithm of the Management of Pediatric Pulmonary Arterial Hypertension. Children who respond acutely to vasodilator testing with nitric oxide or epoprostenol should be treated initially with calcium channel blockers, such as nifedipine or diltiazem. Children who do not respond to acute vasoreactivity testing should receive other forms of therapy. When pulmonary vasculature is nonreactive and there is right-sided heart failure, continuous intravenous epoprostenol should be strongly considered. In the absence of right-sided heart failure, other agents may be tried first. Bosentan, treprostinil, sildenafil, and iloprost have been studied and approved for management of adult pulmonary arterial hypertension. Other drugs that are investigational, such as sitaxsentan, are being assessed. For patients with severe disease, combination therapy may be considered but has not been well studied.

setting, ideally in the cardiac catheterization unit. A positive response is defined by a fall in mean pulmonary artery pressure by more than 10 mmHg to a value less than 40 mmHg, with no change or an increase in cardiac output.[7,36] The younger the child at the time of testing, the greater is the likelihood of acute pulmonary vasodilation in response to vasoreactivity testing.[6] Many intravenous and inhaled vasodilators have been used for testing of vasodilator responsiveness, including inhaled nitric oxide or iloprost and intravenous epoprostenol or adenosine. Inhaled nitric oxide is the agent used most frequently in the pediatric population.[37,38]

Newer vasodilator agents, particularly inhaled nitric oxide, have been an important advance in safely determining vasoreactivity. Inhaled nitric oxide therapy improves gas exchange and selectively lowers pulmonary vascular resistance in several clinical diseases, including idiopathic pulmonary hypertension and congenital heart disease.[37-47] Inhaled nitric oxide diffuses to the adjacent smooth muscle cell, where it activates soluble guanylate cyclase, resulting in an increase in cyclic guanine monophosphate (cGMP) and vasodilation. Inhaled nitric oxide is recommended as the agent of choice for evaluating pulmonary vasoreactivity (see FIGURE 18-1).

Studies have explored the role of long-term inhaled nitric oxide for managing pulmonary hypertensive disorders.[41,48,49] Although it causes sustained decreases in pulmonary vascular resistance, adverse hemodynamic effects may occur after abrupt withdrawal.[50,51] Inhibition of phosphodiesterase type 5, which degrades cGMP within vascular smooth muscle, causes vasodilation and may attenuate this rebound effect.[52,53]

Using calcium channel antagonists to evaluate vasoreactivity is problematic, because these drugs can cause a decrease in cardiac output or a marked drop in systemic blood pressure.[6] Such deleterious effects may be prolonged because of the relatively long half-life of calcium channel blockers. Consequently, elevated right atrial pressure and low cardiac output are contraindications to acute or long-term calcium channel blockade.

It is recommended that an acute trial of calcium channel blocker therapy be performed only in those patients who are acutely responsive to either nitric oxide or epoprostenol. Patients who do not have an acute vasodilatory response are unlikely to benefit from this form of therapy.[36] At least 60 percent of children with severe pulmonary hypertension are not responsive to acute vasodilator testing and therefore require therapy other than calcium channel antagonists.

Children who respond acutely to calcium channel antagonists risk management failure when maintained long-term on these agents. Calcium channel antagonist use has been associated with a 5-year survival rate of 97 percent for acute responders.[36] However, after 10 years the survival rate was only 81 percent and management success only 47 percent.[3] Therefore, close follow-up is required, including serial vasodilator testing and possible transplant evaluation before clinical deterioration develops.[3]

Adults with IPAH and children with congenital heart disease demonstrate an imbalance in the biosynthesis of thromboxane A_2 and prostacyclin[53a,53b]. Likewise, adults and children with severe pulmonary hypertension show diminished prostacyclin synthase expression in the lung vasculature.[54] Long-term administration of prostacyclin as intravenous epoprostenol has been shown to improve survival and quality of life in adults and children with IPAH, whereas previously many such patients would have been poor candidates for calcium channel antagonist treatment and would have required lung transplantation, with its attendant poor long-term outcomes (FIGURE 18-2).[3,7,36,55] Using long-term epoprostenol, the 5-year survival in children with idiopathic pulmonary hypertension who were not candidates for calcium channel blocker therapy may be higher than 80 percent.[36]

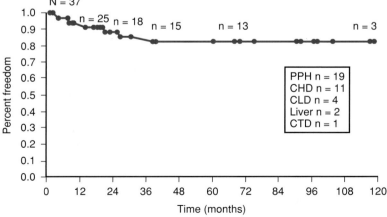

Figure 18-2. Kaplan-Meier Curves of Long-term Prostacyclin Treatment in Children With Pulmonary Hypertension at the Children's Hospital Heart Institute, Pediatric Heart Lung Center, Denver, Colorado. *CHD,* congenital heart disease; *CLD,* chronic lung disease; *CTD,* connective tissue disease; *Liver,* liver disease; *PPH,* primary pulmonary hypertension.

Epoprostenol use in patients with congenital heart disease and other nonidiopathic etiologies of PAH has shown significant benefits on hemodynamics, symptoms, and exercise capacity.[56,56a] Side effects of prostacyclin analogues are dosage dependent and include nausea, anorexia, jaw pain, diarrhea, and musculoskeletal aches and pains. Other adverse events are related to intravenous delivery through a central venous catheter, and thus include thrombosis, hemorrhage, cellulitis, and line sepsis. Abrupt cessation may cause acute deterioration and, in some cases, death. In patients with residual right-to-left shunting, continuous prostacyclin occasionally may worsen shunt physiology and may cause complications such as cerebrovascular accident from paradoxical embolism.[56a]

Alternative Delivery Routes for Prostacyclin Analogues

The effectiveness of epoprostenol therapy coupled with the problems inherent in its delivery has led to the use of prostacyclin analogues with alternative delivery routes. Treprostinil, a subcutaneous prostacyclin analogue, has a half-life of 45 minutes with a side effect profile similar to that of prostacyclin. Importantly, it can cause pain and erythema around the infusion site, thus limiting its usefulness in young children. Treprostinil was tested in a multicenter international placebo-controlled, randomized study and had beneficial effects on hemodynamics and exercise tolerance, the latter being dosage dependent.[57] Studies of intravenous and inhaled treprostinil in both adults and children are ongoing, with the former licensed for use in the United States in 2004.

An inhaled prostacyclin analogue, iloprost, has undergone initial trials with significant beneficial effects on symptomatology and quality of life. Iloprost has a half-life of 20-25 minutes and 6 to 9 inhalations a day are required if it is to be clinically effective. The advantage of an inhaled prostanoid is that it can cause selective pulmonary vasodilation without affecting systemic blood pressure. Additionally, inhaled prostacyclin analogues can improve gas exchange and intrapulmonary shunt in cases of impaired ventilation-perfusion by redistributing pulmonary blood flow from nonventilated to ventilated, aerosol-accessible lung regions.[58] In children with congenital heart disease and PAH, inhaled iloprost may be as effective in lowering pulmonary artery pressure and resistance as inhaled nitric oxide, and thus may be useful in evaluation of acute vasoreactivity.[37,59] One random-

ized controlled trial of aerosolized prostacyclin therapy in children with acute lung injury demonstrated improved oxygenation.[60]

Inhaled iloprost has been available in Europe for a number of years and was approved in the United States in late 2004. The U.S. Food and Drug Administration noted at the time of approval that the drug "has not been studied in children under the age of 18"; nonetheless, it appears to have promise in this population provided that the logistics of reliably undertaking 6-9 inhalations per day are not prohibitive.[61]

Beraprost is an orally active prostacyclin analogue with a half-life of 35-40 minutes. Although beneficial effects have been noted in short-term trials, these may be attenuated with prolonged use.[62] Concerns have been raised regarding its overall risk-to-benefit ratio, and the medication is not licensed for use in the United States.

Endothelin Receptor Antagonists

Another target for management of pulmonary hypertension is the vasoconstrictor peptide, endothelin (ET).[63] The endothelins are a family of isopeptides consisting of ET-1, ET-2, and ET-3. ET-1 is a potent vasoactive peptide produced primarily in vascular endothelial cells, but it also may be produced by smooth muscle cells. Two receptor subtypes, ET_A and ET_B, mediate the activity of ET-1. ET_A and ET_B receptors on vascular smooth muscle mediate vasoconstriction, whereas ET_B receptors on endothelial cells cause release of nitric oxide and prostacyclin (PGI_2), and act as clearance receptors for circulating ET-1. Endothelin-1 expression is increased in the pulmonary arteries of patients with pulmonary hypertension.

Bosentan, a dual ET receptor antagonist, lowers pulmonary artery pressure and resistance and improves exercise tolerance in adults with pulmonary arterial hypertension.[64] In children with IPAH or pulmonary arterial hypertension related to congenital heart disease, bosentan lowers pulmonary pressure and resistance and is well tolerated.[65] Bosentan also has been used in adults with Eisenmenger physiology with good effect.[66]

Bosentan has been used successfully in children treated with long-term epoprostenol.[67,67a] Concomitant use of bosentan allowed for a decrease in epoprostenol dosage and its associated side effects, and it allowed for the discontinuation of epoprostenol in some children.[67] More recent work indicates that bosentan or other ET receptor antagonists may be used as a first-line agent for advanced pulmonary

CHANGE IN WHO FUNCTIONAL CLASS

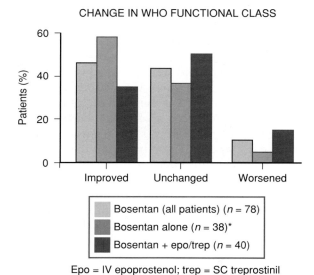

Epo = IV epoprostenol; trep = SC treprostinil

Figure 18-3. World Health Organization functional class at the initiation of bosentan therapy and after at least 8 weeks of management. Patients who died were assigned functional class IV. (From Ref. 69.)

VITAL AND TREATMENT STATUS: 1 YEAR

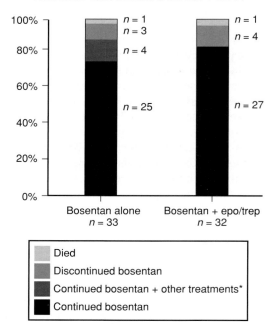

Epo = IV epoprostenol; trep = SC treprostinil
* = additional PAH therapy, septostomy, or transplant

Figure 18-4. Patient Survival and Treatment Status After 1 Year of Management With Bosentan. (From Ref. 69.)

hypertension, resulting in prolonged survival in many cases.[68] One study evaluated bosentan in 86 children,[69] using a dosing strategy developed in earlier studies.[65] Bosentan as monotherapy appeared to be more effective than bosentan as an add-on to prostacyclin or treprostinil. Furthermore, children treated with bosentan as part of a targeted strategy experienced longer survival than did historical controls. Bosentan therapy improved World Health Organization functional class in 46% of children and stabilized functional class in 44% of children (FIGURE 18-3). Sixty-five of the 86 children (76 percent) were followed for at least 1 year. Patient survival and treatment status after 1 year of bosentan management are shown in FIGURE 18-4.

Sitaxsentan and ambrisentan are selective ET_A receptor antagonists with high oral bioavailability and a long duration of action. These agents may benefit patients with pulmonary arterial hypertension by blocking the vasoconstrictor effects of ET_A receptors while maintaining the vasodilator clearance functions of ET_B receptors, although differences in clinical outcomes as compared with nonselective endothelin antagonists have not been demonstrated.[70] Sitaxsentan given orally for 12 weeks improved exercise capacity and cardiopulmonary hemodynamics in patients with pul-

monary arterial hypertension that was idiopathic or related to connective tissue or congenital heart disease.[71] Selective ET_A receptor blockade has also been reported in the management of postoperative congenital heart disease.[72,73]

Phosphodiesterase 5 Inhibitors

Specific phosphodiesterase 5 inhibitors, such as sildenafil,[74-78] promote an increase in cGMP levels and thus promote pulmonary vasodilation and remodeling (see FIGURE 18-5). Sildenafil is as effective an acute pulmonary vasodilator as inhaled nitric oxide.[79] Sildenafil or other phosphodiesterase 5 inhibitors may also be useful in inhaled nitric oxide therapy withdrawal,[52,53] in postoperative pulmonary hypertension,[80,81] or in pulmonary hypertension related to chronic lung disease.[82] However, in the acute postoperative setting, sildenafil may worsen oxygenation in some cases,[80,83] possibly due to impaired ventilation-perfusion matching.

Studies examining the use of oral phosphodiesterase 5 inhibitors in children are ongoing.[78,84] In 14 children with PAH, sildenafil was given at

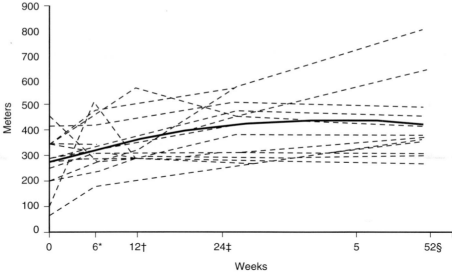

Figure 18-5. Six-minute Walk Distance Following Management With Oral Sildenafil in 14 Children With Pulmonary Artery Hypertension. Distance walked increased between baseline and 24 weeks, with a sustained plateau between 24 and 52 weeks. Mean distance walked after 6 weeks, 12 weeks, 6 months, and 1 year was 331 ± 112, 335 ± 91, 443 ± 107, and 432 ± 156 meters, respectively. (From Ref. 84.)

dosages of 0.25-1.0 mg/kg 4 times daily. During sildenafil therapy, the mean distance walked in 6 minutes increased from 278 to 443 meters over 6 months (P = .02), and this benefit was largely maintained after 12 months.[84]

Anticoagulation

In retrospective trials in adults with IPAH, warfarin use has been associated with improved survival. Although long-term anticoagulation has not been studied widely in children, it usually is recommended. In IPAH, the aim is to maintain an International Normalized Ratio between 1.5 and 2.0. The use of anticoagulation in patients with Eisenmenger syndrome is controversial, and the potential risks and benefits must be weighed carefully.

Surgery

The timing of surgery in patients with congenital heart disease is beyond the scope of this book but depends upon a number of factors. These include age, lesion, vasoreactivity during cardiac catheterization, findings from lung biopsy, and pulmonary wedge angiography.[37,47,85]

Atrial Septostomy

General indications for atrial septostomy include pulmonary hypertension, syncope and intractable heart failure refractory to long-term vasodilator management,[86,86a] and symptomatic low-cardiac output states. Risks associated with this procedure include worsening of hypoxemia with resultant right ventricular ischemia, worsening right ventricular failure, increased left atrial pressure, and pulmonary edema.

Transplantation

For patients who do not respond to prolonged vasodilator treatment, or with certain lesions, such as pulmonary vein stenosis, lung transplantation should be considered.[87–92] Cystic fibrosis accounts for most pediatric lung transplants. IPAH is an indication for transplantation in approximately 15 percent of patients. Heart-lung transplantation may be necessary for certain patients, including those with complex congenital heart disease. A retrospective study found similar outcomes for children with congenital heart disease undergoing repair of congenital heart lesions combined with lung transplantation as compared with combined heart-lung transplantation.[91] However, a report analyzed the United Network for Organ Sharing/International

Society for Heart and Lung Transplantation Joint Thoracic Registry to determine predictors of survival in those with Eisenmenger syndrome. There was a highly significant benefit of heart-lung transplantation over lung transplantation with defect closure for patients with ventricular septal defects (P = .0001).[92]

Conclusion

Advances in the understanding of the pulmonary vasculature have led to improved survival in children with severe pulmonary hypertension. The timely diagnosis of pediatric pulmonary hypertension is of paramount importance, because management strategies can improve both morbidity and mortality. An extensive evaluation is performed in children with severe pulmonary hypertension, because the most successful strategy involves management of underlying causative or associated disorders. A targeted approach includes acute vasodilator testing during cardiac catheterization to determine long-term therapy. In patients reactive to acute vasodilator testing with short-acting agents such as inhaled nitric oxide, calcium channel blockers may provide effective therapy. In those patients not reactive to acute vasodilator testing, one should consider other forms of therapy, such as prostanoids, endothelin antagonists, or phosphodiesterase inhibitors.

References

1. Thilenius OG, Nadas AS, Jockin H: Primary pulmonary vascular obstruction in children. *Pediatrics* 36:75-87, 1965.
2. Sandoval J, Bauerle O, Gomez A, et al: Primary pulmonary hypertension in children: Clinical characterization and survival. *J Am Coll Cardiol* 25:466-474, 1995.
3. Yung D, Widlitz AC, Rosenzweig EB, et al: Outcomes in children with idiopathic pulmonary arterial hypertension. *Circulation* 110:660-665, 2004.
4. Rich S, editor: Primary pulmonary hypertension. Executive summary from the world symposium. 1998, Geneva: World Health Organization.
5. Barst RJ: Recent advances in the treatment of pediatric pulmonary artery hypertension. *Pediatr Clin North Am* 46:331-345, 1999.
6. Widlitz A, Barst RJ: Pulmonary arterial hypertension in children. *Eur Respir J* 21:155-176, 2003.
7. Rashid A, Ivy DD: Severe paediatric pulmonary hypertension: New management strategies. *Arch Dis Child* 90:92-98, 2005.
8. Das BB, Wolfe RR, Chan KC, et al: High-altitude pulmonary edema in children with underlying cardiopulmonary disorders and pulmonary hypertension living at altitude. *Arch Pediatr Adolesc Med* 158:1170-1176, 2004.
9. Condino AA, Ivy DD, O'Connor JA, et al: Portopulmonary hypertension in pediatric patients. *J Pediatr* 147:20-26, 2005.
10. Barst RJ, Abenhaim L: Fatal pulmonary arterial hypertension associated with phenylpropanolamine exposure. *Heart* 90:e42, 2004.
11. Yetman AT, Taylor AL, Doran A, et al: Utility of cardiopulmonary stress testing in assessing disease severity in children with pulmonary arterial hypertension. *Am J Cardiol* 95:697-699, 2005.
12. Beghetti M: Congenital heart disease and pulmonary hypertension. *Rev Port Cardiol* 23:273-281, 2004.
13. McMahon CJ, Penny DJ, Nelson DP, et al: Preterm infants with congenital heart disease and bronchopulmonary dysplasia: Postoperative course and outcome after cardiac surgery. *Pediatrics* 116:423-430, 2005.
14. Berman EB, Barst RJ: Eisenmenger's syndrome: Current management. *Prog Cardiovasc Dis* 45:129-138, 2002.
15. Perloff JK, Marelli AJ, Miner PD: Risk of stroke in adults with cyanotic congenital heart disease. *Circulation* 87:1954-1959, 1993.
16. Humbert M, Sitbon O, Simonneau G: Treatment of pulmonary arterial hypertension. *N Engl J Med* 351:1425-1436, 2004.
16a. D'Alonzo GE, Barst RJ, Ayres SM, et al: Survival in patients with primary pulmonary hypertension: results from a national prospective registry. *Ann Intern Med* 115:343-349, 1991.
17. Loyd JE, Butler MG, Foroud TM, et al: Genetic anticipation and abnormal gender ratio at birth in familial primary pulmonary hypertension. *Am J Respir Crit Care Med* 152:93-97, 1995.
18. Harrison RE, Berger R, Haworth SG, et al: Transforming growth factor-β receptor mutations and pulmonary arterial hypertension in childhood. *Circulation* 111:435-441, 2005.
19. Deng Z, Morse JH, Slager SL, et al: Familial primary pulmonary hypertension (gene *PPH1*) is caused by mutations in the bone morphogenetic protein receptor-II gene. *Am J Hum Genet* 67:737-744, 2000.
20. Thomson JR, Machado RD, Pauciulo MW, et al: Sporadic primary pulmonary hypertension is associated with germline mutations of the gene encoding BMPR-II, a receptor member of the TGF-β family. *J Med Genet* 37:741-745, 2000.
21. Lane KB, Machado RD, Pauciulo MW, et al: Heterozygous germline mutations in *BMPR2*, encoding a TGF-β receptor, cause familial primary pulmonary hypertension. The International PPH Consortium. *Nat Genet* 26:81-84, 2000.

22. Newman JH, Wheeler L, Lane KB, et al: Mutation in the gene for bone morphogenetic protein receptor II as a cause of primary pulmonary hypertension in a large kindred. *N Engl J Med* 345:319-324, 2001.

23. Trembath RC, Harrison R: Insights into the genetic and molecular basis of primary pulmonary hypertension. *Pediatr Res* 53:883-888, 2003.

24. Machado RD, Pauciulo MW, Thomson JR, et al: *BMPR2* haploinsufficiency as the inherited molecular mechanism for primary pulmonary hypertension. *Am J Hum Genet* 68:92-102, 2001.

25. Machado RD, Rudarakanchana N, Atkinson C, et al: Functional interaction between BMPR-II and Tctex-1, a light chain of dynein, is isoform-specific and disrupted by mutations underlying primary pulmonary hypertension. *Hum Mol Genet* 12:3277-3286, 2003.

26. Grunig E, Koehler R, Miltenberger-Miltenyi G, et al: Primary pulmonary hypertension in children may have a different genetic background than in adults. *Pediatr Res* 56:571-578, 2004.

27. Roberts KE, McElroy JJ, Wong WP, et al: *BMPR2* mutations in pulmonary arterial hypertension with congenital heart disease. *Eur Respir J* 24:371-374, 2004.

28. Trembath RC, Thomson JR, Machado RD, et al: Clinical and molecular genetic features of pulmonary hypertension in patients with hereditary hemorrhagic telangiectasia. *N Engl J Med* 345:325-334, 2001.

28a. Harrison RE, Berger R, Haworth SG, et al: Transforming Growth Factor-β Receptor Mutations and Pulmonary Arterial Hypertension in Chilhood. *Circulation* 111:435-441, 2005.

29. Vachharajani A, Saunders S: Allelic variation in the serotonin transporter (5HTT) gene contributes to idiopathic pulmonary hypertension in children. *Biochem Biophys Res Commun* 334:376-379, 2005.

30. Davidson A, Bossuyt A, Dab I: Acute effects of oxygen, nifedipine, and diltiazem in patients with cystic fibrosis and mild pulmonary hypertension. *Pediatr Pulmonol* 6:53-59, 1989.

31. Geggel RL, Dozor AJ, Fyler DC, et al: Effect of vasodilators at rest and during exercise in young adults with cystic fibrosis and chronic cor pulmonale. *Am Rev Respir Dis* 131:531-536, 1985.

32. Abman SH, Groothius JR: Pathophysiology and treatment of bronchopulmonary dysplasia. Current issues. *Pediatr Clin North Am* 41:277-315, 1994.

32a. Mourani PM, Ivy DD, Gao D, et al: Pulmonary vascular effects of inhaled nitric oxide and oxygen tension in bronchopulmonary dysplasia. *Am J Resp crit Care Med* 170:1006-1013, 2004.

33. Parker TA, Abman SH: The pulmonary circulation in bronchopulmonary dysplasia. *Semin Neonatol* 8:51-62, 2003.

34. Kinsella JP, Ivy DD, Abman SH: Pulmonary vasodilator therapy in congenital diaphragmatic hernia: Acute, late, and chronic pulmonary hypertension. *Semin Perinatol* 29:123-128, 2005.

35. Auger WR, Channick RN, Kerr KM, et al: Evaluation of patients with suspected chronic thromboembolic pulmonary hypertension. *Semin Thorac Cardiovasc Surg* 11:179-190, 1999.

36. Barst RJ, Maislin G, Fishman AP: Vasodilator therapy for primary pulmonary hypertension in children. *Circulation* 99:1197-1208, 1999.

37. Rimensberger PC, Spahr-Schopfer I, Berner M, et al: Inhaled nitric oxide versus aerosolized iloprost in secondary pulmonary hypertension in children with congenital heart disease: Vasodilator capacity and cellular mechanisms. *Circulation* 103:544-548, 2001.

38. Atz AM, Adatia I, Lock JE, et al: Combined effects of nitric oxide and oxygen during acute pulmonary vasodilator testing. *J Am Coll Cardiol* 33:813-819, 1999.

39. Pepke-Zaba J, Higenbottam TW, Dinh-Xuan AT, et al: Inhaled nitric oxide as a cause of selective pulmonary vasodilatation in pulmonary hypertension. *Lancet* 338:1173-1174, 1991.

40. Ivy DD, Kinsella JP, Wolfe RR, et al: Atrial natriuretic peptide and nitric oxide in children with pulmonary hypertension after surgical repair of congenital heart disease. *Am J Cardiol* 77:102-105, 1996.

41. Ivy DD, Parker D, Doran A, et al: Acute hemodynamic effects and home therapy using novel pulsed nasal nitric oxide delivery system in children and young adults with pulmonary hypertension. *Am J Cardiol* 92:886-890, 2003.

42. Ivy DD, Griebel JL, Kinsella JP, et al: Acute hemodynamic effects of pulsed delivery of low flow nasal nitric oxide in children with pulmonary hypertension. *J Pediatr* 133:453-456, 1998.

43. Berner M, Beghetti M, Spahr-Schopfer I, et al: Inhaled nitric oxide to test the vasodilator capacity of the pulmonary vascular bed in children with long-standing pulmonary hypertension and congenital heart disease. *Am J Cardiol* 77:532-535, 1996.

44. Atz AM, Wessel DL: Inhaled nitric oxide in the neonate with cardiac disease. *Semin Perinatol* 21:441-455, 1997.

45. Wessel DL, Adatia I, Giglia TM, et al: Use of inhaled nitric oxide and acetylcholine in the evaluation of pulmonary hypertension and endothelial function after cardiopulmonary bypass. *Circulation* 88:2128-2138, 1993.

46. Roberts JD, Jr, Lang P, Bigatello LM, et al: Inhaled nitric oxide in congenital heart disease. *Circulation* 87:447-453, 1993.

47. Balzer DT, Kort H, Day RW, Corneli HM, et al: Inhaled nitric oxide as a preoperative test (INOP Test I): The INOP Test Study Group. *Circulation* 106:176-181, 2002.

48. Channick RN, Newhart JW, Johnson FW, et al: Pulsed delivery of inhaled nitric oxide to patients with primary pulmonary hypertension: An ambulatory delivery system and initial clinical tests. *Chest* 109:1545-1549, 1996.

49. Katayama Y, Higenbottam TW, Cremona G, et al: Minimizing the inhaled dose of NO with breath-by-breath delivery of spikes of concentrated gas. *Circulation* 98:2429-2432, 1998.

50. Atz AM, Adatia I, Wessel DL: Rebound pulmonary hypertension after inhalation of nitric oxide. *Ann Thorac Surg* 62:1759-1764, 1996.

51. Pearl JM, Nelson DP, Raake JL, et al: Inhaled nitric oxide increases endothelin-1 levels: A potential cause of rebound pulmonary hypertension. *Crit Care Med* 30:89-93, 2002.

52. Ivy DD, Kinsella JP, Ziegler JW, et al: Dipyridamole attenuates rebound pulmonary hypertension after inhaled nitric oxide withdrawal in postoperative congenital heart disease. *J Thorac Cardiovasc Surg* 115:875-882, 1998.

53. Atz AM, Wessel DL: Sildenafil ameliorates effects of inhaled nitric oxide withdrawal. *Anesthesiology* 91:307-310, 1999.

53a. Adatia I, Barrow SE, Stratton PD, et al: Thromboxane A2 and prostacyclin biosynthesis in children and adolescents with pulmonary vascular disease. *Circulation* 88:2117-2122, 1993.

53b. Christman BW, McPherson CD, Newman JH, et al: An imbalance between the excretion of thromboxane and prostacyclin metabolites in pulmonary hypertension. *N Engl J Med* 327:70-75, 1992.

54. Tuder RM, Cool CD, Geraci MW, et al: Prostacyclin synthase expression is decreased in lungs from patients with severe pulmonary hypertension. *Am J Respir Crit Care Med* 159:1925-1932, 1999.

55. Sitbon O, Humbert M, Nunes H, et al: Long-term intravenous epoprostenol infusion in primary pulmonary hypertension: Prognostic factors and survival. *J Am Coll Cardiol* 40:780-788, 2002.

56. Rosenzweig EB, Kerstein D, Barst RJ: Long-term prostacyclin for pulmonary hypertension with associated congenital heart defects. *Circulation* 99:1858-1865, 1999.

56a. Fernandes SM, Newburger JW, Lang P, et al: Usefulness of epoprostenol therapy in the severely ill adolescent/adult with Eisenmenger physiology. *Am J Cardiol* 91:632-635, 2003.

57. Simonneau G, Barst RJ, Galie N, et al: Continuous subcutaneous infusion of treprostinil, a prostacyclin analogue, in patients with pulmonary arterial hypertension: A double-blind, randomized, placebo-controlled trial. *Am J Respir Crit Care Med* 165:800-804, 2002.

58. Max M, Rossaint R: Inhaled prostacyclin in the treatment of pulmonary hypertension. *Eur J Pediatr* 158:S23-S26, 1999.

59. Hallioglu O, Dilber E, Celiker A: Comparison of acute hemodynamic effects of aerosolized and intravenous iloprost in secondary pulmonary hypertension in children with congenital heart disease. *Am J Cardiol* 92:1007-1009, 2003.

60. Dahlem P, van Aalderen WM, de Neef M, et al: Randomized controlled trial of aerosolized prostacyclin therapy in children with acute lung injury. *Crit Care Med* 32:1055-1060, 2004.

61. Olschewski H, Simonneau G, Galie N, et al: Inhaled iloprost for severe pulmonary hypertension. *N Engl J Med* 347:322-329, 2002.

62. Barst RJ, McGoon M, McLaughlin V, et al: Beraprost therapy for pulmonary arterial hypertension. *J Am Coll Cardiol* 41:2119-2125, 2003.

63. Beghetti M, Black SM, Fineman JR: Endothelin-1 in congenital heart disease. *Pediatr Res* 57:16R-20R, 2005.

64. Rubin LJ, Badesch DB, Barst RJ, et al: Bosentan therapy for pulmonary arterial hypertension. *N Engl J Med* 346:896-903, 2002.

65. Barst RJ, Ivy D, Dingemanse J, et al: Pharmacokinetics, safety, and efficacy of bosentan in pediatric patients with pulmonary arterial hypertension. *Clin Pharmacol Ther* 73:372-382, 2003.

66. Gatzoulis MA, Rogers P, Li W, et al: Safety and tolerability of bosentan in adults with Eisenmenger physiology. *Int J Cardiol* 98:147-151, 2005.

67. Ivy DD, Doran A, Claussen L, et al: Weaning and discontinuation of epoprostenol in children with idiopathic pulmonary arterial hypertension receiving concomitant bosentan. *Am J Cardiol* 93:943-946, 2004.

67a. Maiya S, Hislop A, Flynn, et al: Response to bosentan in children with pulmonary hypertension. *Heart* online: 10.1136/hrt.2005.072314

68. McLaughlin VV, Sitbon O, Badesch DB, et al: Survival with first-line bosentan in patients with primary pulmonary hypertension. *Eur Respir J* 25:244-249, 2005.

69. Rosenzweig EB, Ivy DD, Widlitz AC, et al: Effects of long-term bosentan in children with pulmonary arterial hypertension. *J Am Coll Cardiol* 46:697-704, 2005.

70. Ivy DD, McMurtry IF, Colvin K, et al: Development of occlusive neointimal lesions in distal pulmonary arteries of endothelin B receptor-deficient rats: A new model of severe pulmonary arterial hypertension. *Circulation* 111:2988-2996, 2005.

71. Barst RJ, Langleben D, Frost A, et al: Sitaxsentan therapy for pulmonary arterial hypertension. *Am J Respir Crit Care Med* 169:441-447, 2004.

72. Schulze-Neick I, Li J, Reader JA, et al: The endothelin antagonist BQ123 reduces pulmonary vascular resistance after surgical intervention for congenital heart disease. *J Thorac Cardiovasc Surg* 124:435-441, 2002.

73. Prendergast B, Newby DE, Wilson LE, et al: Early therapeutic experience with the endothelin antagonist BQ-123 in pulmonary hypertension after congenital heart surgery. *Heart* 82:505-508, 1999.

74. Prasad S, Wilkinson J, Gatzoulis MA: Sildenafil in primary pulmonary hypertension. *N Engl J Med* 343:1342, 2000.

75. Kumar S: Indian doctor in protest after using Viagra to save "blue babies." *BMJ* 325:181, 2002.

76. Michelakis ED, Tymchak W, Noga M, et al: Long-term treatment with oral sildenafil is safe and improves functional capacity and hemodynamics in patients with pulmonary arterial hypertension. *Circulation* 108:2066-2069, 2003.

77. Abrams D, Schulze-Neick I, Magee AG: Sildenafil as a selective pulmonary vasodilator in childhood primary pulmonary hypertension. *Heart* 84:E4, 2000.

78. Karatza AA, Bush A, Magee AG: Safety and efficacy of sildenafil therapy in children with pulmonary hypertension. *Int J Cardiol* 100:267-273, 2005.

79. Michelakis E, Tymchak W, Lien D, et al: Oral sildenafil is an effective and specific pulmonary vasodilator in patients with pulmonary arterial hypertension: Comparison with inhaled nitric oxide. *Circulation* 105:2398-2403, 2002.

80. Schulze-Neick I, Hartenstein P, Li J, et al: Intravenous sildenafil is a potent pulmonary vasodilator in children with congenital heart disease. *Circulation* 108:II167-173, 2003.

81. Atz AM, Lefler AK, Fairbrother DL, et al: Sildenafil augments the effect of inhaled nitric oxide for postoperative pulmonary hypertensive crisis. *J Thorac Cardiovasc Surg* 124:628-629, 2002.

82. Ghofrani HA, Wiedemann R, Rose F, et al: Sildenafil for treatment of lung fibrosis and pulmonary hypertension: A randomised controlled trial. *Lancet* 360:895-900, 2002.

83. Stocker C, Penny DJ, Brizard CP, et al: Intravenous sildenafil and inhaled nitric oxide: A randomised trial in infants after cardiac surgery. *Intensive Care Med* 29:1996-2003, 2003.

84. Humpl T, Reyes JT, Holtby H, et al: Beneficial effect of oral sildenafil therapy on childhood pulmonary arterial hypertension: Twelve-month clinical trial of a single-drug, open-label, pilot study. *Circulation* 111:3274-3280, 2005.

85. Rabinovitch M: Pulmonary hypertension: Pathophysiology as a basis for clinical decision making. *J Heart Lung Transplant* 18:1041-1053, 1999.

86. Sandoval J, Gaspar J, Pulido T, et al: Graded balloon dilation atrial septostomy in severe primary pulmonary hypertension. A therapeutic alternative for patients nonresponsive to vasodilator treatment. *J Am Coll Cardiol* 32:297-304, 1998.

86a. Micheletti A, Hislop A, Lammers A, et al: Role of atrial septostomy in the treatment of children with pulmonary arterial hypertension. *Heart* online: 10.1136/hrt.2005.077669

87. Mallory GB, Spray TL: Paediatric lung transplantation. *Eur Respir J* 24:839-845, 2004.

88. Boucek MM, Edwards LB, Keck BM, et al: Registry of the International Society for Heart and Lung Transplantation: Eigth official pediatric report. *J Heart Lung Transplant* 24:968-982, 2005.

89. Gaynor JW, Bridges ND, Clark BJ, et al: Update on lung transplantation in children. *Curr Opin Pediatr* 10:256-261, 1998.

90. Clabby ML, Canter CE, Moller JH, et al: Hemodynamic data and survival in children with pulmonary hypertension. *J Am Coll Cardiol* 30:554-560, 1997.

91. Choong CK, Sweet SC, Guthrie TJ, et al: Repair of congenital heart lesions combined with lung transplantation for the treatment of severe pulmonary hypertension: A 13-year experience. *J Thorac Cardiovasc Surg* 129:661-669, 2005.

92. Waddell TK, Bennett L, Kennedy R, et al: Heart-lung or lung transplantation for Eisenmenger syndrome. *J Heart Lung Transplant* 21:731-737, 2002.

19 Chapter

High Altitude Pulmonary Edema

Giora Netzer, MD,

Darren B. Taichman, MD, PhD

Introduction

High altitude disease includes the syndromes of acute mountain sickness (AMS), high altitude pulmonary edema (HAPE), and high altitude cerebral edema (HACE). Each appears to result, at least in part, from alterations in vascular homeostasis. Although incompletely understood, these conditions share many clinical and apparent pathophysiologic features. Management is largely supportive, although a growing understanding of these syndromes has permitted more effective means of prevention and the identification of those at risk.

History of High Altitude Medicine

Climbing to high altitudes and understanding and overcoming its hazards have fascinated scientists and explorers for over a century. High altitude places the body under significant physiologic stress. In 1920, the British physiologist Alexander M. Kellas predicted that "Mount Everest could be ascended by a man of excellent physical and mental constitution in first-rate training, without adventitious aids if the difficulties are not too great."[1] The oxygen content of inhaled gas falls with increasing altitude. Considering that alveolar gas samples taken at the summit of Mount Everest (8,848 meters) showed an alveolar PO_2 of just 35 torr, the "difficulties" Kellas foresaw were indeed significant.[2] Yet, the summit was reached only 33 years later by Sir Edmund Hillary and Tenzing Norgay, and in 1978 by Reinhold Messner and Peter Habeler without

supplemental oxygen—achievements at the body's outer limits.

That high altitude can have deleterious effects on the body has been long recognized. Perhaps the first reference to illness associated with altitude was recorded nearly 2,000 years ago by Tseen Hanshoo, who described "Great and Little Headache" mountains on the journey along the Silk Road.[3] A description of a monk foaming at the mouth during the ascent of a mountain pass in 403 AD is believed to have been a form of altitude sickness.[4] Later, the emergence of hot-air ballooning provided a more convenient mechanism to explore the effects of altitude. Within a month of the first balloon flight by the Montgolfier brothers in 1783, the French physicist Jacques Charles described pain he ascribed to the expansion of gas in his right ear.[5] By 1862, James Glaisher and Henry Coxwell had reached heights in excess of 8,800 meters in an open hot-air balloon. Glaisher described the effects of altitude on himself, including transient loss of vision, paralysis, and then loss of consciousness. In 1895, tachypnea and tachycardia were recognized as symptoms brought on by altitude when Tissandier described the deaths of his flying companions Croce-Spinelli and Sivel.[6]

Growing interest and accomplishment in mountaineering similarly resulted in recognition of altitude-related illness. Climbing to progressively higher altitudes without supplemental oxygen, mountaineers astounded physiologists by continually surpassing what was believed the limits of endurance.[7] These exposures also offered an opportunity to study the physiologic and pathologic consequences of high altitude. Indeed, likely the first postmortem description of HAPE is that of Jacottet, a physician who died during the construction of an observatory on Mont Blanc in 1891.[8] It described a normal heart and lungs but bilateral pulmonary edema.[9] By the end of the nineteenth century, Angelo Mosso, an Italian physiologist and climber, had built the advanced Regina Margherita on Monte Rosa in the Italian Alps (4,559 meters), where he conducted pioneering experiments on the physiologic effects of altitude. Rebuilt by Swiss researchers between 1978 and 1980, experiments at the observatory continue to form the source of much of our understanding of HAPE (FIGURE 19-1).[10]

A landmark paper describing altitude sickness was written in 1913 by T.H. Ravenhill, an English physician working as a medical officer of the Ponderosa Mining Company and La Compania Minera de Collahuasi in Chile. He described the clinical findings of AMS, HAPE, and HACE encountered at altitudes of 4,690-4,840 meters. He described *"puna,"* a term used by Bolivian inhabitants to describe mountain sickness.[11] Darwin had experienced *puna* during his exploration of the Andes in 1835.[12] Altitude sickness continued to be described in the South American medical literature,[13] although Ravenhill's work was overlooked in the English language literature for nearly half a century, and HAPE remained a largely unrecognized diagnosis in most of the world.

This changed in 1960 when Charles Houston, an Aspen internist, reported on a healthy 21-year-old cross country skier who developed pulmonary edema while crossing a 3,650-meter pass. His chest radiograph showed pulmonary edema, while his electrocardiogram displayed nonspecific changes. Although such cases had been

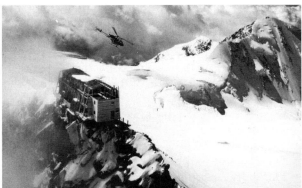

Figure 19-1. The High Altitude Research Laboratory at Capanna Regina Margherita (4,559 Meters). (Reproduced with permission from Scherrer U, Vollenweider L, Delabays A, et al: Inhaled nitric oxide for high-altitude pulmonary edema. *N Engl J Med* 334(10):624-629, 1996.)

termed "high altitude pneumonia," Houston recognized this to be acute pulmonary edema without heart disease. Houston's series of four patients included a 26-year-old physician who "..., undertook a self-examination with the stethoscope and could detect fine, moist rales."[14] Thereafter, several case series described noncardiogenic pulmonary edema developing at altitude,[15-17] and Hultgren performed cardiac catheterization on seven patients with HAPE at the Chulec General Hospital in Peru. The patients had pulmonary hypertension, reduced cardiac outputs, and low-normal pulmonary artery occlusion pressures; oxygen administration caused a fall in pulmonary artery pressure and an increase in occlusion pressure.[18] The large number of Indian troops stationed in the Himalayas provided further for description of HAPE in otherwise healthy young men.[19,20] In one study of 1925 soldiers with AMS, frank pulmonary edema was found in approximately one-third.[21]

Interest in altitude-related disease continued to grow, with increasing exposure in the English language medical literature. In 1991, a group of experts met to define criteria for the diagnosis of illnesses associated with altitude: acute mountain sickness, high altitude pulmonary edema, and high altitude cerebral edema. These definitions, named after the location of this meeting, are known as the Lake Louise Criteria (TABLE 19-1).

High Altitude Physiology

The driving force behind the physiologic stress of altitude is hypobaric hypoxia. This was recognized as early as 1820, when the Russian climber Joseph Hamel suggested the use of supplemental oxygen in his attempt to ascend Mont Blanc.[22] During the mid-nineteenth century, Bert first demonstrated that the low partial pressure of oxygen associated with low barometric pressure was responsible for the deleterious effects of altitude.[5]

As altitude increases, barometric pressure (and thus oxygen tension) decreases (FIGURE 19-2). The resultant effects are embodied in the ideal gas-law equation:

$$PV = nRT$$

where P = pressure, V = volume, n = number of molecules of gas, R = universal gas constant, and T = absolute temperature. The barometric pressure at sea level is 760 mmHg but decreases to 608 mmHg at

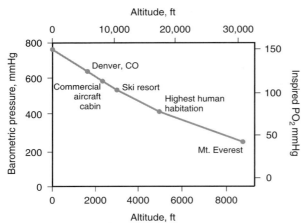

Figure 19-2. The Relationship Between Altitude, Barometric Pressure, and Inspired Oxygen Pressure (PO₂). (Reproduced with permission from West JB: The physiologic basis of high-altitude diseases. *Ann Intern Med* 141(10):789-800, 2004.)

1,829 meters and 380 mmHg at 5,486 meters. Although the fraction of inspired oxygen remains proportionally constant at 21 percent, the decrease in barometric pressure means that the inspired oxygen tension decreases. The effect is dramatic: at 5,486 meters, the inspired O_2 tension (PIO_2) is one-half that at sea level (80 mmHg versus 160 mmHg), and at 7,315 meters, the PIO_2 is only 62 mmHg.[3] Additionally, as altitude increases, the relative effect of water vapor on inspired oxygen tension increases. Inspired air is warmed and saturated with water vapor in the upper airways by a constant amount determined by body temperature and independent of barometric pressure. At sea level, the water vapor pressure of approximately 47 mmHg accounts for only 6 percent of total barometric pressure, while at the summit of Mount Everest it accounts for 19 percent.[23] This increase in water vapor pressure effectively lowers the partial pressure of inspired oxygen even further.

High Altitude Illnesses

Exposure to high altitude is associated with several clinical syndromes that can occur independently or simultaneously, including AMS, HACE, and HAPE. Each of these entities is believed to result from altered responses to hypoxia and hypobaria, with HACE and HAPE representing extreme effects in the brain and lung, respectively. Each, however, can occur without preceding symptoms of AMS.

Acute Mountain Sickness

AMS is the most common of the illnesses associated with exposure to altitude. Estimates of incidence vary with the population studied and the length and level of exposure. In one study of tourists visiting altitudes from 1,900 to 2,950 meters, AMS occurred in 25 percent.[24] A study of mountaineers at 4,559 meters reported the incidence of AMS following rapid ascent to be 58 percent among those with and 31 percent in those without a history of AMS. The risk was lower when a significant amount of time had been spent at high altitude during the previous 2 months ("preexposure"), lower still with a slow ascent, and lowest with both preexposure and slow ascent.[25] In another study, approximately 50 percent of trekkers in the Mount Everest region developed symptoms while trekking to areas higher than 4,000 meters over 5 days.[26]

Risk factors for AMS include younger age and poorer physical conditioning; no consistent difference between women and men has been found. A history of AMS and preexisting lung disease are each significant risk factors, and it is rare among those who live at high altitude.[24] Exercise may increase both the risk and severity of AMS.[27] One study simulating altitude with a hypobaric chamber suggested that obesity is associated with AMS,[28] although this study did not define the incidence and severity of sleep-disordered breathing in its subjects. A history of neck irradiation or surgery has also been suggested,[29] but rapid ascent and history of AMS are the most consistently noted risk factors for the syndrome.

Although the pathophysiology of AMS is not fully understood, it appears to involve hypoxemia-induced changes in vascular permeability and vasodilation. Ultimately, swelling of cerebral tissues appears to be an important cause of symptoms and mortality.[3,30-34]

AMS is a clinical diagnosis. In the setting of a recent ascent, AMS is defined by the presence of headache and at least one of the following[35]:

- Gastrointestinal symptoms (anorexia, nausea, or vomiting)
- Fatigue or weakness
- Dizziness or lightheadedness
- Difficulty sleeping

This definition was adopted in the Lake Louise Criteria in 1991 and has been useful in standardizing reports and research (TABLE 19-1). These symptoms are aggravated by wintry weather and by significant physical activity soon after arrival at high altitudes, and they can be worse after air travel.[21] Symptoms typically occur 6-10 hours after ascent, although they have been reported as early as within 1 hour.[31]

No specific laboratory abnormalities are associated with AMS. However, one study compared 10 previously healthy subjects who developed AMS with 22 controls at 2,216 meters and 4,700 meters. All subjects had normal electrocardiograph and chest radiograph findings at the lower altitude. Although diffusing capacity increased in both groups at higher altitude, the increase in diffusing capacity was smaller in the group that suffered AMS. Additionally, subjects with AMS had a lower vital capacity and a greater alveolar-arterial gradient than those without AMS criteria.[36]

High Altitude Cerebral Edema

HACE likely represents the consequences of hypoxia on the cerebral vasculature. According to the Lake Louise consensus group, HACE occurs with a recent ascent, and the diagnosis requires either a change in mental status or ataxia in a person with AMS or, alternatively, the presence of both mental status changes and ataxia in the absence of AMS.[35] Physical examination may reveal papilledema, retinal hemorrhages, and occasionally cranial nerve palsy. Generalized encephalopathy is more common than focal findings. Stupor follows drowsiness, and the illness progresses over hours to days. Death can occur from tonsillar herniation.[31]

High Altitude Pulmonary Edema

HAPE is a potentially fatal pulmonary vasculopathy following exposure to high altitude and hypoxia. Worldwide, approximately 20 deaths occur each year as a result of HAPE.[13] The clinical manifestations have been well described, and numerous risk factors and pathogenetic mechanisms identified. Certain preventive strategies are accepted, and management involves removal of the patient from high altitude, reversal of hypoxemia, and supportive measures.

In 1991, the Lake Louise consensus group defined HAPE as involving at least two essential symptoms and two essential signs after a recent gain in altitude (TABLE 19-1). The severity of HAPE can be graded either on the basis of symptoms and the activity required to precipitate them[13] or upon vital signs and chest radiographic findings.[37] Although these grading systems have been useful in describing the severity of disease, studies evaluating their predictive value on outcome have not been conducted.

TABLE 19-1
Lake Louise Consensus Definitions of Altitude Illness

Acute Mountain Sickness (AMS)

In the setting of a recent gain in altitude, the presence of headache and at least one of the following symptoms:

- gastrointestinal (anorexia, nausea or vomiting)
- fatigue or weakness
- dizziness or lightheadedness
- difficulty sleeping

High Altitude Cerebral Edema (HACE)

Can be considered "end stage" or severe AMS. In the setting of a recent gain in altitude, either:

- the presence of a change in mental status and/or ataxia in a person with AMS
- or, the presence of both mental status changes and ataxia in a person without AMS

High Altitude Mountain Sickness (HAPE)

In the setting of a recent gain in altitude, the presence of the following:

Symptoms, at least two of:
- dyspnea at rest
- cough
- weakness or decreased exercise performance
- chest tightness or congestion

Signs, at least two of:
- crackles or wheezing in at least one lung field
- central cyanosis
- tachypnea
- tachycardia

Definitions were adopted at the 1991 International Hypoxia Symposium at Lake Louise, Alberta, Canada. Reproduced with permission from The Lake Louise Consensus on the Definition and Quantification of Altitude Illness. In: Sutton JR, Coates G, Houston CS, editors: Hypoxia and mountain medicine, Burlington, VT, 1992, Queen City Printers.

The clinical picture of HAPE can be quite striking. One physician described a stricken Sherpa as, "... unconscious, with eyes closed, writhing around the floor and moaning. From across the tent I could hear rales—bubbling sounds coming from his lungs. He didn't respond to his name or anything else except painful stimulation. When I pushed my knuckles hard into his sternum, it caused him to change the pitch of his moans and make a vague arm gesture to push me away. His pulse and respirations were rapid and shallow. His skin was clammy and pale."[38]

Symptoms of HAPE most often occur 48-96 hours following exposure to high altitude and frequently develop at night.[12] The first symptoms are usually dyspnea on exertion and a reduced exercise tolerance felt to be out of proportion to the altitude.[26] This may be noted as breathlessness in excess of that experienced by one's climbing or expedition companions.[39] An initially nonproductive cough often will become severe, persistent, and may progress to stridor and dyspnea. The cough can become productive of copious, pinkish sputum.[12] These symptoms also appear to occur more commonly at night.[40] Orthopnea is uncommon, as is frank hemoptysis.[31]

Physical examination reveals tachycardia and tachypnea.[26] On auscultation, a right ventricular heave and accentuated second heart sound occasionally are heard.[39] Crackles are common, most often first appreciated in the right mid-lung field and subsequently becoming more widespread.[26] A predilection for the right middle lobe may be due to its collateral ventilation and an accentuated pulmonary vascular response to hypoxia.[12,26] Marked cyanosis of the lips and nail beds also can be seen.[18]

Up to 14 percent of patients with HAPE may have concomitant signs and symptoms of HACE, and one-half of those who die have evidence of HACE at autopsy.[31] Findings of HACE in these patients include retinal hemorrhages, papilledema, difficulty in ambulation, and coma.[40]

LABORATORY FINDINGS. Patients with HAPE have more profound hypoxemia than unaffected individuals at the same altitude. Depending upon the altitude and disease severity, PaO_2 values as low as 23 mmHg have been reported.[3] Arterial blood gas analysis typically reveals a respiratory alkalosis, with $PaCO_2$ between 30-40 mmHg.[31] Most patients display leukocytosis, an increased hemoglobin concentration, and higher red blood cell counts. Creatine kinase levels frequently are elevated. Serum protein, albumin, and iron values can be low. Most patients also have albuminuria.[14,40]

The electrocardiogram typically shows sinus tachycardia; right heart strain, right bundle branch block, and right ventricular hypertrophy can also be seen.[12]

Chest radiography often shows findings consistent with pulmonary edema (FIGURE 19-3). One reader-blinded study of 60 posteroanterior radiographs from patients with HAPE found that the classic "bat wing" appearance of pulmonary edema occurred in only 25 percent of patients. More often, the air space disease was homogenous. This study showed that Kerley B lines occur 15 percent of the time but that all patients had peribronchial and perivascular cuffing, and nearly all had perihilar "haziness." Pleural effusions were not seen. Typically changes appeared most prominently at the bases, especially the right lower lung field. Radiographic appearance correlated with the severity of HAPE but did not differ based on concomitant HACE.[41] Computerized tomography can demonstrate many small, confluent airspace consolidations, with sparing of the apices and the lung cortex.[42]

Pulmonary hypertension is an essential feature of HAPE, but it is reversible. Right heart catheterizations performed on patients with HAPE have revealed elevated pulmonary arterial pressures with normal pulmonary capillary wedge pressures (PCWP). In Hultgren's study at 12,300 feet of seven

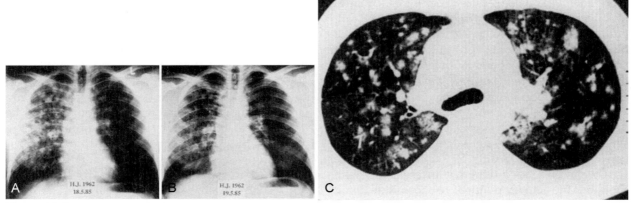

Figure 19-3. Plain radiographs showing patchy alveolar edema at initial visit (**A**) and reduction after the administration of oxygen (**B**) in a 23-year-old man with HAPE developing at 4,559 meters. Computerized tomography similarly demonstrates patchy, nonconfluent pulmonary edema in a 29-year-old patient with HAPE (**C**). (Reproduced with permission from Bartsch P: High altitude pulmonary edema. *Med Sci Sports Exerc* 31(1 Suppl):S23-S27, 1999.)

patients at first contact and again after recovery, systolic pulmonary arterial pressures were elevated initially (range 41-144 mmHg), increased further with exercise, and normalized with administration of 100 percent oxygen to the range of acclimatized residents at that altitude.[18] PCWPs were low or normal.[18] A series of five patients similarly found pulmonary arterial hypertension with a mean pulmonary artery pressure of 62 mmHg and PCWP of 5 mmHg.[13] Another study found essentially normal values in patients evaluated after descent to 610 meters.[41]

PATHOLOGIC CHANGES. Gross pathologic findings in HAPE include airways filled with frothy, pink fluid and heavy lung congestion. Microscopic examination revealed proteinaceous fluid and hyaline membranes. Increases in both macrophages and neutrophils are seen. This bronchiolitis or pneumonitis may be patchy or consolidated. Other findings less consistently noted are capillary and arteriolar thrombi, fibrin deposits, as well as hemorrhage and infarct.[12]

INCIDENCE AND RISK FACTORS. The exact incidence of HAPE is unknown. Estimates of incidence range from around 1-10 percent. One study in 1976 found that among climbers in Nepal at an altitude of 4,243 meters, the incidence of HAPE was 2.5 percent.[43] A study of 97 subjects living at 3,750 meters found that 0.6 percent of 1,157 ascents to higher altitude resulted in HAPE. These events occurred in 6 percent of the subjects studied. The rates were higher in younger subjects, approximately double among children 2-12 years old than the rates seen in those over 21.[44] Because this study evaluated persons acclimatized to altitude ascending even higher, however, it might not be applicable to travelers, trekkers, and climbers unaccustomed to high altitude in whom rates might be even higher.

HAPE may be underdiagnosed. In one study of 262 climbers of Monte Rosa, only 1 subject developed symptomatic HAPE, but 15 percent of the climbers (n = 40) developed either rales heard on examination or interstitial edema on chest radiograph. Closing volume increased in 74 percent of the subjects, also suggesting an increase in extravascular fluid.[45] Houston noted rales in 24 percent of asymptomatic climbers at an altitude of 4,394 meters on Mount Rainier.[12]

A history of HAPE appears to place one at significant risk for recurrence. In a study of mountaineers at 4,559 meters evaluated with daily examinations, chest radiographs, and blood gas measurements, the rate of HAPE was 62 percent among those with a prior episode as

compared with 6 percent in those without.[46] Additional reported risk factors include cold weather[47] and a history of pulmonary hypertension.[48,49] Because exposure to altitude usually occurs in those participating in sporting activities such as climbing and trekking, most reported cases have followed at least moderate physical exertion.[13] The risk may increase at higher altitudes. In a simulated climb of Mount Everest using a hypobaric chamber, six of seven subjects developed significant defects in gas exchange.[50] Although no single threshold altitude has been established clearly under controlled study, HAPE generally occurs above 2,500 meters.[51] The potential effects of genetic variables influencing physiologic responses to hypoxia and thus altering the risk of HAPE are discussed below.

PATHOPHYSIOLOGY. Hypoxia at high elevations, rather than the altitude itself, is believed to be the main inciting factor for HAPE. Indeed, the hypoxemic exposure at high altitudes can be profound. Oximetry of subjects at 19,000 feet, for example, revealed an average resting arterial oxygen saturation of 67 percent and desaturation to an average of 56 percent during intense exertion.[52] Abnormalities in any of the several normal pulmonary, neurohumoral, and cardiovascular responses to hypoxia have been implicated in the pathogenesis of HAPE.

HYPOXIC VENTILATORY RESPONSE. The hypoxic ventilatory response (HVR) increases minute ventilation in response to hypoxia and its magnitude is influenced by hypercapnea.[39] The increase in ventilation at altitude can be quite striking: subjects on Mount Everest (at 6,300 meters) have been reported to achieve a maximal minute ventilation over 200 liters at peak exercise.[53] By preventing hypoxemia, this augmented HVR may be a determinant of certain individuals' superior physical performance at high altitude, although data are not conclusive.[54-56] Conversely, an insufficient HVR has been implicated in the pathogenesis of HAPE. In one study on Mount McKinley (4,400 meters), subjects with HAPE had a lower HVR than unaffected controls, and patients with the lowest HVR the most hypoxemic.[57] Similarly, at a simulated altitude of 4,800 meters, patients with a history of HAPE who once again developed symptoms had both a lower HVR and lower minute ventilation than unaffected individuals.[33] In a meta-analysis of 91 subjects, 77 percent of HAPE-susceptible subjects had a low HVR, while 75 percent of nonsusceptible individuals had a normal HVR.[9] Body habitus may contribute to the observed differences in HVR, because

HAPE-susceptible individuals have shorter chests and smaller lung volumes than those without such a history.[58]

Genetic factors might also influence the hypoxemic ventilatory response. Marked differences among ethnic groups have been noted in studies of HVR and exercise capacity at altitude. For example, native Tibetans have a higher resting HVR at altitude than do their neighbors of Han Chinese ancestry.[59] Lowland-dwelling Tibetans also show better acclimatization at altitude than well-conditioned white lowlanders.[60] Sherpas, of highland Tibetan ancestry, live at altitudes of 2,800-3,500 meters in the Solu Khumbu region of Nepal, and are famous for their skills as guides on Himalayan expeditions. Compared with their lowland-dwelling Tibetan ancestors living at 1,300 meters, the Sherpas show superior peak aerobic performance ($\overset{\circ}{V}O_2$ max) at altitude.[60] Although it is tempting to ascribe the Sherpa's apparent resistance to HAPE, at least in part, to some genetic advantage, confirmatory studies are lacking.[61]

Sleep-disordered breathing might also contribute to HAPE. Cheyne-Stokes respiration at altitude is well described.[3] Polysomnograms performed at 4,559 meters demonstrated periodic breathing to be more common among individuals with a history of HAPE than those with either a history of AMS or no altitude illness.[34] Whether HAPE and its resultant hypoxemia exacerbate the periodic breathing or vice versa is not clear. Although the administration of either acetazolamide or theophylline to stimulate ventilation have been shown to decrease periodic breathing at altitude and to reduce the risk of AMS,[62-64] a similar role in HAPE has not been reported.

VASOCONSTRICTION AND PULMONARY HYPERTENSION. Pulmonary arterial hypertension has been found consistently in hemodynamic studies of patients with HAPE.[17,18,65,66] The risk of HAPE is higher in those with preexisting pulmonary arterial hypertension (both idiopathic and other forms).[48,49,67] Susceptible individuals have higher pulmonary arterial pressures than nonsusceptible controls,[68-72] as well as higher pulmonary artery pressures following exercise.[69,70,73,74] Further, in HAPE-susceptible men evaluated at altitude, pulmonary hypertension occurs before pulmonary edema develops.[74] Finally, susceptible individuals have consistently had higher pulmonary artery pressures under hypoxic conditions.[58,68-72,75,76] This may be exacerbated by the cold weather that characterizes high altitude, as pulmonary artery pressures increase at lower temperatures in both animal and human studies.[12,43,47]

Elevated pulmonary arterial pressures under hypoxic conditions suggest that abnormalities in the control of hypoxic pulmonary vasoconstriction may be involved in the development of HAPE. Hypoxic pulmonary vasoconstriction is a normal regulatory mechanism by which regional blood flow is directed away from poorly ventilated (and thus hypoxic) alveolar units toward better oxygenated areas. Such "ventilation-perfusion matching" is a critical means of preventing hypoxemia and is controlled by numerous mediators and genetic factors (see Chapter 1).

Abnormalities in factors normally involved in the control of pulmonary vasodilation and constriction have been identified in patients with HAPE. A deficiency in nitric oxide-mediated vasodilation, for example, has been observed in studies performed both at high altitude (4,559 meters) and using hypoxia-inducing gas mixtures. Reductions in exhaled nitric oxide are found in HAPE-susceptible individuals and the levels inversely related to pulmonary artery pressures.[77,78] Administration of inhaled nitric oxide to HAPE-susceptible climbers results in both a greater incremental increase in arterial oxygenation and decrease in pulmonary artery pressures than is seen in HAPE-resistant subjects.[75] Genetic factors may influence these differences in nitric oxide-mediated vasodilation. In one study of Japanese climbers, polymorphisms in the endothelial nitric oxide synthase gene (involved in nitric oxide production) were associated with the risk of developing HAPE.[79]

Endothelin-1, a potent pulmonary vasoconstrictor, might also be important in the development of HAPE. Plasma levels of endothelin-1 rise with higher altitude in healthy volunteers.[80] An abnormally augmented endothelin response is seen among HAPE-susceptible individuals, and levels correlate with the observed increase in pulmonary artery pressures.[81]

Alterations in sympathetic nervous system activity might also influence vascular tone and the development of HAPE. Indeed, sympathetic responses are altered in normal subjects at high altitude: nearly all subjects become presyncopal in a head-up tilt test.[82] Sympathetic activity increases in response to hypoxia (particularly in the presence of hypocapnia).[83] Chronic hypoxemia, as seen in advanced lung disease, also alters sympathetic nervous system activity.[84] Healthy individuals who normally reside at sea level develop an average increase of 28 percent in mean systemic blood pressure and have higher plasma epinephrine and norepinephrine concentrations when exposed to altitude.[85] During hypoxia-inducing exercise, seven mountaineers with a history of HAPE had dramatically higher rates of sympathetic nervous discharge as compared with seven HAPE-resistant controls, despite similar degrees of hypoxemia in the two groups. This augmented sympathetic response preceded pulmonary edema.[86] Genetic differences may influence sympathetic nervous system activity in the development of HAPE. Specifically, polymorphisms in the gene for angiotensin-converting enzyme have been linked to differences in exercise capacity and oxygenation at altitude.[87] Angiotensin-converting enzyme, as well as polymorphisms for the angiotensin receptor genes, have been linked to HAPE susceptibility in several populations,[79,88-90] although the exact relationship remains unclear.

HAPE may result in part from pulmonary hypertension-induced damage to the capillary and alveolar membrane. Such damage is thought to be worsened by hypoxia-induced redistribution of blood flow, and to result in extravasation of fluid and protein into the alveolar space.[3,12,13,31,43,91-94] Several factors have been implicated in the capillary-alveolar membrane disruption seen in HAPE. In addition to elevated pulmonary artery pressures, increased pulmonary capillary pressures have been demonstrated at high altitude in HAPE-susceptible patients using an arterial occlusion technique during right heart catheterization. This increase in capillary pressure precedes the development of pulmonary edema.[95] It has been hypothesized that certain alveolar units are subjected to greater increases in vascular pressure than others, owing to a disruption in the normal distribution of blood flow. This is supported by the observation in normal subjects that under hypoxic conditions, exercise results in a worsening of ventilation-perfusion mismatch,[96] and the degree of redistribution of blood flow varies from host to host.[97] Pressure-induced "stress failure" of the capillary-alveolar membrane in these over-perfused regions is thought to result in the radiographically apparent patchy distribution of edema. In HAPE-susceptible subjects, patterns of redistributed flow from basilar to apical (and vice versa) have been observed.[72,98] This heterogeneity in perfusion as compared with that of HAPE-resistant individuals is also seen on magnetic resonance imaging.[99] Uneven perfusion might also explain the disease pattern when HAPE occurs in patients with anatomic disruptions to flow (such as congenital absence of a pulmonary artery or occlusion secondary to thromboembolism).[100-104] Regional differences in perfusion alone, however, do not appear to be sufficient for the development of HAPE, because such changes have been observed at altitude in subjects who do not develop HAPE.[105]

Investigators using animal models of elevated capillary pressure and of HAPE have noted findings consistent with such "stress failure." In rabbits, high capillary transmural pressures cause disruption of the capillary epithelium and the alveolar epithelium, while the basement membrane remains intact (FIGURE 19-4).[106,107] At even higher pressures, all three layers of the blood-gas barrier are affected and interstitial edema develops. Extravasation of red blood cells can be seen in the alveolar spaces[108] and increased levels of protein, albumin, and leukotriene B_4 found on bronchoalveolar lavage.[109] This stress failure worsens when lung volumes are increased.[110] Reversibility of such defects can occur when transmural pressures are lowered, as evidenced by a reduction in the number of endothelial and epithelial defects.[111] Similar ultrastructural abnormalities have been found in a rat model of HAPE.[112]

Bronchoalveolar lavage fluid from patients with HAPE has similarly suggested a disruption of the alveolar-capillary barrier, as elevated levels of protein, albumin, leukotriene B_4, and the presence of erythrocytes and hemosiderin-laden macrophages

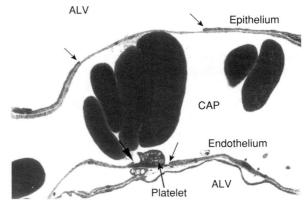

Figure 19-4. Electron micrograph demonstrating ultrastructural changes in the pulmonary capillary of a rabbit when hydrostatic pressure is elevated ("stress failure"). Disruption of the alveolar epithelial layer (*arrow at top*) and capillary endothelial layer (*arrows at bottom*) are seen. *ALV,* alveolus; *CAP,* capillary lumen. (Reproduced with permission from West JB: The physiologic basis of high-altitude diseases. *Ann Intern Med* 141(10): 789-800, 2004.)

are observed.[113-115] Vascular damage has also been suggested by elevated serum levels of endothelial-specific selectins.[116] Elevated levels of interleukin (IL)-1β, IL-6, IL-8, urinary leukotrienes, C-reactive protein, tumor necrosis factor-α, and other markers of inflammation at high altitude or with HAPE have suggested the involvement of an active inflammatory response.[117-120] Furthermore, elevated levels of inflammatory cytokines correlate with the increased pressure gradient (pulmonary artery pressure minus wedge pressure) "driving" fluid from the intravascular to extravascular spaces.

To assess the temporal sequence of capillary disruption (due to elevated pressures) and inflammation, Swenson and colleagues performed an elegant study of HAPE-susceptible and resistant climbers, both before and after rapid ascent. As in other studies, they found no difference in pulmonary artery pressures (estimated by echocardiography) or bronchoalveolar lavage findings between the patients and the controls at low altitude. Following ascent, however, pulmonary artery pressures were increased in subjects early in the development of HAPE. Compared with controls, subjects at this early stage of HAPE also had protein-rich and mildly hemorrhagic bronchoalveolar lavage fluid, indicative of alveolar-capillary leakage. Levels of leukocytes, cytokines, or eicosanoids (markers of inflammation), however, were normal and no different from those of control subjects despite the early stages of HAPE. Thus, it appears that alveolar-capillary leak in early HAPE is not due to inflammation, but rather due to increased hydrostatic pressures.[71] An inflammatory reaction ensues during later stages, likely initiated by the endothelial-epithelial disruption and extravasation of fluid and cells.[12,31] Indeed, markers of inflammation such as urinary leukotriene E_4 remain at normal levels in the early stage of the disease but subsequently rise with progression.[121] The resulting inflammatory reaction might worsen the clinical manifestations. In addition, prior inflammatory conditions (such as respiratory infection) have been noted frequently in studies of pediatric patients with HAPE.[122] Viral respiratory infection predisposes rats to pulmonary edema under hypoxic conditions.[123] HAPE susceptibility has also been associated with the human leucocyte antigen (HLA)-DR6 and HLA-DQ4 alleles, which might promote an inflammatory response via their expression on antigen-presenting cells.[98,124]

It remains unclear why HAPE usually occurs only within the first 4-5 days spent at high altitude.

Cannot the hypothesized capillary failure occur at any time? West has postulated that delayed development of "stress failure" is prevented by rapid remodeling of the vasculature that occurs in response to vasoconstriction. Within hours, collagen and elastin synthesis increase as does the expression of several growth factors. Rapid remodeling of the pulmonary vascular smooth muscle protects the delicate capillaries downstream.[125] Hence, HAPE usually will not develop, unless altitude is gained.

The rate at which extravasated fluid is removed from the alveolar space may be an important determinant of clinically apparent HAPE. Insufficient transport of alveolar fluid is important to the development of various forms of acute lung injury, including acute respiratory distress syndrome.[126] Fluid is pumped out of the interstitium by transepithelial sodium channels on Type 1 and Type 2 cells. In acute respiratory distress syndrome, as in other forms of pulmonary edema, fluid moves across the pulmonary blood-gas barrier faster than it can be pumped out, and more rapid fluid clearance is associated with better outcomes.[127] Similar abnormalities in fluid transport might be important in the pathogenesis of HAPE. In animal models, hypoxia has been shown to decrease alveolar sodium transport.[128] In humans, HAPE-resistant climbers have larger increases in nasal epithelial potential (a marker of sodium channel activity) than HAPE-susceptible individuals.[129,130] In experimental models, β-adrenergic agonists seemed to improve fluid clearance,[131] including capillary leak from high pressures.[132] This might explain the results of a double-blind, randomized, placebo-controlled trial, in which salmeterol (a β-adrenergic agonist) reduced the incidence of HAPE.[133]

Prevention and Management

ACUTE MOUNTAIN SICKNESS. As the number of travelers and workers at high altitude increases, HAPE and other altitude-related illness are becoming more common causes of morbidity and mortality, and numerous strategies for prevention and management have been explored. One of the most time-honored practices for prevention is acclimatization. The dictum, "climb high and sleep low," is well known and respected by experienced climbers.[134] The altitude at which one sleeps is associated more closely with the subsequent development of HAPE than is the maximum altitude exposure during the day. For this reason, it is generally recommended that sleeping elevation be increased only slowly, with incremental nightly increases of not more than 300 meters.[3] A rest day every 2 or 3 days is also recommended.[125]

As discussed previously, the driving force behind altitude illness is hypoxia: low inspired oxygen tension resulting from reduced barometric pressure. Not surprisingly, therefore, administration of supplemental oxygen is one of the most important interventions for the prevention of AMS and other high altitude illness. This is not new; the first significant use of supplemental oxygen with climbing occurred on a Mount Everest expedition in 1922.[22] Supplemental oxygen, however, is not always practical, and relatively few promote its routine use with skiing at moderate altitudes despite the not-so-infrequent development of AMS. As hypoxia worsens at higher altitudes, however, more serious consideration should be given to the use of supplemental oxygen to prevent HAPE and HACE.

As noted above, a blunted HVR is associated with AMS and HAPE. Alcohol blunts the HVR, and it is therefore prudent to minimize or eliminate alcohol use at altitude.[135] In contrast, acetazolamide, a carbonic anhydrase inhibitor, increases minute ventilation and alveolar PO_2 at altitude and under hypoxic conditions, and is often used prophylactically.[63,136] Acetazolamide also improves high-altitude sleep-disordered breathing.[137] Theophylline has been found to be of benefit in AMS,[138] although acetazolamide has been better studied.[64] Although exercise capacity may actually decrease with acetazolamide use,[62,139] it remains one of the mainstays of pharmacotherapy. A 500-mg total daily dose of acetazolamide appears more effective than 250 mg, and a 750-mg dose is likely the most effective.[64,140,141] The addition of medroxyprogesterone may potentiate the respiratory stimulatory effects, but inadequate data exist to support its routine use at high altitude.[142] Dexamethasone is also of benefit as prophylaxis against AMS at a dosage of 4 mg orally every 12 hours.[143,144] It may be important for those intolerant of the side effects of acetazolamide, allergic to its sulfa moiety, or those who need to reach high altitude rapidly (e.g., search and rescue missions by helicopter).[145]

A variety of food-based and herbal substances have been evaluated for AMS prophylaxis including antioxidants[146] (ascorbic acid, α-tocopherol and α-lipoic acid), gingko biloba, garlic, and red wine.[147-149] The potential benefit of these agents in AMS prophylaxis, however, has not been clearly established.

High Altitude Pulmonary Edema

PREVENTION. Prevention of excessive increases in pulmonary artery pressures with vasodilators has been studied extensively in HAPE prophylaxis. The most effective pulmonary vasodilator in this setting remains oxygen. Tested head-to-head against oral agents, supplemental oxygen is an essential means of preventing HAPE.[150] Nifedipine also is effective and commonly is used on mountaineering expeditions, where its use by climbers with a history of HAPE has dramatically reduced recurrence.[151] It should be noted, however, that nifedipine is not effective as prophylaxis against AMS.[152] Amlodipine, a newer calcium channel blocker, has also been evaluated under simulated high altitude conditions; although it reduced pulmonary artery pressures, subjects experienced greater breathlessness during exercise.[153] The phosphodiesterase inhibitor sildenafil potentiates the vasodilatory effects of nitric oxide. Sildenafil has been used to manage pulmonary arterial hypertension[154,155] and can prevent hypoxia-induced pulmonary hypertension.[156] In a placebo-controlled, crossover study of 14 mountaineers with no history of HAPE, sildenafil reduced hypoxic pulmonary hypertension during both rest and exercise at the Mount Everest base camp (5,425 meters). Exercise capacity under hypoxia-inducing conditions at low altitude and at the Mount Everest base camp were also increased.[157] There was no significant effect on systolic blood pressure or cardiac output. HAPE-susceptible individuals, however, were not studied, nor was the use of sildenafil in HAPE management. A double-blind, placebo-controlled trial of 37 mountaineers with a history of HAPE found that the long acting β-adrenergic agonist salmeterol reduced the incidence of HAPE by over 50 percent.[133] Volume expansion has not been found to be of significant benefit at high altitude.

MANAGEMENT. Management of HAPE involves the reversal of hypoxemia and the use of vasodilators. As the symptoms of severe AMS (or HACE) can overlap with HAPE, and many patients suffer from a combination of these entities, management of both is often required. Mild cases of AMS can be managed symptomatically with nonsteroidal antiinflammatory medications, such as ibuprofen and naproxen, or with acetaminophen.[145] Dexamethasone is also effective for AMS management[158,159] at an initial dose of 8 mg and then 4 mg every 6 hours, which can be given orally, intramuscularly, or intravenously. It is recommended for those with HACE while awaiting hyperbaric management or descent.[39,160] Rapid descent and dexamethasone are now the standard of care for cases of HACE. Dexamethasone for isolated HAPE, however, has not been proven effective, and glucocorticoids should be reserved for patients with both HACE and HAPE.

Supplemental oxygen is a cornerstone of management for altitude-related illness. Oxygen reduces pulmonary artery pressures[161] and usually reverses the symptoms of HAPE rapidly.[31] It has also been shown to improve the symptoms of AMS.[162] Supplemental oxygen rapidly increases inspired oxygen tension, although descent from high altitude is the preferred and definitive management. Prompt descent or supplemental oxygen, however, may not be feasible or available. In such cases, an alternative means of support is hyperbaric management. One mechanism of such support is the Gamow bag (FIGURE 19-5). This recompression chamber is highly portable and can be inflated in 2 minutes using a foot pump.[163] It has been found effective for management of both AMS and HAPE.[134,159,164,165] In addition to the early recognition of HAPE or other high altitude-related illness, management of hypoxia at altitude with descent, a hyperbaric chamber, or supplemental oxygen, is the single most important therapeutic intervention.

Other ventilatory modalities may be of benefit, as well. In one study, expiratory positive airway pressure improved oxygenation in patients with HAPE,[166] and a portable device for this purpose has been developed.[26] This has not been as practical, however, for most expeditions, and a Gamow bag is more likely to be available than an expiratory positive airway pressure device.

In addition to oxygen, other agents to promote vasodilation have been evaluated. These include inhaled nitric oxide, which has been shown to improve arterial oxygenation in patients with HAPE, but its administration is often impractical under the limiting conditions of high altitude.[75,161] Nifedipine reduces pulmonary artery pressures and pulmonary vascular resistance, and improves oxygenation and relieves symptoms.[150,167] Nifedipine is used commonly for HAPE at an initial single dose of 10 mg orally, followed by 20 to 30 mg of a sustained release form orally every 12-24 hours. Caution must be used to monitor for hypotension.

Additional vasodilators that have been evaluated include hydralazine and the α-adrenergic blocker phentolamine. Hydralazine and phentolamine reduce both pulmonary artery pressures and pulmonary vascular resistance.[150] In one trial, acetazolamide was also effective in increasing arterial oxygenation, though this was in an AMS population and not studied specifically for HAPE.[62]

Although diuresis is appropriate for cardiogenic pulmonary edema, it must be stressed that HAPE is a form of noncardiogenic pulmonary edema, and attempts at diuresis may prove harmful. Although some series have described using loop diuretics to manage HAPE,[21] their role is not clearly established, and compelling literature to support their use is lacking.[31] Although it may seem of theoretical benefit to manage concomitant HACE with diuretics, volume depletion commonly is found among climbers, as is hypotension caused by the vasodilators used to manage HAPE. Diuretic use, therefore, cannot be recommended and in most situations is best avoided. Similarly, although opiates can relieve pulmonary edema in patients with volume overload, their use in patients with HAPE might decrease HVR and thus worsen hypoxemia.[3]

Conclusion

Altitude-related illness is precipitated by hypobaric hypoxia, which initiates deleterious pulmonary vascular responses including vasoconstriction and pulmonary hypertension. Variations in the HVR appear to be determinants of susceptibility, as do differences in the degree of pulmonary hypertension seen in HAPE-susceptible individuals. Pulmonary hypertension can lead to vascular damage exacerbated by heterogenous flow and resultant overperfusion of some capillary beds. When these "stressed" capillaries fail, fluid extra-

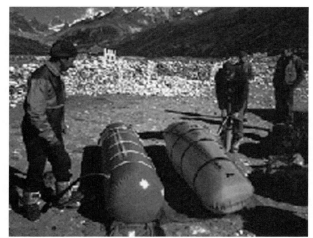

Figure 19-5. Recompression Chambers. Gamow bag is at left, Certec at right being inflated by foot or hand for management of altitude-related illness. (Reproduced with permission from Chinook Medical Gear.)

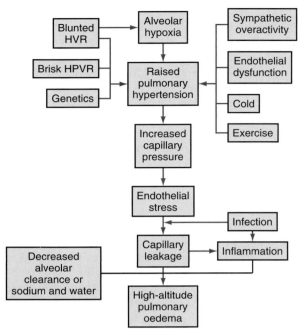

Figure 19-6. Summary of Proposed Pathophysiologic Mechanisms Contributing to HAPE. HVR, hypoxic ventilatory response; HPVR, hypoxic pulmonary vascular response. (Reproduced with permission from Basnyat B, Murdoch DR: High-altitude illness. *Lancet* 361(9373): 1967-1974, 2003.)

vasates and pulmonary edema ensues. Deficiencies in epithelial sodium-potassium pump action appear to slow resolution of edema, thereby contributing to the pathogenesis of HAPE (FIGURE 19-6).

Symptoms typically occur within 48 to 96 hours after exposure to high altitude, and the risk of developing HAPE is increased by a more rapid rate of ascent and a history of altitude-related illness. A measured rate of ascent and minimization of daily incremental increases are important preventative strategies. Supplemental oxygen is also an important means of prevention. Nifedipine (and potentially other vasodilators administered orally) can also reduce the incidence of HAPE. Management requires reversal of hypoxia with supplemental oxygen or portable hyperbaric chambers, or both, while rapid descent is arranged. Judicious use of additional vasodilators may be of further benefit. Advances in the understanding of genetic and other factors that increase susceptibility will help to better target efforts at prophylaxis. As high altitude becomes more easily accessible to a broader range of travelers, altitude-related illness including HAPE will likely become a more frequently encountered problem.

References

1. West JB: Alexander M. Kellas and the physiological challenge of Mt. Everest. *J Appl Physiol* 63:3-11, 1987.
2. West JB, Hackett PH, Maret KH, et al: Pulmonary gas exchange on the summit of Mount Everest. *J Appl Physiol* 55:678-687, 1983.
3. Krieger BP, de la Hoz RE: Altitude-related pulmonary disorders. *Crit Care Clin* 15:265-280, viii, 1999.
4. Rennie D: The great breathlessness mountains. *JAMA* 256:81-82, 1986.
5. West JB: Man at extreme altitude. *J Appl Physiol* 52:1393-1399, 1982.
6. Doherty MJ: James Glaisher's 1862 account of balloon sickness: Altitude, decompression injury, and hypoxemia. *Neurology* 60:1016-1018, 2003.
7. Bailey DM: The last "oxygenless" ascent of Mt. Everest. *Br J Sports Med* 35:294-296, 2001.
8. Gensini GF, Conti AA: A historical perspective on high altitude pulmonary edema. *Monaldi Arch Chest Dis* 60:45-47, 2003.
9. Richalet JP: High altitude pulmonary oedema: Still a place for controversy? *Thorax* 50:923-929, 1995.
10. Hackett P, Rennie D: High-altitude pulmonary edema. *JAMA* 287:2275-2278, 2002.
11. West JB: TH Ravenhill and his contributions to mountain sickness. *J Appl Physiol* 80:715-724, 1996.
12. Schoene RB: Pulmonary edema at high altitude. Review, pathophysiology, and update. *Clin Chest Med* 6:491-507, 1985.
13. Hultgren HN: High-altitude pulmonary edema: Current concepts. *Annu Rev Med* 47:267-284, 1996.
14. Houston CS: Acute pulmonary edema of high altitude. *N Engl J Med* 263:478-480, 1960.
15. Hultgren HN, Spickard W, Hellriegel K, et al: High altitude pulmonary edema. *Medicine (Baltimore)* 40: 289-313, 1961.
16. Stewart L: Acute pulmonary edema of high altitude. *N Z Med J* 60:79, 1961.
17. Fred H, Schmidt AM, Bates T, et al: Acute pulmonary edema of altitude. *Circulation* 25:929-937, 1962.
18. Hultgren HN, Lopez CE, Lundberg E, et al: Physiologic studies of pulmonary edema at high altitude. *Circulation* 29:393-408, 1964.
19. Singh I, Kapila CC, Khanna PK, et al: High-altitude pulmonary oedema. *Lancet* 191:229-234, 1965.
20. Menon ND: High-altitude pulmonary edema: A clinical study. *N Engl J Med* 273:66-73, 1965.
21. Singh I, Khanna PK, Srivastava MC, et al: Acute mountain sickness. *N Engl J Med* 280:175-184, 1969.
22. West JB: George I. Finch and his pioneering use of oxygen for climbing at extreme altitudes. *J Appl Physiol* 94:1702-1713, 2003.

23. Mason N: The physiology of high altitude: An introduction to the cardio-respiratory changes occurring on ascent to altitude. *Curr Anaesth Crit Care* 11:31-41, 2000.

24. Honigman B, Theis MK, Koziol-McLain J, et al: Acute mountain sickness in a general tourist population at moderate altitudes. *Ann Intern Med* 118:587-592, 1993.

25. Schneider M, Bernasch D, Weymann J, et al: Acute mountain sickness: Influence of susceptibility, preexposure, and ascent rate. *Med Sci Sports Exerc* 34:1886-1891, 2002.

26. Basnyat B, Murdoch DR: High-altitude illness. *Lancet* 361:1967-1974, 2003.

27. Roach RC, Maes D, Sandoval D, et al: Exercise exacerbates acute mountain sickness at simulated high altitude. *J Appl Physiol* 88:581-585, 2000.

28. Ri-Li G, Chase PJ, Witkowski S, et al: Obesity: Associations with acute mountain sickness. *Ann Intern Med* 139:253-257, 2003.

29. Basnyat B: Neck irradiation or surgery may predispose to severe acute mountain sickness. *J Travel Med* 9:105, 2002.

30. Roach RC, Hackett PH: Frontiers of hypoxia research: Acute mountain sickness. *J Exp Biol* 204:3161-3170, 2001.

31. Hackett PH, Roach RC: High-altitude illness. *N Engl J Med* 345:107-114, 2001.

32. Morocz IA, Zientara GP, Gudbjartsson H, et al: Volumetric quantification of brain swelling after hypobaric hypoxia exposure. *Exp Neurol* 168:96-104, 2001.

33. Moore LG, Harrison GL, McCullough RE, et al: Low acute hypoxic ventilatory response and hypoxic depression in acute altitude sickness. *J Appl Physiol* 60:1407-1412, 1986.

34. Eichenberger U, Weiss E, Riemann D, et al: Nocturnal periodic breathing and the development of acute high altitude illness. *Am J Respir Crit Care Med* 154:1748-1754, 1996.

35. Hackett P, Oelz O: The Lake Louise Consensus on the Definition and Quantification of Altitude Illness. In: Sutton JR, Coates G, Houston CS, editors: *Hypoxia and mountain medicine,* Burlington, VT, 1992, Queen City Printers.

36. Ge RL, Matsuzawa Y, Takeoka M, et al: Low pulmonary diffusing capacity in subjects with acute mountain sickness. *Chest* 111:58-64, 1997.

37. Hackett P: High altitude medicine. In: Auerbach P, editor: *Wilderness medicine: Management of wilderness and environmental emergencies,* St Louis, 1995, Mosby.

38. Kammler K: *Doctor on Everest: Emergency medicine at the top of the world—A personal account including the 1996 disaster.* New York, 2000, Lyons Press.

39. Lahiri S, Milledge JS: Pulmonary adaption and clinical disorders related to high altitude. In: Fishman AP, editor: *Pulmonary diseases and disorders,* ed 3, New York, 1998, McGraw Hill.

40. Kobayashi T, Koyama S, Kubo K, et al: Clinical features of patients with high-altitude pulmonary edema in Japan. *Chest* 92:814-821, 1987.

41. Vock P, Brutsche MH, Nanzer A, et al: Variable radiomorphologic data of high altitude pulmonary edema. Features from 60 patients. *Chest* 100:1306-1311, 1991.

42. Gluecker T, Capasso P, Schnyder P, et al: Clinical and radiologic features of pulmonary edema. *Radiographics* 19:1507-1531; discussion 1532-1533, 1999.

43. Peacock AJ: High altitude pulmonary oedema: Who gets it and why? *Eur Respir J* 8:1819-1821, 1995.

44. Hultgren HN, Marticorena EA: High altitude pulmonary edema. Epidemiologic observations in Peru. *Chest* 74:372-376, 1978.

45. Cremona G, Asnaghi R, Baderna P, et al: Pulmonary extravascular fluid accumulation in recreational climbers: A prospective study. *Lancet* 359:303-309, 2002.

46. Vock P, Fretz C, Franciolli M, et al: High-altitude pulmonary edema: Findings at high-altitude chest radiography and physical examination. *Radiology* 170:661-666, 1989.

47. Reeves J, Wagner J, Zafren K, et al: Seasonal variation in barometric pressure and temperature in Summit County: Effect on altitude illness. In: Sutton JR, Houston CS, Coates G, editors: *Hypoxia and molecular medicine,* Burlington, VT, 1993, Queen City Printers.

48. Naeije R, De Backer D, Vachiery JL, et al: High-altitude pulmonary edema with primary pulmonary hypertension. *Chest* 110:286-289, 1996.

49. Durmowicz AG: Pulmonary edema in 6 children with Down syndrome during travel to moderate altitudes. *Pediatrics* 108:443-447, 2001.

50. Wagner PD, Sutton JR, Reeves JT, et al: Operation Everest II: Pulmonary gas exchange during a simulated ascent of Mt. Everest. *J Appl Physiol* 63:2348-2259, 1987.

51. Raymond LW: Altitude pulmonary edema below 8,000 feet: What are we missing? *Chest* 123:5-7, 2003.

52. West JB, Lahiri S, Gill MB, et al: Arterial oxygen saturation during exercise at high altitude. *J Appl Physiol* 17:617-621, 1962.

53. West JB, Boyer SJ, Graber DJ, et al: Maximal exercise at extreme altitudes on Mount Everest. *J Appl Physiol* 55:688-698, 1983.

54. Moore LG: Comparative human ventilatory adaptation to high altitude. *Respir Physiol* 121:257-276, 2000.

55. Schoene RB, Lahiri S, Hackett PH, et al: Relationship of hypoxic ventilatory response to exercise

performance on Mount Everest. *J Appl Physiol* 56: 1478-1483, 1984.

56. Oelz O, Howald H, Di Prampero PE, et al: Physiological profile of world-class high-altitude climbers. *J Appl Physiol* 60:1734-1742, 1986.

57. Hackett PH, Roach RC, Schoene RB, et al: Abnormal control of ventilation in high-altitude pulmonary edema. *J Appl Physiol* 64:1268-1272, 1988.

58. Viswanathan R, Jain SK, Subramanian S, et al: Pulmonary edema of high altitude. II. Clinical, aero-hemodynamic, and biochemical studies in a group with history of pulmonary edema of high altitude. *Am Rev Respir Dis* 100:334-341, 1969.

59. Curran LS, Zhuang J, Sun SF, et al: Ventilation and hypoxic ventilatory responsiveness in Chinese-Tibetan residents at 3,658 m. *J Appl Physiol* 83:2098-2104, 1997.

60. Marconi C, Marzorati M, Grassi B, et al: Second generation Tibetan lowlanders acclimatize to high altitude more quickly than Caucasians. *J Physiol* 556:661-671, 2004.

61. Hanaoka M, Droma Y, Hotta J, et al: Polymorphisms of the tyrosine hydroxylase gene in subjects susceptible to high-altitude pulmonary edema. *Chest* 123: 54-58, 2003.

62. Grissom CK, Roach RC, Sarnquist FH, et al: Acetazolamide in the treatment of acute mountain sickness: Clinical efficacy and effect on gas exchange. *Ann Intern Med* 116:461-465, 1992.

63. Schoene RB, Bates PW, Larson EB, et al: Effect of acetazolamide on normoxic and hypoxic exercise in humans at sea level. *J Appl Physiol* 55:1772-1776, 1983.

64. Basnyat B, Gertsch JH, Johnson EW, et al: Efficacy of low-dose acetazolamide (125 mg BID) for the pro-phylaxis of acute mountain sickness: A prospective, double-blind, randomized, placebo-controlled trial. *High Alt Med Biol* 4:45-52, 2003.

65. Roy SB, Guleria JS, Khanna PK, et al: Haemo-dynamic studies in high altitude pulmonary oedema. *Br Heart J* 31:52-58, 1969.

66. Penaloza D, Sime F: Circulatory dynamics during high altitude pulmonary edema. *Am J Cardiol* 23:369-378, 1969.

67. Das BB, Wolfe RR, Chan KC, et al: High-altitude pulmonary edema in children with underlying cardiopulmonary disorders and pulmonary hyper-tension living at altitude. *Arch Pediatr Adolesc Med* 158:1170-1176, 2004.

68. Yagi H, Yamada H, Kobayashi T, et al: Doppler assess-ment of pulmonary hypertension induced by hypoxic breathing in subjects susceptible to high altitude pul-monary edema. *Am Rev Respir Dis* 142:796-801, 1990.

69. Grunig E, Mereles D, Hildebrandt W, et al: Stress Doppler echocardiography for identification of susceptibility to high altitude pulmonary edema. *J Am Coll Cardiol* 35:980-987, 2000.

70. Kawashima A, Kubo K, Kobayashi T, et al: Hemodynamic responses to acute hypoxia, hypo-baria, and exercise in subjects susceptible to high-altitude pulmonary edema. *J Appl Physiol* 67: 1982-1989, 1989.

71. Swenson ER, Maggiorini M, Mongovin S, et al: Pathogenesis of high-altitude pulmonary edema: Inflammation is not an etiologic factor. *JAMA* 287:2228-2235, 2002.

72. Viswanathan R, Subramanian S, Lodi ST, et al: Further studies on pulmonary oedema of high alti-tude. Abnormal responses to hypoxia of men who had developed pulmonary oedema at high altitude. *Respiration* 36:216-222, 1978.

73. Eldridge MW, Podolsky A, Richardson RS, et al: Pulmonary hemodynamic response to exercise in subjects with prior high-altitude pulmonary edema. *J Appl Physiol* 81:911-921, 1996.

74. Hultgren HN, Grover RF, Hartley LH: Abnormal circulatory responses to high altitude in subjects with a previous history of high-altitude pulmonary edema *Circulation* 44:759-770, 1971.

75. Scherrer U, Vollenweider L, Delabays A, et al: Inhaled nitric oxide for high-altitude pulmonary edema. *N Engl J Med* 334:624-629, 1996.

76. Vachiery JL, McDonagh T, Moraine JJ, et al: Doppler assessment of hypoxic pulmonary vasoconstriction and susceptibility to high altitude pulmonary oedema. *Thorax* 50:22-27, 1995.

77. Duplain H, Sartori C, Lepori M, et al: Exhaled nitric oxide in high-altitude pulmonary edema: Role in the regulation of pulmonary vascular tone and evi-dence for a role against inflammation. *Am J Respir Crit Care Med* 162:221-224, 2000.

78. Busch T, Bartsch P, Pappert D, et al: Hypoxia decreases exhaled nitric oxide in mountaineers sus-ceptible to high-altitude pulmonary edema. *Am J Respir Crit Care Med* 163:368-373, 2001.

79. Hotta J, Hanaoka M, Droma Y, et al: Polymorphisms of renin-angiotensin system genes with high-alti-tude pulmonary edema in Japanese subjects. *Chest* 126:825-830, 2004.

80. Goerre S, Wenk M, Bartsch P, et al: Endothelin-1 in pulmonary hypertension associated with high-alti-tude exposure. *Circulation* 91:359-364, 1995.

81. Sartori C, Vollenweider L, Loffler BM, et al: Exaggerated endothelin release in high-altitude pulmonary edema. *Circulation* 99:2665-2668, 1999.

82. Blaber AP, Hartley T, Pretorius PJ: Effect of acute exposure to 3660 m altitude on orthostatic responses and tolerance. *J Appl Physiol* 95:591-601, 2003.

83. Somers VK, Mark AL, Zavala DC, et al: Influence of ventilation and hypocapnia on sympathetic nerve

responses to hypoxia in normal humans. *J Appl Physiol* 67:2095-2100, 1989.

84. Heindl S, Lehnert M, Criee CP, et al: Marked sympathetic activation in patients with chronic respiratory failure. *Am J Respir Crit Care Med* 164:597-601, 2001.

85. Calbet JA: Chronic hypoxia increases blood pressure and noradrenaline spillover in healthy humans. *J Physiol* 551:379-386, 2003.

86. Duplain H, Vollenweider L, Delabays A, et al: Augmented sympathetic activation during short-term hypoxia and high-altitude exposure in subjects susceptible to high-altitude pulmonary edema. *Circulation* 99:1713-1718, 1999.

87. Woods DR, Pollard AJ, Collier DJ, et al: Insertion /deletion polymorphism of the angiotensin I-converting enzyme gene and arterial oxygen saturation at high altitude. *Am J Respir Crit Care Med* 166:362-366, 2002.

88. Rupert JL, Kidd KK, Norman LE, et al: Genetic polymorphisms in the renin-angiotensin system in high-altitude and low-altitude Native American populations. *Ann Hum Genet* 67:17-25, 2003.

89. Aldashev AA, Sarybaev AS, Sydykov AS, et al: Characterization of high-altitude pulmonary hypertension in the Kyrgyz: Association with angiotensin-converting enzyme genotype. *Am J Respir Crit Care Med* 166:1396-1402, 2002.

90. Dehnert C, Weymann J, Montgomery HE, et al: No association between high-altitude tolerance and the ACE I/D gene polymorphism. *Med Sci Sports Exerc* 34:1928-1933, 2002.

91. Fraser R, Muller NL, Colman N, et al: Pulmonary edema. In: Fraser R, editor: *Fraser and Pare's diagnosis of diseases of the chest,* Philadelphia, 1999, WB Saunders, pp 1946-2015.

92. Schuster D: Pulmonary edema. In: AP Fishman, Elias JA, Kaiser LR, et al, editors: *Fishman's pulmonary diseases and disorders,* New York, 1998, McGraw Hill, pp 1331-1356.

93. Barry PW, Pollard AJ: Altitude illness. *BMJ* 326:915-919, 2003.

94. West JB: Cellular response to mechanical stress invited review: Pulmonary capillary stress failure. *J Appl Physiol* 89:2483-2489, 2000.

95. Maggiorini M, Melot C, Pierre S, et al: High-altitude pulmonary edema is initially caused by an increase in capillary pressure. *Circulation* 103:2078-2083, 2001.

96. Wagner PD, Gale GE, Moon RE, et al: Pulmonary gas exchange in humans exercising at sea level and simulated altitude. *J Appl Physiol* 61:260-270, 1986.

97. Kuwahira I, Moue Y, Urano T, et al: Redistribution of pulmonary blood flow during hypoxic exercise. *Int J Sports Med* 22:393-399, 2001.

98. Hanaoka M, Tanaka M, Ge RL, et al: Hypoxia-induced pulmonary blood redistribution in subjects with a history of high-altitude pulmonary edema. *Circulation* 101:1418-1422, 2000.

99. Hopkins SR, Garg J, Bolar DS, et al: Pulmonary blood flow heterogeneity during hypoxia and high-altitude pulmonary edema. *Am J Respir Crit Care Med* 171:83-87, 2005.

100. Hackett PH, Creagh CE, Grover RF, et al: High-altitude pulmonary edema in persons without the right pulmonary artery. *N Engl J Med* 302:1070-1073, 1980.

101. Nana-Sinkam P, Bost TW, Sippel JM: Unilateral pulmonary edema in a 29-year-old man visiting high altitude. *Chest* 122:2230-2233, 2002.

102. Torrington KG: Recurrent high-altitude illness associated with right pulmonary artery occlusion from granulomatous mediastinitis. *Chest* 96:1422-1424, 1989.

103. Mokta JK, Mahajan SK, Prashar BS, et al: Life threatening unilateral pulmonary oedema at moderate altitude. *Indian J Chest Dis Allied Sci* 46:113-116, 2004.

104. Nakagawa S, Kubo K, Koizumi T, et al: High-altitude pulmonary edema with pulmonary thromboembolism. *Chest* 103:948-950, 1993.

105. Richalet JP, Merlet P, Bourguignon M, et al: MIBG scintigraphic assessment of cardiac adrenergic activity in response to altitude hypoxia. *J Nucl Med* 31:34-37, 1990.

106. West JB, Tsukimoto K, Mathieu-Costello O, et al: Stress failure in pulmonary capillaries. *J Appl Physiol* 70:1731-1742, 1991.

107. Costello ML, O. Mathieu-Costello, West JB: Stress failure of alveolar epithelial cells studied by scanning electron microscopy. *Am Rev Respir Dis* 145:1446-1455, 1992.

108. Tsukimoto K, Mathieu-Costello O, Prediletto R, et al: Ultrastructural appearances of pulmonary capillaries at high transmural pressures. *J Appl Physiol* 71:573-582, 1991.

109. Tsukimoto K, Yoshimura N, Ichioka M, et al: Protein, cell, and LTB_4 concentrations of lung edema fluid produced by high capillary pressures in rabbit. *J Appl Physiol* 76:321-327, 1994.

110. Fu Z, Costello ML, Tsukimoto K, et al: High lung volume increases stress failure in pulmonary capillaries. *J Appl Physiol* 73:123-133, 1992.

111. Elliott AR, Fu Z, Tsukimoto K, et al: Short-term reversibility of ultrastructural changes in pulmonary capillaries caused by stress failure. *J Appl Physiol* 73:1150-1158, 1992.

112. West JB, Colice GL, Lee YJ, et al: Pathogenesis of high-altitude pulmonary oedema: Direct evidence of stress failure of pulmonary capillaries. *Eur Respir J* 8:523-529, 1995.

113. Schoene RB, Swenson ER, Pizzo CJ, et al: The lung at high altitude: Bronchoalveolar lavage in acute

mountain sickness and pulmonary edema. *J Appl Physiol* 64:2605-2613, 1988.

114. Schoene RB, Hackett PH, Henderson WR, et al: High-altitude pulmonary edema. Characteristics of lung lavage fluid. *JAMA* 256:63-69, 1986.

115. Grissom CK, Albertine KH, Elstad MR: Alveolar haemorrhage in a case of high altitude pulmonary oedema. *Thorax* 55:167-169, 2000.

116. Grissom CK, Zimmerman GA, Whatley RE: Endothelial selectins in acute mountain sickness and high-altitude pulmonary edema. *Chest* 112:1572-1578, 1997.

117. Kubo K, Hanaoka M, Yamaguchi S, et al: Cytokines in bronchoalveolar lavage fluid in patients with high altitude pulmonary oedema at moderate altitude in Japan. *Thorax* 51:739-742, 1996.

118. Kubo K, Hanaoka M, Hayano T, et al: Inflammatory cytokines in BAL fluid and pulmonary hemodynamics in high-altitude pulmonary edema. *Respir Physiol* 111:301-310, 1998.

119. Kaminsky DA, Jones K, Schoene RB, et al: Urinary leukotriene E_4 levels in high-altitude pulmonary edema. A possible role for inflammation. *Chest* 110:939-945, 1996.

120. Hartmann G, Tschop M, Fischer R, et al: High altitude increases circulating interleukin-6, interleukin-1 receptor antagonist and C-reactive protein. *Cytokine* 12:246-252, 2000.

121. Bartsch P, Eichenberger U, Ballmer PE, et al: Urinary leukotriene E levels are not increased prior to high-altitude pulmonary edema. *Chest* 117:1393-1398, 2000.

122. Durmowicz AG, Noordeweir E, Nicholas R, et al: Inflammatory processes may predispose children to high-altitude pulmonary edema. *J Pediatr* 130:838-840, 1997.

123. Carpenter TC, Reeves JT, Durmowicz AG: Viral respiratory infection increases susceptibility of young rats to hypoxia-induced pulmonary edema. *J Appl Physiol* 84:1048-1054, 1998.

124. Hanaoka M, Kubo K, Yamazaki Y, et al: Association of high-altitude pulmonary edema with the major histocompatibility complex. *Circulation* 97:1124-1128, 1998.

125. West JB: The physiologic basis of high-altitude diseases. *Ann Intern Med* 141:789-800, 2004.

126. Sartori C, Matthay MA, Scherrer U: Transepithelial sodium and water transport in the lung. Major player and novel therapeutic target in pulmonary edema. *Adv Exp Med Biol* 502:315-338, 2001.

127. Ware LB, Matthay MA: Alveolar fluid clearance is impaired in the majority of patients with acute lung injury and the acute respiratory distress syndrome. *Am J Respir Crit Care Med* 163:1376-1383, 2001.

128. Hoschele S, Mairbaurl H: Alveolar flooding at high altitude: Failure of reabsorption? *News Physiol Sci* 18:55-59, 2003.

129. Mairbaurl H, Weymann J, Mohrlein A, et al: Nasal epithelium potential difference at high altitude (4,559 m): Evidence for secretion. *Am J Respir Crit Care Med* 167:862-867, 2003.

130. Mason NP, Petersen M, Melot C, et al: Serial changes in nasal potential difference and lung electrical impedance tomography at high altitude. *J Appl Physiol* 94:2043-2050, 2003.

131. Sakuma T, Folkesson HG, Suzuki S, et al: β-Adrenergic agonist stimulated alveolar fluid clearance in *ex vivo* human and rat lungs. *Am J Respir Crit Care Med* 155:506-512, 1997.

132. Parker JC, Ivey CL: Isoproterenol attenuates high vascular pressure-induced permeability increases in isolated rat lungs. *J Appl Physiol* 83:1962-1967, 1997.

133. Sartori C, Allemann Y, Duplain H, et al: Salmeterol for the prevention of high-altitude pulmonary edema. *N Engl J Med* 346:1631-1636, 2002.

134. Peacock AJ: ABC of oxygen: Oxygen at high altitude. *BMJ* 317:1063-1066, 1998.

135. Roeggla G, Roeggla H, Roeggla M, et al: Effect of alcohol on acute ventilatory adaptation to mild hypoxia at moderate altitude. *Ann Intern Med* 122:925-927, 1995.

136. Cain SM, Dunn JE, II: Low doses of acetazolamide to aid accommodation of men to altitude. *J Appl Physiol* 21:1195-1200, 1966.

137. Fischer R, Lang SM, Leitl M, et al: Theophylline and acetazolamide reduce sleep-disordered breathing at high altitude. *Eur Respir J* 23:47-52, 2004.

138. Fischer R, Lang SM, Steiner U, et al: Theophylline improves acute mountain sickness. *Eur Respir J* 15:123-127, 2000.

139. Garske LA, Brown MG, Morrison SC: Acetazolamide reduces exercise capacity and increases leg fatigue under hypoxic conditions. *J Appl Physiol* 94:991-996, 2003.

140. Carlsten C, Swenson ER, Ruoss S: A dose-response study of acetazolamide for acute mountain sickness prophylaxis in vacationing tourists at 12,000 feet (3,630 m). *High Alt Med Biol* 5:33-39, 2004.

141. Dumont L, Mardirosoff C, Tramer MR: Efficacy and harm of pharmacological prevention of acute mountain sickness: Quantitative systematic review. *BMJ* 321:267-272, 2000.

142. Wright AD, Beazley MF, Bradwell AR, et al: Medroxyprogesterone at high altitude. The effects on blood gases, cerebral regional oxygenation, and acute mountain sickness. *Wilderness Environ Med* 15:25-31, 2004.

143. Rock PB, Johnson TS, Larsen RF, et al: Dexamethasone as prophylaxis for acute mountain

sickness. Effect of dose level. *Chest* 95:568-573, 1989.

144. Ellsworth AJ, Meyer EF, Larson EB: Acetazolamide or dexamethasone use versus placebo to prevent acute mountain sickness on Mount Rainier. *West J Med* 154:289-293, 1991.

145. Ellsworth A: Pharmacology for altitude-related illness. *J Pharm Practice* 16:68-75, 2003.

146. Askew EW: Work at high altitude and oxidative stress: Antioxidant nutrients. *Toxicology* 180:107-119, 2002.

147. Gertsch JH, Seto TB, Mor J, et al: Ginkgo biloba for the prevention of severe acute mountain sickness (AMS) starting one day before rapid ascent. *High Alt Med Biol* 3:29-37, 2002.

148. Bailey DM, Davies B: Acute mountain sickness; prophylactic benefits of antioxidant vitamin supplementation at high altitude. *High Alt Med Biol* 2:21-29, 2001.

149. Gertsch JH, Basnyat B, Johnson EW, et al: Randomised, double blind, placebo controlled comparison of ginkgo biloba and acetazolamide for prevention of acute mountain sickness among Himalayan trekkers: The prevention of high altitude illness trial (PHAIT). *BMJ* 328:797, 2004.

150. Hackett PH, Roach RC, Hartig GS, et al: The effect of vasodilators on pulmonary hemodynamics in high altitude pulmonary edema: A comparison. *Int J Sports Med* 13(Suppl 1):S68-S71, 1992.

151. Bartsch P, Maggiorini M, Ritter M, et al: Prevention of high-altitude pulmonary edema by nifedipine. *N Engl J Med* 325:1284-1289, 1991.

152. Hohenhaus E, Niroomand F, Goerre S, et al: Nifedipine does not prevent acute mountain sickness. *Am J Respir Crit Care Med* 150:857-860, 1994.

153. Watt M, Peacock AJ, Newell J, et al: The effect of amlodipine on respiratory and pulmonary vascular responses to hypoxia in mountaineers. *Eur Respir J* 15:459-463, 2000.

154. Ghofrani HA, Schermuly RT, Rose F, et al: Sildenafil for long-term treatment of nonoperable chronic thromboembolic pulmonary hypertension. *Am J Respir Crit Care Med* 167:1139-1141, 2003.

155. Ghofrani HA, Wiedemann R, Rose F, et al: Sildenafil for treatment of lung fibrosis and pulmonary hypertension: A randomised controlled trial. *Lancet* 360:895-900, 2002.

156. Zhao L, Mason NA, Morrell NW, et al: Sildenafil inhibits hypoxia-induced pulmonary hypertension. *Circulation* 104:424-428, 2001.

157. Ghofrani HA, Reichenberger F, Kohstall MG, et al: Sildenafil increased exercise capacity during hypoxia at low altitudes and at Mount Everest base camp: A randomized, double-blind, placebo-controlled crossover trial. *Ann Intern Med* 141:169-177, 2004.

158. Levine BD, Yoshimura K, Kobayashi T, et al: Dexamethasone in the treatment of acute mountain sickness. *N Engl J Med* 321:1707-1713, 1989.

159. Keller HR, Maggiorini M, Bartsch P, et al: Simulated descent v dexamethasone in treatment of acute mountain sickness: A randomised trial. *BMJ* 310:1232-1235, 1995.

160. Klocke DL, Decker WW, Stepanek J: Altitude-related illnesses. *Mayo Clin Proc* 73:988-992; quiz 992-993, 1998.

161. Anand IS, Prasad BA, Chugh SS, et al: Effects of inhaled nitric oxide and oxygen in high-altitude pulmonary edema. *Circulation* 98:2441-2445, 1998.

162. Kasic JF, Yaron M, Nicholas RA, et al: Treatment of acute mountain sickness: Hyperbaric versus oxygen therapy. *Ann Emerg Med* 20:1109-1112, 1991.

163. A'Court CH, Stables RH, Travis S: Doctor on a mountaineering expedition. *BMJ* 310:1248-1252, 1995.

164. Bartsch P, Merki B, Hofstetter D, et al: Treatment of acute mountain sickness by simulated descent: A randomised controlled trial. *BMJ* 306:1098-1101, 1993.

165. King S, Greenlee R: Successful use of the Gamow hyperbaric bag in the treatment of altitude illness on Everest. *J Wilderness Med* 1:193-202, 1990.

166. Schoene RB, Roach RC, Hackett PH, et al: High altitude pulmonary edema and exercise at 4,400 meters on Mount McKinley. Effect of expiratory positive airway pressure. *Chest* 87:330-333, 1985.

167. Oelz O, Maggiorini M, Ritter M, et al: Nifedipine for high altitude pulmonary oedema. *Lancet* 2:1241-1244, 1989.

168. Bartsch P: High altitude pulmonary edema. *Med Sci Sports Exerc* 31(1 Suppl):S23-S27, 1999.

Chapter 20

Embolism of Fat, Air, or Amniotic Fluid

Alix Ashare, MD,

James Carroll, MD

Fat Embolism

Symptoms consistent with fat embolism were described as early as 1861 by F.A. Zenker in a railroad worker who suffered a thoracolumbar crush injury. However, the fat embolism syndrome was not defined until it was described by Von Bergman in 1873 in a patient with a femoral fracture. The diagnosis was confirmed by postmortem examination. Although the disease has been recognized for over a century, it still remains a significant diagnostic challenge for physicians.

The term "fat embolism" refers to globules of free fat within the vasculature (FIGURE 20-1). The disease typically occurs following long bone fracture or orthopedic surgery. However, it has also been described as a complication of liposuction, pancreatitis, and osteomyelitis.[1-3] Findings of dyspnea and hypoxemia vary from mild to extremely severe, and fat globules in the pulmonary circulation can pass into the systemic circulation to embolize to the brain and skin. The classic onset of fat embolism syndrome consists of an asymptomatic interval followed by pulmonary, neurologic, and dermatologic manifestations.

Epidemiology

Fat embolism occurs in nearly all patients with bone fractures and during many orthopedic procedures.[4,5] However, most patients with fat emboli are asymptomatic, and less than 20 percent develop overt fat embolism syndrome.[5] The true incidence of fat embolism syndrome remains unknown, because many mild cases go unrecognized.

Fat embolism syndrome is most likely to occur after severe trauma. Multiple skeletal fractures increase the risk of fat embolism syndrome, because a larger amount of fat is released into the marrow vessels.[5] In individuals with significant trauma, the incidence of fat embolism syndrome is estimated at 20 percent when multiple fractures are present, and 0.5 to 20 percent with a single fracture.[5,6] Fat embolism syndrome is more likely to occur after closed, rather than open, fractures and in patients with fractures involving the middle and proximal parts of the femoral shaft. However, fat embolism syndrome can occur following minor injury, particularly in patients with underlying pulmonary vascular disease.

In addition to trauma, fat embolism can occur following liposuction or in patients with pancreatitis, fatty liver, or osteomyelitis.[1-3] Furthermore, fat emboli may be a cause of acute chest syndrome associated with sickle cell disease[7] (see Chapter 12).

Clinical Picture and Diagnosis

The classic triad of fat embolism syndrome consists of hypoxemia, neurologic abnormalities, and a petechial rash. The syndrome typically follows a biphasic course. Most patients are asymptomatic for 12 to 24 hours following embolization, and in some cases symptoms can be delayed as long as 3 days.[8] The clinical picture may be subclinical, mild, or fulminant.

Pulmonary manifestations, including dyspnea, tachypnea, and hypoxemia, occur in 90 percent of patients with fat embolism and are often the earliest findings. Arterial hypoxemia in these patients has been attributed to ventilation-perfusion mismatch and intrapulmonary shunting. Cough,

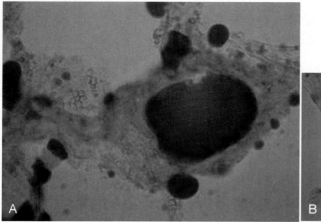
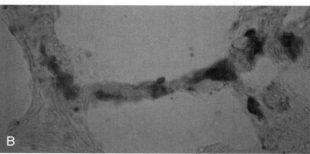

Figure 20-1. High-power photomicrographs reveal numerous fat emboli within pulmonary capillaries. The patient was an unrestrained driver in a high speed motor vehicle accident and suffered multiple fractures. (Sudan III stain.) (Courtesy of Dr. Giuseppe G. Pietra.) (See Color Plate 11).

hemoptysis, and pleuritic chest pain may develop but are less common. On physical examination, inspiratory crackles are a common finding. A pleural rub occasionally can be heard. Approximately 50 percent of patients with fat embolism secondary to a long bone fracture develop acute respiratory distress syndrome (ARDS) and require mechanical ventilation.[9]

Neurologic symptoms develop in up to 85 percent of patients with pulmonary manifestations.[6] Symptoms typically occur after the onset of respiratory symptoms. Patients usually become confused, followed by an altered level of consciousness. Seizures and focal neurologic deficits have also been described. In most cases, the neurologic findings are reversible and resolve in tandem with the respiratory manifestations.

Skin involvement is also frequent, occurring in 20 to 50 percent of patients with pulmonary manifestations.[6] Skin disease typically appears as a petechial rash. It is often a late and transient finding and occurs 2 to 3 days after embolization. The petechiae result from the occlusion of skin capillaries by fat globules, resulting in the extravasation of erythrocytes. Petechiae are most prominent along the axillary folds, conjunctiva, and retina.

The diagnosis of fat embolism syndrome usually is made on the basis of clinical characteristics: respiratory and neurologic symptoms following long bone fracture are suggestive of fat embolism. The petechial rash is considered pathognomonic, but it occurs in less than 50 percent of cases. Gurd and Wilson[10] established a set of diagnostic criteria for fat embolism syndrome, but these criteria have not been well validated and rarely are used clinically.[11]

The chest radiograph usually is not helpful in establishing the diagnosis. A minority of patients' radiographs demonstrate patchy airspace disease, but most have normal chest radiograph findings. Ventilation-perfusion scans may show subsegmental perfusion defects with normal ventilation. High-resolution computed tomography (CT) of the chest may show ground glass infiltrates,[12] but this is not a specific finding.

No laboratory test is specific for the diagnosis of fat embolism syndrome. Thrombocytopenia and anemia are common findings, and disseminated intravascular coagulation (DIC) and hemolytic anemia may occur. Hypocalcemia can develop because of the affinity of calcium ions for free fatty acids. Lipiduria occurs commonly. Circulating fat levels have not been found to correlate with the presence or severity of fat embolism syndrome.

Several studies have suggested that recovery of fat globules from wedged pulmonary artery catheter or bronchoalveolar lavage specimens may assist in establishing the diagnosis. However, fat globules are present in the blood in patients with long bone fractures independent of whether the fat embolism syndrome develops.[9] Similarly, lipid-laden macrophages in bronchoalveolar lavage fluid can be found in a variety of conditions, and the sensitivity and specificity of their presence for the diagnosis of fat embolism syndrome is not known.[13-15]

In summary, the diagnosis of fat embolism syndrome is based upon pulmonary, neurologic, and dermatologic manifestations in the appropriate clinical setting. Physicians should have a high index of suspicion in any patient who develops dyspnea or hypoxia after experiencing trauma or undergoing orthopedic surgery.

Pathophysiology

Marrow contents commonly enter the circulation following a fracture or when the medullary cavity is reamed during placement of an internal fixation device. Both of these cause increased pressure within the medullary cavity, thereby permitting entry of marrow fat into torn vessels. However, the mechanism by which fat in the blood produces the severe clinical manifestations of the syndrome is not entirely clear.[5] Two main hypotheses have been advanced:

1. The "mechanical" theory suggests that fat from traumatized marrow is forced into torn venous channels that remain open because they are attached to the surrounding bone. The increased intramedullary pressure pushes the marrow into the sinusoid. From there, fat travels to the pulmonary circulation and mechanically occludes the pulmonary capillaries. Evidence supporting the mechanical theory includes visualization of marrow fat in the femoral vein within seconds of intramedullary manipulation.[5] In addition, transesophageal echocardiograms performed during orthopedic procedures have demonstrated that echogenic material passes through the heart at the time a guide wire is inserted into the bone marrow canal for intramedullary nailing.[16] The main criticism of this theory is that the events related to mechanical obstruction appear to occur at the time of injury, while the symptoms of fat embolism syndrome are delayed 12-24 hours.

2. The "toxic mediator" theory hypothesizes that fat embolism syndrome occurs as a result of hydrolysis of fat to more toxic free fatty acids and other species. Circulating free fatty acids are directly toxic to pneumocytes and capillary endothelium in the lung.[17] In animal models, free fatty acids have been associated with ARDS. This theory is supported by the delayed appearance of rash, neurologic dysfunction, and progressive respiratory failure.

It is likely that both mechanisms contribute to fat embolism syndrome. The initial mild respiratory symptoms may be caused by mechanical obstruction by multiple fat globules that are too large to traverse the pulmonary capillaries. Because fat globules are deformable, they may not occlude the vasculature completely and, therefore, the obstruction may be incomplete. The later onset of neurologic, dermatologic, and severe respiratory symptoms may be a result of hydrolysis of fat to free fatty acids. These free fatty acids can then migrate to other organs via the systemic circulation.

Management and Prevention

Management of fat embolism syndrome is usually supportive, including maintenance of intravascular volume and mechanical ventilation as required. Mortality is estimated to be 15 percent or less with meticulous supportive care.[5]

The risk for developing fat embolism syndrome is thought to be reduced by early immobilization and operative correction of long bone fractures.[18,19] Limiting elevation of intraosseous pressure during orthopedic surgery via a number of techniques may reduce the release of intramedullary fat into the circulation and decrease the risk of fat embolism syndrome.[20] Glucocorticoids have been effective in preventing fat embolism syndrome in several trials,[21,22] but their routine prophylactic use remains controversial due to the risk of steroid-related complications. There is no evidence that glucocorticoids are beneficial in managing established fat embolism syndrome.

Air Embolism

Gas embolism occurs as a result of entrainment of gas, typically air, into the vasculature. The first clinical report of air embolism dates from 1821 and resulted in death.[23] Most cases are related to medical procedures or rapid ascent during underwater diving.

Air embolism can be divided further into venous air embolism and arterial air embolism. The two are distinguished both by the mechanism of air entry into the vasculature and the vascular site where the emboli lodge. This chapter will focus on venous air embolism because of its greater relevance to the pulmonary circulation.

Epidemiology

The most common risk factor for air entry into the venous circulation is a procedure involving the incision or puncture of large, non-collapsed veins when the pressure within those veins is subatmospheric.[24] Many surgical procedures have been implicated, including neurosurgical, gynecologic, and orthopedic interventions. Neurosurgical procedures performed in the sitting position have the greatest incidence of venous air embolism, estimated as high as 80 percent for posterior fossa surgery in this orientation.[25] Venous air embolism also may occur during neurosurgical procedures in the lateral, supine, or prone positions. Similarly, air may enter the veins of the myometrium during delivery, and one study reported the incidence of venous air embolism in women undergoing cesarean section to be 40 percent.[26] During hip replacement surgery, the incidence of venous air embolism is as high as 30 percent.[27]

Venous air embolism can occur during placement, maintenance, or removal of a central venous catheter.[28] A spontaneously breathing patient generates negative intrathoracic pressure during inspiration, and pressure within the central veins may be subatmospheric, particularly if the veins are above the heart and the patient is hypovolemic. In such a situation, significant quantities of air can rapidly enter the venous circulation.

Although gas embolism usually is caused by entrainment of air, other gases also can gain access to the venous circulation. During laparoscopic procedures, insufflation of carbon dioxide maintains intraabdominal pressure greater than venous pressure. If there is venous injury during the procedure, carbon dioxide can gain entry into the venous circulation.[27] The precise incidence of this complication is unknown.

During diving, air embolism can result from distention and rupture of the alveoli by expanding gases during ascent. An individual who has airflow obstruction and cannot exhale fully on ascent has an increased likelihood of barotrauma on ascent, which can result in an arterial or venous air embolism.[29] Pulmonary air embolism can also be a manifestation of decompression sickness, resulting from the formation of nitrogen bubbles following rapid ascent from a dive. This form of decompression sickness is commonly referred to as "the chokes."

Clinical Manifestations and Diagnosis

Clinical manifestations of air embolism are nonspecific. In a conscious patient, air embolism is accompanied by symptoms of dyspnea and chest pain. Signs of mild air embolism include tachypnea and diaphoresis. A more severe air embolism can cause hypotension, cardiac arrest, or electrocardiographic changes such as tachyarrhythmias, atrioventricular block, or right ventricular strain.[27] On physical examination, a "mill wheel" or "mill pond" murmur may be auscultated. This is a splashing sound caused by air in the cardiac chambers and is typically a late sign.[24] These findings in a patient at risk should prompt the physician to consider air embolism. Because definitive diagnostic measures require time, management should begin as soon as air embolism is suspected.

The definitive diagnosis of air embolism can be made by echocardiography, and intraoperative transthoracic echocardiography should be considered during high-risk surgeries, such as seated neurosurgical procedures. A properly positioned precordial Doppler ultrasound device can detect as little as 0.25 mL of air injected into the venous circulation.[30] Transesophageal echocardiography is a more sensitive technique, although it is a more invasive procedure and its intraoperative utility is limited by its expense. Although radiographs may be normal in patients with air embolism, CT may show small amounts of air in the in the pulmonary arteries or right side of the heart.[31] Chest radiographs are relatively insensitive.

Pathophysiology

Factors that determine the severity of illness following venous air embolism include the volume of air entrained, the rate of air entrainment, the position of the patient at the time, and the patient's underlying cardiopulmonary reserve. The lethal volume of air in animals depends on the rate of injection. When injected rapidly, injection of 7.5 mL/kg of air into dogs has been uniformly fatal.[27] However, dogs are able to tolerate 1,400 mL of air injected over a period of hours. The absolute volume of air tolerated in humans is not known; however, there have been case reports demonstrating that accidental injection of 300 mL of air can be fatal.

The most common cause of death from massive air embolism is circulatory collapse due to right ventricular outflow obstruction. The rate of entrainment appears to be critical in this process. Rapid entrainment of air into the venous circulation causes an acute rise in pulmonary artery pressures within 60 seconds.[27] In addition, the large volume of air trapped in the pulmonary vasculature may obstruct the right ventricular outflow tract. Both the increased pulmonary artery pressures and the right ventricular outflow obstruction put increased strain on the right ventricle and decrease pulmonary venous return. This results in decreased left ventricular preload and decreased cardiac output. The occluded pulmonary vasculature can cause ventilation-perfusion mismatch, resulting in hypoxemia. When air is entrained more slowly, the pulmonary artery pressures increase less rapidly. Typically, pulmonary artery pressures peak after 10 minutes and then slowly decline. Tachyarrhythmias occur commonly, and their severity is related to the volume of air entrained. Bradycardia can occur and is considered an ominous sign.

The position of the patient is an important factor in air entrainment. Procedures performed with the patient in the seated position are associated with the highest risk for air embolism. A greater pressure gradient between the procedural site and the right atrial pressure is associated with a greater potential for entrainment of air. Hypovolemia will exacerbate this by further reducing the right atrial pressure.

Another related factor is whether the patient is breathing spontaneously. A spontaneously breathing person generates negative intrathoracic pressure during inspiration that can draw air into the vessel if a catheter or other route of air entry is open. In addition, air entrainment may cause chest pain and dyspnea and lead the patient to gasp, resulting in even greater negative intrathoracic pressure and further air entrainment.

Air embolism can cause ARDS. Entrapment of air bubbles in the pulmonary circulation may lead to release of vasoactive mediators, increasing alveolar capillary permeability and resulting in pulmonary edema. Furthermore, these mediators may recruit activated neutrophils to the pulmonary vasculature, resulting in inflammation and further lung damage.[23]

In diving, the mechanism is slightly different. In deep water divers breathe compressed air at greater-than-ambient pressure, and excess air dissolves in blood and tissue. If the diver ascends too rapidly, gas emerges from solution and forms small bubbles. Nitrogen bubbles are the slowest to be cleared and can cause air embolism in the manner discussed above.

Every venous air embolism has the potential to develop into an arterial air embolism. If the filtering capacity of the pulmonary capillary bed is overwhelmed, air bubbles can pass to the arterial circulation. This can also occur due to the presence of a right-to-left shunt, including a patent foramen ovale. When air bubbles enter the systemic circulation, they distribute to nearly all organs. Embolization to the cerebral or coronary circulation may result in focal ischemia with significant morbidity and mortality.

Management and Prevention

Prevention is critical during procedures that place patients at high risk for air embolism. There are two key ways to prevent venous embolism. First, it is important to take measures to decrease the pressure gradient between the procedural site and the right atrium. Maintaining adequate intravascular volume by intravenous hydration will help prevent further

decline in right atrial pressure. Using the Trendelenburg position for central line insertion and other procedures also can help prevent air entrainment.

Second, minimizing the amount of time that the vessel is open to atmospheric pressure will decrease the opportunity for entrainment of air. During central line insertion, the needle and catheter should be occluded at all times. During removal of a central line, the patient should exhale to prevent air entry on inspiration.

Once air embolism has occurred, the primary management is prevention of further air entrainment. A secondary goal is to decrease the volume of air within the body. If the air embolism occurs intraoperatively, the surgeon should flood the operative field with saline to help prevent further air entry. Volume expansion is recommended to increase right atrial pressure. If possible, the patient should be positioned with the operative site below the level of the heart. It may be helpful to place the patient in the left lateral decubitus position to prevent obstruction of the right ventricular outflow tract. Aspiration of 50 percent of the air entrained from an appropriately placed right atrial catheter has been described,[27] but achieving these results in an emergency situation is challenging.

Supportive therapy for cardiovascular compromise, dysrhythmias, and respiratory failure should be initiated. Many patients require mechanical ventilation. Catecholamines may be required to maintain blood pressure. Supplemental oxygen should be given to produce adequate oxygenation. In the case of decompression sickness, supplemental oxygen may reduce the severity of the air embolism by allowing more rapid nitrogen egress from bubbles.[24]

Hyperbaric oxygen therapy may be employed as adjunctive therapy in severe cases of venous air embolism to help decrease the size of air bubbles in the bloodstream. However, its use usually is reserved for patients with arterial air embolism who have neurologic or cardiac findings.

Amniotic Fluid Embolism

Amniotic fluid embolism is a rare clinical entity, with devastating consequences at a time of anticipated joy. Timely diagnosis can be challenging and requires a high index of suspicion. The syndrome was first described in 1926, when Meyer reported fetal cellular debris within the maternal circulation in a patient who experienced peripartum dyspnea and hypotension.[32] Steiner and Lushbaugh published a landmark autopsy case series in 1941. They found squamous cells, mucin, and amorphous debris within the pulmonary vasculature and concluded that maternal death resulted from the systemic embolization of fetal products and amniotic fluid.[33]

More recent work has called to question the mechanism underlying the severe hypotension characteristic of this syndrome. The term "anaphylactoid syndrome of pregnancy" has been suggested to emphasize the cytokine-mediated mechanisms for systemic hypotension and coagulopathy.[34]

Epidemiology

Amniotic fluid embolism has a reported incidence between 1 in 8,000 to 1 in 10,000 pregnancies. Mortality from amniotic fluid embolism in symptomatic women has been estimated as high as 80 percent. The syndrome may be responsible for 15 percent of maternal deaths.[35] The incidence of subclinical amniotic fluid embolism is unknown.

Because the syndrome is so rare, no single institution (let alone practitioner) has had sufficient experience to define the risk factors or the precise clinical course of amniotic fluid embolism. Review of a national registry of amniotic fluid embolism cases failed to disclose predisposing factors,[34] although earlier reports had suggested advancing maternal age, multiparity, large fetal size, vigorous labor, the use of oxytocic drugs, and second trimester dilation and curettage procedures as potential associations. Seventy percent of cases of amniotic fluid embolism occur during labor, with 11 percent following vaginal delivery and 19 percent following cesarean section.[34]

Clinical Picture and Diagnosis

Patients with amniotic fluid embolism classically have a sudden onset of progressive dyspnea, hypoxia, and cyanosis, and a cough progressively productive of frothy sputum. Oxygen saturation monitoring and arterial blood gas analysis demonstrate hypoxemia. Mental status changes may occur, with up to 20 percent of patients developing seizures. This is followed rapidly by progressive hypotension (out of proportion to blood loss) leading to cardiopulmonary arrest.[34,36] Radiographic findings are nonspecific and can span the spectrum from clear lung fields to diffuse abnormalities consistent with ARDS.

Up to 40 percent of those who recover from hemodynamic collapse develop a coagulopathy, ranging from mild (subclinical laboratory abnormalities) to clinically severe, with fulminant DIC developing in 10 percent.[37] Laboratory abnormalities are consistent with DIC, including elevated fibrin degradation product levels, elevated D-dimer values, decreased fibrinogen levels, thrombocytopenia, and prolonged prothrombin and activated partial thromboplastin times. This coagulopathy, when superimposed upon ongoing uterine blood loss, can be immediately life threatening.

Sufficient multiorgan hypoperfusion may occur during amniotic fluid embolism to result in multiorgan system failure. Survivors of the syndrome often face prolonged lung injury secondary to ARDS. A high percentage of survivors face permanent neurologic damage.[34]

The diagnosis of amniotic fluid embolism is clinical, with a particularly high degree of suspicion at times of greatest risk: during labor, within 30 minutes of delivery, or during a second trimester dilation and curettage. Clues to the diagnosis include acute hypoxia, acute hypotension (out of proportion to blood loss), cardiopulmonary arrest, or worsening coagulopathy. The differential diagnosis includes hemorrhagic shock, sepsis, placental abruption, pulmonary thromboembolism, aspiration of gastric contents, eclampsia, and the syndrome of hemolysis, elevated liver enzymes, and thrombocytopenia (HELLP). Rarely, anaphylaxis, anesthetic drug effect, peripartum myocardial infarction, or a stroke may occur in a similar fashion.[36]

Laboratory testing is rarely helpful in diagnosing amniotic fluid embolism. No abnormalities on common laboratory tests are specific. A monoclonal antibody, TKH-2, has been developed against amniotic fluid-derived mucin[38] and can be applied to blood from the maternal pulmonary artery to help diagnose amniotic fluid embolism. However, its limited availability precludes the clinical utility of this test.[35] Likewise, cytologic examination from pulmonary arterial catheter wedge aspirate is unlikely to provide a timely diagnosis, and amniotic debris can be found in the absence of clinical manifestations of amniotic fluid embolism.

Pathophysiology

The pathophysiology of this syndrome remains poorly understood. Initially, embolization of amniotic fluid and fetal products to the pulmonary vasculature with mechanical obstruction causing acute cor pulmonale and subsequent hemodynamic collapse was thought to be a sufficient explanation. Early autopsy studies revealed mucin, squamous cells, and cellular debris within the pulmonary vasculature.[33] Subsequent studies using a wedged pulmonary artery catheter isolated squamous cells in pulmonary arterial blood aspirates.[39] However, hemodynamic profiles in women suffering from amniotic fluid embolism demonstrated reduced left (rather than right) ventricular ejection fraction and elevated pulmonary capillary wedge pressure, inconsistent with pure mechanical obstruction of the pulmonary arteries and acute right-sided heart failure.[40]

Fetal products within the pulmonary vasculature may not be enough to cause respiratory failure and hemodynamic collapse, because fetal products have been identified within the pulmonary circulation of women who have died during labor of other medical causes, without clinical evidence of amniotic fluid embolism. Cytologic confirmation relies upon the identification of fetal squamous cells, yet distinguishing between maternal and fetal squamous cells can be difficult.[41,42]

Pathogenesis is believed related to the embolization of cytokines, which are present in amniotic fluid at higher concentration than in maternal blood. Two cytokines appear to be key in pathogenesis: endothelin-1 (a potent vasoconstrictor of pulmonary and coronary arterial beds) and tissue factor (an activator of the extrinsic coagulation pathway). Endothelin-1 is present in amniotic fluid at concentrations 10 to 100 times higher than in simultaneously measured maternal plasma levels,[43] while tissue factor is present in amniotic fluid at concentrations up to 45 times higher than in maternal blood plasma.[44]

The initiating step in amniotic fluid embolism is thought to be entry of amniotic fluid into maternal circulation. Throughout gestation, the fetal membranes isolate amniotic fluid from the maternal circulation. At delivery, uterine vessels are exposed. Incomplete collapse of these vessels or tears in the lower uterine segment and endocervix provide portals for entry of amniotic fluid into maternal circulation.[45]

Once in the maternal circulation, amniotic fluid and fetal products travel through the circulation to the pulmonary arteries. Acutely increased endothelin-1 levels within the pulmonary vasculature may cause pulmonary artery vasoconstriction, resulting in acute pulmonary hypertension, severe hypoxia, and right heart strain. A goat model of amniotic fluid embolism supports this theory.[46] Human data are not available, because of delays in pulmonary artery catheter placement during this transient event.[47] Alternatively, it has been suggested that hypoxia from amniotic fluid embolism could, itself, serve as a stimulus for endogenous production of endothelin-1 by the pulmonary vasculature.[48]

Hemodynamic collapse quickly follows. This may be due to coronary artery vasoconstriction from elevated levels of circulating endothelin-1. As a result of coronary artery vasoconstriction, left ventricular systolic function is impaired, resulting in decreased cardiac output and elevated left atrial and pulmonary capillary wedge pressures. These hemodynamic findings are reported in humans and animals.[40]

Survivors of acute hypoxia and hemodynamic collapse face severe DIC, which occurs in up to 40 percent of patients.[34] Amniotic tissue factor enters the systemic circulation through breaks in the fetal-maternal barrier. Once in the maternal circulation, the balance between tissue factor and tissue factor pathway inhibitor shifts to cause activation of the extrinsic coagulation pathway. Coagulopathy can range from mild changes in laboratory tests to severe DIC. Postpartum uterine atony may worsen blood loss.

Management and Prevention

No specific therapy has been proven beneficial in the management or prevention of amniotic fluid embolism. The rapid progression from acute dyspnea to fatal hemodynamic collapse requires prompt and vigorous resuscitation. Adequate support is rarely available outside of an intensive care unit; transfer to an intensive care unit is warranted as soon as the diagnosis is suspected. Resuscitation should proceed with basic and advanced cardiac life support algorithms, with an awareness that the patient is at risk for sudden hemodynamic collapse.

The initial goal of therapy is to maintain oxygenation and perfusion of vital organ systems. An experienced practitioner should rapidly initiate endotracheal intubation and mechanical ventilation if hypoxia persists despite high-concentration oxygen supplementation or if the normal airway protective reflexes are impaired. Airway hyperemia during pregnancy may complicate airway management, and the increased vascularity may predispose to bleeding. Vocal cord and airway edema also may hinder endotracheal tube insertion, and a smaller-than-usual endotracheal tube should be used for intubation.[49]

Because patients frequently have elements of hypovolemia from blood loss, as well as both cardiogenic and noncardiogenic pulmonary edema, pulmonary artery catheterization may be required to help guide resuscitative efforts. Hypovolemia should be corrected with isotonic crystalloid fluid to maintain a mean arterial pressure adequate for vital organ perfusion. Vasopressor agents such as dobutamine, dopamine, or norepinephrine may be required if hypotension does not resolve with crystalloid fluid infusion. Initial goals of therapy should be to maintain a mean arterial pressure of 60 mmHg and urine output of 50 mL per hour.[47] The gravid uterus can impair venous return to the heart through compression of the inferior vena cava.[50] In a patient with critical hypotension or hypoxia, emergent cesarean delivery should be considered.

Use of inhaled nitric oxide or other inhaled pulmonary vasodilators during the hypoxic phase of amniotic fluid embolism has been proposed to manage acute pulmonary hypertension and thus improve gas exchange and cardiac function. However, experience in this population is limited, and no firm recommendations can be given in this regard.[51]

Management of the DIC associated with amniotic fluid embolism is supportive in nature. Frequent serial monitoring of blood counts and DIC parameters is appropriate, with use of blood products when necessary. There are no data to support the routine use of glucocorticoids, although they may be considered if acute adrenal insufficiency is suspected in the hypotensive patient with severe coagulopathy.[47,52] Uterine atony may contribute to ongoing hemorrhage, and oxytocin or similar agents may be useful in diminishing blood loss.[35]

References

1. Laub DR, Jr, Laub DR: Fat embolism syndrome after liposuction: A case report and review of the literature. *Ann Plast Surg* 25:48-52, 1990.

2. Guardia SN, Bilbao JM, Murray D, et al: Fat embolism in acute pancreatitis. *Arch Pathol Lab Med* 113:503-506, 1989.

3. Broder G, Ruzumna L: Systemic fat embolism following acute primary osteomyelitis. *JAMA* 199:150-152, 1967.

4. Palmovic V, McCarroll JR: Fat embolism in trauma. *Arch Pathol* 80:630-635, 1965.

5. Levy D: The fat embolism syndrome. A review. *Clin Orthop Relat Res* Dec; (261):281-286, 1990.

6. Dudney TM, Elliott CG: Pulmonary embolism from amniotic fluid, fat, and air. *Prog Cardiovasc Dis* 36:447-474, 1994.

7. Dang NC, Johnson C, Eslami-Farsani M, et al: Bone marrow embolism in sickle cell disease: A review. *Am J Hematol* 79:61-67, 2005.

8. Burgher LW, Dines DE, Linscheid RL, et al: Fat embolism and the adult respiratory distress syndrome. *Mayo Clin Proc* 49:107-109, 1974.

9. King MB, Harmon KR: Unusual forms of pulmonary embolism. *Clin Chest Med* 15:561-580, 1994.

10. Gurd AR, Wilson RI: The fat embolism syndrome. *J Bone Joint Surg Br* 56B:408-416, 1974.

11. Lindeque BG, Schoeman HS, Dommisse GF, et al: Fat embolism and the fat embolism syndrome. A double-blind therapeutic study. *J Bone Joint Surg Br* 69:128-131, 1987.

12. Malagari K, Economopoulos N, Stoupis C, et al: High-resolution CT findings in mild pulmonary fat embolism. *Chest* 123:1196-1201, 2003.

13. Stanley JD, Hanson RR, Hicklin GA, et al: Specificity of bronchoalveolar lavage for the diagnosis of fat embolism syndrome. *Am Surg* 60:537-541, 1994.

14. Mimoz O, Edouard A, Beydon L, et al: Contribution of bronchoalveolar lavage to the diagnosis of post-traumatic pulmonary fat embolism. *Intensive Care Med* 21:973-980, 1995.

15. Chastre J, Fagon JY, Soler P, et al: Bronchoalveolar lavage for rapid diagnosis of the fat embolism syndrome in trauma patients. *Ann Intern Med* 113:583-588, 1990.

16. Pell AC, Hughes D, Keating J, et al: Brief report: Fulminating fat embolism syndrome caused by paradoxical embolism through a patent foramen ovale. *N Engl J Med* 329:926-929, 1993.

17. Peltier LF: Fat embolism. III. The toxic properties of neutral fat and free fatty acids. *Surgery* 40:665-670, 1956.

18. Riska EB, Myllynen P: Fat embolism in patients with multiple injuries. *J Trauma* 22:891-894, 1982.

19. Behrman SW, Fabian TC, Kudsk KA, et al: Improved outcome with femur fractures: Early vs. delayed fixation. *J Trauma* 30:792-797; discussion 7-8, 1990.

20. Pitto RP, Koessler M: The risk of fat embolism during cemented total hip replacement in the elderly patient. *Chir Organi Mov* 84:119-128, 1999.

21. Kallenbach J, Lewis M, Zaltzman M, et al: "Low-dose" corticosteroid prophylaxis against fat embolism. *J Trauma* 27:1173-1176, 1987.

22. Schonfeld SA, Ploysongsang Y, DiLisio R, et al: Fat embolism prophylaxis with corticosteroids. A prospective study in high-risk patients. *Ann Intern Med* 99:438-443, 1983.

23. van Hulst RA, Klein J, Lachmann B: Gas embolism: Pathophysiology and treatment. *Clin Physiol Funct Imaging* 23:237-246, 2003.

24. Muth CM, Shank ES: Gas embolism. *N Engl J Med* 342:476-482, 2000.

25. Papadopoulos G, Kuhly P, Brock M, et al: Venous and paradoxical air embolism in the sitting position. A prospective study with transoesophageal echocardiography. *Acta Neurochir (Wien)* 126:140-143, 1994.

26. Malinow AM, Naulty JS, Hunt CO, et al: Precordial ultrasonic monitoring during cesarean delivery. *Anesthesiology* 66:816-819, 1987.

27. Palmon SC, Moore LE, Lundberg J, et al: Venous air embolism: A review. *J Clin Anesth* 9:251-257, 1997.

28. McGee DC, Gould MK: Preventing complications of central venous catheterization. *N Engl J Med* 348:1123-1133, 2003.

29. Melamed Y, Shupak A, Bitterman H: Medical problems associated with underwater diving. *N Engl J Med* 326:30-35, 1992.

30. Edmonds-Seal J, Prys-Roberts C, Adams AP: Air embolism. A comparison of various methods of detection. *Anaesthesia* 26:202-208, 1971.

31. Han D, Lee KS, Franquet T, et al: Thrombotic and nonthrombotic pulmonary arterial embolism: Spectrum of imaging findings. *Radiographics* 23:1521-1539, 2003.

32. Meyer J: Embolia pulmonar amnio caseosa. *Bras Medico* 2:301, 1926.

33. Steiner PE, Lushbaugh CC: Landmark article, Oct. 1941: Maternal pulmonary embolism by amniotic fluid as a cause of obstetric shock and unexpected deaths in obstetrics. By Paul E. Steiner and C.C. Lushbaugh. *JAMA* 255:2187-2203, 1986.

34. Clark SL, Hankins GD, Dudley DA, et al: Amniotic fluid embolism: Analysis of the national registry. *Am J Obstet Gynecol* 172:1158-1167; discussion 67-69, 1995.

35. Locksmith GJ: Amniotic fluid embolism. *Obstet Gynecol Clin North Am* 26:435-444, vii, 1999.

36. McDougall RJ, Duke GJ: Amniotic fluid embolism syndrome: Case report and review. *Anaesth Intensive Care* 23:735-740, 1995.

37. Morgan M: Amniotic fluid embolism. *Anaesthesia* 34:20-32, 1979.

38. Kobayashi H, Ooi H, Hayakawa H, et al: Histological diagnosis of amniotic fluid embolism by monoclonal antibody TKH-2 that recognizes NeuAc α 2-6GalNAc epitope. *Hum Pathol* 28:428-433, 1997.

39. Masson RG, Ruggieri J: Pulmonary microvascular cytology. A new diagnostic application of the pulmonary artery catheter. *Chest* 88:908-914, 1985.

40. Clark SL, Montz FJ, Phelan JP: Hemodynamic alterations associated with amniotic fluid embolism: A reappraisal. *Am J Obstet Gynecol* 151:617-621, 1985.

41. Giampaolo C, Schneider V, Kowalski BH, et al: The cytologic diagnosis of amniotic fluid embolism: A critical reappraisal. *Diagn Cytopathol* 3:126-128, 1987.

42. Lee KR, Catalano PM, Ortiz-Giroux S: Cytologic diagnosis of amniotic fluid embolism. Report of a case with a unique cytologic feature and emphasis on the difficulty of eliminating squamous contamination. *Acta Cytol* 30:177-182, 1986.

43. Casey ML, Brown CE, Peters M, et al: Endothelin levels in human amniotic fluid at mid-trimester and at term before and during spontaneous labor. *J Clin Endocrinol Metab* 76:1647-1650, 1993.

44. Uszynski M, Zekanowska E, Uszynski W, et al: Tissue factor and tissue factor pathway inhibitor (TFPI) in amniotic fluid and blood plasma: Implications for the mechanism of amniotic fluid embolism. *Eur J Obstet Gynecol Reprod Biol* 95:163-166, 2001.

45. Davies S: Amniotic fluid embolus: A review of the literature. *Can J Anaesth* 48:88-98, 2001.

46. Hankins GD, Snyder RR, Clark SL, et al: Acute hemodynamic and respiratory effects of amniotic fluid embolism in the pregnant goat model. *Am J Obstet Gynecol* 168:1113-1129; discussion 29-30, 1993.

47. Aurangzeb I, George L, Raoof S: Amniotic fluid embolism. *Crit Care Clin* 20:643-650, 2004.

48. Khong TY: Expression of endothelin-1 in amniotic fluid embolism and possible pathophysiological mechanism. *Br J Obstet Gynaecol* 105:802-804, 1998.

49. Munnur U, Suresh MS: Airway problems in pregnancy. *Crit Care Clin* 20:617-642, 2004.

50. Chesnutt AN: Physiology of normal pregnancy. *Crit Care Clin* 20:609-615, 2004.

51. Tanus-Santos JE, Moreno H, Jr: Inhaled nitric oxide and amniotic fluid embolism. *Anesth Analg* 88:691, 1999.

52. Siu SC, Kitzman DW, Sheedy PF, II, et al: Adrenal insufficiency from bilateral adrenal hemorrhage. *Mayo Clin Proc* 65:664-670, 1990.

Practical Nursing Issues in the Outpatient Management of Pulmonary Vascular Disease

Christine Archer-Chicko, MSN, CRNP,

Traci Housten-Harris, RN, MS,

Harold I. Palevsky, MD

Introduction

Nurses play a key role in coordinating the care of patients with all forms of pulmonary hypertension (PH). From the patient's initial referral to a pulmonary vascular disease program through the diagnostic evaluation and the initiation of medical therapies and the ongoing assessment of a patient's response to therapy, nurses are integral in guiding and managing patient care. Nurses also participate in end-of-life decision making and planning.

Two key aspects of this patient treatment are communication and education. Nurses frequently are more accessible via the telephone (or e-mail) than are physicians. In addition, patients may feel more at ease calling and speaking with a nurse. As a result of such frequent contact, the nurse becomes very attuned to the patient's medical condition and psychosocial needs. This knowledge provides nurses with the opportunity to support and to advocate for patients and their families as they confront the various phases of chronic illness.

Nurses also spend a great deal of time educating patients, their family members, and other significant individuals. Medical therapy for pulmonary arterial hypertension (PAH) can be complex and quite technically challenging. Patients need to understand their disease, how to follow prescribed medical regimens, and to identify early and overt signs and symptoms of disease exacerbation and progression. Through education, frequent communication, and emotional support, nurses help patients learn to care for themselves independently and to monitor their care on an ongoing basis.

This chapter will highlight practical issues of management coordination for patients with pulmonary vascular disease. Issues will be addressed chronologically from initial referral for evaluation of PH through ongoing care. Patient communication and education issues will be highlighted specifically.

Initial Referral and Evaluation

Referrals to a pulmonary vascular disease program may be initiated from a variety of sources: patients themselves, family members, or physicians, including primary care practitioners, cardiologists, pulmonologists, rheumatologists, and gynecologists. Data from the National Institutes of Health Primary Pulmonary Hypertension Registry suggest that the average time from onset of symptoms to diagnosis was approximately 2 years.[1] Although this time may be shorter, patients frequently have been evaluated by multiple providers and undergone numerous tests before evaluation at a pulmonary vascular disease program. It is thus essential that patients come to their first appointment with all available medical records and test results (or forward these materials to the center before the first appointment) to facilitate assessment.

The standard evaluation for PAH is outlined in Chapter 6. In our program, medical records are requested and reviewed before scheduling an initial appointment, and referring physicians are contacted to request any outstanding testing or missing reports. This serves two purposes. First, having complete medical records gives the PH program the ability to prioritize appointments and gain an idea of how quickly a patient may need to move through the system. Second, complete medical records provide the patient, the PH physician, and the nurse specialist the ability to optimally utilize the first visit by building trust, correcting any misinformation, educating the patient about his or her specific condition, discussing the need for right heart catheterization and an acute vasodilator trial, and reviewing management options. This is particularly beneficial when the patient has traveled a significant distance for evaluation at the PH center.

Each test in the evaluation is important. It is not uncommon for an initial diagnosis of collagen vascular disease or human immunodeficiency virus (HIV) infection to be made at the PH center. Most patients with previously undiagnosed HIV infection reported having had negative HIV test results in the past or described no obvious risk factors. Many patients with newly recognized collagen vascular disease have been without overt clinical findings. In addition to HIV and collagen vascular disease, it is our policy to screen for thyroid and liver disease (including hepatitis virus serologies).

Patients are instructed to bring all radiographs and ventilation-perfusion radionuclide scan reports for review. This helps clarify vague or unusual reports, particularly ventilation-perfusion radionuclide scan reports. Review of chest x-rays and computed tomography images can give the PH team a better understanding of the extent of interstitial or other lung disease, for example, than written reports alone.

Data from the National Institutes of Health registry suggest that 6-10 percent of patients who have been diagnosed with idiopathic pulmonary arterial hypertension (IPAH) have family members with disease (i.e., familial pulmonary arterial hypertension [FPAH]). It is therefore important to elicit a detailed family history, including several generations if possible, and request the records of family members who may have recognized or occult pulmonary vascular disease.

Cardiac Catheterization

In virtually all PH programs, right heart catheterization remains the gold standard diagnostic tool for confirming the diagnosis of PAH, evaluating the hemodynamic severity of the disease, and aiding in the selection of appropriate medical therapies.[2,3]

Each patient has a catheterization procedure planned based upon his or her clinical situation and diagnosis. For example, a patient with congenital heart disease may require serial oxygen saturation measurements to evaluate the direction and magnitude of intracardiac shunting. Likewise, a patient with a question of concomitant left-sided heart dysfunction may also require a left heart catheterization to evaluate the coronary arteries and left heart function.

During a cardiac catheterization, several physiologic parameters may be assessed: right-sided hemodynamics (right atrial pressure, right ventricular pressure, pulmonary artery pressure [systolic, diastolic, and mean], pulmonary capillary wedge pressure, mixed venous oxygen saturation, cardiac output, cardiac index, and pulmonary vascular resistance), left-sided hemodynamics, left ventricular ejection fraction, the extent and location of coronary artery disease, and evaluation of intracardiac shunting through a patent foramen ovale or as a consequence of congenital heart disease. Patients who demonstrate normal pulmonary hemodynamics at rest should be exercised with the right heart catheter in place to assess hemodynamics with activity. Arm exercise (e.g., lifting saline bags), serial leg raises, recumbent and upright stationery bicycle riding are forms of exercise that can be used during right heart catheterization.

Pulmonary vasoreactivity testing may also be performed at the time of right heart catheterization. Testing with a short-acting vasodilator (intravenous adenosine, intravenous prostacyclin, inhaled nitric oxide, or inhaled prostacyclin) remains a crucial step in the evaluation. Perhaps 10 percent of patients with PAH will demonstrate acute vasoreactivity. The current definition of acute vasoreactivity is a fall of mean pulmonary artery pressure of at least 10 mmHg to less than 40 mmHg with an increased or unchanged cardiac output.[4] Only patients who demonstrate an acute response to short-acting vasodilators during a right heart catheterization (i.e., "responders") are appropriate for treatment with oral calcium channel blockers. Although these represent a minority of patients seen at PH centers, their treatment regimens and prognoses differ dramatically from those of nonresponders.[5]

Preparing the patient to undergo the cardiac catheterization and pulmonary vasodilator testing frequently falls to the PH nurse. Patients need to be informed of the specifics of the procedure and how the catheterization and drug testing fit into their treatment plans.

Many PH centers perform right heart catheterization and vasoreactivity testing as an outpatient procedure. Whether the right heart catheterization is performed through the internal jugular or femoral vein, the procedure and recovery time take a few hours. If the patient requires oral vasodilator therapy, it may be initiated and adjusted on an outpatient basis. Should the patient require initiation of a therapy that is more intensive and invasive (e.g., subcutaneous treprostinil, intravenous prostacyclin, intravenous treprostinil, or inhaled iloprost), and depending on the patient's clinical status, this may be done immediately, or the patient may be scheduled for an elective admission.

Other PH centers schedule the catheterization as an inpatient procedure, leaving the right heart catheter in place for continuous hemodynamic monitoring and vasodilator trials. To schedule a heart catheterization and pulmonary vasodilator studies as an inpatient procedure, there are typically three steps to securing the admission:

1. Contact the patient's insurance provider and obtain precertification for the procedure and 1 inpatient day with concurrent review. Often, a nurse case reviewer from the insurer will need to know why the catheterization is being done on an inpatient basis. We explain there will be continuous hemodynamic monitoring to test various vasodilator agents. In some rare instances, the physician may have to speak directly with the insurer's medical director to secure precertification. Once the patient has been admitted, the hospital case management team can update the insurer as to patient's condition and obtain approval for the rest of the patient's hospital stay.
2. Schedule the catheterization with your hospital's inpatient services, such as the admissions department, precatheterization unit, cardiac catheterization lab, and inpatient heart failure or intensive care unit where the patient will spend the remainder of the stay while hemodynamic monitoring is required. We prepare a packet of clinical and demographic information and fax it to the various departments so that each is prepared for the patient's admission.
3. Next, we confirm with the patient that the admission has been scheduled and precertified

by the insurance company. In some instances, patients may need to obtain a written referral from a primary care physician for the admission, depending on the insurance company's policy. Patients are instructed to call the insurance company to clarify the policy. We speak directly with each patient and review directions for the admission over the telephone. Each patient is reminded that the catheterization will be performed on the first hospital day and that the catheter will remain in the neck for the next several days while the physician assesses various agents to find the medication that best reduces pulmonary artery pressures or best improves heart function. We take time to allow patients and their family members to ask questions and voice concerns. Then we send a detailed letter, which again reviews all the directions for the admission:

- Date, time, and location of arrival at the hospital are included.
- Bring insurance cards.
- Type of heart catheterization procedure to be performed is outlined.
- Take nothing by mouth from midnight the night before the procedure.
- Warfarin (Coumadin) must be held for 4 days before the procedure.
- Use no aspirin or aspirin-containing products for 1 week before the admission.
- Medications that must be held the morning of the catheterization procedure are specified.
- Bring all current medications to the hospital.
- Bring any continuous positive airway pressure (CPAP) or bilevel positive airway pressure (BiPAP) equipment for nighttime use.

Right heart catheterizations may be repeated on a periodic basis or at the discretion of the physician when there has been a change in the patient's clinical status, a need to evaluate a patient's response to interventions, or to optimize medical therapies.

Conventional Medical Therapies

Several common medical therapies are used routinely in PH management.

Oxygen

The true first-line medical therapy used for managing PH is supplemental oxygen. Patients who are hypoxemic are at risk for hypoxic pulmonary vaso-constriction, which elevates pulmonary artery pressures and thereby increases right heart strain and failure.[4] We generally attempt to maintain an oxyhemoglobin saturation of over 90 percent. However, in patients with congenital heart disease, Eisenmenger physiology, patent foramen ovale, or interstitial lung disease, this may not be feasible with achievable oxygen flow rates.

Patients typically are reluctant when told they need supplemental oxygen. They are embarrassed to be seen wearing a nasal cannula, or they do not want to deal with handling the cylinders or tanks. We instruct patients to consider supplemental oxygen as a vital medication. It requires a prescription from a physician or nurse practitioner. Likewise, patients who have been diagnosed with sleep apnea for whom CPAP or BiPAP therapy has been prescribed should demonstrate compliance. We generally will not evaluate additional medical therapies to manage PH unless a patient has been using prescribed oxygen therapy consistently or CPAP/BiPAP reliably for a minimum of 3 months. Patients should use oxygen as prescribed, and such prescriptions should state specific flow rates in liters per minute and whether the oxygen is to be used with activity, during sleep, or continuously.

It is important that the supplemental oxygen system meet the patient's needs. We prefer an ambulatory system that is lightweight and refillable so that patients can get out of the house and remain as physically active as possible. A conserving device (if tolerated) is also helpful to make a patient's portable oxygen supply last longer. The oxygen supplier should be able to discuss several equipment options with the patient and recommend a system that meets the patient's needs.

Patients should be informed of necessary safety precautions with the use of supplemental oxygen. It should never be used near an open flame, such as that of a gas cook stove. Although oxygen is not explosive, it does potentiate and accelerate combustion. Unfortunately, some of our patients have used their oxygen improperly and suffered severe burns.

It is important to reevaluate periodically whether oxygen requirements have changed. We check oxyhemoglobin saturation at each outpatient clinic visit. An oxygen desaturation exercise study may be required to titrate oxygen requirements during activity, or an overnight record of oximetry may be needed to assess requirements during sleep. Most insurers require an annual reevaluation of oxygen needs in order for patients to requalify for equipment.

Digoxin

Digoxin (Lanoxin) is an inotropic agent prescribed in many pulmonary vascular disease centers. Digoxin improves left ventricular function in patients with left-sided congestive heart failure. Similarly, it generally is felt to be beneficial in supporting the right side of the heart in patients with PH.[4] Dosing is usually 0.125 mg to 0.25 mg daily and is monitored periodically with serum digoxin levels. Patients with renal insufficiency may require a lower dosage, because digoxin is cleared by the kidney; these patients should have blood digoxin levels checked more frequently and the dosage adjusted to avoid toxicity. Toxic side effects of digoxin include nausea, anorexia, diarrhea, abdominal pain, headache, confusion, hallucinations, depression, changes in vision (yellow-green halos), and bradycardia or other disturbances in heart rhythm, and may occur at any blood digoxin level.[6]

Diuretics

Diuretics are important for patients with PH. Managing the intravascular volume status is critical to reduce cor pulmonale and right heart strain. Careful and appropriate use of diuretics can dramatically improve a patient's symptoms, functional class, and perhaps survival. Nurses must be prepared to assist patients in managing their fluids. Patients must understand the need to limit intake of salt and fluids, to comply with diuretic regimens, and to participate in monitoring their electrolytes and renal function.

Patients should be instructed to weigh themselves daily and to learn to identify edema (swelling of their feet, legs) and ascites (abdomen). They should be instructed to call the office when their weight has increased by 3-4 pounds rather than after they have retained larger amounts of fluid. Nurses can alter the diuretic regimen over the telephone and have patients call back in a few days to report on progress with diuresis. Nurses can also send the patient for blood tests to monitor electrolytes (sodium, potassium, magnesium) and replace them as needed, and to monitor renal function (blood urea nitrogen (BUN), creatinine). Patients should be instructed to consume a no-added-salt diet, including refraining from table salt and avoiding foods high in sodium, such as pickles, processed meats, salty snack foods, and soy sauce. We generally recommend a diet with no more than 1,200 mg of sodium per day. For patients who experience persistent edema despite diuretic therapy and compliance with a no-added-salt diet, we frequently advise a fluid restriction.

There are several types of diuretics, including loop, potassium-sparing, and thiazide diuretics. Spironolactone (Aldactone®) is often the initial agent chosen for two reasons. First, it is a mild diuretic that spares potassium and may reduce the need for potassium supplementation. Second, it can effectively reduce fluid retention in patients who are beginning to develop ascites.[7] In addition, spironolactone is believed to have beneficial effects of modulating neurohormonal responses that develop as a consequence of ventricular decompensation.[7] Many patients require more than one type of diuretic to maintain an acceptable fluid balance and to minimize electrolyte abnormalities. When patients are beginning to deteriorate clinically, we often alter the maintenance diuretic regimen with by using higher dosages of furosemide (Lasix®) or metolazone (Zaroxolyn®) or both. If patients appear to have excessive edema not adequately responsive to oral diuretics, we admit them to the hospital for intravenous diuretic administration, possible use of short-term inotropic agents, and frequent monitoring of electrolytes and renal function. In adjusting diuretics on an outpatient basis, nurses need to monitor patients closely; overzealous diuresis can cause hypotension, renal insufficiency, electrolyte derangements, orthostasis, or syncope.[4]

Anticoagulation

Warfarin (Coumadin®) has been associated in several observational studies with improved survival of patients with PAH.[4] It is theorized that warfarin reduces the formation of microthrombi within small pulmonary vessels that occurs as a consequence of shear stress, turbulent flow, and endothelial injury. Dosing is individualized and monitored by prothrombin time (PT) and International Normalized Ratio (INR). The target INR is typically 1.5-2.5, but this may vary among centers. Patients with a history of atrial fibrillation, cardiac valve replacement surgery, or deep vein thrombosis or pulmonary emboli have a higher target INR.

Nurses play an important role in monitoring therapy and educating patients. Blood work should be performed every 4-8 weeks in patients who have had stable INRs and more frequently in patients with fluctuating INRs. The nurse can confirm that blood work is being done, monitor a patient's INR and, in conjunction with the physician, adjust the warfarin dosage as needed.

Patients require substantial education about warfarin therapy.[8] Topics of particular importance include:

- Patients are instructed in self-assessment for excessive bleeding (e.g., nosebleeds, bleeding gums, blood in stool or urine, easy bruising, prolonged bleeding from venipuncture sites, heavy menstrual periods, coughing or vomiting blood) and to report such problems to the program office nurse.
- Nurses reinforce the importance of scheduled blood work for PT and INR to ensure therapeutic and safe dosage.
- Diet modifications: Some physicians tell patients to avoid foods containing vitamin K (e.g., leafy green vegetables, fish, canola oil, soybean oil), because they can alter warfarin requirements. Other physicians advise patients to eat a consistent, healthy diet that should remain relatively stable once the warfarin dosage is adjusted.
- Numerous drugs interact with warfarin. We advise patients to call the program office of any changes in their medication regimen.
- Patients are instructed to hold warfarin if undergoing dental work (including dental cleaning), surgical procedures, or other procedures such as colonoscopy or endoscopy. Patients should be instructed to contact the office for instructions for warfarin dosing when procedures are scheduled.
- Patients should notify their nurse or physician of a fall or injury while taking warfarin.
- Patients should wear a medic alert bracelet while they are taking warfarin.

Calcium Channel Antagonists

Calcium channel antagonists are considered only for patients who have demonstrated a significant vasoreactivity response to short-acting vasodilators. Nifedipine (Procardia XL®), diltiazem (Cardizem CD®), and amlodipine (Norvasc®) are used most frequently. The choice often is based on the patient's heart rate; those with relative bradycardia often receive nifedipine while those with relative tachycardia may be treated with diltiazem. Calcium channel antagonists with a significant negative inotropic effect, such as verapamil (Calan®), should be avoided.[4] Although patients typically require higher dosages for PAH management than those used for systemic hypertension, most physicians initiate calcium channel antagonists cautiously and titrate the dosage upward gradually. Long-acting forms of these agents are used frequently to help eliminate the risk of rebound symptoms if a dose is late or missed, and the total daily dosage is often divided into two or three long-acting pills to minimize the side effects of peak serum levels.

Patients treated with calcium channel antagonists generally should have a repeat right heart catheterization after several months of therapy to confirm that the pulmonary hemodynamics are significantly improved. If pulmonary hemodynamics remain suboptimal at the time of right heart catheterization (even if improved over pretreatment values), an acute vasodilator trial should be repeated to assess for additional reactivity and the benefit of a higher dosage of calcium channel antagonists.

Patients should be educated about the need to take calcium channel antagonists on a regular schedule and never to stop the medication without discussion with the pulmonary vascular disease program staff. Abrupt discontinuation in a responsive patient can result in rebound pulmonary vasoconstriction, increased symptoms, and possibly syncope or death.

Endothelin Receptor Antagonist Therapy

Endothelin-1 is a potent vasoconstrictor and smooth muscle mitogen important in the development of pulmonary arterial hypertension.[9] Bosentan (Tracleer®) was the first oral endothelin receptor antagonist approved by the U.S. Food and Drug Administration (FDA) for PAH management in patients with World Health Organization (WHO) functional class III or IV symptoms. It is manufactured by Actelion Pharmaceuticals and was approved in November 2002. Bosentan inhibits both endothelin-A and endothelin-B receptors.

Bosentan improves hemodynamics and exercise capacity, and slows the rate of clinical deterioration[10] while being generally well tolerated. Side effects observed in a 1-year follow-up safety study included headache, upper respiratory tract infection, dyspnea, chest pain, sinusitis, bronchitis, palpitations, dizziness, fatigue, cough, arthralgia, dyspepsia, epistaxis, influenza-like illness, nausea, and lower limb edema.[11] In our practice, new or worsened lower extremity edema is the most frequent troubling side effect and usually responds promptly to the addition or adjustment of diuretic therapy. Elevated liver transaminase levels up to 3 times normal have occurred in

12.7 percent of patients studied; higher elevations occur less frequently.[12] Some patients may also experience a decrease in hemoglobin values (an average of 0.9 g/dl), usually during the first few weeks of treatment. Patients must have their liver function tests checked monthly while taking bosentan and a complete blood count checked every third month.

Women of childbearing age must be informed that bosentan can have serious teratogenic effects and be counseled to use adequate protection from pregnancy. The efficacy of hormonal contraceptives may be altered when taken in conjunction with bosentan, so women are required to also use two barrier forms of birth control such as a condom and diaphragm.

Before starting therapy, baseline liver function tests must be drawn and recorded. In addition, women of childbearing age should have a negative serum pregnancy test documented. Bosentan is initiated at 62.5 mg by mouth every 12 hours. It may be taken with food. Liver function test are redrawn after 1 month and, if normal, the dosage of bosentan increased to 125 mg by mouth twice daily. Thereafter, liver function is monitored monthly and complete blood count every 3 months. If liver transaminase levels are elevated, they are either rechecked for confirmation and a dosage adjustment made, or therapy is discontinued depending upon the severity of the abnormality (TABLE 21-1).[13]

If a patient must discontinue bosentan therapy because of insurance issues, we do not stop treatment abruptly. Rather, we instruct patients to wean bosentan over several days to avoid rebound effects.

Sitaxsentan

Sitaxsentan (Thelin®), a more selective endothelin-A receptor antagonist manufactured by Encysive Pharmaceutical, is undergoing FDA review at the time of this writing. It is likely to become available during the first half of 2006. In clinical trials, sitaxsentan demonstrated improvement in mean 6-minute walk distance comparable to that seen with bosentan. Which endothelin receptor antagonist should be used for an individual patient remains to be determined.

Phosphodiesterase Inhibitor Therapy

Sildenafil citrate (Revatio®) was approved by the FDA for PAH management in June 2005. It is a phosphodiesterase 5 inhibitor that inhibits the breakdown

TABLE 21-1

Recommended Action for Abnormal Liver Function with Bosentan Therapy

ALT / AST Level	Action
>3 to ≤5 × ULN	Repeat, confirm If confirmed, reduce dosage or interrupt medication; repeat every 2 wks Restart after return to normal
>5 to ≤8 × ULN	Repeat, confirm If confirmed, stop and monitor q 2 weeks Consider restart after return to normal
>8 × ULN	Stop bosentan therapy

ALT, *alanine aminotransferase*; AST, *aspartate aminotransferase*; ULN, *upper limits of normal*.

of cyclic guanosine monophosphate, which promotes the relaxation of smooth muscle cells of the vascular bed, thus resulting in vasodilation.[14]

In a 12-week double-blind, placebo-controlled study, 278 patients were randomized by taking placebo or sildenafil 20 mg, 40 mg, or 80 mg by mouth 3 times daily. Sildenafil improved the exercise capacity in patients with WHO functional class II, III, and IV symptoms, and 20 mg 3 times daily by mouth was an effective initial dosage.[15] Sildenafil was well tolerated, with few minor side effects (headache, back pain, dyspepsia, flushing, diarrhea, limb pain, myalgia, and cough).[15] Early reports show promising results regarding its efficacy in long-term PH management. Additional studies, however, are needed to compare its efficacy with that of other therapies or to assess combination therapy.

Prostanoid Therapies

Three forms of prostanoid therapy are available: inhaled, intravenous, and subcutaneous.

Inhaled Iloprost

Inhaled iloprost (Ventavis®) was approved by the FDA in December 2004 for PAH in patients with WHO functional class III or IV symptoms.[16] It is a synthetic analogue of prostacyclin that dilates the systemic and pulmonary vascular beds. It also inhibits platelet aggregation. Ventavis is manufactured by Schering-Plough for CoTherix.

Iloprost is available as a clear solution at 10 mcg/ml for inhalation via the Prodose AAD (adaptive aerosol delivery) system or the I-neb AAD system. Each glass ampule contains 2 ml (20 mcg) of iloprost, and a single treatment is set to deliver either 2.5 mcg or 5.0 mcg (the remaining drug is "lost" in the delivery system).

The patient is instructed to draw the iloprost solution into a small pipette and to place the medication in the I-neb AAD system or the Prodose AAD device medication chamber. The patient then engages the device and takes the treatment. Each inhalational treatment lasts 6-12 minutes while the patient breathes with steady and regular breaths. Specialty pharmacies (e.g., Accredo Therapeutics or Cora Script Pharmacy, inc.) are available for educating patients, nurses, and respiratory therapists.

The initial treatment is 2.5 mcg, which is then increased and maintained at 5.0 mcg. A patient may receive a maximum dosage of 45 mcg per day. The serum half-life of iloprost is 20-25 minutes. Because of this short duration of action, 6-9 inhaled treatments are required each day during waking hours.[4,17] Because inhaled iloprost is administered on an intermittent basis, patients are instructed to administer a morning treatment immediately upon awakening (before performing any activities) to prevent syncope or other symptoms. Patients taking bosentan or sildenafil may require fewer doses per day.[18]

Before inhaled iloprost therapy can be initiated, a patient must sign consent to release insurance information and clinical evaluation to one of the specialty pharmacies. The clinical evaluation documents (to be submitted by the prescribing PH center) indicate the diagnosis of PAH and WHO functional class. It should include the results of an echocardiogram, cardiac catheterization, ventilation-perfusion scan, computed tomography scan of the chest, pulmonary function testing, and relevant collagen vascular disease serology results. The specialty pharmacy will then pursue insurance clearance. Coverage for this inhalational therapy falls under the patient's medical insurance, not the pharmaceutical coverage.

Iloprost therapy may be initiated in the outpatient clinic or in the hospital, where vital signs are monitored closely. Patients who participated in the U.S. clinical trial of iloprost were all initiated as outpatients. Inhaled iloprost should not be started on a patient who is hypotensive (systolic BP <85 mmHg). Physicians and nurses should be aware of concomitant conditions or medications that may increase the risk of hypotension or syncope. When inhaled iloprost is initiated, patients should be watched closely for signs of pulmonary edema. If they occur, the treatment should be stopped immediately, because this may be a sign of pulmonary venous hypertension (e.g., pulmonary veno-occlusive disease).

In a long-term study, inhaled iloprost treatments were well tolerated. Mild coughing, headache, and jaw pain occurred in some patients.[17] Patients who receive excessive dosing may develop side effects like those seen with prostacyclin, such as a severe headache, chest pain, flushing, dizziness, jaw pain, nausea, vomiting, or diarrhea. We instruct patients to notify us if any adverse effects occur.

Patients are instructed by the specialty pharmacy, nurses, or respiratory therapists. Patients are taught about iloprost, itself, how to administer the inhaled treatments and care for the equipment, and signs to report to the physician or nurse. Additional points emphasized include:

- Iloprost solution should not come in contact with skin or eyes. It should not be taken orally.
- Patients should rinse their mouths after each inhaled treatment is completed.
- The I-neb AAD system and Prodose AAD system devices are not nebulizers. Patients should not mix any other medications (e.g., β-agonist solutions) with iloprost in either device. Similarly, other medications cannot be administered with the I-neb AAD system or Prodose AAD device.
- Patients should wash the mouthpiece with soap and water after each treatment.
- When taking a treatment, other persons (especially babies and pregnant women) should not be exposed to the iloprost.

If therapy is initiated in the hospital, the patient is discharged when clinically stable and independent in administering treatments. A follow-up nursing visit from the specialty pharmacy is scheduled within 1 week of discharge to reinforce teaching and evaluate the patient's status.

Intravenous Epoprostenol

Epoprostenol sodium (prostacyclin [Flolan®]) was developed by what is now GlaxoSmithKline and approved for treatment of PAH by the FDA in 1996. It is a potent systemic and pulmonary vasodilator indicated for PAH patients with WHO class III or IV symptoms. Epoprostenol inhibits platelet aggregation and may also have significant inotropic effects on the right heart.[4]

Epoprostenol sodium is available as a lyophilized white powder in glass vials of 0.5 mg (blue-top vials) or 1.5 mg (red-top vials). It must be reconstituted with a specially formulated alkaline diluent into a small 100-ml medication cassette. It is relatively unstable in solution and must be kept cold to remain effective; even when cold it will last no longer than 48 hours once reconstituted. Epoprostenol has a circulating half-life of only 2-3 minutes and thus requires a continuous intravenous infusion. If drug delivery is interrupted or stopped, the patient will rapidly lose the beneficial effects and there is a significant risk of rebound PH, clinical deterioration, and even death.[4] Epoprostenol is administered as a continuous infusion with a CADD-Legacy pump through a central venous catheter (e.g., Hickman, Broviac, or peripherally inserted central catheter [PICC line]). It must be prepared daily and kept cold throughout the day with ice packs.

Before initiating therapy with epoprostenol, patient selection must be considered carefully and insurance clearance obtained. Consideration of intravenous epoprostenol therapy requires attention to both medical and psychosocial issues. From a medical standpoint, patients typically fit into one of two scenarios. First are patients who are failing traditional oral therapies and now have more severe symptoms of cor pulmonale (deteriorating exercise capacity, intractable edema, worsening oxygenation) and worsened hemodynamics. In the second scenario are patients who have come to medical attention emergently in severe right-sided heart failure (cardiac index typically <2.0 L/min/m², right atrial pressure >20 mmHg, episodes of syncope).[19] The patient's capacity to manage complicated therapy is an important issue. Nurses need to work with the physician to evaluate physical and a psychosocial issues in determining whether continuous intravenous infusion therapy through a central venous catheter is safe and appropriate.[20] Considerations include:

- Has the patient been compliant with medical therapy in the past?
- Does the patient actively perform self-care or depend upon others?
- Is the patient motivated to prepare the epoprostenol infusion daily and to care for a central venous catheter safely?
- Does the patient have a history of substance abuse or mental illness that may make caring for such a complex system risky on a long-term basis?

- Does the patient have a stable home environment (telephone service, electrical service, etc.)?
- Does the patient possess the cognitive skills to follow a sterile protocol and to troubleshoot alarms?[21]
- Does the patient have physical limitations (loss of digital mobility from severe collagen vascular disease, loss of hearing, poor eyesight) that would make handling the infusion pump or its supplies difficult?
- Will the patient be able to manipulate small drug vials, needles, and syringes in a sterile fashion to prepare the infusion?
- Does the patient have a social support system (spouse, significant other, family, or close friend) committed to assisting with care of the infusion when the patient is unable?

It is important to discuss these issues pertaining to care of an epoprostenol infusion with both the patient and family or support persons before deciding to initiate therapy. All individuals involved need to make a commitment to caring for the infusion. A lack of such ability or commitment may result in a life-threatening complication.

When a patient has been identified as needing and appropriate for intravenous epoprostenol therapy, it is best to initiate the process of obtaining insurance approval immediately. Generally, epoprostenol is covered while the patient is an inpatient, but before discharge, insurance approval must be obtained for the outpatient aspect of ongoing care. This includes all necessary supplies such as epoprostenol medication vials, sterile diluent, needles, syringes, medication cassettes, tubing, central line dressing kits, and rental of two CADD-Legacy infusion pumps.

Epoprostenol therapy is billed under the home infusion benefit of the patient's medical insurance coverage. For patients who have inadequate insurance coverage, an expedited application for state or federal coverage may need to be filed. In these instances, it is helpful to involve a social worker to help guide the nurse with paperwork that must be submitted.

Nurses seeking to obtain insurance approval can make a referral to one of the two specialty pharmacies that provide epoprostenol care (Accredo Therapeutics or Theracom/Caremark). Both pharmacies require the patient's demographic and insurance information. In addition, each pharmacy will need clinical data that confirms the diagnosis of PAH (heart catheterization, echocardiogram, 12-lead electrocardiogram, ventilation-perfusion scan, chest radiograph, computed tomography scan, antinuclear antibody levels, and pulmonary function testing results). In addition, statements regarding WHO functional classification and the result of vasoreactivity testing and response to oral vasodilator agents (if any) are required (e.g., "the patient had worsening symptoms and progression of disease despite being on nifedipine"). Such clinical data support the medical necessity of epoprostenol therapy in the event that the insurer contests the need. The specialty pharmacy will contact the patient's insurance provider and assist in obtaining clearance for the patient. In addition, there is a patient assistance program available from GlaxoSmithKline (makers of epoprostenol), but patients must meet the program's financial criteria.

In most pulmonary vascular disease centers epoprostenol therapy is initiated on an inpatient basis with close clinical monitoring because of its potential for severe side effects, including systemic hypotension and pulmonary edema. PH programs may approach dosing differently, but in general, an intravenous epoprostenol infusion is initiated at a dosage of 2 ng/kg/min and gradually increased, usually over several days, until a balance is achieved between improved symptoms (e.g., dyspnea) and tolerable side effects. We refer to this as the "acute dosing phase."

Adverse effects that occur during the acute or early dosing phase include jaw pain, flushing, nausea, diarrhea, rash, headache, systemic hypotension, and photosensitivity.[19] The jaw pain affects almost all patients at each meal as they take their first few bites of food. As they continue to chew, the pain subsides. Chronic side effects may include anorexia, weight loss, ascites, thrombocytopenia, pancytopenia, leg and foot pain, and high cardiac output failure.[19] Complications may occur related to the central venous catheter, including local catheter site infections, bacteremia, sepsis, thrombosis, catheter line malfunction (hole or tear), obstruction, and catheter line displacement. Complications associated with an infusion pump include incorrect programming, battery failure, pump not turned on, improperly attached medication cassette, or catheter clamp not opened.[19]

Once the patient has demonstrated clinical tolerance with the initial epoprostenol infusion, we begin to focus on teaching the patient how to care for the infusion. Many PH centers have written materials for patients to teach them how to care for their epoprostenol infusion. These materials help patients, family, and support persons to review what they have learned after the teaching session has ended. Both specialty pharmacies also make teaching materials available.

It is important to initiate teaching slowly. Most patients have never worked with needles or syringes and are frightened to handle them. They are often very clumsy in handling the supplies required to prepare the infusion. It is best to watch over them closely and avoid mistakes that can occur easily, such as poking themselves with the needle. In addition, patients are easily overwhelmed with the teaching. To help reduce their anxiety, divide the teaching into several sections:

1. How to mix the medication
2. How to attach the medication cassette to the infusion pump
3. How to set the infusion pump
4. How to care for the central venous catheter
5. What to do in an emergency situation

By focusing on one section at a time, the patient can build self-confidence. It generally takes about 4-7 days for most patients to become proficient with epoprostenol therapy and to become comfortable with the equipment.

Patients learn in different ways. It is important to match your teaching style to your patient's learning style. For instance, some patients learn by a hands-on approach and get easily distracted if trying to refer to written materials. These patients do better by following or mimicking your demonstration of mixing the infusion and handling the supplies. Other patients learn by following step-by-step written instructions similar to following a recipe. Nurses who can assess a patient's style of learning and adjust their teaching style accordingly will provide more effective education. It is also very helpful to have only one or two dedicated nurses teach a patient. When too many nurses teach a patient, each may present a different style to a task and the patient can easily become confused. Consistency with technique makes teaching go more smoothly. Both specialty pharmacies offer inpatient teaching to patients and their support persons. It is important to include a patient's support person in teaching sessions. A trained support person is essential in case of a situation in which the patient cannot mix or manage the epoprostenol infusion alone. In addition to learning while watching the patient, the support person can assist by providing emotional support. Individualized teaching sessions, a slow and repetitive pace of teaching, and emotional support are vital to a successful outcome.

A patient should be discharged only when independent and comfortable caring for the epoprostenol infusion. Following discharge, each patient should have a follow-up visit by a home care nurse from the specialty pharmacy. This home visit is helpful to identify unexpected problems following discharge.

A central venous catheter is placed after insurance clearance is secured and while the patient is focusing on learning. We consult the general surgery service for placement of an adult-size single-lumen Hickman catheter. Typically the catheter is inserted through a small incision near the clavicle and tunneled under the skin to exit near the sternum. The surgical procedure usually takes about 30 minutes. Other centers may use a smaller size catheter, such as a pediatric-size Hickman catheter or Broviac catheter. We avoid placement of multilumen catheters, which require routine flushing of the extra port and thus may increase the risk of infection.

Epoprostenol dosing must be individualized. Once patients are discharged, we begin long-term dosing. Induced metabolism and tachyphylaxis require that dosage is frequently increased at first. Patients must learn to recognize when a slight dosage increase is required to prevent the symptoms of heart failure from returning. Upon discharge, patients may be given a schedule of small increases for their infusion, or they may be instructed to call the office at regular intervals for instructions. They are also instructed to call if they feel the dosage is too low (and they are having signs of PH such as dyspnea, fatigue, or fluid retention) or too high (and they are experiencing signs and symptoms such as tachycardia or skin flushing). The ideal situation is to have the patient increase the epoprostenol infusion without experiencing excessive side effects. Over time, patients may become proficient at adjusting the dosage.

Intravenous Treprostinil

Treprostinil (Remodulin®), in its intravenous form, is a prostacyclin analogue similar to epoprostenol, but it has some advantages. Like treprostinil that is given subcutaneously (discussed below), it is produced by United Therapeutics and was approved by the FDA for intravenous use in November 2004. It has a half-life of approximately 2 hours, which provides a larger safety margin in case of an infusion interruption. Treprostinil is stable at a neutral pH and at room temperature and thus does not require ice packs. Furthermore, because the drug is more stable in solution, treprostinil can last up to 48 hours before a change in medication cassettes is required. These advantages require patients to perform less work to maintain their infusion.

The principles of obtaining intravenous treprostinil from a specialty pharmacy, selecting appropriate patients, initiating therapy, and patient teaching are all similar to those of intravenous epoprostenol therapy. Dosing is also similar, but it appears that patients may require a higher dosage of treprostinil than they would epoprostenol. Less is known regarding the long-term efficacy of intravenous treprostinil than that of epoprostenol.

Subcutaneous Treprostinil

Treprostinil sodium (Remodulin®) is a prostacyclin analog developed as a nonintravenous alternative to epoprostenol by United Therapeutics, a pharmaceutical company founded by a woman whose daughter has IPAH. Treprostinil is available for continuous intravenous or subcutaneous administration. Treprostinil sodium has a longer half-life than epoprostenol of approximately 2 hours when given intravenously and 3-4 hours subcutaneously. It is stable at a neutral pH and at room temperature. Because of these properties, the drug can be administered via a continuous subcutaneous infusion using a small syringe pump.

The FDA approved subcutaneous treprostinil therapy for PAH in May 2002, with an indication for patients in WHO functional classes II, III, and IV. Approximately 75 percent of prescriptions for treprostinil are written for patients who are in WHO class III. Continuous subcutaneous treprostinil generally is used in patients who are not candidates for or have failed oral therapies, or in epoprostenol users who have had recurrent intravenous catheter infections.

Treprostinil is available from three specialty pharmacies. These pharmacies can provide insurance verification, shipment of supplies and medication, patient education, infusion site pain management, and 24-hour on-call assistance. Treprostinil is dispensed in a 30-ml multidose vial in four concentrations. Each vial is quite expensive and contains at least a 2-week supply of medication. For this reason, most hospital pharmacies will not stock treprostinil; instead patients must bring and use their own supply.

Treprostinil is a long-term therapy, and patients must learn to be independent in all aspects of medication delivery. These include operating the portable pump and inserting the subcutaneous catheter. It is the same delivery system used by diabetics for continuous subcutaneous insulin delivery (MiniMed, Medtronic). Patients learn to fill a syringe with medication attached to tubing and the pump, and to insert a small cannula into the skin. The whole system is changed approximately every 3 days, and the injection site is rotated. Patients are given two pumps in case of pump malfunction. The patient should be trained and proficient in care of the delivery system before drug initiation. This can be accomplished by having the patient practice pump operation and injection with sterile saline solution. Because of its potent vasodilatory effects, treprostinil should be initiated in a monitored setting with emergency equipment and staff readily available.

The most significant problem with subcutaneous treprostinil therapy is infusion site pain and reaction. This side effect occurs in nearly all patients. Although this may prompt inadequate dosing, it generally is agreed that there is little or no relationship between infusion site pain and the dosage of treprostinil; severe pain and erythema can occur at very low dosages.[22] There are many strategies to decrease and alleviate pain, ranging from varying the size and shape of the insertion needle to oral analgesics. Patients initiating treprostinil need a great deal of emotional support to continue the therapy during the first several months. For some patients the pain becomes more tolerable after 3-6 months, while in others the pain remains and can become intolerable. In clinical usage of subcutaneous treprostinil, 25-50 percent of patients discontinued therapy due to infusion site pain. The package insert recommends initiating the drug at a dosage of 1.25 ng/kg/min and increasing each week. Most centers are aggressive at titrating the dosage upward as quickly as the patient can tolerate to obtain symptomatic improvement. Patients who achieved a dosage of 13 ng/kg/min or more by the end of a 12-week clinical study were able to walk significantly further than those at lower dosages.[23] For patients to tolerate the injection site pain, it is important that they experience some degree of subjective improvement in their PH symptoms.

Investigational Therapies

Once the only way for patients with PAH to access medical therapy, investigational therapies continue to play an important role in PAH management. The focus and applications of investigational therapies, however, have changed dramatically over the years. Because effective therapies are available, there can be significant ethical issues around enrolling patients in clinical trials conducted with a placebo arm. The gold standard in drug efficacy and safety evaluation is a double-blind, placebo-controlled study. Now that there are five FDA-approved therapies, subjecting patients to trials that may randomize them to receive placebo, and thus withhold therapy for several months, is of great concern. Even with the ability to remove deteriorating patients from a placebo treatment arm, all placebo-controlled trials done in PAH have demonstrated that the placebo group worsens over a period of 3-4 months. Patients enrolling in studies frequently are limited to those who cannot access approved therapies because of insurance issues, thus reducing the number of available subjects. In addition, it can be difficult to identify patients who meet the strict inclusion criteria. In the future it might be possible only to develop new drugs that add on to conventional FDA-approved therapies. Enrollment of patients in clinical studies, however, is essential to further advances in therapy for PAH.

As of this writing, several therapies are in development for PAH management, some of which may receive FDA approval before publication. Although not discussed here, they include:

- Sitaxsentan (Thelin®)
- Tadalafil (Cialis®)
- Simvastatin (Zocor®)
- Ambrisentan
- Inhaled or oral treprostinil (Remodulin®)
- Vasoactive intestinal peptide

Telephone Triage

One of the most time-consuming activities for the nurse in a pulmonary vascular disease program is speaking with patients on the telephone; however, it is one of the most important ways a nurse can care for patients. Communication with patients and their families is vital to provide them with education and emotional support as they deal with the unpredictable and often frustrating nature of chronic disease. Patients and their families call on the nurse for help when they are overwhelmed. Nurses are an important resource for patients, because they are available to spend time on the phone explaining issues surrounding PH and assisting in solving day-to-day problems and concerns. This section will discuss typical phone calls received by nurses at a PH center and offer some recommendations for handling calls efficiently.

Because of the high volume, we recommend a formal or informal method of prioritizing calls. Some centers have a telephone menu from which patient calls go directly to the nurse, while prescription requests are sent to a separate, dedicated prescription refill line. Other centers have a voicemail message directing patients with emergencies to contact a secretary who can page the nurse or physician immediately; nonurgent calls are left for the voicemail line.

Emergency calls can be intimidating, particularly if the nurse is new to caring for patients with PH or to managing a particular therapy. Patients often panic when they call and reveal only a few details of the emergency because they are so frightened. Keeping yourself calm and eliciting the necessary information can make the situation easier. Patients will often relax when they hear your voice; if you stay calm, they will. Try to obtain as much information about the problem as possible. Ask the patient: When did this start? How bad is the symptom or problem? Ask questions to ascertain quality, quantity, location, and duration of the symptom or problem. What makes it worse or better? Have you ever had this symptoms or problem before?

After you have assessed the situation, consider if this is a medical problem that can be managed over the telephone or one that requires that the patient be seen. Should the patient who needs to be seen come to your office or go to the local emergency room? If your patient with PH is experiencing severe chest pain and some nausea, going to the nearest emergency room for evaluation is appropriate. The patient would be best served by being evaluated by a physician, with scrutiny of vital signs, pulse oximeter readings, an electrocardiogram, chest radiograph, and blood work as indicated. If necessary, the patient can then be transferred to your center. If the patient has recently had a heart catheterization demonstrating normal coronary arteries and is felt to be experiencing musculoskeletal pain, suggesting something for pain is appropriate. Collaborating and working closely with a physician to discuss such calls can be helpful.

Emergency calls about technical issues with epoprostenol or treprostinil therapy are common. Patients should have received extensive teaching regarding these therapies but may call to report problems because of fear, anxiety, or the need for direction or emotional support. Patients who lose function of their central intravenous access (e.g., the catheter falls out or has a hole) are instructed to seek emergency care immediately in order to reestablish intravenous (peripheral) access promptly for immediate resumption of therapy. This is especially critical for patients newly on epoprostenol who are at highest risk for developing acute cor pulmonale secondary to the drug's short half-life.

Patients may forget to clamp the central venous access catheter and then call reporting profuse bleeding all over their clothing. Such patients are reminded that the catheter is in a large blood vessel and reassured. It is one mistake they will likely not make again. Catheter site infections are managed with antibiotics according to the institution's protocol. Typically, cephalexin (Keflex®) or dicloxacillin is used as initial therapy for skin and catheter tract infections. A patient who is febrile or for whom there is concern about catheter infection with bacteremia is instructed to go to the local emergency room for blood cultures and possible intravenous antibiotic therapy. In general, if bacteremia persists, the central line should be removed and a temporary central venous access (such as a double-lumen PICC line) should be established for both the prostacyclin or treprostinil and intravenous antibiotics. Before replacement of the tunneled central venous catheter, the patient should have negative blood culture results for at least 2 weeks following a completed course of antibiotics.

Examples of Emergency Calls

New or Worsening Symptoms
"I'm more short of breath."
"I'm having chest pain."
"I coughed up blood."
"I'm dizzy and light-headed. I passed out this morning and woke up on the kitchen floor."
"I fell on my right knee and being on warfarin it's really bruised and swollen."
"My legs are very swollen and my weight is up 8 pounds."

Technical Problems
"My Hickman catheter fell out."
"My Hickman catheter has a hole in it."
"I forgot to clamp my Hickman catheter when I changed the tubing and I bled all over my shirt. It really scared me."
"My Hickman catheter looks infected."

Several types of less urgent or routine calls come into a PH center. These calls should be handled after emergency calls. Patients may call to report new or worsened symptoms. Once you assess the situation, decide if the patient needs to be seen or can be advised over the phone. On many occasions, we consider enlisting the support of the primary care physician or family physician, especially if the patient lives far from the PH center. As an example, if a patient calls reporting a new cough with yellow sputum production and low-grade fever, we may request the patient be seen by the local physician to evaluate the need for a chest radiograph or antibiotic therapy. We resist ordering antibiotic therapy unless we are sure the patient requires it. Patients frequently call to report "cold" symptoms. PH patients cannot take most over-the-counter cold preparations, because the decongestant component may worsen PH. Therefore, patients are treated with antihistamines and nasal spray (such as ipratropium [Atrovent®] nasal spray), and acetaminophen or ibuprofen to ease symptoms.

Another type of patient call is for anxiety or depression. Patients are often so overwhelmed with their symptoms and lack of control over disease progression that they often cannot think to ask all of their questions at an office appointment. Frequently patients call the very next day to ask the same question, because they were so anxious or upset that they need to hear again what was discussed at the appointment. Nurses can take the time the next day to reexplain what was discussed and to answer any new questions when the patient is more relaxed. We encourage patients to bring family or other support persons to their office appointments to ask questions, hear the ongoing discussions, and to participate in the patient's care. We also tell patients to make a list of items they wish to discuss or questions they wish to ask so that all areas of concern are addressed. Similarly, patients may call complaining of feeling tired or depressed. They express frustration over not feeling well, frequent hospitalizations, or poor quality of life.[24] Although antidepressants and antianxiety agents are available, we like to initially recommend alternative solutions such as talking with other patients and getting out on good-weather days. In our patients' experience, sunshine goes a long way toward reducing depressive feelings. There are local support groups and PH Web sites where a patient can interact with other patients and families for additional support. (See Web sites listed at end of this chapter.)

Patients frequently call for medication refills. We return these calls as soon as possible, because patients typically wait until they have only a few pills left before calling to request a refill. On occasion, medications must be authorized by the insurance company. Usually these are the specialized and costly medications that a pharmacy coverage plan attempts to limit. When requesting an authorization, try to get it for as long as possible (e.g., 6 months or a year).

Insurance issues are another type of incoming call that PH nurses handle. These calls range from questions about coverage, to insurance changes, to loss of coverage. When there is a change of insurance, patients are instructed to notify their physician's office so that their records can be updated. This important step can prevent erroneous billing for future outpatient physician visits. For patients losing a portion of their coverage (e.g., pharmacy coverage), we advise them to shop around via internet or telephone for supplemental coverage. To help patients with the cost of medications, most pharmaceutical companies offer a limited financial assistance program for certain drugs. These programs require a financial application and then re-enrollment on an annual basis. Bosentan is now covered by many Medicare Part D prescription programs. However, due to the high cost of bosentan, the monthly patient co-pay associated is prohibitively high for most patients. A co-pay assistance program has been developed and is currently administrated by the Caring Voices Coalition at 888-267-1440. The manufacturers of epoprostenol, treprostinil, iloprost, bosentan and sildenafil all have patient assistance programs for patients without medical insurance. Information about these programs is available from the specialty pharmacy distributors.

Patients may also call to ask about applying for disability payments. They usually have many questions specific to their circumstances. We encourage each patient to discuss disability coverage with the physician. For appropriate patients, we recommend a free program called ACCESS (Advocating for Chronic Conditions and Social Services), which is offered by Accredo Therapeutics. This program also helps patients who are still working to maintain their benefits. They can educate and advise patients on their benefit options and help patients apply for Social Security Disability, Medicare, Medicaid, and Supplemental Security Income. They have a free booklet called "ACCESS: Helping Families Cope" that explains medical and disability entitlements. Patients can call (888) 700-7010 to reach this valuable service.

Questions regarding preventive care are another type of call. We recommend that patients with PH receive annual influenza vaccines. Pneumococcal vaccine should be administered every 5 years. We teach patients that handwashing is very important to decrease the risk of colds and flu. We instruct them to get appropriate rest, eat healthy and well-balanced meals, and to exercise regularly.

Examples of Non-Urgent Calls

New or Worsened Symptoms
"I can't get rid of this cough."
"I can't sleep."
"My ankles are more swollen at the end of the day."
"I have a cold. What can I take?"

Anxiety, Depression
"What did the doctor say about this treatment?"
"I am so tired all the time. I just can't take this anymore."

Medication Refills or Reauthorizations
"My insurance company needs to be called to reauthorize my drug therapy for another 6 months."

Other Insurance Issues
"I am changing my coverage."
"I am losing my prescription coverage and I can't afford this therapy."

Work Versus Disability
"Should I keep working?" "Am I hurting myself?"
"Will I qualify for disability?" "How do I apply for disability?" (short term, long term)

Prevention Calls

"Do I need an influenza vaccine?"
"How often should I get a pneumococcal vaccine?"
"Is it okay if I exercise?"
"Do I need to take antibiotics for dental work?"

Patients with PAH face many ups and downs. They require support and education as they learn about their PH, possible complications, medical therapies, and as they strive to achieve the best quality of life possible. Nurses are well qualified and well positioned to work as patient educators, patient advocates, and providers of emotional support.

Special Note Regarding the Pulmonary Hypertension Association

The authors of this chapter recommend the resources of the Pulmonary Hypertension Association to all health care providers caring for patients with PH and their families. This nonprofit organization was initiated by a handful of patients as a resource for individuals who, like themselves, were diagnosed with PH and wanted to learn more about their disease and treatment options. Over the years, it has grown to become the leading organization in the PH community involving patients, doctors, nurses, and researchers. It offers an informative and up-to-date Web site, a biennial international conference, support groups, fund-raising activities, a telephone support help line, a physician registry, a nursing and allied health network (Pulmonary Hypertension Resource network), a peer-reviewed journal called *Advances in Pulmonary Hypertension*, and "Pathlight" (a newsletter).

Web Sites for Reference

Pulmonary Hypertension Association: *www.phassociation.org*. Accessed January 8, 2006.

Pulmonary Hypertenision Central: *www.PHCentral.org*. Accessed January 8, 2006.

National Registry for Familial Primary Pulmonary Hypertension: *http:www.mc.Vanderbilt.edu/root/Vumc/php?site=vupphstudy*. Accessed February 15, 2006.

International Registry of Primary Pulmonary Hypertension (IRPPH): *http:/irpph.cineca.it/*. Accessed February 15, 2006.

PPH Cure Foundation: *http://www.pphcure.org*. Accessed February 15, 2006.

National Organization for Rare Disorders (NORD): *http://www.rarediseases.org/*. Accessed February 15, 2006.

Medicare Approved Lung and Heart-Lung Transplant Centers: *http://www.cms.hhs.gov/ApprovedTransplant Centers/*. Accessed February 15, 2006.

Second Wind Lung Transplant Association, INC: *www.2ndwind.org*. Accessed January 8, 2006.

Transplant Recipients International Organization (TRIO): *www.TRIOweb.org*. Accessed January 8, 2006.

United Network for Organ Sharing (UNOS): *www.unos.org*. Accessed January 8, 2006.

Scleroderma Foundation: *http://www.scleroderma.org/*. Accessed February 15, 2006.

Also useful: *Pulmonary Hypertension: A Patient's Survival Guide*, 3rd Ed. (A publication of the Pulmonary Hypertension Association).

http://www.phassociation.org/learn/Survival-Guide/index.asp. Accessed February 15, 2006.

Bring a pad of paper to write down the issues discussed during the appointment.

We encourage significant others or family members to attend clinic appointments to hear what is discussed and to understand the treatment plan.

Bring a current medication list to the appointment and know what medications need to be reordered when you visit your physician or nurse. If you do not have an accurate list, bring the pill boxes of all the medicines you are taking.

- When providing patients with a set of specific and important directions, such as details pertaining to a hospital admission or outpatient procedure, it is helpful to provide written directions as a backup to your verbal instructions.

- Patients should consider supplemental oxygen as a drug prescribed by a physician. It should be used as prescribed including the correct flow rate (liters/minute), with activity, rest, and sleep.

- Nurses and physicians shouldn't be afraid to learn from patients. They can be quite ingenious. One patient and her husband found lightweight pipe-insulating material that could be cut into 6-inch squares and used to keep ice packs frozen longer for cooling her epoprostenol (Flolan®) infusion.

- Patients are encouraged to get a medic alert bracelet that lists allergy and medication (such as warfarin) information that may be critical in the event of an emergency.

- We recommend that patients carry a wallet card with their current medication list, drug allergies, and physician and nurse contact phone numbers.

- Patients with pulmonary hypertension are advised to obtain an influenza vaccination annually and a pneumococcal vaccination every 5 years.

- Patients with pulmonary hypertension are cautioned to avoid over-the-counter decongestants when experiencing cold symptoms. Decongestants are vasoconstrictors that can elevate pulmonary vascular pressures and worsen symptoms. Patients are advised to use antihistamines, nasal sprays (e.g., ipratropium [Atrovent®] nasal spray), acetaminophen, or ibuprofen to ease cold symptoms.

Clinical Pearls

- Patients are encouraged to get the most from their clinic appointments:
  Bring a list of questions you want to ask the nurse and physician.

References

1. D'Alonzo GE, Barst RJ, Ayres SM, et al: Survival in patients with primary pulmonary hypertension. Results from a national prospective registry. *Ann Intern Med* 115:343-349, 1991.

2. Rubin LJ: Diagnosis and management of pulmonary arterial hypertension: ACCP evidence-based clinical practice guidelines. *Chest* 126(1 Suppl):7S-10S, 2004.

3. McGoon M, Gutterman D, Steen V, et al: Screening, early detection, and diagnosis of pulmonary arterial hypertension: ACCP evidence-based clinical practice guidelines. *Chest* 126(1 Suppl):14S-34S, 2004.

4. Badesch DB, Abman SH, Ahearn GS, et al: Medical therapy for pulmonary arterial hypertension: ACCP evidence-based clinical practice guidelines. *Chest* 126(1 Suppl):35S-62S, 2004.

5. Rich S, Kaufmann E, Levy PS: The effect of high doses of calcium-channel blockers on survival in primary pulmonary hypertension. *N Engl J Med* 327:76-81, 1992.

6. Gheorghiade M, Adams KF, Jr, Colucci WS: Digoxin in the management of cardiovascular disorders. *Circulation* 109:2959-2964, 2004.

7. Gerbes AL: Medical treatment of ascites in cirrhosis. *J Hepatol* 17 (Suppl 2):S4-S9, 1993.

8. *http://www.coumadin.com.* Accessed January 8, 2006.

9. Channick RN, Simonneau G, Sitbon O, et al: Effects of the dual endothelin-receptor antagonist bosentan in patients with pulmonary hypertension: A randomised placebo-controlled study. *Lancet* 358:1119-1123, 2001.

10. Rubin LJ, Badesch DB, Barst RJ, et al: Bosentan therapy for pulmonary arterial hypertension. *N Engl J Med* 346:896-903, 2002.

11. Sitbon O, Badesch DB, Channick RN, et al: Effects of the dual endothelin receptor antagonist bosentan in patients with pulmonary arterial hypertension: A 1-year follow-up study. *Chest* 124: 247-254, 2003.

12. Actelion Pharmaceuticals US, I, Package insert: Bosentan. South San Francisco, 2001.

13. Taichman DB, Palevsky HI: Treatment of pulmonary arterial hypertension with the endothelin receptor antagonist bosentan. *Clin Pulm Med* 12:121-127, 2005.

14. Stiebellehner L, Petkov V, Vonbank K, et al: Long-term treatment with oral sildenafil in addition to continuous IV epoprostenol in patients with pulmonary arterial hypertension. *Chest* 123:1293-1295, 2003.

15. Badesch DB, Burgess G, Papira T, et al: Sildenafil citrate in patients with pulmonary arterial hypertension (PAH): Results of a multicenter, multinational, randomized, double-blind, placebo-controlled trial by WHO functional class. *Proc Am Thorac Soc* 2:A206, 2005 (abstracts).

16. Olschewski H, Simonneau G, Galie N, et al: Inhaled iloprost for severe pulmonary hypertension. *N Engl J Med* 347:322-329, 2002.

17. Hoeper MM, Schwarze M, Ehlerding S, et al: Long-term treatment of primary pulmonary hypertension with aerosolized iloprost, a prostacyclin analogue. *N Engl J Med* 342:1866-1870, 2000.

18. Hoeper MM, Taha N, Bekjarova A, et al: Bosentan treatment in patients with primary pulmonary hypertension receiving nonparenteral prostanoids. *Eur Respir J* 22:330-334, 2003.

19. Fortin TA, Tapson VF: Intravenous prostacyclin for pulmonary arterial hypertension. In: A.J.a.R. Peacock, L.J, editor: *Pulmonary circulation: Diseases and their treatment,* 2004, Oxford University Press, pp 255-267.

20. Severson CJ, McGoon MD: Continuous intravenous epoprostenol for pulmonary arterial hypertension: Highlighting practical issues, specials considerations. *Adv Pulm Hypertension* 1:4–8, 2002.

21. Taichman DB, Christie J, Biester R, et al: Validation of a brief telephone battery for neurocognitive assessment of patients with pulmonary arterial hypertension. *Respir Res* 6:39, 2005.

22. Simonneau G, Barst RJ, Galie N, et al: Continuous subcutaneous infusion of treprostinil, a prostacyclin analogue, in patients with pulmonary arterial hypertension: A double-blind, randomized, placebo-controlled trial. *Am J Respir Crit Care Med* 165:800-804, 2002.

23. Sitbon O, Humbert M, Nunes H, et al: Long-term intravenous epoprostenol infusion in primary pulmonary hypertension: Prognostic factors and survival. *J Am Coll Cardiol* 40:780-788, 2002.

24. Taichman DB, Shin J, Hud L, et al: Health-related quality of life in patients with pulmonary arterial hypertension. *Respir Res* 6:92, 2005.

22 Chapter

Patient and Family Perspectives on Pulmonary Hypertension

The goal of this text has been to provide a reference that will ultimately benefit patients by helping those who care for them. It is thus fitting that we end with a view of pulmonary vascular disease from its most important vantage point—that of the patients and families who battle its effects daily at the most personal level. The importance of such an emphasis is best stated by Jerry Wojciechowski, a patient with pulmonary arterial hypertension and the father of two sons lost to the ravages of this disease. Jerry Wojciechowski has lived with the triumphs and tragedies of both clinical research and care. He, like other patients and families, has shouldered the advances—and deteriorations—that become the published outcomes of clinical trials. As he puts it, "I am a living end point."

Angela Eldam

Angela Eldam is a nurse and mother, diagnosed with idiopathic ("primary") pulmonary hypertension at age 29. Following treatment with intravenous epoprostenol, she underwent lung transplantation. She lives with her family in Sugar Land, Texas.

In May of 1990, I was 29 years old. I was a nurse and the mother of three, planning for my eldest child's kindergarten graduation. My daughter was 4 months old, I was able to work 40 hours most weekends, enabling me to stay home during the week and be a "stay-at-home" mom, and everything was perfect in the world.

I remember a close friend telling me that I seemed out of breath while carrying my daughter, but I dismissed it and reminded her that I had three children, ages 5 and under, still had my "baby fat," and that when I stopped breastfeeding I was going to get in shape. The following month, while driving my sons home from karate class, I felt my left

arm go numb. I thought I was going to have a migraine headache, which was not unusual for me, but then it moved up my left neck and felt like an "egg white" had dried on my skin. I suspected it had something to do with my heart and prayed to God to please let me get my kids home. Once safe in my driveway, I turned off the car and just sat there. My husband had been visiting with a neighbor, and he came over and asked me what was wrong. I tried to explain what I was feeling, and he helped me into the house and called a cardiologist that we knew. He instructed us to come to the office in the morning, but to go to the emergency room if it got worse. It subsided and I went to see him.

He ran many tests including, an echocardiogram, which showed my right ventricle enlarged and ordered a lung scan to see if I had blood clots in my lungs. He was going on vacation the following week, the test turned out negative, and we were relieved. Looking back I realize that blood clots would have been a relief. Upon return, he performed a heart catheterization and diagnosed primary pulmonary hypertension (now called idiopathic pulmonary arterial hypertension [IPAH]). I was a licensed vocational nurse but had never heard of this condition, so I asked what medication he would prescribe. With my husband by my side and my baby in my arms, he instructed me to "put my affairs in order." He prescribed warfarin, a blood thinner.

Six months later, following fainting spells, I was admitted to the hospital. I told my doctor that it was impossible to keep up with my toddler because of the fainting spells, so he contacted a pediatric cardiologist who specialized in pulmonary hypertension. He explained that my fainting spells were caused by the left side of my heart not having enough volume to keep my systemic blood pressure normal, and that this was because the blood vessels in my lungs were being constricted. He mentioned a surgical procedure that he could perform to help increase the volume of blood to the left side of my heart by putting a hole in my heart.

The procedure was called an atrial septostomy, but it too had risks. He said I would either improve or not make it off the table. He gave me a week to think about it. I asked my son, then 5 years old, to sit on the hospital bed with me. I looked into his eyes and told him, "Mommy needs to have surgery, but it's dangerous. The doctor said I could die." He looked at me and his eyes got as big as saucers. He didn't say anything. I told him, "You need to go home and pray about it." The following morning he came to visit me and he jumped up on my bed and said, "You're not going to die, Mommy!" The decision was made. The following week I had the surgery. It was successful except for a tremendous drop in my oxygen saturations. I had no more fainting spells and was able to take care of my toddler.

I recall one clinic visit when my oxygen saturation was checked and it was at 52%. The nurse asked me if I was OK. I told her I was fine, that my body was used to it and I had driven myself to the clinic alone. Once when my daughter was going up the stairs, she stopped and was just standing there. I asked her what was wrong. She said, "I'm catching my breath." It tore my heart out that she had to learn this from me.

After about 3 years, I was getting progressively weaker. My children's pediatrician mentioned that he had seen, on a TV program, a new drug called epoprostenol, administered through a central line into the heart that was used to treat pulmonary hypertension. He had written down the number of the doctor using the drug. I called his office and the nurse was so attentive that she called the manufacturer and found a doctor who was involved in the study of the drug locally. It was a miracle! I used epoprostenol for about 18 months and met three patients also on the drug, so we started meeting at the local restaurant once a month. I circulated flyers to see if more patients wanted to come, and they did. We had about 10-12 patients during those first few years. Only about four of the original are left. We still have this support group today, now meeting every other month, and we have quite a few new patients. I also provide support to patients via telephone or e-mail if they prefer.

On April 11, 1995, the day of the Oklahoma City bombing, I had developed a low-grade fever and excruciating pain in both of my feet. I was hospitalized and put on IV antibiotics and had my central line changed. They eventually diagnosed a fungal infection in my blood. I spent 3 months in the hospital and was discharged in June. I had always told my doctor that as long as I could laugh, I wasn't ready for a transplant. I stopped laughing. Each and every breath was an effort. Sometimes I would be thirsty, but I wouldn't get myself a drink because it was too much effort to get it. My wonderful husband, along with my children, had turned into caregivers. It was so hard for me to watch them taking care of me when I should be the one taking care of them. I was listed for a transplant.

I had three "false alarms" to have my transplant, each time saying goodbye to my children; they knew that they might never see me alive again. No one should ever have to endure such pain. Finally, on the evening of October 5th, 1995, it was a go. Afterward it took me almost 2 weeks to get off the ventilator and 6 weeks to get out of the hospital. I was terrified of going home; I was used to being in charge, after all I was a nurse!! Nonetheless, I was discharged on November 11, but my legs were so weak that I was unable to lift myself up off the commode. On November 25th, my son's tenth birthday, I felt as though I was getting stronger from the occupational therapy treatments. I leaned over and grabbed my ankles, then I pushed myself off the sofa and walked my hands up my legs and stood up. Just then, my son entered the room and said, "That's the best birthday present I could ever get," and we embraced.

After that day, I haven't stopped moving! By January, I was giving my daughter a birthday party with thirty 6 year olds without having to stop to rest. One day, my daughter and I were in a hurry at the local supermarket and she told me, "Slow down Mommy, I can't keep up!" I stopped and looked at her and said, "What did you say?" We burst out laughing so hard that other customers looked at us, but we didn't care. We knew.

I was able to meet my donor's family on my 1-year anniversary. We have kept in touch and we spend some holidays with them. They know that they can give their daughter's lungs a hug anytime they want to. I went 3 years without spending the night at the hospital. I had some rejection in 1998, but once they treated it, I have not had any since. On October 6, 2003, it will be 8 years. I have watched my children grow up. My eldest is now in his second year of college, another is a senior in high school, and my daughter is now Student Council President in the eighth grade. I have enjoyed baseball and soccer games, school band concerts, vacationing with the family, helping my son move off to college and into an apartment, and tending to illnesses and broken bones. All those

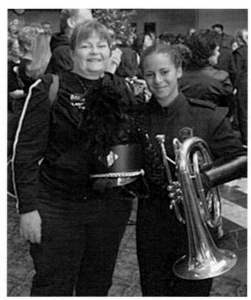

Figure 22-1. Angie, following her transplant, celebrating with her daughter at a high school marching band competition.

wonderful things a mother's life affords. I recently celebrated my forty-third birthday and thank God for each and every day (FIGURE 22-1).

Bonnie Dukart

Bonnie Dukart was a mother, wife, banker, and volunteer. Following her diagnosis with idiopathic ("primary") pulmonary arterial hypertension, she became an active member of the Pulmonary Hypertension Association, serving as its second president. Bonnie died on January 19, 2001, and is survived by her husband, Gary, and her son, Brian.

I was diagnosed with PPH in January of 1982. I knew that I got more short of breath than my friends, but had no idea that I suffered from a fatal disease. A snowstorm and chest pains brought me into the emergency room.

Within a week, the diagnosis of primary pulmonary hypertension was confirmed. I was 25 years old and I was given approximately 2 years to live. At first, nothing brought down my pulmonary artery pressures. The doctor then came in and told me about a very new drug called nifedipine. He asked me whether I wanted to try it and told me that the drug might help me or it might kill me.

I decided to try the drug, and it worked. My pulmonary artery pressure went down and my cardiac output went up. We had no idea how long this would last.

Over the next few years I worked as a banker for a large New York bank, becoming one of the youngest female vice presidents at the age of 31.

I worked in operations and then in marketing. I managed with this disease by using flextime, so that I could get a seat on the bus or train and by working smarter, not harder. I didn't have the stamina of my colleagues, so I had to make sure that I worked efficiently. I used the weekends to rest.

Because my PPH was stable, we decided to adopt a baby. I worked until our son was 18 months old and then decided to stay home and enjoy being a mother. A variety of volunteer work in community services and a part-time job assisting the comptroller of a local organization was a good mix with motherhood.

My PPH was stable on certain tests, but I knew that I wasn't doing as much as I had been. I was very worried, because I didn't know of anything else that could help me. It was the early 1990s and my son was in nursery school. My husband has always been supportive, but it was still a scary time.

In 1992, I started researching PPH on the internet. I found United Patient Association for Pulmonary Hypertension (Pulmonary Hypertension Association [PHA] under its old name) and a wealth of information on this disease. I had spent 10 years thinking that I was almost the only PPH survivor. We had read articles that stated that nifedipine hadn't worked for very many people and that if it worked, it was only for a short time. I was pleased to find other people like myself, long-term survivors with this disease. After a few months of phone calls and correspondence with other patients, I flew to Chicago for my first support group meeting. I had been diagnosed for $10\frac{1}{2}$ years and I was about to meet other patients for the very first time. When everyone told their story in the support group, I felt like I had come home. I wasn't alone anymore. Here were people who understood exactly what I was going through. I was also pleased to find out about a then experimental drug called epoprostenol and the possibility of lung transplants.

At least there were other options.

I went back to New Jersey and started a support group there. People came from as far away as Philadelphia just to meet other patients. We were a small, but close, group. We were a very lucky group, too. Four out of the first six members are still alive. The other two died because epoprostenol didn't work and transplants just weren't readily available or very successful.

I switched my medical care to a specialist in Chicago. After a week of those "fun" tests and discussions with my husband and myself, it was decided that I would try a new calcium channel blocker called amlodipine.

The drug was absolutely wonderful for 6 years. I studied martial arts, rode a bicycle, traveled, and was able to do a multitude of household tasks each day. As my husband noted, I had very few "couch days," those days when all IPAH patients want to do is sit on the couch and do nothing.

I also started volunteering for United Patient Association for Pulmonary Hypertension. In the beginning I took calls from patients, set up the mechanics of our hotline, and did a limited amount of public relations work. As the years went on, I cochaired two of our conferences, got volunteers to set up our first Web site and set the pieces in motion for volunteers to write and review the book, *Pulmonary Hypertension: A Patient's Survival Guide*. I also raised money for our first leadership training seminar, hired our first employee, and in general brought the association from a kitchen table organization to the point where we needed, and hired, an executive director. In 1999, after finishing as president of PHA, I began PHA's fundraising and research program with the help of many able volunteers. In 1 year we raised enough money to award three grants to researchers in the field. This year we hope to do even better.

My health started failing after the 1998 PHA conference. At first the decline was slow, but after a number of months the deterioration was rapid. In August of 1999, I entered a clinical trial for a new drug, treprostinil. Unfortunately, I was placed on a placebo and my health declined. Most of my days were couch days. I couldn't cook, clean, or even go to the store. My husband did everything. My son helped out as he struggled with the reality of having a sick mother.

In October of 1999, I finally got the real stuff, the real treprostinil. And, it worked! I was so thankful. The improvement was very slow, but steady. After a little more than 5 months on the new drug, I can cook, shop, take classes, take care of my son, and lead a somewhat normal life. I have very few couch days. I am looking forward to the time when I can do everything again. We are anxious to take my bicycle down from the hooks and get it geared up for the nice spring weather. We hope to resume traveling this summer and have already begun to entertain and socialize again. My son is finishing his first year of middle school and looking forward to a great summer. My husband can finally be a husband again, instead of a caretaker.

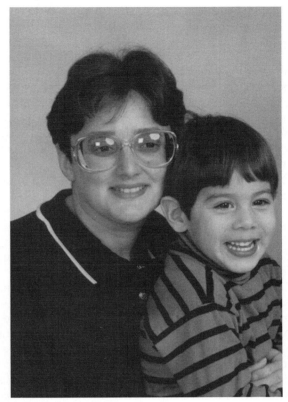

Figure 22-2. Bonnie with her son, Brian.

I am very grateful to be able to see each sunrise and enjoy the little surprises of each day. Even doing the laundry is a pleasure. With all of the new treatments on the horizon, I am also looking forward to the day when this disease is cured and the day when I can ride a bicycle with my yet-to-be born grandchildren (FIGURE 22-2).

Jean March

The following was written by Jean March in January 2001. She wrote this passage expressing her feelings toward the caregivers of PH patients. It was first presented to her PH support group at a meeting in Tampa, Florida. Jean March succumbed to her illness on January 29, 2002.

The Plight of the Caregiver

It is devastating to be diagnosed with pulmonary hypertension. It changes our lives. We live with constant reminders of the disease.

But, I believe the plight of the caregiver is much worse.

When I am sick, I go to the hospital and someone takes care of me. I feel bad but medication helps.

When I am sick my husband comes to the hospital, also. He worries about me. He makes sure I am receiving the best of care. He brings me whatever I need and helps me mix the epoprostenol. He follows the nurse to the refrigerator to make sure she places the ice packs in the freezer and the cassettes in the refrigerator and not vice versa. He calls me several times a day to make sure I am OK. If I have a procedure, he is there waiting for me when I return to my room. He visits every day. He loves me.

He also has to go to work and take care of everything at home. He has to explain to the dog that not only has she been home all day long but now he's too tired to spend much time with her. If he has any time left, he takes care of himself.

PH affects the caregivers more than anyone can realize. They live in constant awareness that their loved ones may be ill or in need of their help. They make important decisions based upon what the doctors think may happen. They live their lives under a tremendous amount of PH stress.

Perhaps those researchers can come up with a much-needed cure for the PH caregiver. Perhaps this cure should help them sleep better, give them more hours in the day, and help them worry less. Perhaps it can give them wisdom to make important decisions based upon supreme knowledge of what this disease will do with their loved ones.

To all the caregivers out there, we salute you! (FIGURE 22-3).

Denise Vigue

Denise Vigue lost two sisters, Dee Dee Topczewski and Velma ("Val") Borla, to pulmonary hypertension. She organizes local support groups and educational programs for patients with pulmonary hypertension in Wisconsin.

Pulmonary Hypertension... "What Little We Know"

Today's woman has many stresses in her life, including balancing career and family. In her care and work for others, oftentimes she may neglect her own physical health. Exercise and fitness clubs abound with women rushing from work then rushing home to cook and care for their families. Even for the single woman, taking time out from her busy schedule to work out doesn't always take priority.

So one day she feels a little breathless climbing the stairs at work. She may think she is simply out of shape, and mentally reminds herself to get back to the gym. Then a few weeks go by and she may experience that same breathless feeling just getting up in the morning.

A trip to the doctor oftentimes leads to a cursory exam. With the usual culprits ruled out, like a thyroid condition, anemia, diabetes, a virus or "women's problems," she feels better and her doctor tells her to eat a healthier diet, relax a little more, and take vitamins.

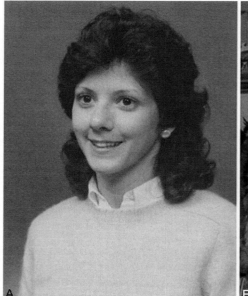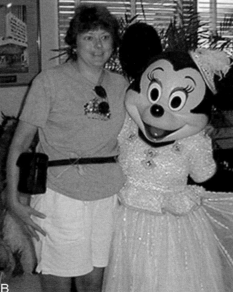

Figure 22-3. **A**, Jean at age 42 and (**B**) with Minnie Mouse and her CADD infusion pump.

She may have a cough and think a cold is coming on. With all the symptoms of a cold, she takes it easy, bed rest, fluids, TLC from family, and cold remedies. After a few more weeks, she goes to the doctor again. "Some viruses can have you down for weeks," her doctor tells her. "It's not uncommon. Take it easy." So she gets antibiotics and goes back to work.

With that pesky cough hurting her chest, she still feels run down and still has that heavy feeling in her chest, so yet another doctor visit. By this time she, her family, and the doctor are becoming a bit concerned. A full blood workup and complete physical are done, but nothing out of the ordinary shows up. Finally, the doctor suggests she see a psychiatrist. Perhaps she has some mental problems that need to be dealt with that may be affecting her health.

Feeling depressed about being so tired, she goes to see the recommended psychiatrist. By this time she also thinks, "Maybe something is wrong with my mind." Of course, the psychiatrist knows she has gone through a complete physical, so they talk about her feelings. She is definitely depressed. She agrees to an antidepressant prescription and begins weekly visits to discuss her feelings. She is too tired to work, so she takes some time off.

Then one day at home, while attempting with great effort to clean her house, she faints. Her doctor and psychiatrist make joint referrals to a series of specialists, but nothing out of ordinary shows up.

Finally, many months later one specialist says, "I believe you have pulmonary hypertension." Relief at last. She is not crazy and everyone is so happy! So what now? What medicine can she take? More tests are taken. Relief turns to horror and incomprehension when the doctor confirms the diagnosis and tells her and her family that indeed she has PH. A rare fatal condition with no known cure.

"But I'm only 37!" she cries. "How can this be? No one in my family has such a thing." "What causes this and why me?" Frustration ensues because the cause is unknown. Dread grips the family when they are told most patients live only a few years after diagnosis.

She goes home with her family and they cry and they cry and prepare for her death—with no where to turn for support or hope. Day after day they watch her as she slowly gets weaker. Her breathing becomes more labored and painful. Although some of the medications give her a little relief, she suffers from extreme leg cramps, muscle weakness, anemia, syncope, labored breathing, depression, and fear.

Two months before her thirty-ninth birthday she dies. Her mother still cannot understand why the doctors couldn't save her (FIGURE 22-4).

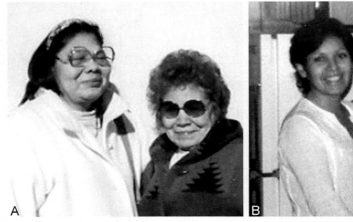

Figure 22-4. **A**, Velma Borla with her mother, Viola Ortiz. **B**, Dee Dee Topczewski several years after being diagnosed with primary pulmonary hypertension.

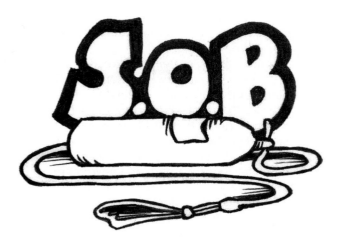

Art by Leslie Polss, a patient with idiopathic pulmonary arterial hypertension

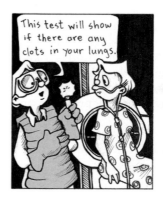

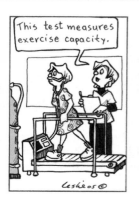

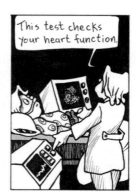

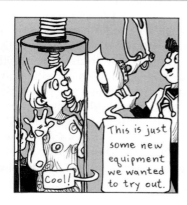

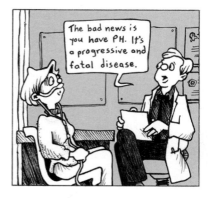

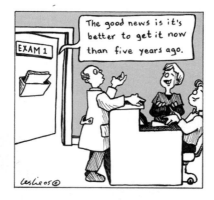

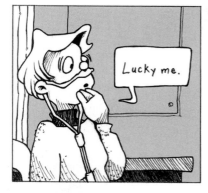

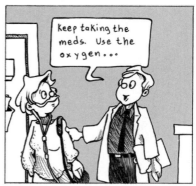

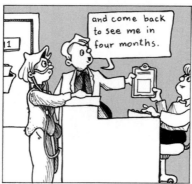

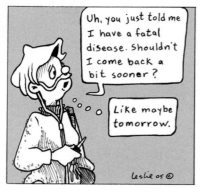

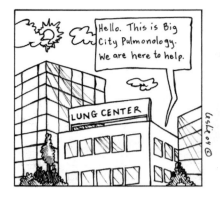

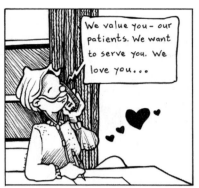

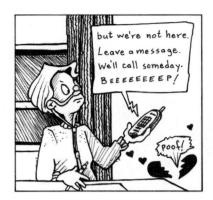

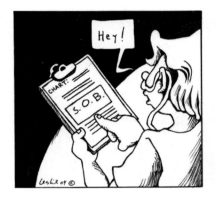

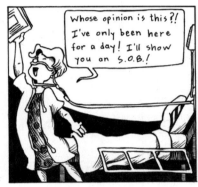

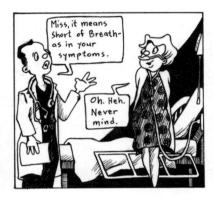

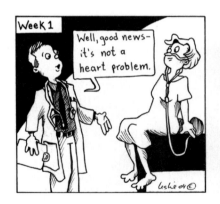

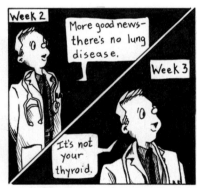

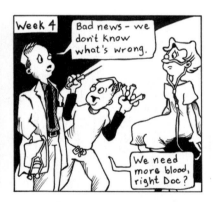

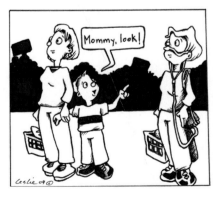

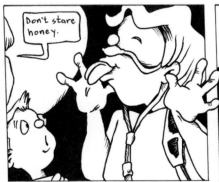

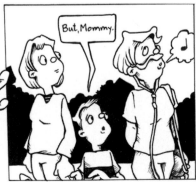

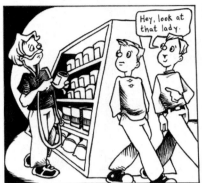

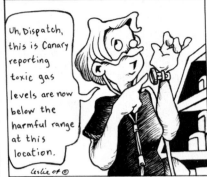

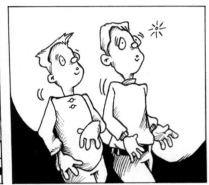

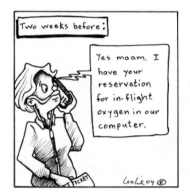

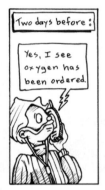

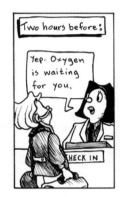

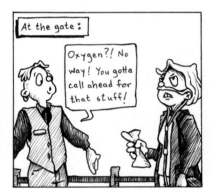

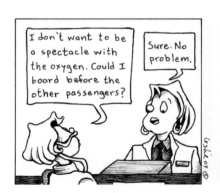

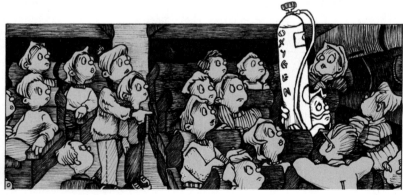

Subject Index